MEDICAL RADIOLOGY

Diagnostic Imaging and Radiation Oncology

Late Sequelae in Oncology

Contributors

H. Alheit · M. Bamberg · M. Baumann · J.D. Beck · C. Behles · W. Berberich
M.R. Berger · A. Besserer · S. Bielack · A. Binder · S. Birkenhake · E.A. Bleher
C. Bokemeyer · J. Boos · M. Buchfelder · H. G. Dörr · J. Dunst · M. Engel
R. Erttmann · D. Felsenberg · M. Flentje · B. Frank · H. Frommhold · M. Galanski
U. Gatzemeier · J. Grab · G. Grabenbauer · R.H. Greiner · S. Hartmann
K. Henne · T. Herrmann · C.F. Hess · N. Hodapp · F. Kamprad · L. Keilholz
A. Koch · A. Koch · R. Korinthenberg · R.D. Kortmann · H.-J. Krämling
E.-D. Kreuser · M. Landthaler · S.H. Levitt · M. Molls · G. Moog · R.-P. Müller
P.E. Mullis · M. Niewald · L. Plasswilm · R. Rathmann · S. Reitz · M. Riepl
H.P. Rodemann · R. Rossi · C. Rübe · H. Sauer · T. Sauerwald · M. Schabet
C. Schaefer-Prokop · C. Schlichting · H.-J. Schmoll · K. Schnabel · J. Schorcht
H. Schünemann · S. Schultz-Hector · J. Slanina · V. Strnad · E. Thiel
K.-R. Trott · A. Uhrig · H. Völler · H. J. Weh · R. Wilkowski · N. Willich

Edited by

J. Dunst and R. Sauer

Foreword by

Luther W. Brady and Hans-Peter Heilmann

Springer-Verlag

Berlin Heidelberg New York
London Paris Tokyo
Hong Kong Barcelona
Budapest

Professor Dr. JÜRGEN DUNST

Strahlentherapeutische Klinik
Martin-Luther-Universität Halle-Wittenberg
Dryanderstraße 4–7
06097 Halle/Saale, FRG

Professor Dr. ROLF SAUER

Klinik und Poliklinik für Strahlentherapie
der Universität Erlangen-Nürnberg
Universitätsstraße 27
91054 Erlangen, FRG

MEDICAL RADIOLOGY · Diagnostic Imaging and Radiation Oncology

Continuation of
Handbuch der medizinischen Radiologie
Encyclopedia of Medical Radiology

With 80 Figures and 104 Tables

ISBN-13: 978-3-642-46796-7 e-ISBN-13: 978-3-642-46794-3
DOI: 10.1007/978-3-642-46794-3

Library of Congress Cataloging-in-Publication Data. Late sequelae in oncology/contributors, H. Alheit ··· [et al.]; edited by J. Dunst and R. Sauer; foreword by Luther W. Brady and Hans-Peter Heilmann. p. cm.–(Medical radiology) Includes bibliographical references and index. ISBN 3-540-56936-7: DM198.00 1. Cancer–Treatment–Complications. I. Alheit, H. II. Dunst, J. (Jürgen), 1958- . III. Sauer, Rolf. IV. Series. [DNLM: 1. Neoplasms–radiotherapy. 2. Neoplasms–drug therapy. 3. Radiotherapy–adverse effects. 4. Drug Therapy–adverse effects. QZ 269 L351 1995] RC270.8.L38 1995 616.99'406–dc20 DNLM/DLC for Library of Congress 94-45370

Softcover reprint of the hardcover 1st edition 1995

Typesetting: Thomson Press (India) Ltd., New Delhi

SPIN: 10122139 21/3130/SPS – 5 4 3 2 1 0 – Printed on acid-free paper

Foreword

The basic premise in treating a cancer patient is to maximize the potential for cure and to do so in the manner least likely to cause complications. In modern oncology, major progress has been made in the last decade by the utilization of combined multimodal integrated programs of management, more aggressively conceived in order to improve the cure rate. This is particularly true for tumors where the cure rates in the past have been poor, such as carcinomas of the colon, rectum, anus, bladder, etc. The combination of surgical management by either biopsy or curative resection with continuous infusion chemotherapy and radiation therapy has clearly led to a better outlook in terms of cure rates as well as in terms of organ preservation. With this more aggressive management program, sequelae of cancer treatment will be greater and more frequent.

In this context, the present volume *Late Sequelae in Oncology* is particularly appropriate, both by defining these risks by virtue of its comprehensive overview, and by insuring that all the parameters relative to the treatment program in terms of its concept, justification, complications, and potential for cure be discussed in detail with the patient.

As more experience is gained in combined integrated multimodal treatment, concomitant efforts can be directed toward reducing the complications to the greatest degree possible. Therefore, the value of this volume is clearly set forth in defining late sequelae.

Philadelphia/Hamburg,
January 1995

LUTHER W. BRADY
HANS-PETER HEILMANN

Preface

Prior to the era of modern medicine, most life-threatening diseases were incurable. "Nil nocere", the principle of doctors in antiquity, derived from the inefficacy of their therapies and reminded them of thoroughly weighting of treatment risks against the minimal chances of effective palliation. During the last one hundred years, however, curative therapies for cancer have been developed, the discovery of X-rays by Wilhelm Conrad Röntgen in 1895 being just one milestone. Modern oncological therapy has become more and more effective in terms of cure, disease prolongation, and even palliation. The risk of lethal complications has also decreased during the last decades.

Nevertheless, high cancer cure rates have confronted oncologists with a new range of side effects: chronic morbidity in long-term survivors. Sophisticated multimodality treatment strategies offer us the chance of curing the majority of patients with advanced lymphomas or childhood sarcomas, for example. With longer follow-up, however, these patients may develop certain therapy-related diseases, such as cardiac morbidity or second tumors. Improvement of cancer therapy must, therefore, include strategies to minimize these long-term effects to make sure that an increase in early disease-free survival will be maintained in the long-run.

The most reliable results concerning late effects of therapies derive from follow-up examinations of long-term survivors. Other approaches include the use of special examinations to detect subclinical morphological or functional abnormalities that might progress to clinically relevant changes over years. This requires cooperation between oncologists and those working in other disciplines and integrated efforts by various specialists in the routine follow-up of cancer patients.

This volume would like to provide an up-to-date overview of our rapidly growing knowledge about late effects. Our objective is to sensitize physicians in clinical practice for the problem of long-term effects and to stimulate clinical and experimental investigators to increase research in this area of oncology.

Halle/Erlangen,
December 1994

Jürgen Dunst
Rolf Sauer

Contents

1 Individual Variation of Radio- and Chemosensitivity

1.1 Impact of Endogenous and Exogenous Factors on Radiation Sequelae
M. BAUMANN 3

1.2 Endogenous and Exogenous Factors Modifying Chemosensitivity to Cytostatic Drugs
H. SAUER 13

2 Neurotoxicity

2.1 Radiation-Induced Injury of the Central Nervous System
R.-P. MÜLLER 23

2.2 Cytostatic-Induced Central Nervous System Abnormalities
R. KORINTHENBERG 29

2.3 Radiation Myelopathy
L. KEILHOLZ and J. DUNST 35

2.4 Acute and Late Toxicity on Peripheral Nerves After Radiotherapy
C.F. HESS, R.D. KORTMANN, M. SCHABET, and M. BAMBERG 43

2.5 Acute and Late Toxicity on Peripheral Nerves After Chemotherapy – A Review
C. BOKEMEYER, B. FRANK, and H.-J. SCHMOLL 51

2.6 Endocrine Dysfunction After Brain Tumor Therapy in Children
H.G. DÖRR, A. KOCH, T. SAUERWALD, and J.D. BECK 59

2.7 Endocrine Dysfunction in Adults After Radiotherapy for Pituitary Adenomas and Suprasellar Tumors
M. BUCHFELDER and G. GRABENBAUER 65

2.8 Late Sequelae Affecting the Ear
S. BIRKENHAKE 73

2.9 Ototoxicity in Pediatric Oncology
S. HARTMANN 81

3 Skin and Mucosal Toxicity

3.1 Biological Basis for Skin and Mucosal Toxicity
K.-R. TROTT 89

3.2 Radiation-Induced Fibrosis: Experimental Studies
H.P. RODEMANN, A. BINDER, and M. BAMBERG 93

3.3 Lymphedema of the Arm After Treatment of Breast Cancer
H. SCHÜNEMANN and N. WILLICH 99

3.4 Skin and Mucosal Damage After Radiotherapy
for Head and Neck Tumors
M. NIEWALD, W. BERBERICH, C. SCHLICHTING, M. ENGEL, A. KOCH,
and K. SCHNABEL 105

3.5 Mucosal Toxicity After Radiochemotherapy
L. PLASSWILM and V. STRNAD 111

3.6 Complications of the Small Intestine and the Pancreas
After Intraoperative Radiotherapy
C. RÜBE, H.-J. KRÄMLING, N. WILLICH, J. GRAB, and R. WILKOWSKI 121

3.7 Skin Toxicity
M. LANDTHALER 127

4 Lung Toxicity

4.1 Radiation Pneumopathy – Experimental and Clinical Data
T. HERRMANN, J. SCHORCHT, and M. MOLLS 135

4.2 Lung Toxicity of Chemotherapeutic Agents
U. GATZEMEIER 141

4.3 Differential Diagnosis of Treatment Sequelae in the Lung
M. GALANSKI, R. RATHMANN, and C. SCHAEFER-PROKOP 151

5 Cardiotoxicity

5.1 Evaluation of Late Cardiotoxicity by Pulsed Doppler
Echocardiography in Patients Treated for Hodgkin's Disease
E.-D. KREUSER, H. VÖLLER, A. UHRIG, A. BESSERER, and E. THIEL 163

5.2 Anthracycline-Induced Cardiotoxicity in Children:
Pathophysiology and Prevention
S. BIELACK and R. ERTTMANN 175

5.3 Radiation-Induced Cardiotoxicity: Experimental Data
S. SCHULTZ-HECTOR 181

5.4 Cardiotoxicity After Megavoltage Irradiation and Chemotherapy
for Hodgkin's Disease with Special Emphasis on Coronary Heart
Disease Mortality – The Freiburg Experience 1940–1992
J. SLANINA, K. HENNE, N. HODAPP, G. MOOG,
and H. FROMMHOLD 191

5.5 Cardiac Morbidity and Mortality Followig Radiotherapy
S.H. LEVITT 197

6 Nephrotoxicity

6.1 Nephrotoxicity of Ifosfamide in Children
R. ROSSI and J. BOSS 207

6.2 Radiation Nephritis
M. FLENTJE 215

7 Gonadal Toxicity

7.1 Long-Term Gonadal Dysfunction and Its Impact on Bone Mineralization in Patients Following COPP/ABVD Chemotherapy for Hodgkin's Disease
E.-D. KREUSER, D. FELSENBERG, C. BEHLES, and E. THIEL 227

7.2 Gonadal Dysfunction After Radiotherapy
M. RIEPL and S. REITZ 235

8 Disturbances of Sceletal Growth

8.1 Dose-Time Considerations for Skeletal Growth Disturbances After Radiotherapy
H. ALHEIT 245

8.2 Disturbances in Growth of Bone, Muscle, and Fat Tissue Following Irradiation in Childhood
F. KAMPRAD 251

8.3 Growth Failure Secondary to Radiotherapy of Brain Tumors in Childhood
R.H. GREINER, E.A. BLEHER, and P.E. MULLIS 255

9 Cancerogenesis

9.1 Experiments on the Carcinogenic Potential of Antineoplastic Agents
M.R. BERGER 263

9.2 Secondary Malignancies Following Cytotoxic Chemotherapy
H.J. WEH 273

9.3 Secondary Malignancies After Radiotherapy
S.H. LEVITT 279

Subject Index 291

List of Contributors 295

1 Individual Variation of Radio- and Chemosensitivity

1.1 Impact of Endogenous and Exogenous Factors on Radiation Sequelae

MICHAEL BAUMANN

CONTENTS

1	Introduction	3
2	Impact of Radiosensitive Subsets of Patients on Tolerance Doses	4
3	Clinical Consequences of Decreased Acute and Late-Occurring Normal Tissue Tolerance	5
4	Evidence for "Intrinsically" Radiosensitive Patients	5
5	Clinically Important Factors Other Than Genetics That May Increase Radiation Sensitivity of Normal Tissues	6
5.1	Smoking and Abuse of Alcohol	6
5.2	Infections	7
5.3	Surgery	7
5.4	Chemotherapeutic Agents and Other Drugs	8
5.5	Age	8
5.6	Preexisting Disease in Irradiated Organs	8
5.7	Hypertension	8
5.8	Diabetes Mellitus	8
5.9	Hyperthyroidism	8
5.10	Hemoglobin Level	8
5.11	Diet	9
5.12	Skin Pigmentation and Hair Color	9
6	Summary and Conclusions	9
	References	9

1 Introduction

The aim of curative radiation therapy is to achieve uncomplicated local tumor control, that is to destroy all clonogenic tumor cells without producing major damage to surrounding normal tissue. This principle was illustrated by Hermann Holthusen, who used data on control of skin carcinoma and development of telangiectasia as an indicator of late-occurring normal tissue damage (Fig. 1). Both the probability of local tumor control and the development of normal tissue damage increased as sigmoid functions of radiation dose. The probability of uncomplicated local tumor control at each dose level was given as the product of the probability to achieve local tumor control and the probability of preventing normal tissue damage (HOLTHUSEN 1936; BUSCH 1987).

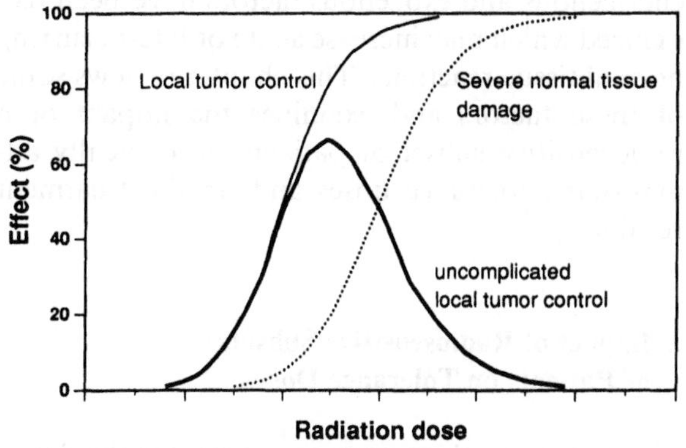

Fig. 1. Relationship of uncomplicated local tumor control by radiation therapy to local tumor control probability and severe normal tissue damage. (After Holthusen 1936)

Parameters such as tumor histology and grade, tumor size and site, and hemoglobin level, age, and general condition of the patient are widely used in clinical radiation therapy to determine the relative position on the tumor response curve and to predict the probability of achieving local tumor control for a given dose in individual patients (WETTERER 1913–1914; HOLTHUSEN 1936; PATERSON 1948; FLETCHER 1966; PETERS et al. 1982, 1986, 1988; RUBIN et al. 1974; SUIT and WALKER 1988; BENTZEN et al. 1991). Recently, considerable research efforts have been made to supplement these clinical parameters by quantitative predictors of the radiation response of individual tumors (PETERS et al. 1982, 1986, 1988; BAUMANN et al. 1993; HORSMAN 1993; WILSON 1993).

To minimize severe normal tissue reactions, the total dose given to the tumor in clinical practice is limited by the tolerance doses of the surrounding normal tissues (PATERSON 1948; RUBIN and CASARETT 1968, 1974; EMAMI et al. 1991). These tolerance doses represent estimates at which a certain percentage of all patients will develop specified normal tissue damage. For a given tissue, the toler-

MICHAEL BAUMANN, Dr., Radiologische Klinik, Abteilung für Strahlentherapie, Universitätsklinikum Eppendorf, Martinistraße 52, 20251 Hamburg, FRG ance dose depends critically on the fractionation schedule and on the volume of normal tissue irradiated. For severe, late-occurring, normal tissue damage many radiooncologists consider the tolerance dose 5% (TD5) as the maximum dose which should be administered. For especially devasting sequelae, e.g. radiation myelitis, doses are generally limited to well below the TD1.

During the history of radiation therapy several endogenous and exogenous factors have been recognized which may increase acute or late-occurring normal tissue reactions. This chapter reviews some of these factors and examines the impact of a radiosensitive subset of patients on clinically administered tolerance doses and on the treatment results.

2 Impact of Radiosensitive Subsets of Patients on Tolerance Doses

Figure 2 shows dose-response curves for the development of severe normal tissue damage in both patients with normal radiosensitivity and in a radiosensitive subset of patients. The composite curve for the clinically observed incidence of normal tissue damage in the mixed population is progressively skewed toward lower doses when the proportion of radiosensitive patients increases. This is especially apparent at low probabilities of normal tissue damage, that is at dose levels that are clinically used for the definition of TD5 and TD1 values. Table 1 gives a simplified numerical example to illustrate this effect. A TD5 value of 62.5 Gy has been assumed for the normal population. This value is in the order of magnitude of TD5 values given for development of late-occurring damage after *partial* irradiation of a variety of normal tissues in humans such as skin, brain, brachial plexus, heart, esophagus, and bone (Rubin and Casarett 1968, 1972; Rubin 1989; Emami et al. 1991). For the relative steepness of the dose-incidence curves, a $\gamma 50$ value of 4 was chosen, that is a 4% increase in probability of normal tissue damage for a 1% increase in dose on the linear part of the dose-response curve (Brahme 1984). Turesson (1991) reported $\gamma 50$ values between approximately 2 and 8 for the development of telangiectasia, necrosis and death from complication after radiation therapy of breast and head and neck cancer. Table 1 shows that with decreasing TD5 values in the radiosensitive patients (by factors of 1.25–2 compared to the normal patients) the TD5 for the mixed population also decreases rapidly. This effect is more pronounced when the proportion of radiosensitive patients among all patients is high; however, small subsets of radiosensitive patients may also impact the overall TD5 significantly.

Table 1. Example of the impact of radiosensitive subsets of patients on clinically observed tolerance doses

TD5 normal (Gy)	TD5 sensitive (Gy)	TD5 normal/ TD5 sensitive	TD5 composite (Gy)
62.5	50	1.25	58
62.5	42	1.5	50
62.5	31	2.0	38

TD5, tolerance dose 5%.
Dose-response curves for normal and sensitive patients were constructed on logit-log dose grids for different TD5 values, a $\gamma 50$ value of 4, and a proportion of 10% sensitive patients. The dose-response curve of the composite, that is, the clinically observed population, was constructed from the sum of the incidence of both groups multiplied with their respective proportion.

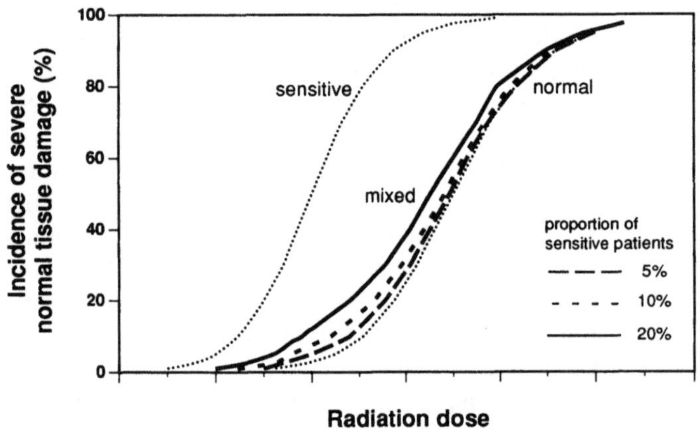

Fig. 2. Incidence of severe normal tissue damage after radiation therapy in a mixed population of radiosensitive and normal patients. Proportions of 5%–20% radiosensitive patients were considered

3 Clinical Consequences of Decreased Acute and Late-Occurring Normal Tissue Tolerance

Since acute normal tissue damage occurs during or shortly after completion of radiation treatment, severe acute reactions most likely will result in an interruption of treatment. This interruption of treatment will generally be necessary only for radiosensitive patients, whereas in patients with normal radiosensitivity the treatment can be completed without delay. Treatment gaps (OVERGAARD et al. 1988; WÜRSCHMIDT et al. 1991) and prolongation of treatment may result in a decreased probability of local tumor control due to repopulation of clonogenic tumor cells (WITHERS 1993; TROTT and KUMMERMEHR 1993). It is therefore anticipated that increased acute toxicities will worsen the prognosis of affected patients, but – as a first approximation – will not affect the prognosis of patients with normal radiosensitivity.

This is in contrast to late-occurring normal tissue damage. Since these reactions occur months or even years after completion of therapy, the treatments of radiosensitive patients cannot be modified based on an individual basis. Therefore empirical data, that is TD values, are used in treatment planning to limit the doses to surrounding normal tissues. Since these TD values may be influenced by radiosensitive subsets of patients (Fig. 2), the limitation of the total dose to the tumor may decrease the chance to control the tumor not only in the sensitive subset but in all patients undergoing radiation therapy (NORMAN et al. 1988; SUIT et al. 1989; HÜBENER et al. 1993).

4 Evidence for "Intrinsically" Radiosensitive Patients

In the first decade of radiation therapy it was widely believed that the radiation sensitivity of individual patients varied by wide margins and that a considerable proportion of so-called idiosynchratic X-ray sensitive patients suffered from severe radiation damage at doses that did not evoke the slightest effect in other individuals. This believe was strongly challenged by WETTERER (1913–1914), who quoted several authors and concluded that most reported cases of severe normal tissue damage were caused by uncertainties in dosimetry. The classification of patients as idiosynchratic X-ray sensitive was discussed by WETTERER as a convenient way for physicians to transfer some of the responsibility for radiation sequelae back to the patient. Nevertheless, it was clearly recognized at that time that some degree of variability of skin reaction was present among radiotherapy patients even when the dosimetry was carefully controlled.

Even today, most clinicians follow some patients in whom severe early- or late-occurring normal tissue damage developed that was unanticipated based on experience with the same treatment in other patients. There are only sparse reports on such unusually sensitive patients in the literature. The data suggest that their proportion among all patients is well below 1% (SMITH et al. 1980; LOEFFLER et al. 1990). Comparing such low incidences to the values assumed in Table 1, it might be argued that the impact of heterogeneity of normal tissue response on tolerance doses is of little importance in clinical practice. However, the clinically used tolerance doses may already be based on heterogeneous populations (Fig. 2), and the unusually sensitive patient would be that patient whose response lies even outside these tolerance levels.

Recently much interest has been directed toward an increased radiosensitivity associated with hereditary diseases. Several clinical reports have shown an enhanced toxicity of radiation therapy in patients suffering from ataxia telangiectasia (AT), an autosomal recessive disorder (GOTOFF et al. 1967; MORGAN et al. 1968; CUNLIFFE et al. 1975; PRITCHARD et al. 1982; ABADIR and HAKAMI 1983; HART et al. 1987). Two of these reports also suggest a higher sensitivity of tumors arising in these patients (ABADIR and HAKAMI 1983; HART et al. 1987). In 1975 it was demonstrated by TAYLOR et al. that skin fibroblasts of patients with AT are, by a factor of approximately 3, more radiosensitive than skin fibroblasts of normal donors. AT is a rare disease, the incidence of homozygotes is about 1 in 40 000. However, the radiosensitivity of fibroblasts of heterozygotes appears to lie between homozygotes and normal donors (DESCHAVANNE et al. 1986; ARLETT et al. 1988). The incidence of heterozygotes for AT has been estimated to be approximately 1% of the US white population and, because of an increased risk to develop malignancies, the incidence of AT heterozygotes among cancer patients may constitute between 5% and 10% (SWIFT et al. 1987, 1991). In addition some other genetic disorders including Fanconi's anemia, 5-oxoprolinuria, Cockayne's syndrome and Gardner's syndrome have been associated with a higher radiation sensitivity in vitro (DESCHAVANNE et al. 1986). Thus, based on epidemiological estimates and on the assumption that the radiation sensitivity of skin fibroblasts in vitro reflects the radiation response of normal tissues in vivo, it has been suggested that a considerable subset of all radiotherapy patients might be genetically radiosensitive. If so, TD values selected in clinical practice might depend almost exclusively on the incidence of severe damage in the genetically sensitive subgroup and virtually not on the dose-effect relationship in normal patients (NORMAN et al. 1988; SUIT et al. 1989).

There is considerable hope among clinicians and radiobiologists to detect genetically radiosensitive patients prior to treatment by detemination of the radiation sensitivity of normal tissue cells in vitro. This approach is supported by correlations reported between the radiosensitivity of skin fibroblasts in vitro and clinically observed skin reactions (SMITH et al. 1980; LOEFFLER et al. 1990; BURNET et al. 1992). However, the studies reported to date are very small and many problems such as different radiosenstivities among different cell types of the same individual (GEARA et al. 1992; GREEN et al. 1991; KUSHIRO et al. 1990), different results obtained for the same cells by different experimentors (LITTLE et al. 1988), and differences between assay techniques remain to be solved before the impact of radiosensitivity testing of normal cells on clinical practice can be assessed.

In carefully designed studies on skin reactions in breast cancer patients who received differently fractionated radiation therapy to the right and left internal mammary node fields, (TURESSON 1989, 1990; TURESSON and THAMES 1989) found a considerable individual variation of the progression rate and the peak score of telangiectasia of the skin. Reanalysis of these data and of data on acute skin reactions in the same patients indicated that dose effects were not sufficient to explain fully the patient-to-patient differences (TUCKER et al. 1992). The authors concluded that their data provide evidence for the existence of individual variability in the radiation response of human skin, both for early and late effects. However, the fact that no clear-cut correlations were observed between acute and late endpoints suggests that individual differences in radiosensitivity are not dominated by a single factor common to all tissues and all cells of the same individual. Similar data were reported by BENTZEN et al. (1993), who compared the degree of telangiectasia and subcutaneous fibrosis in postmastectomy patients treated with an anterior photon field covering the axillary, infraclavicular and superaclavicular nodes and an electron field covering the chest wall. The authors found a highly significant correlation that patients experiencing stronger than expected reactions in one treatment field did so in the second treatment field as well. However, when telangiectasia and subcutaneous fibrosis were compared, there was no significant within-patient correlation, again suggesting that there is no common factor that determines increased radiosensitivity of all tissues in individual patients.

Thus, despite the fact that dose-response relationships of many normal tissues are steep (RUBIN and CASARETT 1968, 1972; THAMES et al. 1989; TURRESON 1991; BURMAN et al. 1991; BENTZEN and OVERGAARD 1993) there is growing evidence of individual differences in radiosensitivity. More detailed data on this variability are necessary before sound estimates on the proportion of radiosensitive patients among all radiotherapy patients can be made. Since a variety of factors other than genetics may increase normal tissue reactions it appears essential to control for these factors in studies addressing this question.

5 Clinically Important Factors Other Than Genetics That May Increase Radiation Sensitivity of Normal Tissues

5.1 Smoking and Abuse of Alcohol

Many cancer patients, in particular those presenting with malignancies of the upper aerodigestive tracts and the lungs, have been heavy smokers and drinkers for years. Not only do both factors play a significant role in the etiology of cancer, they may also increase normal tissue reactions during and after radiation therapy. In a study on patients enrolled in the continuous hyperfractionated accelerated radiation therapy (CHART) program, RUGG and colleagues (1990) showed that the time necessary for complete resolution of mucositis was clearly increased in smokers compared to nonsmokers and those who had quit smoking. A relationship between acute normal tissue reactions and smoking was also found by WHITTET et al. (1991), who used serum cotinine, the major metabolite of nicotine, as a biochemical marker of smoking behavior during radiotherapy of patients with laryngeal carcinoma. Six of the 31 patients studied continued to smoke and all of them exhibited normal tissue reaction scores greater than the average. Of the remaining 25 patients another five developed significant complicating symptoms during radiotherapy; four of these patients had evidence of a high alcohol intake during treatment. KLUTH et al. (1988) found that approximately 90% of all patients who developed osteoradionecrosis of the jaw as late-occurring normal tissue damage after radiation therapy had continued heavy use of alcohol and tobacco. The authors suggested that these strong tissue irritants could have either directly contributed to the breakdown of mucosa and exposure of bone, or that these factors may be associated with other negative factors such as poor oral hygiene. Different results have been reported by BROWMAN et al. (1993), who investigated mucositis and dermatitis in smoking and nonsmoking patients treated by radiation therapy with or without chemotherapy for carcinoma of the head and neck, found that acute normal tissue reactions did not differ between groups.

Performing bronchoalveolar lavage in a small group of smoking and nonsmoking patients treated with postoperative radiation therapy for breast cancer, FRANZEN et al. (1989) observed a significant reduction in inflammatory parameters in the smokers. Furthermore, radiological signs of pneumonitis were exclusively seen in the nonsmoking group of patients. The authors suggested that ongoing smoking during treatment may reduce the level of pneumonitis. Nevertheless, increased late-occurring effects associated with smoking were reported by SLANINA (1977) and JENSEN et al. (1989, 1990), who found a decreased diffusion capacity in smokers compared to nonsmokers treated with mantle field irradiation with or without chemotherapy for Hodgkin's disease.

KUCERA et al. (1987) studied the frequency of side effects in patients with carcinoma of the cervix and found significantly increased, severe, irreversible gastrointestinal complications in smokers compared to nonsmokers. They suggested that this increased rate of side effects may be caused by a deficient capacity for regeneration of the tissue surrounding the tumor.

Even if not directly related to radiation sequelae in normal tissues it should be noted that there is increasing clinical and experimental evidence that local tumor control rates are lower in smoking than in nonsmoking patients (SIEMAN et al. 1978; BROWMAN et al. 1993; KUCERA et al. 1987; GRAU et al. 1992).

5.2 Infections

It is well recognized that infections may increase the risk of acute or late radiation damage to normal tissue. Mucositis in patients treated for head and neck cancer, for example, is often aggravated by moniliasis, and the incidence of osteoradionecrosis of the jaws and soft tissue necrosis is significantly enhanced in patients with dental caries and other intraoral infections (NG et al. 1959; DALY 1980; MARCIAL 1989; WANG 1990). Several oral hygiene programs have been developed that, if meticulously followed, clearly decrease the risk of radiation induced normal tissue damage (KEYS and CASLAND 1976; JANSMA et al. 1992).

Another clinically important example of an interaction between radiation and infection is the development of chronic bowel ulcerations which may be increased as a consequence of mechanical and infectious damage to the chronically atrophic mucosa (TROTT et al. 1986; HAUER-JENSEN 1990).

Recently it has been found that mucosal reactions are enhanced in AIDS patients receiving oropharyngeal irradiation for lymphoma or Kaposi's sarcoma (WATKINS et al. 1987). The mechanisms underlying this phenomenon are poorly understood; however, it has been suggested that opportunistic infections, concurrent treatment with drugs, and deficiencies in repair of radiation damage in AIDS patients may all be involved.

5.3 Surgery

Surgery before or after radiation therapy may considerably enhance complications in normal tissues. One of the best studied clinical examples is the development of lymphedema of the arm in patients with mammary carcinoma after dissection of the axilla and radiation therapy, which, for a given radiation dose, is clearly dependent on the extent of surgery (LARSON et al. 1986; RYOO et al. 1989; BENTZEN et al. 1989). Other well established examples are the high complication rates of salvage surgery following radiation therapy of head and neck cancers (DONALD 1978; FLETCHER et al. 1980; GALLI et al. 1987; RUGG et al. 1991). Increased gastrointestinal toxicity of radiation therapy was observed after staging laparotomy or lymph node dissection in patients with abdominal or pelvic malignancies. The underlying mechanism of this phenomenon is probably a fixation of intestinal loops due to adhesions (POTISH et al. 1983; GUNDERSON et al. 1985; COIA and HANKS 1988; DALY et al. 1989; POTISH and DUSENBERY 1990; MAMEGHAN et al. 1990).

5.4 Chemotherapeutic Agents and Other Drugs

Many chemotherapeutic agents are known to increase acute and late-occurring normal tissue toxicity due to radiation therapy. Among these interactions are enhanced mucosal reactions in patients receiving fluoroaracil, increased lung toxicity after bleomycin, renal toxicity after cisplatin, bladder toxicity after cyclophosphamide, bone marrow toxicity after alkylating agents, skin toxicity after actinomycin D, and central nervous system toxicity after intrathecal application of methotrexate. Several excellent reviews are available that discuss the mechanisms of these toxicities in detail (e.g., RUBIN 1984; PHILLIPS 1989; STEWART 1991).

Another drug that has been associated with increased normal tissue toxicity is amiodarone, an antiarrhythmic which may increase acute reactions of mucosa and skin (DEMANGE et al. 1987; TOPHAM et al. 1988; HERCBERGS 1989, DE NEVE et al. 1992).

5.5 Age

Several tissues in children are more sensitive to irradiation than in adults, among the most prominent of these are brain, growing bone, and mammary gland (RUBIN and CASARETT 1968; MOLLS and STUSCHKE 1991). Beside differences in radiosensitivity between children and adults, age has been suggested by some investigators to also be predictive for the development of radiation damage in normal tissues among adult patients (CASARETT 1972; BENTZEN et al. 1989; MAMEGHAN et al. 1990; JENSEN et al. 1990; GREVEN et al. 1991; BUJKO et al. 1993).

5.6 Preexisting Disease in Irradiated Organs

Preexisting disease may limit the capacity of organs to withstand the trauma of irradiation. For example, a past history of gastrointestinal disease including duodenal ulcer, regional enteritis and colitis was shown to be a significant risk factor for intestinal complications after paraaortic or pelvic radiation therapy (HAMILTON et al. 1987; COIA and HANKS 1988; SMIT et al. 1990). Even if not studied in detail it appears safe to assume that preexisting disease in other organs such as emphysema of the lung, cardiomyopathy, nephritis, and osteoporosis may decrease the functional reserve of the organ to compensate for radiation damage.

5.7 Hypertension

Hypertension has been shown to enhance radiation induced vascular damage in the central nervous system of laboratory animal (ASSCHER and ANSON 1962) and in the retina in humans (BROWN et al. 1982). Radiation damage of the kidney in both humans and laboratory animals is known to be at least partly the result of secondary hypertension (WACHHOLZ and CASARETT 1970; STEWART and WILLIAMS 1991). Hypertension was not a significant predictor of gastrointestinal (GREVEN et al. 1991; LAWTON et al. 1991; MAMEGHAN et al. 1990) and soft tissue toxicity of radiation therapy (BUJKO et al. 1993).

5.8 Diabetes Mellitus

Several case reports suggest that diabetes mellitus may enhance the toxicity of radiation therapy to normal tissues including soft tissues (LIVENGOOD et al. 1991), brainstem (SMITH et al. 1979), and retina (BROWN et al. 1982; DHIR et al. 1982; VIEBAHN and BARRICKS 1993). An accumulative damaging effect on the structure and function of the retinal vasculature was also clearly demonstrated in diabetic rats (ARCHER et al. 1991). However, the question whether diabetes mellitus is an important predictor of radiation damage other than retinopathy remains unsettled. Recent studies on irradiation of carcinoma of the cervix (KUCERA et al. 1987), endometrium (GREVEN et al. 1991), and sarcoma of soft tissues (BUJKO et al. 1993) did not reveal a significant impact of diabetes mellitus on complications of radiation therapy.

5.9 Hyperthyroidism

Hyperthyroidism has been shown to enhance acute normal tissue damage of radiation therapy in humans and in laboratory animals. It has been suggested that this potentiating effect depends on an increased mitotic rate of the irradiated tissues (STEIN and GRIEM 1958; GRIEM et al. 1961).

5.10 Hemoglobin Level

In an analysis of patients treated for carcinoma of the bronchus DISCHE et al. (1986) reported an increased risk of radiation myelopathy in patients with hemoglobin levels higher than 13.0 g%. The authors suggest that higher hemoglobin concentrations result in an increased oxygen tension in the spinal cord at the time of radiotherapy, thereby increasing the radiosensitivity of this normal tissue.

5.11 *Diet*

Bacterial flora, bile, pancreatic enzymes, and mechanical-dietary facors have been found to increase the risk of acute and late-occurring radiation enteropathy. Several strategies including administration of special diets, bile acid sequestering resins, and enteroprotective drugs have been recommended to minimize this problem (MULHOLLAND et al. 1984; TROTT et al. 1986; HAUER-JENSEN 1990; MESTER et al. 1990).

5.12 *Skin Pigmentation and Hair Color*

It is widely believed that fair skinned patients express more severe skin damage than pigmented patients (WETTERER 1913–1914; RUBIN and CASARETT 1968). However, careful clinical studies on this subject indicate that skin reactions in differently pigmented patients are not different (GLICKSMAN et al. 1960).

6 Summary and Conclusions

Several endogenous and exogenous factors can increase the acute and late-occurring toxicity of radiation therapy. Even if sound data on the prevalence of these risk factors among radiation therapy patients are not available to date, it appears likely that a considerable proportion of all patients is at risk. Factors that exclusively increase acute normal tissue reactions will primarily worsen the prognosis of affected patients, whereas factors that increase late-occurring normal tissue damage are more likely to decrease via tolerance doses the probability of local tumor control in all patients. Recent evidence suggests that genetic factors may play an important role in individual differences of radiosensitivity, and some genetically radiosensitive patients might be detectable by laboratory tests in the near future. However, several factors other than genetics may also importantly impact the radiosensitivity of individual patients. Many of these factors can be easily detected by careful history taking and physical examination. Efforts should be made to identify and abolish such factors to reduce radiation induced morbidity in affected patients. Nevertheless, at least as important as reducing individual risk, is diminishing the impact of confounding factors on clinically administered tolerance doses, which may affect the chance of local tumor control in all radiotherapy patients. Since these tolerance doses are based on published experience, it appears essential to evaluate and report confounding factors in all clinical studies on normal tissue damage.

References

Abadir R, Hakami N (1983) Ataxia telangiectasia with cancer. An indication for reduced radiotherapy and chemotherapy doses. Br J Radiol 56: 343–345

Archer DB, Amoaku WM, Gardiner TA (1991) Radiation retinopathy-clinical, histopathological, ultrastructural and experimental correlations. Eye 5: 239–251

Arlett CF, Green MHL, Priestley A, Harcourt SA, Mayne LV (1988) Comparative human cellular radiosensitivity: I. The effect of SV40 transformation and immortilization on the gamma-irradiation survival of skin derived fibroblasts from normal individuals and from ataxia-telangiectasia patients and heterozygotes. Int J Radiat Biol 54: 911–928

Asscher AW, Anson SG (1962) Arterial hypertension and irradiation damage to the nervous system. Lancet 1343–1346

Baumann M, Taghian A, Budach W (1993) Radiosensitivity of tumor cells: the predictive value of SF2. In: Beck-Bornholdt HP (ed) Current topics in clinical radiobiology of tumors, medical radiology, Springer, Berlin Heidelberg New York, pp 87–98

Bentzen SM, Overgaard M (1993) Early and late normal tissue injury after postmastectomy radiotherapy. In: Hinkelbein W, Bruggmoser G, Frommhold H, Wannenmacher M (eds) Acute and Long-term side-effects of radiotherapy. Springer, Berlin Heidelberg New York, pp 59–78

Bentzen SM, Overgaard M, Thames HD (1989) Fractionation sensitivity of a clinical endpoint: impaired shoulder movement after post-mastectomy radiotherapy. Int J Radiat Oncol Biol Phys 17: 531–537

Bentzen SM, Johansen L, Overgaard J, Thames HD (1991) Clinical radiobiology of squamous cell carcinoma of the oropharynx. Int J Radiat Oncol Biol Phys 20: 1197–1206

Bentzen SM, Overgaard M, Overgaard J (1993) Clinical correlations between late normal-tissue endpoints after radiotherapy: implication for predictive assays of radiosensitivity. Eur J Cancer 29: 1373–1376

Brahme A (1984) Dosimetric precision requirements in radiation therapy. Acta Oncol 23: 379–391

Browman GP, Wong G, Hodson I, Sathya J, Russell R, McAlpine L, Skingley P, Levine MN (1993) Influence of cigarette smoking on the efficacy of radiation therapy in head and neck cancer. NEJM 328: 159–163

Brown GC, Shields JA, Augsburger JJ, Savino PJ, Schatz NJ (1982) Radiation retinopathy. Ophthalmology 89: 1494–1501

Bujko K, Suit HD, Springfield DS, Convery K (1993) Wound healing after preoperative radiation for sarcoma of soft tissues. Surg Gynecol Obstet 176: 124–134

Burman C, Kutcher GJ, Emami B, Goitein M (1991) Fitting of normal tissue tolerance data to an analytic fucntion. Int J Radiat Oncol Biol Phys 21: 123–135
Burnet NG, Nyman J, Turresson I, Wurm R, Yarnold JR, Peacock JH (1992) Prediction of normal tissue tolerance to radiotherapy from in vitro cellular radiation sensitivity. Lancet 339: 1570–1571
Busch M (1987) Risiken und Heilungschancen bei der Tumortherapie. In: Scherer E (ed) Strahlentherapie, 3rd edn. Springer, Berlin Heidelberg New York, pp 299–317
Casarett (1972) Aging. In Vaeth JM (ed) Radiation effects and tolerance, normal tissue, Karger, Basel, pp 479–485 (Frontiers of radiation therapy and oncology, vol 6)
Coia LR, Hanks GE (1988) Complications from large field intermediate dose infradiaphragmatic irradiation: an analysis of the patterns of care outcome studies for Hodgkin's disease and seminoma. Int J Radiat Oncol Biol Phys 15: 29–35
Cuncliffe PN, Mann R, Cameron AH, Roberts K (1975) Radiosensitivity in ataxia telangiectasia. Br J Radiol 48: 374–376
Daly TE (1980) Dental care in the irradiated patient. In: Fletcher GH (ed) Textbook of radiotherapy. Lea and Fabinger, Philadelphia, pp 229–237
Daly NJ, Izar F, Bachaud JM, Delannes M (1989) The incidence of severe chronic ileitis after abdominal and/or pelviv external irradiation with high energy photon beams. Radiother Oncol 14: 287–295
Demange L, Marechal F, Nguyen TD (1987) Could amiodaron increase acute cutaneous and mucosal toxicity of radiotherapy. Int J Radiat Oncol Biol Phys 13: 289
De Neve W, Fortan L, Storme G (1992) Increased acute mucosal and cutaneous toxicity in two patients taking amiodaron. Int J Radiat Oncol Biol Phys 22: 224
Deschavanne PJ, Debieu D, Fertil B, Malaise EP (1986) Reevaluation of in vitro radiosensitivity of human fibroblasts of different genetic origins. Int J Radiat Biol 50: 279–293
Dhir SP, Joshi AV, Banerjee AK (1982) Radiation retinopathy in diabetes mellitus. A case report Acta Radiol Oncol 21: 111–113
Dische S, Saunders M, Warburton MF (1986) Hemoglobin, morbidity and survival. Int J Radiat Oncol Biol Phys 12: 1335–1337
Donald PJ (1978) Complications of combined therapy in head and neck carcinomas. Arch Otolaryngol 104: 329–332
Emami B, Lyman J, Brown A, Coia L, Goitein M, Munzenrider JE, Shank B, Solin LJ, Wesson M (1991) Tolerance of normal tissue to therapeutic irradiation. Int J Radiat Oncol Biol Phys 11: 1685–1699
Fletcher GH (1966)) Basic parameters of radiotherapy. In: Fletcher GH (ed) Textbook of radiotherapy, 1st edn. Lea and Febinger, Philadelphia, pp 103–114
Fletcher GH, Westbrook KC, Jesse RH (1980) Interaction of surgery and irradiation in head and neck cancers. In: Fletcher GH (ed) Textbook of radiotherapy, 3rd edn. Lea and Febinger, Philadelphia, pp 237–249
Franzen L, Bjermer L, Hendrikson R, Littbrand B, Nilsson K (1989) Does smoking protect against radiation-induced pneumonitis. Int J Radiat Biol 56: 721–724
Galli A, Berrino P, Rainero ML, Santi P (1987) Present day role of plastic surgery in management of chronic radiation wounds: our experience. Eur J Surg Oncol 13: 239–246
Geara FB, Peters LJ, Ang KK, Wike JL, Brock WA (1992) Radiosensitivity measurements of keratinocytes and fibroblasts from radiotherapy patients. Int J Radiat Oncol Biol Phys 24: 287–293
Glicksman AS, Chu FCH, Bane HN, Nickson JJ (1960) Quantitative and qualitative evaluation of skin erythema. II. Clinical study in patients on a standardized irradiation schedule. Radiology 75: 411–415
Gotoff SP, Amiromokri E, Liebner E (1967) Ataxia telangiectasia: neoplasia, untoward response to x-irradiation and tuberous sclerosis. Am J Dis Child 114: 617–625
Grau C, Horsman MR, Overgaard J (1992) Influence of carboxyhemoglobin level on tumor growth, blood flow, and radiation response in an experimental model. Int J Radiat Oncol Biol Phys 22: 421–424
Green MHL, Arlett CF, Cole J, Harcourt SA, Priestley A, Waught APW, Stephens G, Beare DM, Brown NAP, Shun-Shin GA (1991) Comparative human cellular radiosensitivity: III. γ-radiation survival of cultured skin fibroblasts and resting T-lymphocytes from the peripheral blood of the same individual. Int J Radiat Biol 59: 749–765
Greven KM, Lanciano RM, Herbert SH, Hogan PE (1991) Analysis of complications in patients with endometrial carcinoma receiving adjuvant irradiation. Int J Radiat Oncol Biol Phys 21: 919–923
Griem ML, Stein JA, Reinertson RP, Reinertson R, Brown BR (1961) Comparison of Effects of 1-131-induced hypothyroidism and L-triiodothyronine on irradiated hair roots in Mice. Radiat Res 15: 202–210
Gunderson LL, Russell AH, Llewellyn HJ, Doppke KP, Tepper JE (1985) Treatment planning for colorectal cancer: radiation and surgical techniques and value of small-bowel films. Int J Radiat Oncol Biol Phys 11: 1379–1393
Hamilton CR, Horwich A, Bliss JM, Peckham MJ (1987) Gastrointestinal morbidity of adjuvant radiotherapy in stage I malignant teratoma of the testis. Radiother Oncol 10: 85–90
Hart RM, Kimler BF, Evans RG, Park CH (1987) Radiotherapeutic management of medulloblastoma in a pediatric patient with ataxia telangiectasia. Int J Radiat Oncol Biol Phys 13: 1237–1240
Hauer-Jensen M (1990) Late radiation injury of the small intestine. Acta Oncol 29: 401–415
Hercbergs A (1989) Early onset acute radiation toxicity and amiodaron. Int J Radiat Oncol Biol Phys 16: 525
Holthusen H (1936) Erfahrungen über die Verträglichkeitsgrenze für Röntgenstrahlen und deren Nutzanwendung. Strahlentherapie 57: 254–269
Horsman MR (1993) Hypoxia in tumours: its relevance, identification, and modification. In: Beck-Bornholdt HP (ed) Current topics in clinical radiobiology of tumors, medical radiology. Springer, Berlin Heidelberg New York, pp 99–112
Hübener KH, Baumann M, Krüll A, Schwarz R (1993) Clinically important factors modifying the response of tumors and normal tissue to radiation therapy. In Hinkelbein W, Bruggmoser G, Frommhold H, Wannenmacher M (eds) Acute and long-term side-effects of radiotherapy. Springer, Berlin Heidelberg New York, pp 41–47
Jansma J, Vissink A, Bouma J, Vermey A, Panders AK, Gravenmade EJ (1992) A survey of prevention and treatment regimens for oral sequelae resulting from head and neck radiotherapy used in Dutch radiotherapy institutes. Int J Radiat Oncol Biol Phys 24: 359–367
Jensen BV, Carlsen NLT, Groth S, Nissen NI (1989) Late effects on pulmonary function of mantle-field irradiation, chemotherapy or combined modality therapy for Hodgkin's disease. Eur J Haematol 44: 165–171
Jensen BV, Carlsen NLT, Nissen NI (1990) Influence of age and duration of follow-up on lung function after combined

chemotherapy for Hodgkin's disease. Eur Respir J 3: 1140–1145
Keys HM, Casland JP (1976) Techniques and results of a comprehensive dental care program in head and neck cancer patients. Int J Radiat Oncol Biol Phys 1: 859–865
Kluth EV, Jain PR, Stuchell, Frich JC (1988) A study of factors contributing to the development of osteoradionecrosis of the jaws. J Prosthet Dent 59: 194–201
Kucera H, Engelsberger H, Eppel W, Weghaupt K (1987) The influence of nicotine abuse and diabetes mellitus on the results of primary irradiation in the treatment of carcinoma of the cervix. Cancer 60: 1–4
Kushiro JI, Nakamura N, Kyoizumi S, Nishiki M, Dohi K, Akiyma M (1990) Absence of correlations between radiosensitivities of human T-Lymphocytes in G0 and skin fibroblasts in log phase. Radiat Res 122: 326–332
Larson D, Weinstein M, Goldberg I, Silver B, Recht A, Cady B, Silen W, Harris JR (1986) Edema of the arm as a function of the extent of axillary surgery in patients with stage I–II carcinoma of the breast treated with primary radiotherapy. Int J Radiat Oncol Biol Phys 12: 1575–1582
Lawton CA, Won M, Pilepich MV et al. (1991) Long-term treatment sequelae following external beam irradiation for adenocarcinoma of the prostate: analysis of RTOG studies 7506 and 7706. Int J Radiat Oncol Biol Phys 21: 935–939
Little JB, Nove J, Strong LC, Nichols WW (1988) Survival of human diploid skin fibroblasts from normal individuals after x-irradiation. Int J Radiat Biol 54: 899–910
Livengood CH, Soper JT, Clarke-Pearsson DL, Addison WA (1991) Necrotizing fasciitis in irradiated tissue from diabetic women. A report of two cases. J Reprod Med 36: 455–458
Loeffler JS, Harris JR, Dahlberg WK, Little JB (1990) In vitro radiosensitivity of human diploid fibroblasts derived from women with unusual sensitive clinical responses to definite radiation therapy for breast cancer. Radiat Res 121: 227–231
Mameghan H, Fisher R, Mameghan J, Watt WH, Tynan A (1990) Bowel complications after radiotherapy for carcinoma of the prostate: the volume effect. Int J Radiat Oncol Biol Phys 18: 315–320
Marcial VA (1989) The oral cavity and oropharynx. In: Moss WT, Cox JD (eds) Radiation oncology: rationale, technique, results. Mosby, St Louis, pp 112–163
Mester M, Hoover HC, Compton CC, Willett CG (1990) Experimental aspects of elimentary diets as radioprotectors. Arq Bras Cir Dig 5: 17–26
Molls M, Stuschke M (1991) Radiotherapy in Children: normal tissue injuries and carcinogenesis. In: Scherer E, Streffer C, Trott KR (eds) Radiopathology of organs and tissues. Springer, Berlin Heidelberg New York, pp 461–481
Morgan JL, Holcomb TM, Morrissey RW (1968) Radiation reaction in ataxia telangiectasia. Am J Dis Child 116: 557–558
Mulholland MW, Levitt SH, Song CW, Potish RA, Delaney JP (1984) The role of luminal contents in radiation enteritis. Cancer 54: 2396–2402
Ng E, Chambers FW, Odgen HS, Coggs GC, Crane JT (1959) Osteomyelitis of the mandible following irradiation. Radiology 72: 68–74
Norman A, Kagan RA, Chan SL (1988) The importance of genetics for the optimization of radiation therapy. Am J Clin Oncol (CCT) 11: 84–88
Overgaard J, Hjelm-Hansen M, Vendelbo-Johansen L, Andersen AP (1988) Comparison of conventional and split-course radiotherapy as primary treatment in carcinoma of the larynx. Acta Oncol 27: 147–152
Paterson R (1948) The treatment of malignant disease by radium and x-rays. Arnold, London
Peters LJ, Withers HR, Thames HD, Fletcher GH (1982) Keynote address. The problem: tumor radioresistance in clinical radiotherapy. Int J Radiat Oncol Biol Phys 8: 101–108
Peters LJ, Brock WA, Johnston T, Meyn RE, Tofilon PJ, Milas L (1986) Potential methods for predicting tumor radiocurability. Int J Radiat Oncol Biol Phys 12: 459–467
Peters LJ, Brock WA, Chapman JD, Wilson G (1988) Predictive assays of tumor radiocurability. Am J Clin Oncol 11: 275–285
Phillips TL (1989) Chemical modifiers of normal-tissue radiation injury. In: Vaeth JM, Meyer JL (eds) Radiation tolerance of normal tissues. Karger, Basel, pp 177–184 (Frontiers of radiation therapy and oncology, vol 23)
Potish RA, Dusenbery KE (1990) Enteric morbidity of postoperative pelvic external beam and brachytherapy for uterine cancer. Int J Radiat Oncol Biol Phys 18: 1005–1010
Potish RA, Twiggs L, Adcock LL, Prem KA (1983) Logistic models for prediction of enteric morbidity in the treatment of ovarian and cervical cancers. Am J Obstet Gynecol 147: 65–72
Pritchard J, Sandland MR, Breatnach FB, Pincott JR, Cox R, Husband P (1982) The effects of radiation therapy for Hodgkin's disease in a child with ataxia telangiectasia. Cancer 50: 877–886
Rubin P (1984) The Franz Buschke Lecture: Late effects of chemotherapy and radiation therapy: a new hypothesis. Int J Radiat Oncol Biol Phys 10: 5–34
Rubin P (1989) The law and order of radiation sensitivity, absolute versus relative. In: Vaeth JM, Meyr JL (eds) Radiation tolerance of normal tissues. Karger, Basel, pp 7–40 (Frontiers of radiation therapy and oncology, vol 23)
Rubin P, Cassarett G (1968) Clinical radiation pathology. Saunders, Philadelphia
Rubin P, Casarett G (1972) A direction for clinical radiation pathology. In: Vaeth JM (ed) Radiation effect and tolerance, normal tissue. Karger, Basel, pp 1–16 (Frontiers of radiation therapy and oncology, vol 6)
Rubin P, Keller B, Quick R (1974) The range of prescribed tumor lethal doses in the treatment of different human tumors. In: Friedman M (ed) The biological and clinical basis of radiosensitivity. Thomas, Springfield, pp 435–484
Rugg T, Saunders M, Dische S (1990) Smoking and mucosal reaction to radiotherapy. Br J Radiol 63: 554–556
Rugg T, Lartigau E, Sanders R, Glover G, Saunders M, Dische S (1991) The morbidity of salvage surgery following conventional radiotherapy and continuous, hyperfractionated accelerated radiotherapy (CHART) Int J Radiat Oncol Biol Phys 20: 581–586
Ryoo MC, Kagan AR, Wollin M, Tome MA, Tedeschi MA, Rao AR, Hintz BL, Kuruvilla AM, Nussbaum H, Streeter OE, Jabola BR, Miller MJ (1989) Prognostic factors for recurrence and cosmesis in 393 patients after radiation therapy for early mammary carcinoma. Radiology 172: 555–559
Sieman DW, Hill RP, Bush RS (1978) Smoking: the influence of carboxyhemoglobin (HbCO) on tumor oxygenation and response to irradiation. Int J Radiat Oncol Biol Phys 4: 657–662
Slanina J (1977) Untersuchungen über somatische Späts-

chäden nach ausgedehnter Strahlentherapie. Habilitationsschrift, University of Freiburg

Smit WGJM, Helle PA, van Putten WLJ, Wijnmaalen AJ, Seldenrath JJ, van der Werf-Messing BHP (1990) Late radiation damage in prostae cancer patients treated by high dose external radiotherapy in relation to rectal dose. Int J Radiat Oncol Biol Phys 18: 23–29

Smith BM, Mc Ginnis W, Cook J, Latourette H (1979) Central nervous system changes complicating the use of radiotherapy for the treatment of a nasopharyngeal neoplasm in a diabetic patient. Cancer 43: 2239–2242

Smith KC, Hahn GM, Hoppe RT, Earle JD (1980) Radiosensitivity in vitro of human fibroblasts derived from patients with a severe skin reaction to radiation therapy. Int J Radiat Oncol Biol Phys 6: 1573–1575

Stein JA, Griem ML (1958) Effect of triiodothyronine on radiosensitivity. Nature 182: 1681–1682

Stewart FA (1991) Keynote address: modulation of normal tissue toxicity by combined modality therapy: considerations for improving the therapeutic gain. Int J Radiat Oncol Biol Phys 20: 319–325

Stewart FA and Williams MV (1991) The Urinary tract. In: Scherer E, Streffer C, Trott KR (eds) Radiopathology of organs and tissues. Springer, Berlin Heidelberg New York, pp 405–431

Suit HD, Walker AM (1988) Predictors of radiation response in use today: criteria for new assays and methods of verification. In: Chapman JD, Peters LJ, Withers HR (eds) Prediction of tumor treatment response. Pergamon, New York, pp 3–19

Suit HD, Baumann M, Skates S, Convery K (1989) Clinical interest in determinations of cellular radiation sensitivity. Int J Radiat Biol 56: 725–737

Swift M, Reitnauer PJ, Morrell D, Chase C (1987) Breast and other cancers in families with ataxia-telangiectasia. N Engl J Med 316: 1289–1294

Swift M, Morrell D, Massey RB, Chase CL (1991) Incidence of cancer in 161 families affected by ataxia telangiectasia. N Engl J Med 325: 1831–1836

Taylor AMR, Harnden DG, Arlett CF, Harcourt SA, Lehmann AR, Stevens S, Bridges BA (1975) Ataxia telangiectasia: a human mutation with abnormal radiation sensitivity. Nature 258: 427–429

Thames HD, Hendry JH, Moore JV, Ang KK, Travis EL (1989) The high steepness of dose response curves for late responding normal tissues. Radiother Oncol 15: 49–53

Topham C, Brierley J, Tomlinson H (1988) Toxicity and amiodaron. Int J Radiat Oncol Biol Phys 14: 1056

Trott KR, Kummermehr J (1993) The time factor and repopulation in tumors and normal tissues. Semin Radiat Oncol 3: 115–125

Trott KR, Breiter N, Spiethoff A (1986) Experimental studies on the pathogenesis of the chronic radiation ulcer of the large bowel in rats. Int J Radiat Oncol Biol Phys 12: 1637–1643

Tucker SL, Turresson I, Thames HD (1992) Evidence for individual differences in the radiosensitivity of human skin. Eur J Cancer 11: 1783–1791

Turreson I (1989) The progression rate of late radiation effects in normal tissue and its impact on dose-response relationships. Radiother Oncol 15: 217–226

Turreson I (1990) Individual variation and dose dependency in the progression rate of skin telangiectasia. Int J Radiat Oncol Biol Phys 29: 1569–1574

Turesson I (1991) Characteristics of dose-response relationships for late radiation effects: an analysis of skin telangiectasia and of head and neck morbidity. Radiother Oncol 20: 149–158

Turreson I, Thames H (1989) Repair capacity and kinetics of human skin during fractionated radiotherapy: erythema, desquamation and telangiectasia after 3 and 5 years follow up. Radiother Oncol 15: 169–188

Viebahn M, Barricks ME (1993) Potentiating effect of diabetes in radiation retinopathy. Int J Radiat Oncol Biol Phys 25: 379–380

Wachholz BW, Casarett GW (1970) Radiation hypertension and nephrosclerosis. Radiat Res 41: 39–56

Wang CC (1990) Radiation therapy for head and neck neoplasms: indications, techniques, and results. Year Book Medical Publishers, Chicago

Watkins EB, Findlay P, Gelman E, Lane HC, Zabell A (1987) Enhanced mucosal reactions in AIDS patients receiving orophgaryngeal irradiation. Int J Radiat Oncol Biol Phys 13: 1403–1408

Wetterer J (1913–1914) Handbuch der Röntgentherapie, 2nd edn. Nemnich, Leipzig

Wilson GD (1993) Limitation of the bromodeoxyuridine technique for measurement of tumour proliferation. In: Beck-Bornhold HP (ed) Current topics in clinical radiobiology of tumors, medical radiology. Springer, Berlin Heidelberg New York, pp 27–44

Withers HR (1993) Treatment-induced accelerated human tumor growth. Semin Radiat Oncol 3: 135–143

Whittet HB, Lund VJ, Brockbank M, Feyerabend C (1991) Serum cotinine as an objective marker for smoking habit in head and neck malignancy. J Laryngol Otol 105: 1036–1039

Würschmidt F, Beck-Bornholdt HP, Vogler H, Jung H (1991) Radiotherapy of the rhabdomyosarcoma R1H of the rat: split course versus continuous fractionation. Strahlenther Onkol 167: 26–30

1.2 Endogenous and Exogenous Factors Modifying Chemosensitivity to Cytostatic Drugs

HANS-JÖRG SAUER

CONTENTS

1 Introduction 13
2 Drug Interaction 13
3 Organ Dysfunctions 14
4 Resistance Mechanisms 14
5 Metabolic Polymorphism 15
6 Chromosomal Aberrations 15
7 Inborn Enzyme Defects 16
8 DNA Repair Defects 16
9 Biorhythm 17
10 Summary and Conclusions 17
References 18

Table 1. Endogenous and exogenous factors modifying chemosensitivity to cytostatic drugs

Drug interactions (with cytostatics and/or noncytostatics)
Organ dysfunctions (e.g., liver, kidneys)
Expression of resistance mechanisms (e.g., multiple drug resistance)
Metabolic polymorphism (e.g., cytochrome P-450 enzyme systems, low/high carboxylators)
Chromosomal aberrations (e.g., Down's syndrome, fragile X syndrome)
Inborn metabolic errors (e.g., DNA repair defects, enzyme defects)
Biorhythm (e.g., DNA synthesis, enzyme activities)

1 Introduction

It is well known that, with respect to cytostatic drug, there is a small therapeutic range between the dose with the desired antitumor activity and the dose which can cause severe side effects. Side effects occur usually in rapidly proliferating self-regenerating tissues such as bone marrow and mucosae.

There are numerous exogenous and endogenous factors which can modify the pharmacokinetics, metabolism and pharmacodynamics of cytostatic drugs. These interactions may lead to an increased (or decreased) activity of the respective drug. Indeed, even a minor increase in activity may cause severe bone marrow suppression or mucositis. In this context, several clinically relevant aspects will be discussed (Table 1).

2 Drug Interactions

Combinations of different cytostatic drugs are often used in the treatment of cancer patients in order to generate an increased antitumor effect without a substantial accumulation of toxic side effects. One example is the combination of alkylating agents (e.g., ifosfamide) with inhibitors of the enzyme topoisomerase II (e.g., etoposide). This causes an increased antitumor effect by decreasing the efficacy of the repair mechanisms at the alkylated sites in the DNA (CLARK and SLEVIN 1987; MISER et al. 1987). Another example is the sequential administration of methotrexate and 5-fluorouracil which results in an increased activation of 5-fluorouracil to the cytostatically active forms 5-fluorodeoxyuridine (5-FUdR) and 5-fluorouraciltriphosphates (5-FUTP, 5-dFUTP).

The numerous other cytostatic-cytostatic interactions cannot be described here in detail (e.g., cytarabine and fludarabine, vincristine and methotrexate, methotrexate and L-asparaginase, hydroxyurea and cytarabine). Rather, in this review it seems more interesting to point out the interactions of cytostatic drugs with other, primarily noncytostatic, agents. A review of the recent literature (SAUER 1992a) revealed at least 160 different such combinations which can provoke increased cytostatic activity and more than 60 combinations which lead to a reduction of the activity of specified antiproliferative agents. A complete listing of all these phenomena cannot be given here. Table 2 shows some of the well known interactions.

Practically, when treating patients, these combinations should be avoided or the dose of the cytostatic drug should be reduced (e.g., only 25% of 6-mercaptopurine when in combination with allopurinol). However, such combinations can also be

HANS-JÖRG SAUER, Prof. Dr., Medizinische Klinik III, Klinikum Großhadern, Ludwig-Maximilians-Universität München, Marchioninistraße 15, 81377 München, FRG

Table 2. Interactions between cytostatic and noncytostatic drugs (Sauer 1992a)

Cytostatic drug	Activity intensification	Activity reduction
Bleomycin	Caffeine	Thiols
Cyclophosphamide	Cimetidine	Thiols
Daunorubicin	Cyclosporin A	Copper ions
Doxorubicin	Verapamil	Phenobarbital
Etoposide	Dipyridamole	Phenytoin
Fluorouracil	Folinic acid Dipyridamole	Allopurinol
Mercaptopurine	Allopurinol	
Methotrexate	NSAID Cotrimoxazole	Folinic acid
Mitoxantrone	Diazepam	Heparin
Platinum derivatives	DMSO	Thiols
Vinca alkaloids	Verapamil Cyclosporin A	Folinic acid(?)

used with the intention to make a standard dose of a cytostatic drug more effective (e.g., 5- fluorouracil and folinic acid) or to overcome resistance mechanisms (e.g., anthracyclines and verapamil) or to antagonize a drug selectively (e.g., methotrexate and folinic acid, cisplatin and sodium thiosulfate).

3 Organ Dysfunctions

Impaired kidney and liver function can lead to a slower elimination or inactivation of many substances. Table 3 gives the main mechanisms of elimination of some important cytostatic drugs.

Table 3. Renal and hepatic elimination of cytostatic drugs (Sauer and Wilmanns 1991)

Mainly renal	Mainly hepatic
Alkylating agents	Anthracyclines and antibiotics
Cyclophosphamide	Doxorubicin
Ifosfamide	Daunorubicin
Cisplatin	Epirubicin
Carboplatin	Mitoxantrone
Antimetabolites	Mitomycin C
Methotrexate	Actinomycin D
Fluorouracil	
	Vinca alkaloids
Nitrosoureas	Vincristine
BCNU (carmustine)	Vinblastine
CCNU (lomustine)	Vindesine
ACNU (nimustine)	
	Podophyllotoxins
	Etoposide
	Teniposide
	Others
	Dacarbazine
	Procarbazine

Information regarding dose reduction according to the results of serum creatinine, renal clearance or liver function tests are given in detail in the literature, in handbooks and in product information material. (Sauer 1992a; Sauer and Wilmanns 1991).

4 Resistance Mechanisms

Many different mechanisms can lead to resistance against individual cytostatic drugs or even groups of them:

1. Alteration of pharmacokinetics
2. Alteration of metabolism
3. Alteration of target
4. Alteration of membrane transport

Only the last of these four points will be described here in greater detail. The multiple drug resistance (*mdr*-1) gene, located on chromosome 7, can be induced by some cytostatic drugs. A glycoprotein (GP-170) is expressed which is activated by protein kinase C (PKC) and which serves as a membrane associated transport system for the efflux of cytostatic drugs (see Table 4). Thus, the intracellular drug concentration and its cytostatic efficacy are reduced.

The expression of GP-170 may also be important for the integrity of normal tissues. Table 5 lists the relative GP-170 content of different tissues. High concentrations are found in the epithelial cells of excretory organs. This could be a physiological rescue mechanism against the accumulation of toxic substances. By contrast, tissues and other structures which do not express GP-170, including bone marrow, mucosae and hair follicles, are more susceptible to toxic substances such as the cytostatic drugs listed in Table 4.

Table 4. Cytostatic drugs with increased efflux by GP-170 (*mdr*-1) (Volm et al. 1990)

Anthracyclines and antibiotics
Doxorubicin
Daunorubicin
Mitomycin C
Actinomycin D
Vinca alkaloids
Vincristine
Vinblastine
Vindesine
Podophyllotoxins
Etoposide
Teniposide

Table 5. Glycoprotein GP-170 in normal tissues (Volm et al. 1990)

Higher levels	Lower levels
Epithelium of:	
Stomach	Bronchi
Small intestine	Blood vessels
Colon	Renal tubuli
Biliary system	Superarenal glands
Gallbladder	Heart
Pancreas	Spleen
Salivary glands	Lymph nodes
Female breast	Muscles
Sweat glands	

Many substances can directly or indirectly inhibit the function of GP-170 (e.g., verapamil and other calcium antagonists, cyclosporin A, quinidine, chlorpromazine, trifluperazine, tamoxifen and its derivatives). Thus, combination with the cytostatic drugs given in Table 4 can eventually result in increased toxic effects on susceptible tissues. Clinical therapeutic studies use such combinations to overcome primary or induced P-170 related resistance of malignant tissues (Ford and Hait 1990).

5 Metabolic Polymorphism

Many cytostatic drugs are either directly or indirectly activated or degraded via the cytochrome P-450-dependent hepatic mixed functional oxidative enzyme system (MFOS) (see Table 6). Thus, hepatic drug metabolism can be influenced significantly by inducers or inhibitors of this system. Inducers include barbiturates, diphenylhydantoin, diazepam and its derivatives. Inhibitors include cimetidine, ranitidine, antidepressants (fluoxetine), neuroleptics (chlorpromazine). The latter substances may provoke increased toxicity of cytostatic drugs by alteration of their pharmacokinetics (higher area under the concentration curve or AUC values).

A similar result can occur in "poor metabolizers," i.e., individuals who have a genetically determined deficiency of one of the MFOS subunits (P-450-II-D6 protein). It is assumed that in a healthy human population 5%–10% have such a defect (Gaedigk et al. 1991). Patients with fatty liver degeneration are also reported to have a relative deficiency in MFOS activity (Rodvold et al. 1988). Another drug metabolizing enzymatic step in the liver is via the carboxylating system. Aldophosphamide dehydrogenase (EC 1.2.1.3.) degrades phosphamide mustard, a cytostatically active metabolite of cyclophosphamide, to the renally eliminated product carboxyphosphamide. In about 36% of all cyclophosphamide treated patients an enzymatic polymorphism could be detected. Low carboxylators had twofold increased AUC values for phosphamide mustard and the urotoxic acrolein. This explained the increased bone marrow depression and hemorrhagic cystitis observed after administration of the standard dose of cyclophosphamide (Hadidi et al. 1988).

Table 6. Direct or indirect effects of P-450 enzyme systems on cytostatic drugs (Sauer 1992a)

Drug activation	Drug degradation
Altretamine	Altretamine
Anthracyclines	Amsacrine
Cyclophosphamide	Anthracyclines
Dacarbazine	Bleomycin
Etoposide	Busulfan
Ifosfamide	Chlorambucil
Mitomycin C	Cyclophosphamide
Procarbazine	Dacarbazine
Thio-TEPA	Estramustine
Trofosfamide	Etoposide
	Hydroxyurea
	Ifosfamide
	Lomustine
	Mitoxantrone
	Nimustine
	Prednimustine
	Thio-TEPA
	Vinca alkaloids

6 Chromosomal Aberrations

Down's syndrome (trisomy 21) is connected with an abnormal sensitivity to methotrexate. It is supposed that increased purine biosynthesis requires a greater supply of tetrahydrofolate derivatives. This makes the entire metabolism more susceptible to the action of methotrexate. Thus, in Down's syndrome patients one should reduce the normally prescribed dose by 50%–70% (Lejeune et al. 1991; Peeters and Poon 1987; Ueland et al. 1990).

Fragile X syndrome is an X-linked recessive syndrome. Affected male children display intellectual defects, autism, large testes, big ears and dwarfism. The frequency is 1:1000 (3000) in men and accounts for about 10% of all intellectually disabeled men. In women the frequency is 1:700 (2000), but women are carriers and therefore usually not seriously affected. Expression of the defect is folate sensitive: A deficiency in metabolically active tetrahydrofolate derivatives, e.g., as occurs during treatment with methotrexate or 5-fluorouracil, may worsen the clinical degree of the illness. Thus, methotrexate and 5-fluorouracil should be avoided in fragile X patients. Additionally, patients with fragile X syndrome have a reduced potency to repair bleomycin-induced DNA damage. This results in a higher mutagenic potential of cytostatic drugs (Branda et al. 1984; Glover and Howard-Peebles 1983; Jacky and Sunderland 1983; Kimchi-Sarfaty et al. 1991; Li and Lin 1990; Michels 1985; Schmid 1990).

7 Inborn Enzyme Defects

Several enzymatic defects in the body's biochemical pathways are connected directly or indirectly with purine and pyrimidine de novo synthesis and lead to an increased cytostatic efficacy of the antimetabolites methotrexate, 5-fluorouracil and 6-mercaptopurine (Blau 1988; Evans et al. 1991; Harris et al. 1991; Tuchmann et al. 1985; Zittoun et al. 1987): These defects include:

1. Dihydrofolate reductase (DHFR) deficiency
2. Dihydropteridine reductase (DHPR) deficiency
3. Methionine synthase (MS) deficiency
4. Dihydropyrimidine dehydrogenase (DPD) deficiency (pyridinemia/pyrimidinuria)
5. Thiopurine methyltransferase (TPM) deficiency

The first three defects have a common result, the lack of biologically active tetrahydrofolate derivatives. Consequently, this leads to a higher efficacy of methotrexate. In particular, the MS defect can easily be simulated by administration of the anesthetic gas nitrous oxide (N_2O) in vitro and in vivo. Figure 1 shows the biochemical pathways.

The MS reaction is dependent on reduced vitamin B_{12} in the active center of the enzyme. This oxidized by N_2O whereby the enzymatic activity is blocked totally and irreversibly. Again the resulting deficiency in reduced folates leads to an increased sensitivity to methotrexate. Thus, methotrexate should be avoided at least 3 days before and 3 days after anesthesia with N_2O (Ermens 1990; Ermens et al. 1991; Gillman 1988; Howland 1988; Koblin et al. 1990; Nunn 1988; Waldmann et al. 1990).

Pyrimidinemia is an autosomal recessive defect in pyrimidine catabolism. The accumulation of pyrimidines includes 5-fluorouracil and its derivatives in case of treatment with this drug. Due to the expected higher toxicity, 5-fluorouracil should be avoided in patients with pyrimidinemia.

TPM deficiency is an autosomally inherited defect. It leads to the intracellular accumulation of thiopurine and its derivatives. This also applies for 6-thioguanine nucleotides which are the cytostatically active forms of 6-mercaptopurine. Since severe toxic side effects occur, 6-mercaptopurine should be avoided or reduced to one seventh of the standard close.

8 DNA Repair Defects

One of the important effects of many cytostatic drugs is disturbances to the structure of DNA (Epstein 1990). The resultant defects can be repaired by cellular mechanisms. Small defects are repaired directly in situ, larger defects are repaired by excision, new synthesis and recombination of the defective parts. Figure 2 shows this schematically together with the responsible enzymatic activities.

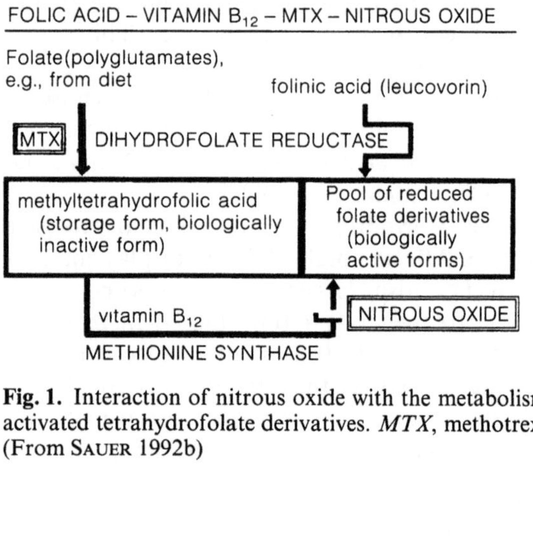

Fig. 1. Interaction of nitrous oxide with the metabolism of activated tetrahydrofolate derivatives. *MTX*, methotrexate. (From Sauer 1992b)

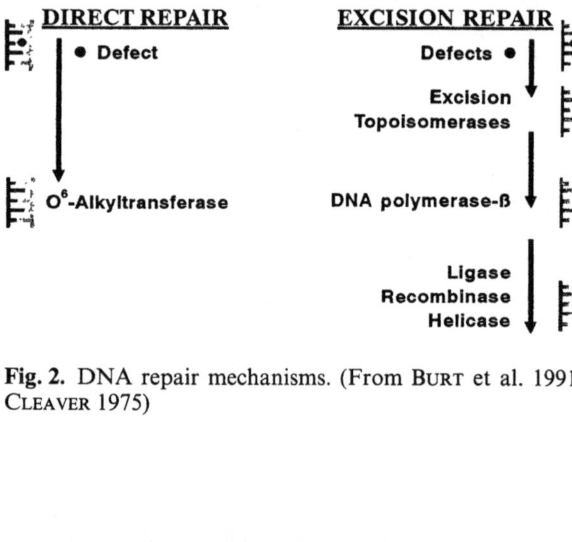

Fig. 2. DNA repair mechanisms. (From Burt et al. 1991; Cleaver 1975)

Table 7. DNA repair defects (GATTI et al. 1991; LINDAHL 1987; TIMME and MOSES 1988)

Syndrome	Signs	Frequency
Ataxia telangiectatica	Ataxia, telangiectasias (skin, conjunctiva), cerebellar dysfunctions, IgA deficiency	$\leqslant$ 1/40000 ($\leqslant$ 7.7% heterozygous)
Xeroderma pigmentosum	Skin hyperkeratosis, telangiectasias, neurological defects, photosensitivity	$\leqslant$ 1/40 000
Fanconi's anemia	Anemia, hypogonadism, dwarfism, bone defects	$\leqslant$ 1/40 000
Bloom syndrome	Immunodeficiency, dwarfism, photosensitivity	1/3 000 000
Cockayne's syndrome	Dwarfism, microcephalia, ataxia, tremor, deafness, photosensitivity	Very seldom

Table 8. Biochemical data on DNA repair defects (CLEAVER 1975; EPSTEIN 1990; LINDAHL 1987; LÖNN et al. 1990; MEREDITH and DODSON 1987; TIMME and MOSES 1988; VUILLAUME et al. 1986)

Syndrome	Supposed biochemical defect	Increased toxicity of drugs or light
Ataxia telangiectasia	DNA recombinase, Glutathione deficiency	Bleomycin, Etoposide
Xeroderma pigmentosum	DNA helicase, DNA ligase catalase	Cisplatin, Ultraviolet light
Fanconi's anemia	Nucleotide metabolism Radical metabolism	Bifunctional alkylating agents
Bloom syndrome	DNA ligase Uracil DNA glycosylase	Bifunctional alkylating agents Fluorouracil
Cockayne's syndrome	Semiconservative DNA replication (?) photosensitivity	Ultraviolet light

Table 7 lists a few of the syndromes which are associated with defects in DNA repair mechanisms. Table 8 lists the supposed biochemical mechanism and some of the cytostatic drugs which may have an increased toxicity in these patients.

Patients with DNA repair defects have a greater mutation rate and a greater risk of getting a malignant disease (MORREU et al. 1990; NARITA and TAGEKI 1984; SWIFT et al. 1987). However, the latter will be difficult to treat with cytostatic drugs, because of their increased toxicity. It is not known if DNA repair defects results also in a higher sensitivity of the tumor tissue.

9 Biorhythm

Several clinical studies are under way to optimally adapt cytostatic chemotherapy regimens to circadian biorhythms. DNA synthesis in normal tissues (e.g., bone marrow, mucosae, epidermis) is most active during daytime and the second half of the night. Thus, if antiproliferative agents are given at times of lower DNA synthesis activity (evening and first half of the night), one could expect less toxicity towards rapidly self-regenerating tissues (BROWN 1991; BUCHI et al. 1991; CANAL et al. 1991; KERR et al. 1990; SMAALAND et al. 1991).

Another possibility is to adapt to the circadian rhythms of enzyme activities. For example, dihydropyrimidine dehydrogenase (DPD) at nighttime has a five fold higher activity. This leads to a rapid degradation of 5-fluorouracil and to five times lower plasma levels during administration at night. This could result in less toxicity but also less therapeutic efficacy (VON ROEMELING 1990).

10 Summary and Conclusions

The pharmacokinetics, metabolism and pharmacodynamics of cytostatic drugs can be influenced by several exogenous and endogenous mechanisms. This can result in better or worse antitumor effects, but also in greater toxicity.

It is difficult to draw practical conclusions. Many defects in cytostatic drug metabolism, such as those listed in Table 1, are "hidden" in "healthy" persons and become overt only during administration of certain cytostatic drugs. One has to be cautious in any patient with a known or supposed error in a biochemical pathways or with a chromosomal abnormality. For these rare cases an extra look at the literature is advisable before any cytostatic chemotherapy is begun.

References

Blau N (1988) Inborn errors of pterin metabolism. Annu Rev Nutr 8: 185–210

Branda RF, Arthur DC, Woods WG, Danzl TJ, King RA (1984) Folate metabolism and chromosomal stability in the fragile X syndrome. Am J Med 77: 602–611

Brown WR (1991) A review and mathematical analysis of circadian rhythms in cell proliferation in mouse, rat, and human epidermis. J Invest Dermatol 97: 273–280

Buchi KN, Moore JG, Hrushesky WJM, Souther RB, Rubin NH (1991) Circadian rhythm of cellular proliferation in the human rectal mucosa. Gastroenterology 101: 410–415

Burt RK, Poirier MC, Link CJ, Bohr VA (1991) Antineoplastic drug resistance and DNA repair Ann Oncol 2: 325–334

Canal P, Sqalli A, Deforni M, Chevreau C, Pujol A, Bugat R, Roche H, Oustrin J, Houin G (1991) Chronopharmacokinetics of doxorubicin in patients with breast cancer Eur J Clin Pharmacol 40: 287–291

Clark PI, Slevin ML (1987) The clinical pharmacology of etoposide and teniposide. Clin Pharmacokinet 12: 223–252

Cleaver JE (1975) Xeroderma pigmentosum: biochemical and genetic characteristics. Annu Rev Genet 9: 19–38

Epstein RJ (1990) Drug-induced DNA damage and tumor chemosensitivity. J Clin Oncol 8: 2062–2084

Ermens AAM (1990) Significance of cobalamin inactivation in normal and malignant hematopoiesis. Pharmaceut Weekbl – Sci Ed 12: 212–214

Ermens AAM, Schoester M, Lindemanns J, Abels J (1991) Effect of nitrous oxide and methotrexate on folate coenzyme pools of blast cells from leukemia patients. Leukor Res 15: 165–171

Evans WE, Horner M, Chu YQ, Kalwinsky D, Roberts WM (1991) Altered mercaptopurine metabolism, toxic effects, and dosage requirement in a thiopurine methyltransferase-deficient child with acute lymphocytic leukemia. J Pediatr 119: 985–989

Ford JM, Hait WN (1990) Pharmacology of drugs that alter multidrug resistance in cancer. Pharmacol Rev 42: 155–199

Gaedigk A, Blum M, Gaedigk R, Eichelbaum M, Meyer UA (1991) Delection of the cytochrome P450 CYP2D6 gene as a cause of impaired drug metabolism in poor metabolizers of the debrisoquine/sparteine polymorphism. Am J Hum Genet 48: 943–950

Gatti RA, Boder E, Vinters HV, Sparkes RS, Norman A, Lange K (1991) Ataxia-telangiectasia – an interdisciplinary approach to pathogenesis. Medicine 70: 99–117

Gillman MA (1988) Anti-neoplastic synergism of nitrous-oxide ant methotrexate. Br J Anaesth 60: 349–350

Glover TW, Howard-Peebles PN (1983) The combined effects of FUdR addition and methionine depletion on the X-chromosome fragile site. Am J Hum Genet 35: 117–122

Hadidi A, Hakam FA, Coulter CEA, Idle JR (1988) Phenotypically deficient urinary elimination of carboxyphosphamide after cyclophosphamide administration to cancer patients. Cancer Res 48: 5167–5171

Harris BE, Carpenter JT, Diasio RB (1991) Severe 5-fluorouracil toxicity secondary to dihydropyrimidine dehydrogenase deficiency – a potentially more common pharmacogenetic syndrome. Cancer 68: 499–501

Howland WL (1988) Methotrexate-associated bone marrow suppression following surgery. Arthritis Rheum. 31: 1586

Jacky PB, Sutherland GR (1983) Thymidylate synthetase und fragile site expression in lymphocytes. Am J Hum Genet 35: 1276–1283

Kerr KJ, Lewis C, O'Neil B, Lawson N, Blackie RG, Newell DR, Boxall F, Cox J, Rinkin EM, Kaye SB (1990) The myelotoxicity of carboplatin is influenced by the time of its administration. Hematol Oncol 8: 59–63

Kimchi-Sarfaty C, Goitein R, Kerem B, Werner M, Meidan B, Schaap T (1991) Endoreduplication and polyploidy in fragile-X cells induced by methotrexate and fluorodeoxyuridine-implications for diagnosis. Am J Med Genet 38: 429–433

Koblin DD, Tomerson BW, Waldman FM, Lampe GH, Wauk LZ, Eger EI (1990) Effect of nitrous oxide on folate and vitamin B12 metabolism in Patients. Anesth Analg 71: 610–617

Lejeune P, Peeters M, Rethore MO, Deblois MC (1991) Homocysteine and the methotrexate toxicity in trisomy-21. Cancer Chemother Pharmacol 27: 331–332

Li SY, Lin JK (1990) Differential bleomycin susceptibility in cultured lymphocytes of fragile X-patients and normal individuals. Hum Genet 85: 267–271

Lindahl T (1987) Regulation and deficiencies in DNA repair. Br J Cancer 56: 91–95

Lönn U, Lönn S, Nylen U, Winblad G (1990) Increased levels of 5-fluorouracil-induced DNA lesions in bloom's syndrome. Int J Cancer 45: 494–499

Meredith MJ, Dodson ML (1987) Impaired glutathione biosynthesis in cultured human ataxia-telangiectasia cells. Cancer Res 47: 4576–4581

Michels VV (1985) Fragile sites on human chromosomes: description and clinical significance. Mayo Clin Proc 60: 690–694

Miser JS, Kinsella TJ, Triche TJ, Tsokos M, Jarosinski P (1987) Ifosfamide with mesna uroprotection and etoposide – an effective regimen in the treatment of recurrent sarcomas and other tumors of children and young adults. J Clin Oncol 5: 1191–1189

Morrell D, Chase CL, Swift M (1990) Cancers in 44 families with ataxia-telangiectasia. Cancer Genet Cytogenet 50: 119–123

Narita T, Tagaki K (1984) Ataxia teleangiectasia with dysgerminoma of right ovary, papillary carcinoma of thyroid, and adenocarcinoma of pancreas. Cancer 54: 1113–1116

Nunn JF (1988) Clinical relevance of the B_{12}/N_2O interaction. A report of a seminar. Anaesthesia 43: 587–589

Peeters M, Poon A (1987) Down syndrome and leukemia: unusual clinical aspects and unexpected methotrexate sensitivity. Eur J Pediat 146: 146–422

Rodvold KA, Rushing DA, Tewksbury DA (1988) Doxorubicin clearance in the obese. J Clin Oncol 6: 1321–1327

Sauer H (1992a) Zytostatische Therapie. In: Wilmanns W, Huhn D, Wilms K (eds) Internistische Onkologie. Thieme, Stuttgart (in press)

Sauer H (1992b) Pharmakodynamik von Methotrexat. In: Rau H (ed) Niedrigdosiertes Methotrexat bei rheumatischen Erkrankungen. Futuramed, Munich (in press)

Sauer H, Wilmanns W (1991) Internistische Therapie maligner Erkrankungen, 3rd edn. Urban and Schwarzenberg, Munich
Schmid F (1990) Das Krankheitsbild: das Fragil-X-Syndrom. Biol Med 394–395
Smaaland R, Laerum OD, Lote K, Sletvold O, Sothern RB, Bjerknes R (1991) DNA synthesis in human bone marrow is circadian stage dependent. Blood 77: 2603–2611
Swift M, Reitnauer PJ, Morrell D, Chase CL (1987) Breast and other cancers in families with ataxia-teleangiectasia. N Engl J Med 316: 1289–1294
Timme TL, Moses RE (1988) Review: diseases with DNA damage-processing defects. Am J Med Sci 295: 40–48
Tuchmann M, Stoeckeler JS, Kiang DT, O'Dea RF, Ramnaraine ML, Mirkin BL (1985) Familial pyrimidinemia and pyrimidinuria associated with severe fluorouracil toxocity N Engl J Med 313: 245–249
Ueland PM, Refsum H, Christensen B (1990) Methotrexate sensitivity in down's syndrome: a hypothesis. Cancer Chemother Pharmacol 25: 384–386
Volm M, Mattern J, Efferth T (1990) P-Glykoprotein als Marker für Multidrug-Resistenz in Tumoren und Normalgewebe. Tumordiagn Ther 11: 189–197
von Roemeling R (1990) Tageszeitspezifische Gabe von Fluoropyrimidinen. Arzneimitteltherapie 8: 210–225
Vuillaume M, Calvayrac R, Best-Belpomme M, Tarroux P, Hubert M, Decroix Y, Sarasin A: Deficiency in the catalase activity of xeroderma pigmentosum cell and simian virus 40-transformed human cell extracts. Cancer Res 46: 538–544
Waldmann FM, Koblin DD, Lampe GH, Wauk LZ, Eger EI (1990) Hematologic effects of nitrous oxide in surgical patients. Anesth Analg 71: 618–624
Zittoun J, Fischer A, Marquet J, Perignon JL, Lagrue A, Griscelli C (1987) Megaloblastic anemia and immune abnormalities in a patient with methionine synthase deficiency. Acta Pediatr Scand 76: 991–998

2 Neurotoxicity

2.1 Radiation-Induced Injury of the Central Nervous System

ROLF-PETER MÜLLER

CONTENTS

1 Introduction 23
2 Pathophysiology 23
3 Acute Reactions 24
4 Early Delayed Reactions 24
5 Late Delayed Reactions 24
5.1 Radionecrosis 24
5.2 Cognitive Dysfunctions 25
6 Radiation-Induced Neoplasms 26
References 26

1 Introduction

Radiation therapy, since its introduction into clinical use, has played an integral part in the treatment and management of various intacranial benign and malignant tumors, and many studies have proven its efficacy. Initially, the central nervous system (CNS) was considered to be relatively radioresistant, but early reports from the 1940s describing severe damage of normal brain tissue and the spinal cord revealed the limited tolerance of the CNS to ionizing radiation (BODEN 1948; GREENFIELD and STARK 1948).

Beside the radiosensitivity of normal tissue, there are additional factors known to be relevant for the development of acute and late toxicity in the brain, including the treatment volume, the radiation dose and fraction size (DROPCHO 1991; LEIBEL and SHELINE 1991). According to the different pathogeneses and prognoses of the injuries, they have been classified as *acute*, *early delayed* and *late delayed* reactions (KRAMER 1968; SHELINE et al. 1980). There are also some other relevant factors, such as age of the patient, known vasculopathy or hypertension and endocrine disorders, which certainly increase the risk of developing radiation injury. Finally, the pretreatment history, including repeated surgery, chemotherapy and infection, are known to be relevant for the amount of toxicity (LEIBEL and SHELINE 1991).

Still, the literature concerning radiation injury to the CNS gives no reliable data about the radiation tolerance of normal brain tissue. The reported data are mostly very fragmentary regarding the description of treatment volume, individual fraction size and number, total radiation dose and the overall treatment time. Moreover, there are only a few more or less systematic investigations, including some experimental and animal data with their well known limited applicability to the actual situation in humans.

This chapter describes only those data concerning damage due to conventional photon and gamma irradiation to the brain, not including heavy particles, neutrons or single dose stereotactic radiation.

Usually CNS injury is caused by direct therapeutic use of ionizing radiation to parts of the brain (or whole brain); a more or less extensive indirect radiation exposure results in patients with mantle field irradiation or for those treated for head and neck tumors.

2 Pathophysiology

Neurones and ganglia are very well differentiated and mature cells, which are not able to proliferate and therefore are relatively radioresistant. Should these cells die, replacement is not possible. Relatively radiosensitive and vulnerable cells are the myelin-producing oligodendrocytes and the vessel-containing nutritive neuroglia. Thus, the white matter is relatively more susceptible to radiation injury than the gray matter. The regions of the brain most sensitive to radiation injury are the sensomotoric centers of the hemispheres and the brain stem, while the frontal, temporal and occipital lobes are less vulnerable (RUBIN 1977).

The molecular mechanisms responsible for the various late toxic effects are still unknown. One

ROLF-PETER MÜLLER, Prof. Dr., Medizinische Einrichtungen der Universität Köln, Klinik und Poliklinik für Strahlentherapie, Joseph-Stelzmann-Strasse 9, 50924 Köln, FRG

must assume that individual patient factors are important and also responsible for development of late radiation toxicity to the brain.

3 Acute Reactions

Acute reactions to cranial irradiation occur within the first hours or days after treatment and consist of headache, nausea and sometimes vomiting, all clinical symptoms of increased intracranial pressure. These symptoms have to be distinguished from an intensification of neurologic signs caused by the tumor itself, which cannot easily be done in most cases. In many patients, a variable amount of tumor- or surgery-associated edema exists before radiation therapy is undertaken. Additionally, in some patients one can observe fever, somnolence and some degree of debility. Using computed tomography, a more or less extensive increase of edema can be seen.

Clinical symptoms tend to be more extensive after irradiation with large single fractions. Clinical and neurological symptoms usually last only for few days, respond well to increased doses of corticosteroids (Sheline et al. 1980) and are completely reversible in almost all cases.

4 Early Delayed Reactions

The early delayed reactions from cranial irradiation occur within a few weeks to a few months after completion of treatment. They can be grouped into two major forms: (1) the somnolence syndrome and (2) the exacerbation of previously existing neurologic deficits.

The *somnolence syndrome* is usually observed in children with acute lymphoblastic leukemia who have received prophylactic cranial irradiation (mostly 18–24 Gy in 10–12 fractions to the whole brain) and intrathecal methotrexate together with systemic chemotherapy. However, the syndrome can occur in any patient undergoing irradiation to extended parts of the brain. Clinical signs are drowsiness, nausea, irritability and, less often, transient papilledema. Symptoms resolve within 3–6 weeks, which also can be documented by the normalization of the electroencephalogram. Corticosteroids support regression of symptoms and even may prevent the syndrome itself if given during the course of irradiation (Berg et al. 1983). There is no clear evidence in the literature whether the somnolence syndrome in children with prophylactic CNS irradiation can be correlated with age (children less than 3 years appear to have more severe symptoms) or total dose and fraction size (Littman et al. 1984; Cecchetti and Brandoli 1979; Parker et al. 1978).

To distinguish early delayed encephalopathy, which clinically is represented by nausea, vomiting and often worsening of focal neurological deficits, from tumor progression or recurrence is especially important in patients treated for primary brain tumors. Computed tomography (CT) or magnetic resonance imaging (MRI) often demonstrate increased enhancement of the affected area and edema. Both clinical and radiographic signs are temporary in most of the cases and usually patients recover within a few weeks completely and remain unrecognized in many cases.

The cause of the symptoms is pathophysiologically attributed to circumscribed demyelinating processes caused by the radiation injury to oligodendroglial cells and commonly is followed by remyelination with complete restoration of the oligodendroglial cells.

5 Late Delayed Reactions

Late delayed complications from cranial irradiation are rare. They occur from months to years after treatment (Sheline et al. 1980) and therefore can only be observed in long-term survivors.

Clinically, late delayed sequelae are characterized by continuous progression of neurologic deficits with lethal outcome in several cases. They can also mimic tumor recurrence or progression, which radiologically cannot be distinguished in some cases. The median time for onset of symptoms is 14 months, and 90% of the cases are observed within the first 2.5 years after treatment.

There are several types of late delayed reactions, including radiologically documented but clinically asymptomatic white matter changes, neuropsychologic impairment, hormonal (pituitary-hypothalamic) dysfunction and radiotherapy-induced second neoplasms. The most common but also most serious form of late radiotherapeutic complication after brain irradiation is radionecrosis.

5.1 Radionecrosis

Cerebral radiation necrosis occurs after whole brain irradiation and after treatment of parts of the brain.

The pathogenesis is attributed as well to a direct effect on the glial cells as to vascular endothelial cell injury of the white matter (MANZ et al. 1979; MARTINS et al. 1977; YOSHII and PHILLIPS 1992). Histopathologically, one can find endothelial proliferation, hyalin wall thickening of vessels, fibrinoid necrosis, amyloid and fatty degeneration and perivascular thrombosis and fibrosis (FIKE et al. 1984, 1988; BURGER et al. 1979; MANZ et al. 1979; MARTINS et al. 1977; MANDYBUR and GORE 1969).

Cerebral radiation necrosis usually occurs only in those patients who received at least 45–50 Gy, conventionally fractionated in 5–6 weeks; and the incidence ranges from 1% to 5%. There is a substantially higher rate of necroses after doses of 55–60 Gy and more and also after high daily fractions (>2Gy/day). It may be impossible to work out the true incidence, because many patients with brain tumors die before they are at risk for cerebral radiation necrosis. There have been some reports about the rare and surprising occurrence of radionecrosis after total doses of not more than 30 Gy.

Recently, new sophisticated methods of radiobiological calculations for different radiation treatment schemes have been published (VAN DER KOGEL 1986, 1991; PEZNER and ARCHAMBEAU 1981; SHELINE et al. 1980; WIGG et al. 1981; WARA et al. 1975; LEIBEL and SHELINE 1990; ANG et al. 1985; MARKS et al. 1981). For a more reliable method to calculate the radiation injury risk, Sheline et al. (1980) created the NSD (neuret) concept. This measurement of *nominal standard dose* calculates the effect of fractionation to normal tissue and was adopted with neuret for the central nervous system.These calculations better reflect the greater importance of the daily administered dose and the less important role of the time to deliver the total radiation dose.

Clinically, patients present with signs of increased intracranial pressure, and sometimes neurological signs are referable to the location of the radionecrosis. Radiologically, on CT or MRI scans, cerebral radionecrosis is typically seen as a contrast-enhancing mass surrounded by a relatively extensive edema in most of the cases. The radiological appearance of the necrosis cannot be distinguished from tumor recurrence. In the future, positron emission tomography (PET) scans may help to differentiate between tumor and radionecrosis, since the latter is hypometabolic (no fluorodeoxyglucose uptake), while recurrent tumor shows hypermetabolic glucose metabolism. In selected cases biopsy may be necessary to establish a correct diagnosis. Treatment of radionecrosis may be conservative, with corticosteroids to reduce the edema and stabilize the clinical symptoms for several months. In some cases there occurs a more or less complete clearance of the necrotic debris by normal body functions. If the radionecrosis is in a surgically accessible region, surgical debulking of necrotic brain tissue is worthwhile and often restores the patient to a prior level of function.

5.2 *Cognitive Dysfunctions*

A very frequent and disturbing neurotoxic effect after cranial irradiation can be described as diffuse cerebral injury. In serial CT scans of adult long-term survivors after irradiation of primary brain tumors with 40–60 Gy whole brain irradiation, a diffuse cortical atrophy, ventricular dilatation and decreased attenuation of hemispheric white matter could be documented in about 50% of the patients (FOO et al. 1986; SEILER 1980; STYLOPOULOS et al. 1988). One can assume that in about half of these patients the changes will progressively worsen (CONSTINE et al. 1988). However, there is a poor correlation between the presence and extent of white matter changes in CT or MRI and cognitive dysfunction (KRAMER et al. 1988).

Not in all, but in a considerable number of patients, clinically-important cognitive impairment develops. Some 30%–50% of adult long-term survivors with malignant gliomas are unable to continue their former employment after treatment with radiation therapy because of marked cortical dysfunction (ASAI et al. 1989), and neuropsychologic testing revealed difficulties with tasks requiring attention or problem solving in many patients (HOCHBERG and SLOTNIK 1980; MAIRE et al. 1987). In some severe cases patients were disabled by progressive dementia and gait disturbance (ASAI et al. 1989; IMPERATO et al. 1990). In patients with progressive dementia, corticosteroids gave only incomplete and temporary remission or stabilization of symptoms. Ventriculoperitoneal shunting did not usually result in marked improvement of the clinical symptoms.

In two patient populations, children receiving prophylactic CNS radiation for acute lymphoblastic leukemia and adults receiving prophylactic cranial irradiation for small cell lung cancer, studies have been performed to document exactly the true extent of cognitive dysfunction (MEADOWS et al. 1981; MUCHI et al. 1987; JOHNSON et al. 1985; CHAK et al.

1986). In these patients, 1–2 years after cranial irradiation, an intellectual decline was diagnosed which was irreversible and no effective treatment could be performed. Most of the studies of children with acute lymphoblastic leukemia have shown that the IQ scores remained in the average range and that the performance IQ was more likely to be affected than the verbal IQ (BLEYER 1988).

Obviously, with the development of more effective treatment regimens, consisting not only of surgery and radiation therapy but also chemotherapy, and with prolonged survival, late complications will become a more common problem.

6 Radiation-Induced Neoplasms

There have been many reports in recent years indicating that radiotherapy-induced cerebral neoplasms are not as uncommon as previously estimated. According to the frequency, meningeomas are the most often radiotherapy-induced cerebral tumors, followed by sarcomas (mostly fibrosarcomas) and gliomas (AL-MEFTY et al. 1990; DEVINSKY 1991). Usually these tumors develop within a long latent period, ranging from 10 to 20 years and more. For meningeomas there are reports of latency from 15–55 years, with a peak between 35 and 40 years (SOFFER et al. 1983; RUBINSTEIN et al. 1984). Also, the induction of gliomas with various degrees of differentiation has been reported in long-term survivors of medulloblastoma, suprasellar tumors and pituitary adenomas (AL-MEFTY et al. 1990; DEVINSKY 1991; SALVATI et al. 1991). The mean time from completion of radiation treatment to diagnosis of the glioma was 10 years. Disturbingly, 40% of radiation-induced gliomas were diagnosed in long-term survivors of childhood acute lymphoblastic leukemia who had received prophylactic cranial irradiation (DEVINSKY 1991; DROPCHO et al. 1987; SHAPIRO et al. 1989). According to MEADOWS et al. (1981) and ALBO et al. (1985), gliomas are the most common, nonhematologic, secondary tumor in patients with acute lymphoblastic leukemia, with an estimated incidence of about 2.3% among 5-year survivors.

References

Albo V, Miller D, Leiken S (1985) Nine brain tumors as a late effect in children "cured" of acute lymphoblastic leukemia from a single pool study (abstract). Proc Am Soc Clin Oncol 4: 172

Al-Mefty O, Kersh JE, Routh A, Smith RR (1990) The long-term side effects of radiation therapy for benign brain tumors in adults. J Neurosurg 73: 502

Ang KK, van der Kogel AJ, van der Schueren E (1985) Lack of evidence for increased tolerance of rat spinal cord with decreasing fraction doses below 2 Gy. Int J Radiat Oncol Biol Phys 11: 105

Asai A, Matsutani M, Kohno T, Nakanira O, Tanaka H, Fujimaki T, Funada N, Matsuda T, Nagata K, Takura K (1989) Subacute brain atrophy after radiation for malignant brain tumors. Cancer 63: 1962

Berg RA, Ch'ien LT, Lancaster W, Wiliams S, Cummins J (1983) Neuropsychological sequelae of postradiation somnolence syndrome. Dev Behav Pediatr 4: 103

Bleyer WA (1988) Hobson's choice in the CNS radioprophylaxis of small cell lung cancer. Int J Radiat Oncol Biol Phys 15: 783

Boden G (1948) Radiation myelitis of the cervical spinal cord. Br J Radiol 21: 464

Burger PC, Mahaly MS Jr, Dudka L, Vogel FS (1979) The morphologic effects of radiation administered therapeutically for intracranial gliomas. Cancer 44: 1256

Cecchetti E, Brandoli V (1979) Cranial irradiation in children with lymphoblastic acute leukemia: results and damages. Int J Radiat Oncol Biol Phys 5: 367

Chak LY, Zatz LM, Wasserstein P, Cox RS, Kushlan PD, Porzig KJ, Sicic BI (1986) Neurologic dysfunction in patients treated for small cell carcinoma of the lung: a clinical and radiological study. Int J Radiat Oncol Biol Phys 12: 385

Constine LS, Konski A, Ekholm S, McDonald S, Rubin P (1988) Adverse effects of brain irradiation correlated with MR and CT imaging. Int J Radiat Oncol Biol Phys 15: 319

DeAngelis L (1991) Radiation induced central and peripheral nervous system complications. In: Poswer FB, Foley MK, Malkin MG, Callaway M (eds) Neurooncology IV: recent developments in the management of neurooncological illnesses. Syllabus (postgraduate course). Memorial Sloane-Kettering Cancer Center, New York

Devinsky O (1991) Radiation-induced tumors of the central and peripheral nervous system. In: Rottenberg DA (ed) Neurological complications of cancer treatment. Butterworth-Heinemann, Boston, p 79

Dropcho EJ (1991) Central nervous system injury by therapeutic irradiation. Neurol Clin 9: 969

Fike JR, Sheline GE, Cann CE, Davis RL (1984) Radiation necrosis. Prog Exp Tumor Res 28: 136

Fike JR, Cann CE, Turowsky K, Higgins RJ, Chan AS, Phillips TL, Davis RL (1988) Radiation dose response of normal brain. Int J Radiat Oncol Biol Phys 14: 63

Foo SH, Hiesinger E, Wise A (1986) Quality of long-term survival of treated patients with malignant glioma (abstract). Proc Am Soc Clin Oncol 5: 136

Greenfield MM, Stark FM (1948) Post-radiation neuropathy. AJR 60: 617

Hochberg FH, Slotnik B (1980) Neuropsychologic impairment in astrocytoma survivors. Neurology 30: 172

Imperato JP, Paleologos NA, Vick NA (1990) Effects of treatment on long-term survivors with malignant astrocytomas. Ann Neurol 28: 818

Johnson BE, Becker B, Goff WB, Petronas N, Krehbiel MA, Makuch RW, McKenna G, Glatstein E, Ihde DC (1985) Neurologic, neuropsychologic and computed tomography scan abnormalities in 2- to 10-years survivors of small-cell lung cancer. J Clin Oncol 3: 1659

Kramer S (1968) The hazards of therapeutic irradiation of the central nervous system. Clin Neurosurgery 15: 301

Kramer JH, Norman D, Brant-Zawatzki M, Ablin A, Moore IM (1988) Absence of white matter changes on magnetic resonance imaging in children treated with CNS prophylaxis for leukemia. Cancer 61: 928

Leibel SA, Sheline GE (1990) Radiotherapy in the cerebral astrocytomas. In: Thomas DGD (ed) Neuro-oncology: primary malignant brain tumors. Arnold, London, p 193

Leibel SA, Sheline GE (1991) Tolerance of the brain and spinal cord to conventional irradiation. In: Gutin PH, Leibel SA, Sheline GE (eds) Radiation injury to the nervous system. Raven, New York, p 239

Littman P, Rosenstock J, Gale G, Krisch RE, Meadows A, Sather H, Coccia P, DeCamargo B (1984) The somnolence syndrome in leukemic children following reduced daily dose fractions of cranial irradiation. Int J Radiat Oncol Biol Phys 10: 1851

Maire JP, Coudin B, Guerin J, Caudry M (1987) Neuropsychological impairment in adults with brain tumors. Am J Clin Oncol 10: 156

Mandybur TI, Gore I (1969) Amyloid in late postirradiation necrosis of brain. Neurology 19: 983

Manz HJ, Woolley PV III, Ornitz RD (1979) Delayed radiation necrosis of brainstem related to fast neutron beam irradiation. Cancer 44: 473

Marks JE, Baglan RJ, Prassad SC, Blank WF (1981) Cerebral radionecrosis: Incidence and risk in relation to dose, time, fractionation and volume. Int J Radiat Oncol Biol Phys 7: 243

Martins AN, Johnston JS, Henry JM, Stoffel TJ, DiChiro G (1977) Delayed radiation necrosis of the brain. J Neurosurgery 47: 336

Meadows AT, Massari DJ, Fergusson J, Gordon J, Littman P, Moss K (1981) Declines in IQ scores and cognitive dysfunction in children with acute lymphcytic leukemia treated with cranial irradiation. Lancet 7: 1015

Muchi H, Satoh T, Yamamoto K, Karube T, Miyao M (1987) Studies on the assessment of neurotoxicity in children with acute lymphoblastic leukemia. Cancer 59: 891

Parker D, Malpas JS, Sandland R, Sheaff PC, Freeman JE, Paxton A (1978) Outlook following "somnolence syndrome" after prophylactic cranial irradiation. Br J Med 4: 554

Pezner RD, Archambeau JO (1981) Brain tolerance unit: a method to estimate risk of radiation brain injury for various dose schedules. Int J Radiat Oncol Biol Phys 7: 397

Rubin P (1977) Radiation toxicology: quantitative radiation pathology for predicting effects. Cancer 39 [Suppl]: 739

Rubinstein AB, Shalit MN, Cohen ML, Zandbank U, Reichenthal E (1984) Radiation-induced cerebral meningioma: a recognizable entity. J Neurosurg 61: 966

Salvati M, Artico M, Caruso R, Rocchi G, Orlando ER, Nucci F (1991) A report on radiation-induced gliomas. Cancer 67: 392

Seiler RW (1980) Late results of multimodality therapy of high-grade supratentorial astrocytomas. Surg Neurol 15: 88

Shapiro S, Mealey J, Sartorius C (1989) Radiation-induced intracranial malignant gliomas. J Neurosurg 71: 77

Sheline GE, Wara WM, Smith V (1980) Therapeutic irradiation and brain injury. Int J Radiat Oncol Biol Phys 6: 1215

Soffer D, Pittaluga S, Feiner M, Beler AJ (1983) Intracranial meningiomas following low-dose irradiation to the head. J Neurosurg 59: 1048

Stylopoulos LA, George AE, de Leon MJ, Miller JD, Foo SH, Hiesiger E, Wise A (1988) Longitudinal study of parenchymal brain changes in glioma survivors. AJNR 9: 517

van der Kogel AJ (1986) Radiation-induced damage in the central nervous system: An interpretation of target cell responses. Br J Cancer (suppl.) 53: 207

van der Kogel AJ (1991) Clinical implications of radiological studies on CNS tolerance. In: Karim ABMF, Laws ER (eds) Glioma. Springer, Berlin Heidelberg New York, p 179

Wara WM, Phillips TL, Sheline GE, Schwade JG (1975) Radiation tolerance of the spinal cord. Cancer 35: 1558

Wigg DR, Koschel K, Hodgson GS (1981) Tolerance of the mature human central nervous system to photon irradiation. Br J Radiol 54: 787

Yoshii Y, Phillips TL (1992) Late vascular effect of whole brain x-irradiation in the mouse. Acta Neurochir (Wien) 64: 87

2.2 Cytostatic-Induced Central Nervous System Abnormalities

RUDOLF KORINTHENBERG

CONTENTS

1 Introduction 29
2 Acute Cytostatic-Induced CNS Toxicity 29
3 Short-Term Effects of Methotrexate 30
4 Chronic Cytostatic-Induced Encephalopathies . . . 31
5 Cytostatic-Induced Neuropsychological Changes . 32
References 33

1 Introduction

Many cytostatic drugs can give rise to side effects in the central nervous system (CNS). These side effects can appear acutely, in which case recovery is generally good, or they may result in a slowly progressive neurological disease with persisting disability.

CNS toxicity can occur as a side effect of treatment for extracerebral tumors. However, it is more frequent and clinically significant as a consequence of treatment for intracranial disease manifestations. This is especially true for children with leukemia or brain tumors. Due to the increasing treatment success and survival rate of these children the question of chronic neurotoxicity is of utmost importance (PACKER et al. 1987).

In the following, I will first discuss the possibility of acute CNS toxicity reactions from various drugs and then deal more closely with the salient problem of chronic toxicity as a result of CNS therapy.

2 Acute Cytostatic-Induced CNS Toxicity

The neurotoxic potential of vincristine (VCR) has been known for a long time. As opposed to the frequent and dose-dependent toxicity in the peripheral nervous system, toxicity in the CNS is fortunately much less common. Seizures, disturbance of consciousness and pareses have been reported in 1%–15% of patients.

There are two mechanisms responsible for these reactions: (1) VCR can cause inappropriate secretion of antidiuretic hormone, resulting in retention of water and hyponatriemia. (2) Although less frequently observed, VCR can also directly induce an encephalopathy. In these cases, with normal serum and CSF sodium values, focal slowing of the EEG and hypodense areas in the cranial computer tomography (CCT) image have been observed. Pathological specimens have shown an enlargement of axons and a dissociation of the neurotubuli, similar to findings in peripheral VCR neurotoxicity.

The acute VCR-related encephalopathies are generally reversible. Persisting neurological defects have rarely been reported (KAPLAN and WIERNIK 1982; HURWITZ et al. 1988).

L-Asparaginase (L-ASP) is an antimetabolite, effective mainly in acute lymphoblastic leukemia. Neurotoxic side effects are observed more often in adults than in children. They present as an acute encephalopathy with changes of mood and consciousness, rarely with seizures. In the EEG diffuse slowing is found. In adults this complication has been reported in 12%–50% of the treatment courses. Usually it is completely reversible after 3–5 days (Fig. 1).

Pathologically, L-ASP is thought to induce hyperammonemia and changes in the amino acid neurotransmitters glutamate and aspartate (KAPLAN and WIERNIK 1982). Independent of these mechanisms, L-ASP can give rise to changes in liver-derived clothing factors, resulting in hypo- or hypercoagulability. Thus, both hemorrhages and thromboses are possible CNS complications which have been observed with L-ASP treatment (OTT et al. 1988).

The neurotoxic potential of corticosteroids is low. However, mood changes and psychotic episodes are known with high dose and long-term treatment. A syndrome of pseudotumor cerebri can occur due to withdrawal of the drug. During

RUDOLF KORINTHENBERG, Prof. Dr., Universitätskinderklinik, Abteilung Neuropädiatrie und Muskelerkrankungen, Mathildenstrasse 1, 79106 Freiburg, FRG

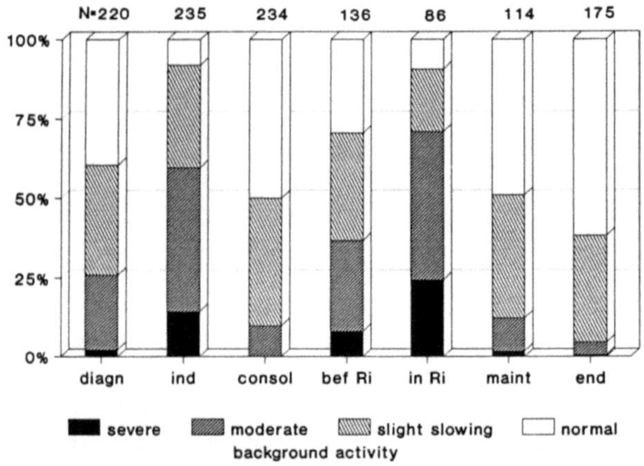

Fig. 1. During treatment of children with acute lymphoblastic leukemia, the electroencephalogram frequently shows diffuse slowing of the background activity as an expression of a generally subclinical encephalopathy. This finding is especially frequent and significant during induction and reinduction treatment, when both vincristine and L-asparaginase are administered. Patients were treated according to protocols BFM76 through BFM83; *diagn*, at diagnosis; *ind*, during induction treatment; *consol*, and of consolidation phase; *bef RI*, before reinduction; *in RI*, during reinduction treatment; *maint*, during maintenance treatment; *end*, at the end of treatment. (Adapted from KORINTHENBERG 1986)

treatment with high dose corticosteroids, in CCT or magnetic resonance imaging (MRI) a shrinkage of the brain parenchyma can be observed. This syndrome is most likely due to a loss of tissue water. Although this reduction of brain volume is generally reversible, the clinical consequences are as yet unknown (KAPLAN and WIERNIK 1982).

Blurring of vision is an infrequent side effect of treatment with cyclophosphamide. Nephrogenic retention of water and hyponatremic seizures can be further consequences. These symptoms usually leave behind no deficits if treated promptly and adequately (KAPLAN and WIERNIK 1982).

Ifosfamide (IFO), generally administered in combination with 2-mercaptoethane sulfonic acid (MESNA) can give rise to an encephalopathy with variable severity in 10%–20% of patients. Somnolence, confusion, hallucinations, extrapyramidal movement disorders and eventually coma have been reported. These effects are usually reversible after 4 days; persisting defects or even death are very rare events. The risk factors of IFO neurotoxicity are advanced age, impaired renal function, oral administration of the drug and pretreatment with cisplatin. The risk is significantly lowered by fractionating the dose and administering it by infusion over 3–4 days (ANDERSON and TANDON 1991; DECHANT et al. 1991).

Cisplatin exerts its main neurotoxic effects at the eighth cranial nerve and at the sensory portion of the peripheral nervous system. An acute encephalopathy with seizures and other signs of cortical dysfunction has been reported in 4%–10% of patients. EEG and CCT presented mainly focal changes.

Various pathological mechanisms, such as a renal loss of magnesium, hyponatremia and an impairment of renal function, have been suggested. However, the real cause of this transient encephalopathy is still unknown (MEAD et al. 1982; HIGHLEY et al. 1992).

High dose, intravenously administered cytosine arabinoside (ARA-C) frequently gives rise to cerebellar ataxia. A further side effect of cerebral dysfunction with somnolence, headaches and seizures is seen less frequently. This complication is dose-dependent and generally reversible. After intrathecal administration of ARA-C, a chemically induced meningitis or an acute encephalomyelopathy can occur within 24 h. Although this is generally reversible, patients suffering from chronic myelopathy, paraplegia and even progressive encephalopathy have also been observed (LAZARUS et al. 1981; SALINSKY et al. 1983).

3 Short-Term Effects of Methotrexate

Due to it's very frequent use in the therapy and prophylactic treatment of CNS tumors and leukemia, the neurotoxic effects of methotrexate (MTX) are of greatest importance. The chemically induced meningitis after intrathecal administration is rarely of any clinical significance. Acute encephalopathy or myelopathy can occur after intrathecal (ith) and after high dose intravenous (HD-iv) administration. In CCT scans one may additionally observe periventricular hypodensity and in MRI an elevation of the periventricular signal. These acute complications are usually associated with increased CSF MTX levels (BLEYER 1981; KAPLAN and WIERNIK 1982; OCHS 1989).

Some 7–14 days after HD-iv administration of MTX, and less frequently after ith administration, a subacute encephalopathy can occur. Similar to a cerebrovascular accident, it commences with a rapidly progressive hemiparesis or with convulsions. Consciousness is generally not impaired. In MRI, distinct changes of the white matter can be found (Fig. 2) (BLEYER 1981; YIM et al. 1991). Due to the apoplectiform onset of this complication and

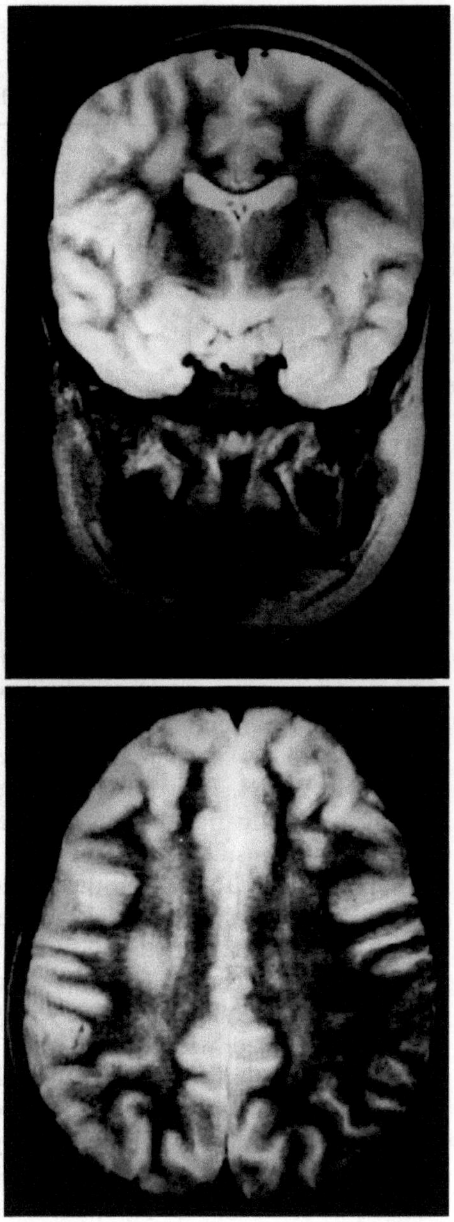

A

B

Fig. 2A, B. Coronal (**A**) and horizontal (**B**) sections of a magnetic resonance image (MRI) of a 5 year old girl who suffered a sudden-onset left hemiparesis 7 days after intrathecal injection of methotrexate for CNS prophylaxis in acute lymphoblastic leukemia. A distinct elevation of the T2 signal is seen in the white matter of the right hemisphere, adjacent to the body of the lateral ventricle. Some months later the paresis resolved completely

its occurrence mainly in osteosarcoma patients, an embolization of tumor particles was initially thought to be the cause. However, the complete recovery in the majority of cases speaks in favor of a metabolic pathology.

HD-iv MTX gives rise to a significant depression of metabolism in the brain parenchyma in both experimental animals and in humans, as documented by 17-fluor-desoxy-glucose positron emission tomography (17-FDG PET) (Phillips et al. 1986, 1987). In prospectively performed MRI, up to 40% of patients receiving HD-iv or ith MTX showed pathological signal changes in the deep white matter, even when no clinical symptoms occurred (Wilson et al. 1991; Asato et al. 1992). In rats and in humans a transient slowing of the EEG background activity after high dose MTX infusion has been observed (Korinthenberg et al. 1982; Phillips et al. 1986).

Although the cytostatic effect of MTX is mediated by an inhibition of the enzyme dihydrofolate reductase, with subsequent depletion of tetrahydrofolate, it is also a potent inhibitor of the biopterin system. As a result, the biosynthesis of the monoaminergic neurotransmitters may also be affected by this drug (Millot et al. 1992).

4 Chronic Cytostatic-Induced Encephalopathies

Chronic chemotherapy-induced encephalopathies develop slowly, usually during ongoing therapy. They are characterized by a progressive change of personality, an atactic or spastic disturbance of gait and a loss of mental abilities. A necrotizing leukoencephalopathy with dystrophic calcification of the white matter has been demonstrated both on CCT and MRI and on postmortem studies.

This serious complication has been observed under high dose and long-term treatment with 5-fluorouracil and its derivatives, ith ARA-C and, most frequently, MTX (Bleyer 1981; Kuzuhara et al. 1987; Hook et al. 1992). The latter can give rise to this complication with either long-term ith or HD-iv treatment. Chronic MTX encephalopathies have even been reported in patients suffering from osteogenic sarcomas without intracranial involvement (Allen et al. 1980). Several factors increase the risk of MTX-encephalopathy: higher dose and longer durations of treatment, a combination of ith and iv administration of MTX and, above all, a preceding radiotherapy of the brain (Bleyer 1981).

Due to the great importance of MTX in the treatment of CNS malignancies, its potential to induce chronic CNS changes has given rise to a great number of investigations. Variable pathological changes have been observed in CCT and

Table 1. Pathological findings in cranial computed tomography after CNS prophylaxis in children suffering from ALL, according to data from OCHS (1989)

Treatment	*N*	Atrophy (%)	Calcification (%)	Hypodensity (%)
With radiotherapy				
24 Gy cr + 5–8 itMTX, or 24 Gy csp	249	15.5	8.5	3.5
24 Gy cr + 35 itMTX	32	25.0	18.7	12.5
18 Gy cr + 5 itMTX	48	35.0	0.0	0.0
18 Gy cr + 18 itMTX	55	1.9	7.2	5.4
Without radiotherapy				
3 × 0.5 g/m2 ivMTX + itMTX	104	3.8	0.0	<1.0
15 × 1 g/m2 ivMTX + itMTX	52	1.9	0.0	19.2
itMTX	82	4.6	0.0	3.5

cr, cranial radiotherapy; csp, craniospinal radiotherapy; ivMTX, intravenous methotrexate; itMTX, intrathecal methotrexate.

MRI studies of children with acute lymphoblastic leukemia who received CNS treatment or prophylaxis. These consist of cortical and subcortical atrophy, multifocal calcifications and white matter hypodensity (BLEYER 1981; OCHS 1989; PÄÄKÖ et al. 1992). However, the frequency of these changes is low and their clinical meaning is far from clear. Referring to her own data and to the literature, OCHS (1989) was able to show that calcifications and brain atrophy most probably are due to radiotherapy of the CNS, while changes of the white matter are due to chemotherapy (Table 1).

PET investigations of regional glucose metabolism in the brain have been performed 3–8 years after treatment for leukemia. In comparison to normal controls, irradiated patients were shown to have a decreased metabolic rate of the white matter and thalamus. The metabolic rate in the thalamus was also decreased in patients who had only been treated with ith MTX (PHILLIPS et al. 1991).

5 Cytostatic-Induced Neuropsychological Changes

Although, with careful treatment, severe acute and chronic encephalopathies remain very infrequent, the possibility of long-term minimal CNS damage in the majority of patients has caused significant concern.

Learning disabilities, slight to moderate impairment of cognitive function and various neuropsychological deficits have been studied in children with leukemia and brain tumors for many years. The majority of the published studies have addressed the question whether prophylactic CNS radiotherapy can give rise to an impairment of later cognitive development. This has been confirmed by most investigations, showing a significantly increased vulnerability in children of younger age and those of the female sex, even with a low radiation dose of 18 or 24 Gy (COUSENS et al. 1988).

Due to these findings, in many presently administered treatment protocols for patients with a standard risk of recurrence, cranial radiotherapy has been replaced by an intensified chemotherapy, mainly with MTX. However, there are only very few studies investigating the long-term effects on the CNS of this intensified chemotherapy. There is in fact some evidence that chemotherapy in very high doses can result in similar deficits in these children as in those who had cranial radiotherapy.

BROWN and coworkers (1992) performed neuropsychological investigations in yearly intervals in children treated with ith ARA-C, MTX and prednisone according to the protocol POG 8602. Even without radiotherapy, they observed a significant decrease of cognitive and neuropsychological abilities.

The Memphis group prospectively compared children treated with 18 or 24 Gy radiotherapy or alternatively with HD-iv and ith MTX. The neuropsychological investigations showed a significant decline of the IQ in all three groups, irrespective of the kind of treatment (MULHERN et al. 1991; OCHS et al. 1991).

Several published studies compared children treated only with chemotherapy with a control group or with the population norm. WHITT and coworkers (1984) reported the neuropsychological function in patients with ith triple therapy and iv MTX to be worse than the population norm, but similar to the function in irradiated patients. MULHERN et al. (1988) reported similar memory deficits in their patients with and without cranial radiotherapy, as compared to the population norms. GIRALT et al. (1992) found a similarly impaired neuropsychological function in patients treated with triple ith therapy and in those treated with cranial irradiation, as compared to healthy siblings and patients with solid extracranial tumors. However, it must be added that SCHLIEPER et al. (1989) and other authors found no difference in cognitive function between their patients treated only with chemotherapy and a control group, whereas their irradiated patients showed significantly reduced abilities.

In several studies, the radiotherapy was kept constant, while randomizing for the kind or dose of chemotherapy. WABER and coworkers (1992) reported that 4 g/m^2 in MTX as compared to 40 mg/m^2 at the start of treatment gave rise to a significant loss of cognitive function in girls. In the study of ROBINSON et al. (1984), patients who received ith MTX in addition to radiation therapy, and those with a longer duration of chemotherapy, performed worse in neuropsychological tests. A similar result was obtained in a study of the Children's Cancer Study Group (BLEYER et al. 1990). CHESSELS et al. (1990) reported lower IQ findings in children after maintenance therapy with intramuscular MTX than in children treated with oral MTX.

In contrast to these reports, investigations in children treated for solid tumors outside the CNS found no cognitive deficits, as compared to normal controls.

Apparently, differing results of neuropsychological investigations after chemotherapy correlate with different drugs, doses and routes of administration. However, it is not possible to delineate this more clearly from the existing literature due to a lack of relevant data about the treatment in many publications.

Intensified chemotherapy regimens with HD-iv and long-term ith administration of MTX can give rise to long-term problems similar to those of cranial radiotherapy with 18 or 24 Gy. An answer to the question as to which cumulative dose can be tolerated without long-term side effects clearly needs more prospective studies with adequate controls.

References

Allen JC, Rosen G, Mehta BM, Horten B (1980) Leukoencephalopathy following high-dose iv methotrexate chemotherapy with leukovorin rescue. Cancer Treat Rep 64: 1261–1273

Anderson NR, Tandon DS (1991) Ifosfamide extrapyramidal neurotoxicity. Cancer 68: 72–75

Asato R, Akiyama Y, Ito M, Kubota M, Okumura R, Miki Y, Konishi J, Mikawa H (1992) Nuclear magnetic resonance abnormalities of the cerebral white matter in children with acute lymphoblastic leukemia and malignant lymphoma during and after central nervous system prophylactic treatment with intrathecal methotrexate. Cancer 70: 1997–1004

Bleyer WA (1981) Neurologic sequelae of methotrexate and ionizing radiation: a new classification. Cancer Treat Rep 65 [Suppl 1]: 89–98

Bleyer WA, Fallavollita J, Robison L, Balsom W, Meadows A, Heyn R, Sitarz A, Ortega J, Miller D, Constine L (1990) Influence of age, sex, and concurrent intrathecal methotrexate therapy on intellectual function after cranial irradiation during childhood: a report from the Children's Cancer Study Group. Pediatr Hematol Oncol 7: 329–338

Brown RT, Madan-Swain A, Pais R, Lambert RG, Sexson S, Ragab A (1992) Chemotherapy for acute lymphocytic leukemia: cognitive and academic sequelae. J Pediatr 121: 885–889

Chessels JM, Cox TCS, Kendall B, Cavanagh NPC, Jannoun L, Richards S (1990) Neurotoxicity in lymphoblastic leukaemia: comparison of oral and intramuscular methotrexate and two doses of radiation. Arch Dis Child 65: 416–422

Cousens P, Waters B, Said J, Stevens M (1988) Cognitive effects of cranial irradiation in leukemia: a survey and meta-analysis. J Child Psychol Psychiatry 29: 839–852

Dechant KL, Brogden RN, Pilkington T, Faulds D (1991) Ifosfamide/Mesna, A review of its antineoplastic activity, pharmakokinetic properties and therapeutic efficacy in cancer. Drugs 42: 428–467

Giralt J, Ortega JJ, Olive T, Verges R, Forio I, Salvador L (1992) Long-term neuropsychologic sequelae of childhood leukemia: comparison of two CNS prophylactic regimens. Int J Radiat Oncol Biol Phys 24: 49–53

Highley M, Meller ST, Pinkerton CR (1992) Seizures and cortical dysfunction following high-dose cisplatin administration in children. Med Pediatr Oncol 20: 143–148

Hook CC, Kimmel DW, Kvols LK, Scheithauer BW, Forsyth PA, Rubin J, Moertel CG, Rodriguez M (1992) Multifocal inflammatory leukoencephalopathy with 5-fluorouracil and levamisole. Ann Neurol 31: 262–267

Hurwitz RL, Mahoney DH, Armstrong DL, Browder TM (1988) Reversible encephalopathy and seizures as a result of conventional vincristine administration. Med Pediatr Oncol 16: 216–219

Kaplan RS, Wiernik PH (1982) Neurotoxicity of antineoplastic drugs. Semin Oncol 9: 103–130

Korinthenberg R (1986) Leukämie und Nervensystem, Das Hirnstrombild im Erkrankungs- und Behandlungsverlauf der akuten Leukämien des Kindesalters. Thieme, Stuttgart

Korinthenberg R, Lükenhöner B, Palm D, Ritter J (1982) EEG-Verlangsamung nach hochdosiertem Methotrexat mit Citrovorumfaktor-Schutz, eine spektralanalytische Untersuchung. Z EEG EMG 13: 22–27

Kuzuhara S, Ohkoshi N, Kanemaru K, Hashimoto H, Nakanishi T, Toyokura Y (1987) Subacute leukoencephalopathy induced by carmofur, a 5-fluorouracil derivative. J Neurol 234: 365–370

Lazarus HM, Herzig RH, Herzig GP, Phillips GL, Roessmann U, Fishman DJ (1981) Central nervous system toxicity of high dose systemic cytosine arabinoside. Cancer 48: 2577–2582

Mead GM, Arnold AM, Green JA, Macbeth FR, Williams CJ, Whitehouse JM (1982) Epileptic seizures associated with cisplatin administration. Cancer Treat Rep 66: 1719–1722

Millot F, Dhondt JL, Hayte JM, Bauters F (1992) Impairment of cerebral biogenic amine synthesis in a patient receiving high-dose methotrexate. Am J Pediatr Hematol Oncol 14: 276–278

Mulhern RK, Wasserman AL, Fairclough D, Ochs J (1988) Memory function in disease-free survivors of childhood acute lymphocytic leukemia given CNS prophylaxis with or without 1,800 cGy cranial irradiation. J Clin Oncol 6: 315–320

Mulhern RK, Fairclough D, Ochs J (1991) A prospective comparison of neuropsychologic performance of children surviving leukemia who received 18-gy, 24-gy, or no cranial irradiation. J Clin Oncol 9: 1348–1356

Ochs J (1989) Neurotoxicity due to central nervous system therapy for childhood leukemia. Am J Pediatr Hematol Oncol 11: 93–105

Ochs J, Mulhern R, Fairclough D, Parvey L, Whitaker J, Ch'ien L, Mauer A, Simone J (1991) Comparison of neuropsychologic functioning and clinical indicators of neurotoxicity in long-term survivors of childhood leukemia given cranial radiation or parenteral methotrexate: a prospective study. J Clin Oncol 9: 145–151

Ott N, Ramsay NKC, Priest JR, Lipton M, Pui C-H, Steinherz P, Nesbit ME (1988) Sequelae of thrombotic or hemorrhagic complications following L-asparaginase therapy for childhood lymphoblastic leukemia. Am J Pediatr Hematol Oncol 10: 191–195

Pääkö E, Vainionpää L, Lanning M, Laitinen J, Pyhtinen J (1992) White matter changes in children treated for acute lymphoblastic leukemia. Cancer 70: 2728–2733

Packer RJ, Meadows AT, Rorke LB, Goldwein JL, D'Angio G (1987) Long-term sequelae of cancer treatment on the central nervous system in childhood. Med Pediatr Oncol 15: 241–253

Phillips PC, Thaler HT, Berger CA, Fleisher M, Wellner D, Allen JC, Rottenberg DA (1986) Acute high-dose methotrexate neurotoxicity in the rat. Ann Neurol 20: 583–589

Phillips PC, Dhawan V, Strother SC, Sidtis JJ, Evans AC, Allen JC, Rottenberg DA (1987) Reduced cerebral glucose metabolism and increased brain capillary permeability following high-dose methotrexate chemotherapy: a positron emission tomographic study. Ann Neurol 21: 59–63

Phillips PC, Moeller JR, Sidtis JJ, Dhawan V, Steinherz PG, Strother SC, Ginos JZ, Rottenberg DA (1991) Abnormal cerebral glucose metabolism in long-term survivors of childhood acute lymhocytic leukemia. Ann Neurol 29: 263–271

Robison LL, Meadows AT, Nesbit ME, Ortega JA, Sather HN, Hammond GD (1984) Factors associated with IQ scores in long-term survivors of childhood acute lymphoblastic leukemia. Am J Pediatr Hematol Oncol 6: 115–121

Salinsky MC, Levine RL, Aubuchon JP, Schutta HS (1983) Acute cerebellar dysfunction with high-dose ARA-C therapy. Cancer 51: 426–429

Schlieper AE, Esseltine DW, Tarshis E (1989) Cognitive function in long survivors of childhood acute lymphoblastic leukemia. Pediatr Hematol Oncol 6: 1–9

Waber DP, Tarbell NJ, Kahn CM, Gelber RD, Sallan SE (1992) The relationship of sex and treatment modality to neuropsychologic outcome in childhood acute lymphoblastic leukemia. J Clin Oncol 10: 810–817

Whitt JK, Wells RJ, Lauria MM, Wilhelm CL, McMillan CW (1984) Cranial radiation in childhood acute lymphocytic leukemia, Neuropsychologic sequelae. Am J Dis Child 138: 730–736

Wilson DA, Nitschke R, Bowman ME, Chaffin MJ, Sexauer CL, Prince JR (1991) Transient white matter changes on MR images in children undergoing chemotherapy for acute lymphoblastic leukemia: correlation with neuropsychologic deficiencies. Radiology 180: 205–209

Yim YS, Mahoney DH, Oshman DG (1991) Hemiparesis and ischemic changes of the white matter after intrathecal therapy for children with acute lymphocytic leukemia. Cancer 67: 2058–2061

2.3 Radiation Myelopathy

LUDWIG KEILHOLZ and JÜRGEN DUNST

CONTENTS

1 Definition 35
2 Pathogenesis and Histological Findings 35
3 Clinical Classification of Radiation Myelitis . . . 37
3.1 Acute Reaction 37
3.2 Subacute Reaction 37
3.3 Chronic Progressive Radiation Myelitis 37
4 Radiation Tolerance of the Spinal Cord 37
4.1 Conventional Fractionation 37
4.2 Impact of Fraction Size 38
4.3 Impact of Interfraction Interval 38
4.4 Impact of Irradiated Volume 39
4.5 Individual Factors 39
4.6 Reirradiation Tolerance 39
5 Latency Period 40
6 Diagnosis and Differential Diagnosis 40
6.1 Clinical Symptoms 40
6.2 Radiological Findings 40
6.3 Diagnostic Procedure and Differential Diagnosis 41
7 Therapy and Prognosis 41
References 41

1 Definition

Radiation myelitis can be defined as radiation-induced injury of the spinal cord with chronic progressive paresis and paralysis. Diagnosis of radiation myelitis requires radiation exposure of the spinal cord and occurrence of neurological symptoms after a symptom-free interval. Radiation exposure may result from direct irradiation of the cord for spinal tumors. More often, irradiation of extraspinal tumors or unintentional exposure is the cause. Radiation myelitis has mainly been observed after treatment for head and neck cancer, bronchogenic carcinoma, thyroid cancer, or malignant lymphomas (BODEN 1948; EICHHORN et al. 1972; WARA et al. 1975; REINHOLD et al. 1976; ABBATUCCI et al. 1978; HATLEVOLL et al. 1983; DISCHE et al. 1981, 1988; MARCUS and MILLION 1990). The underlying changes and the clinical symptoms are irreversible with a poor overall prognosis. The fatal outcome of radiation myelitis requires maximal efforts to avoid it by optimization of biological and physical treatment planning (SAUER 1985).

2 Pathogenesis and Histological Findings

The most important parameters for the development of radiation myelitis are related to the radiation exposure: total dose, single dose, fractionation regimen, treatment time, dose rate, radiation quality, and exposed cord volume. Other parameters such as surgery, chemotherapy, infectious diseases, or accompanying illness, however, may increase the risk of radiation myelitis. Moreover, the tumor itself may damage the spinal cord by direct compression or infiltration and thereby enhance radiation damage.

Several authors have postulated that some areas of the spinal cord, mainly the upper thoracic segments and deep lumbar and sacral segments, may be more disposed to radiation injury than others because of decreased arterial blood supply (JELLINGER and STURM 1971; PISCOL 1972; for review, see BERLIT 1987). This hypothesis has not been confirmed and is in contrast to histological findings, with predominantly capillary and venous, rather than arterial, lesions.

Histologically, three main types of damage can be distinguished (SCHULTHEISS et al. 1988):

1. Damage of glial tissue (type I lesions)
2. Damage of vessels (type II lesions)
3. Combined vessel and glial damage (type III lesions)

Glial damage is characterized by demyelinization and multifocal white matter necrosis. Neurons show swelling of the axon, although this type of damage seems to be less important (MASTAGLIA

LUDWIG KEILHOLZ, Dr., Klinik und Poliklinik für Strahlentherapie, Universität Erlangen-Nürnberg. Universitätsstraße 27, 91054 Erlangen, FRG
JÜRGEN DUNST, Prof., Dr., Martin-Luther-Universität Halle-Wittenberg, Klinik für Strahlentherapie. Dryanderstraße 4-7, 06097 Halle/Saale, FRG

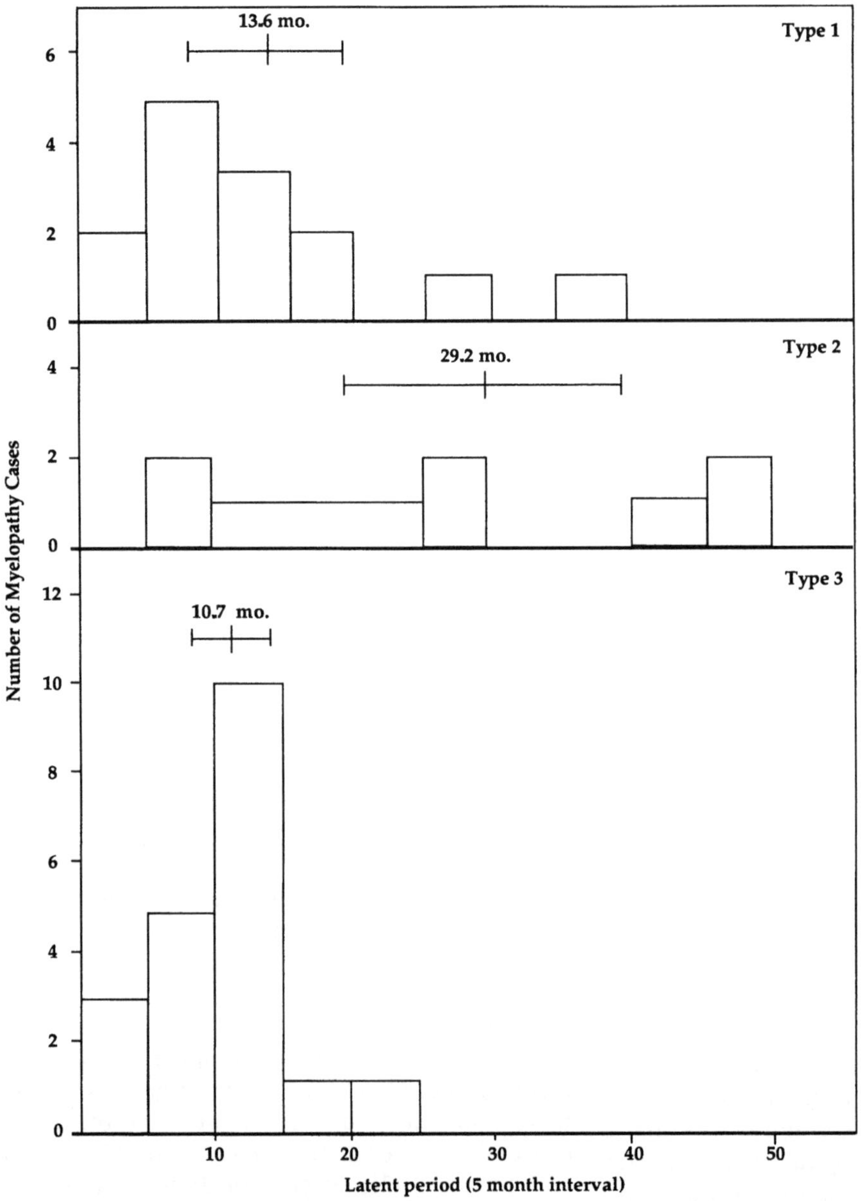

Fig. 1. The distribution of latent periods for humans according to type I–III lesions. (Modified from SCHULTHEISS et al. 1988)

et al. 1976). Capillary endothelial cells swell and perish. An increased cellular permeability results in a perivascular edema. Capillary vessels and small veins show thrombosis. Areas with petechial hemorrhage are found; after high single radiation doses, larger areas with hemorrhagic necrosis are visible.

Type III lesions are often characterized by manifold damage, with necrosis, intra- and intercellular edema, thrombosed capillary and venous vessels, and hemorrhage. Microcalcifications and inflammatory reactions may be present. Depending on the degree of damage, these lesions proceed to segmental atrophy of the spinal cord with irreversible functional disability.

The various types of damage do not only differ with regard to histological findings but also concerning the latency period and the capability of repair (Fig. 1). White matter damage (type I) occurs after a median interval of 13 months, whereas vessel damage (type II) is manifest after a median time of 29 months. Combined type III lesions appear earlier, after 10–12 months. White matter changes occur earlier and seem to have a higher repair capacity than vessel lesions (SCHULTHEISS et al. 1988, 1990).

3 Clinical Classification of Radiation Myelitis

The neurological symptoms of radiation-induced spinal cord injury develop after a latency period of hours to months, depending on radiation parameters and the patient's individual condition. According to the length of the latency period, the severeness of symptoms and the clinical course, three different types of spinal cord reactions can be distinguished.

3.1 Acute Reaction

An early reaction may occur a few hours after radiation exposure. Damage to the cord is not direct but results from edematous swelling in predisposed areas of the cord which have been already compressed by tumor. The symptoms vary depending on the individual situation and the administered radiation dose; transverse myelopathy may rapidly occur. However, acute reactions are generally reversible. Nevertheless, radiation therapy with high single doses to predamaged cord areas is often unavoidable, for example, as emergency treatment for metastatic spinal cord compression. In these cases, prophylactic antiedematous medication with corticoids is required.

3.2 Subacute Reaction

As a subacute reaction, transitory radiation myelopathy occurs after a latency period of 1–6 months (median 3 months). It can be interpreted as an irritation of the spinal cord. The most important clinical findings are paresthesia and dysesthesia in the distal extremities. Lhermitte's sign (electric shock-like sensation on flexion of the neck with stretching of the spinal cord) is a typical finding in transitory radiation myelopathy. Most patients have no complaints and symptoms of transitory radiation myelopathy are often only detected by careful anamnesis and examination. Thus, the literature data on the frequency of transitory radiation myelopathy vary markedly. If longer segments of the cord are irradiated, e.g., as in lymphomas, a substantial subset of patients, in the range of 30%, may develop clinical signs of radiation myelopathy. The prognosis of transitory myelopathy is good. In general, the symptoms disappear without any residual deficit within several weeks to months. However, transitory radiation myelopathy may rarely progress to chronic and fatal radiation myelitis (FISHMAN 1975).

3.3 Chronic Progressive Radiation Myelitis

Chronic radiation myelitis often begins subacutely and insidiously, with batchwise progression. The clinical signs vary depending on the localization and affected segments. The most common findings at the onset of symptoms are spastic and flaccid paralysis and other signs of upper motor neuron dysfunction (hyperreflexia, clonus, Babinski response) resulting from damage of the long cortical spinal tracts, mainly the spinothalamic tract and the pyramidal tract. Posterior column lesions with sensory abnormalities are less frequent. The hemicord syndrome of Brown-Sequard or transverse myelitis and symptoms comparable to an anterior spinal artery syndrome have also been described (GÄNSHIRT 1978). Slight neurological symptoms of chronic radiation myelitis may remain stable over long periods. In most cases, however, the symptoms progress to transverse myelopathy.

4 Radiation Tolerance of the Spinal Cord

In many tumor sites, e.g., lymphomas, head and neck cancer, or bronchogenic carcinoma, the spinal cord is at least partly within the radiation field. As a reasonable number of these patients are cured by radiotherapy, spinal cord tolerance is in fact a matter of major clinical impact. The cord dose administered during routine curative treatment, however, varies markedly from institution to institution. As radiation myelitis is a serious and mostly, in the long run, fatal complication, most radiation therapies operate with conservative tolerance doses and restrict the cord dose in curative treatments to 40–45 Gy or less. Recent experimental and clinical data confirm that the actual cord tolerance is probably much higher (SARTORELLI et al. 1992; MCCUNIFF and LIANG 1989; MARCUS and MILLION 1990; JEREMIE et al. 1991).

4.1 Conventional Fractionation

After conventional fractionation with fraction doses of about 2 Gy, the risk of radiation

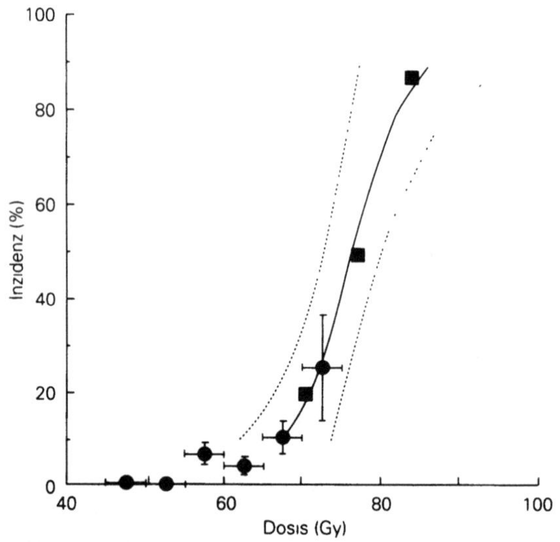

Fig. 2. Dose-effect curves for the incidence of chronic radiation myelopathy after conventional fractionation in humans (●) and rhesus monkeys (■). (From BAUMANN et al. 1994)

myelopathy remains below 1% up to total doses of 50–55 Gy. BAUMANN and coworkers (1994) have recently generated a dose-effect curve on the basis of the literature data. They found a TD 5/5 of about 60 Gy (Fig. 2). There seems to be a steep increase in the incidence of radiation myelopathy after 60–65 Gy, with a 25% risk at about 75 Gy. Their diagram also shows very similar dose-effect curves for human data and experimental data in primates, suggesting that the primate spinal cord may serve as a model for addressing clinical questions.

4.2 Impact of Fraction Size

The spinal cord is a typical late responding tissue, with increasing radiation tolerance if fraction size decreases. For fraction sizes of 2 Gy or more, the linear quadratic model adequately describes the fractionation effect. Large doses per fraction are associated with a highly increased risk of radiation myelopathy (DISCHE et al. 1981; HATLEVOLL et al. 1983). VAN DER SCHUEREN and coworkers (1988) have calculated an α/β-value of 1.7 Gy. Based on their analysis of human data, BAUMANN and coworkers (1994) have suggested lower α/β-values, in the range of 1 Gy. The reason for different α/β-values may be dependent on fraction size, as WONG and coworkers (1993) have demonstrated. They irradiated animals with fraction sizes of 0.85–11.5 Gy and found significantly different α/β-values for the larger vs the smaller fraction sizes (3.41 Gy vs 0.48 Gy, $p < 0.001$).

A major question of clinical importance is whether the sparing effect of smaller doses per fraction is also present if low and very low single doses below 2 Gy are administered. Recent experiments have shown that even very low doses are associated with a pronounced sparing effect (WONG et al. 1993). Contrary data from experiments with twice daily irradiation were probably misleading because the repair kinetics were not taken into account. Thus, radiation doses higher than the generally accepted tolerance dose of 50–55 Gy may probably be tolerated if the fraction size is further decreased, and of the interfraction interval is long enough for to enable complete repair.

4.3 Impact of Interfraction Interval

The use of twice-a-day irradiations schemes with at least moderate acceleration is increasing. In the CHART protocol, an elevated risk of radiation myelitis of 13% was found (DISCHE and SAUNDERS 1989). Two other clinical reports also suggest a higher frequency of radiation myelopathy as expected in case of irradiation with two daily fractions (WONG et al. 1991; DUNST et al. 1993). These clinical data are in contrast to the LQ model, which predicts a sparing effect with lowered fraction sizes. As a possible explanation of this discrepancy, the hypothesis of incomplete repair has been proposed (THAMES et al. 1988). Recent experimental data by ANG and coworkers (1992) in the rat spinal cord support this theory. They found a two-component repair with significantly different repair half-times of 0.7 and 3.8 h. By decreasing the interfraction interval, a lowered spinal cord tolerance results. These experimental data, however, only partially explain the high frequency of radiation myelopathy in the CHART protocol. A 13% incidence of myelopathy as observed in CHART, would require cord doses of more than 60–65 Gy in conventional fractionation. As the CHART patients received less than 50 Gy to the spinal cord, the tolerance of the spinal cord was about 17%–30% lower despite reduced fraction doses. This is higher than the values found in the rat spinal cord by ANG and coworkers (1992). A possible explanation could be a greater impact of the slow repair component in humans than in rats and a longer half-time of repair.

In summary, clinical and experimental data support the finding that the interfraction interval is an important parameter for spinal cord tolerance. The beneficial effect of low fraction sizes may be completely lost or cord tolerance may even decrease if the interfraction interval decreases.

4.4 *Impact of Irradiated Volume*

The impact of the irradiated cord volume on spinal cord tolerance is probably low. Early data from BODEN (1948) have led to the recommendation to reduce the cord dose if the irradiated cord segment is longer than 10 cm (RUBIN 1972; COHEN and CREDITOR 1981). The recent clinical publications on radiation myelopathy have not focused on this problem.

An indirect hint concerning the volume effect may be the fact that subacute cord reactions with Lhermitte's sign are relatively frequent in lymphoma patients after mantle or total nodal irradiation. In these patients half of the cord or the entire cord is included in the radiation volume; the total dose however, is only in the range of 30 Gy with standard treatment techniques. These patients have no elevated risk of late spinal cord sequelae, so that a volume effect may be more pronounced for subacute than late reactions.

Experimental data show that a volume effect in animals is present, especially in the case of high radiation doses. SCHULTHEISS and coworkers (1994) irradiated the spinal cord of rhesus monkeys with 70.4 Gy and found an increase in the frequency of radiation myelopathy from 15% to 38% with cord length in the radiation field of 4 cm and 16 cm, respectively. It should be noted that the cord dose was beyond the TD 5/5. From these experiments it may not be concluded that a significant volume effect exists if the cord dose remains below accepted tolerance doses.

4.5 *Individual Factors*

The impact of individual factors on late sequelae is likely, although not proven, for radiation myelopathy. Several authors have shown a correlation between variation of late radiation response and individual in vitro sensitivity of cultured fibroblasts. Endogenic factors such as diabetes, hypertonus, smoking, renal failure, and chemotherapy probably contributed to radiation myelitis, although their direct impact is not well known (VAN DER KOGEL et al. 1979; BLEYER and GRIFFIN 1980; RUIFROK and VAN DER KOGEL 1993).

4.6 *Reirradiation Tolerance*

The increasing number of patients who achieve cure or even long-term remission after definitive radiotherapy, e.g., in head and neck cancer, raises the problem of retreatment with radiotherapy in case of late recurrence or newly developed second tumors. Clinical data on reirradiation tolerance are rare. Early data of TAN and KHOR (1969) showed that reirradiation may be possible with regard to the former spinal cord dose. SCHULTHEISS et al. (1984) noted a shorter latency period in patients developing radiation myelopathy after two radiation treatments than in patients with one treatment.

Long-term recovery of the spinal cord has been shown in animals in several studies. In guinea-pigs, irradiation of the cord with a single dose of 10 Gy given one day after birth had no impact on the cord tolerance of adult animals (Knowles 1993). Other authors have also shown evidence for long-term recovery (HORNSEY et al. 1982; VAN DER KOGEL et al. 1982; WHITE and HORNSEY 1980). VAN DER KOGEL and coworkers (1982) have shown that the recovery started 56–120 days after treatment and reached a plateau after 140 days.

Recent experimental work by WONG and coworkers (1993) has also demonstrated that repair of the initial damage after the first treatment series depends on the dose of the first treatment. Rats received fractionated irradiation of up to 0%–90% of the cord tolerance and were retreated 20 weeks later with graded single doses. The residual injury of the first treatment was 59%–74% of the initial damage. The greatest recovery of initial damage (41% and 43%) was found for an initial injury representing 50%–70% of the cord tolerance. The recovery rate was smaller after lower and higher initial injury (26% recovery after an initial damage of 25%, 35% recovery after an initial damage of 90%).

MASON and coworkers (1993) have also shown that much of the initial damage after a first radiation treatment can be repaired. In guinea-pigs, nearly complete recovery from the initial treatment was found if the initial dose was lower than 50% of the cord tolerance. By increasing the initial dose, however, the tolerance of the second treatment also decreased.

In summary, recovery from initial damage has been well proven. The amount of recovery seems to be influenced by different factors, mainly the initial damage, as expressed as the percentage of the cord tolerance. The interval between first treatment and retreatment is probably also important. The real total tolerance of the spinal cord may be about 130% of the tolerance dose for the first treatment, as estimated by VAN DER KOGEL (1993). Although the general phenomenon of repair is surely present in humans, as compared to animals, some controversies remain in terms of transferring the experimental animal data to the clinic. First, the histological pattern of radiation myelitis in guinea-pigs differs from that in humans (diffuse demyelinization in animals instead of focal necrosis and vascular damage in humans). Second, the repair kinetics are probably different and it is questionable how long it takes to achieve maximal repair and retolerance in humans.

5 Latency Period

Radiation myelitis is a rare late sequelae after radiotherapy. It occurs in less than 1% of curatively treated patients in whom the spinal cord is within the radiation field. The interval between the end of treatment and onset of symptoms is at least several months. The incidence increases with longer follow-up. In analyzing a series of 300 cases from the literature, SCHULTHEISS and coworkers (1984) found that 50% of all radiation myelopathies develop within 20 months and 75% within 30 months after radiotherapy. It is not sure, whether a plateau is reached after 4–5 years (BAUMANN et al. 1994).

There are some hints that age at the time of treatment may have an impact on the latency period. SCHULTHEISS and coworkers (1984) reported shorter latency intervals in children than in adults. A comparable result was found by MASON et al. (1993) in guinea-pigs. As the data on the impact of age on the incidence of radiation myelopathy are conflicting, it is not clear whether shorter latency periods are a real phenomenon (e.g., by earlier expression of radiation sequele) or not.

6 Diagnosis and Differential Diagnosis

6.1 Clinical Symptoms

The clinical symptoms vary markedly depending on the localization of the affected segment of the spinal cord and the affected volume. Late radiation necrosis may cause irreversible damage of the cord. The main symptoms are progressive, spastic or flaccid paralysis. Sensory abnormalities may be present but are less frequent, especially at the onset of symptoms.

6.2 Radiological Findings

Nowadays, the most sensitive examination procedure is magnetic resonance (MR) tomography. Sagittal scans visualize long segments of the spinal cord and can directly illustrate abnormal areas within the cord. Radiation necrosis can be seen as areas of high signal intensity on T2-weighted images and show contrast enhancement on T1-weighted slices (Fig. 3). An indirect sign of radiation sequelae may be a thinning of the cord.

MR tomography is also very helpful in differential diagnosis, as it may exclude other reasons for spinal cord symptoms, e.g., compression syndromes of the cord.

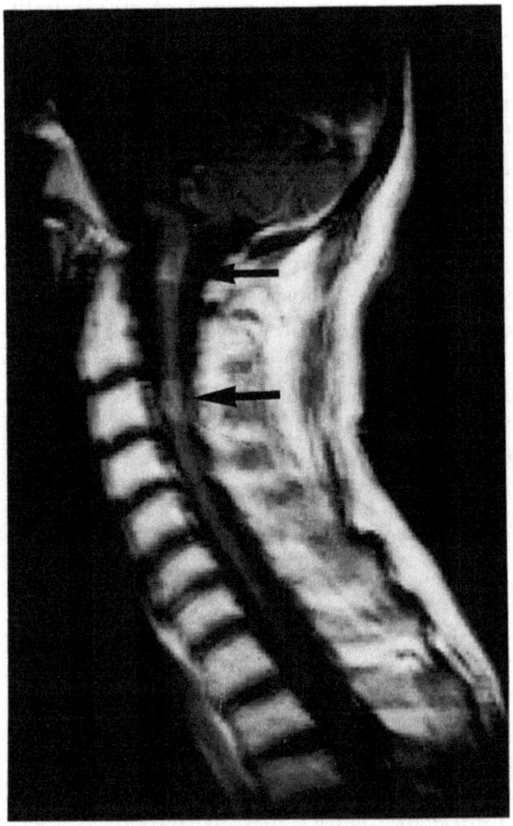

Fig. 3. Radiation myelitis in a 56 year old male after hyperfractionated accelerated radiotherapy for oropharyngeal carcinoma. The T1-weighted sagittal image after Gd application showed two contrast enhancing lesions (*arrows*) of the cervical cord. The patient died 8 months later with progressive symptoms. (From DUNST et al. 1993)

6.3 Diagnostic Procedure and Differential Diagnosis

It is surely unwise to diagnose radiation myelopathy if an irradiated patient develops neurological symptoms compatible with an isolated spinal process. Radiation myelitis is only likely if several basic criteria are fulfilled:

1. Previous irradiation of the spinal cord with a dose of at least 45 Gy in conventional fractionation or an equieffective dose
2. Latency period of at least 3–6 months
3. Neurological finding of spinal cord damage compatible with the irradiated cord segments

Moreover, if radiation myelpathy is diagnosed, additional procedures should be used to directly prove irradiation-induced damage and to exclude other causes:

1. MR tomography of the spinal cord showing necrotic areas within the irradiated cord segment on T2- and Gd-enhanced T1-images
2. Exclusion of an active inflammatory CNS process by cerebrospinal fluid examination

The most important differential diagnosis is tumor recurrence. Recurrence may be difficult to demonstrate and diagnosis may require computed tomography (CT) or MR tomography (Fig. 4). Myelography cannot directly visualize the spinal cord and can only be used to exclude spinal cord compression. Electrophysiological examinations are of minor importance and not helpful in the presence of clinical symptoms. A cerebrospinal fluid examination should always be performed to clearly exclude an inflammatory CNS disease.

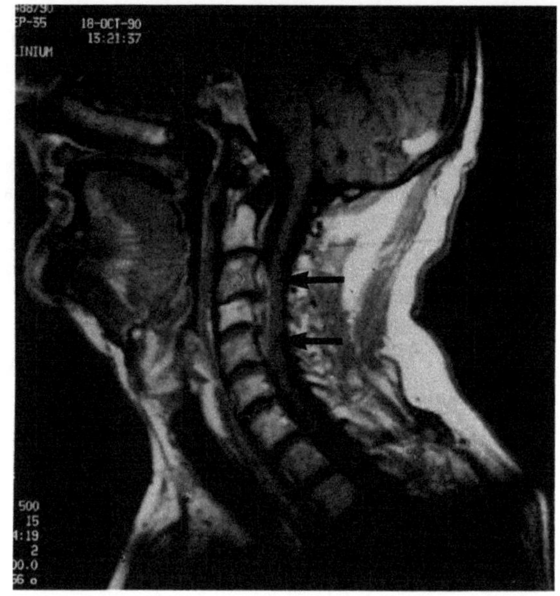

Fig. 4. False diagnosis for radiation myelitis in a 50 year old male after resection and postoperative radiotherapy for oropharyngeal cancer. The T1-weighted contrast-enhanced magnetic resonance tomogram shows intraspinal tumor recurrence (*arrows*) with cord compression

7 Therapy and Prognosis

As for other late sequelae of radiation therapy, specific therapeutic procedures do not exist. As with other CNS diseases with spinal cord affections, antispastic medications and remedial gymnastics may be helpful. Corticosteroids may suppress the necrosis-induced perifocal edema and are normally useful. The prognosis of radiation myelitis is poor. The cord changes normally progress in most cases.

References

Abbatucci JS, Delozier T, Quint R, Roussel A, Brune D (1978) Radiation myelopathy of the cervical spinal cord: time, dose and volume factors. Int J Radiat Oncol Biol Phys 4: 239–248

Ang KK, Jiang GL, Guttenberger R, Thames HD, Stephens LC, Smith CD, Feng Y (1992) Impact of spinal cord repair kinetics on the practice of altered fractionation schedules. Radiother Oncol 25: 287–294

Baumann M, Budach V, Appold S (1994) Strahlentoleranz des menschlichen Rückenmarks. Strahlenther Onkol 170: 131–139

Berlit P (1987) Die Strahlenmyelopathie. Klinische Analyse des Krankheitsbildes. Schriftenreihe Neurologie. Springer, Berlin Heidelberg New York, London, Paris, Tokyo

Bleyer WA, Griffin TW (1980) White matter necrosis, mineralizing microangiopathy, and intellectual abilities in survivors of childhood leukemia: associations with central nervous system irradiation and methotrexate therapy. In: Gilbert HA, Kagan AR (eds) Radiation damage of the nervous system. Raven Press, New York, pp 155–174

Boden G (1948) Radiation myelitis of the cervical spinal cord. Brit J Radiol 21: 464–469

Cohen L, Creditor M (1991) An iso-effect table for radiation tolerance of the human spinal cord. Int J Radiat Oncol Biol Phys 7: 961–966

Dische S, Martin WMC, Anderson P (1981) Radiation myelopathy in patients treated for carcinoma of bronchus using a six fraction regime of radiotherapy. Brit J Radiol 54: 29–35

Dische S, Warburton MF, Saunders M (1988) Radiation myelitis and survival in the radiotherapy of lung cancer. Int J Radiat Oncol Biol Phys 15: 75–81

Dische S, Saunders MI (1989) Continuous, hyperfractionated, accelerated radiotherapy (CHART): an interim report upon late morbidity. Radiother Oncol 16: 65–72

Dunst J, Dunst U, Wittmoser W (1993) Radiogene Myelitis nach akzelerierter Radiotherapie. Strahlenther Onkol 169: 543–544

Eichhorn HJ, Lessel A, Rotte KH (1972) Einfluß verschiedener Bestrahlungsrhythmen auf Tumor- und Normalgewebe in vivo. Strahlentherapie 143: 614–629

Fishman RA (1975) Letter. N Engl J Med 292: 669

Gänshirt H (1978) Strahlenmyelopathie. Med Welt 29: 261–264

Hatlevoll R, Host H, Kaalhus O (1983) Myelopathy following radiotherapy of bronchial carcinoma with large single fractions: a retrospective study. Int J Radiat Oncol Biol Phys 9: 41–44

Hornsey S, Myers R, Warren P (1982) Residual injury in the spinal cord after treatment with X-rays and neutrons. Br J Radiol 55: 516–519

Jellinger K, Sturm KW (1971) Delayed radiation myelopathy in man. Report of twelve necropsy cases. J Neurol Sci 14: 389–408

Jeremie B, Djuric L, Mijatovic L (1991) Incidence of radiation myelitis of the cervical spinal cord at doses of 5500 cGy or greater. Cancer 68: 2138–2141

Knowles JF (1993) The radiosensitivity of the guinea-pig spinal cord to X-rays; the effect of retreatment at one year and the effect of age at the time of irradiation. Int J Radiat Biol 44: 433–442

Marcus RB, Million RR (1990) The incidence of myelitis after irradiation of the cervical spinal cord. Int J Radiat Oncol Biol Phys 19: 3–8

Mason KA, Withers HR, Chiang CS (1993) Late effects of radiation on the lumbar spinal cord of guinea pigs: retreatment tolerance. Int J Radiat Oncol Biol Phys 26: 643–648

Mastaglia FL, McDonald WI, Watson JV, Yogendranm K (1976) Effects of X-radiation on the spinal cord: an experimental study of morphological changes in central nerve fibres. Brain 99: 101–122

McCuniff AJ, Liang MJ (1989) Radiation tolerance of the cervical spinal cord. Int J Radiat Oncol Biol Phys 16: 675–678

Piscol K (1972) Die Blutversorgung des Rückenmarkes und ihre klinische Relevanz. Schriftenreihe Neurologie. Springer, Berlin, Heidelberg, New York

Reinhold HS, Kaalen JGAH, Unger-Gils K (1976) Radiation myelopathy of the thoracic spinal cord. Int J Radiat Oncol Biol Phys 1: 651–657

Rubin P (1972) Radiation effect and tolerance, normal tissue. In: Vaeth JM (ed) Frontiers of radiation therapy and oncology, vol 6. University Park Press, Baltimore

Ruifrok ACC, van der Kogel AJ (1993) The effect of intraspinal cytosine arabinoside on the re-irradiation tolerance of the cervical spinal cord of young and adult rats. Eur J Cancer 29A: 1766–1770

Sartorelli B, Glanzmann C, Cordt-Riehle J (1992) Strahlentoleranz des thorakalen Rückenmarks bei konventioneller Fraktionierung. Abstract 412, Zbl Radiol 146: 157

Sauer R (1985) Klinik der Strahlenfolgen an Hirn- und Nervengewebe. In: Diethelm L, Heuck F, Olsson O et al. (eds) Strahlengefährdung und Strahlenschutz. Springer, Berlin, Heidelberg, New York, pp 317–339 (Handbuch der Medizinischen Radiologie vol 20)

Schultheiss TE, Higgins EM, El-Mahdi AM (1984) The latent period in clinical radiation myelopathy. Int J Radiat Oncol Biol Phys 10: 1109–1115

Schultheiss TE, Clifton-Stephens L, Maor MH (1988) Analysis of the histopathology of radiation myelopathy. Int J Radiat Oncol Biol Phys 14: 27–32

Schultheiss TE, Clifton-Stephens L, Jiang GL, Ang KK, Peters LJ (1990) Radiation myelopathy in primates treated with conventional fractionation. Int J Radiat Oncol Biol Phys 19: 935–940

Schultheiss TE, Stephens LC, Ang KK, Price RE, Peters LJ (1984) Volume effects in rhesus monkey spinal cord. Int J Radiat Oncol Biol Phys 29: 67–72

Tan BC, Khor TH (1969) Radiation myelitis in carcinoma of the nasopharynx. Clin Radiol 20: 329–331

Thames HD, Ang KK, Stewarts FA, van der Schueren E (1988) Does incomplete repair explain the apparent failure of the basic LQ model to predict spinal cord and kidney responses to low doses per fraction? Int J Radiat Biol 55: 27–43

Van der Kogel AJ (1979) Late effects of radiation on the spinal cord. Dose-effect relationships and pathogenesis. Publication of the Radiobiological Institute TNO, Rijswijk, The Netherlands, pp 1–160

Van der Kogel AJ, Sissingh HA, Zostelief J (1982) Effect of X-rays and neutrons on repair and regeneration in the rat spinal cord. Int J Radiat Oncol Biol Phys 8: 2095–2097

Van der Kogel AJ (1993) Retreatment tolerance of the spinal cord. Int J Radiat Oncol Biol Phys 26: 715–717

Van der Schueren E, Landuyt W, Ang KK, van der Kogel AJ (1988) From 2 Gy to 1 Gy per fraction: sparing effect in rat spinal cord? Int J Radiat Oncol Biol Phys 14: 297–300

Wara WM, Phillips TL, Sheline GE, Schwade JG (1975) Radiation tolerance of the spinal cord. Cancer 35: 1558–1562

White A, Hornsey S (1980) Time dependent repair of radiation damage in the rat spinal cord after X-rays and neutrons. Eur J Cancer 16: 957–962

Wong CS, van Dyk J, Simpson WJ (1991) Myelopathy following hyperfractionated accelerated radiotherapy for anaplastic thyroid carcinoma. Radiother Oncol 20: 3–9

Wong CS, Minkin S, Hill RP (1993) Effect of small doses per fraction in rat spinal cord: influence of initial vs final top-up doses. Radiother Oncol 28: 52–56

2.4 Acute and Late Toxicity on Peripheral Nerves After Radiotherapy

Clemens F. Hess, Rolf D. Kortmann, Martin Schabet, and Michael Bamberg

CONTENTS

1 Introduction 43
2 Diagnosis and Differential Diagnosis 43
2.1 Signs and Symptoms 44
2.2 Electrophysiological and Imaging Studies 44
3 Radiation Dose and Fractionation 45
3.1 Fractionated Radiotherapy 45
3.2 Single Dose Radiotherapy 45
4 Histopathological Features 47
5 Additional Effects of Chemotherapy and Surgery 47
6 Treatment of Radiation-Induced Peripheral Neuropathy 47
7 Summary and Therapeutic Recommendations . . 48
References 48

1 Introduction

For many years the peripheral nervous system was thought to be a radioresistant tissue, until it was realized that neurological toxicity took time to become apparent (Bamberg 1987; Hildebrand 1992; Sauer 1985). In particular, it has been demonstrated that radiation-induced brachial and lumbosacral plexopathy may occur in patients irradiated for breast cancer and for pelvic malignancies, respectively (Aho and Sainio 1983; Bagley et al. 1978; Basso-Ricci et al. 1980; Cherubino and Berzero 1983; Kori et al. 1981; Lederman and Wilbourn 1984; Olsen et al. 1990; Salner et al. 1981). Recently, it has been suggested that the peripheral nerve may be the principal, dose-limiting, normal tissue for intraoperative radiotherapy (IORT) in the pelvis (Le Couteur et al. 1989; Shaw et al. 1990).

From these reports increasing data on the radiation tolerance of peripheral nerves have been gathered, generally focussed on late-occurring irreversible damage of nervous tissue. In contrast, little is known about acute reactions of the peripheral nerve occurring early during fractionated radiotherapy. Sauer (1985) reported on breast cancer patients complaining of reversible lancinating pain and paresthesia affecting the inside of the upper arm and, rarely, the forearm and the fingers. Similarly, radiotherapy of carcinoma of the urinary bladder or the prostate has occasionally been found to result in reversible pain and paresthesia in dorsal parts of the thighs (Sauer 1985).

This chapter concentrates on the late-occurring radiation tolerance of peripheral nervous tissue. In particular, the clinical reliability of signs and symptoms and of electrophysiological and imaging studies in the diagnosis and differential diagnosis of radiation-induced peripheral neuropathy (RPN) is discussed. The influence of radiation dose and fractionation, of the extent of additional surgery, and of chemotherapy on the incidence of RPN is reviewed. In addition, the histopathological features and the therapeutic options in treating RPN are addressed.

2 Diagnosis and Differential Diagnosis

The main differential diagnosis in patients with peripheral nerve injury is radiation vs neoplastic injury (NPN) of peripheral nervous tissue (Bagley et al. 1978; Harper et al. 1989; Ledermann and Wilbourn 1984; Thomas et al. 1985). Both are associated with the same malignancies, primarily lung and breast cancer (in brachial plexopathy) and sarcoma and rectal and gynecological cancer (in lumbosacral plexopathy). Most importantly, however, it should be noted that neoplastic lesions are much more frequent than radiation-induced plexopathies (Hildebrand 1992), particularly in patients with proven tumour recurrence elsewhere, for example, in patients with positive chest or bone imaging studies (Table 1).

Clemens F. Hess, Prof., Dr., Strahlentherapentische Klinik, Robert-Koch-Straße 40, 37075, Göttingen, FRG
Rolf D. Kortmann, Dr., med.; Michael Bamberg Prof., Dr., Radiologische Universitätsklinik, Abteilung für Strahlentherapie, Hoppe-Seyler-Straße 3, 72076 Tübingen, FRG
Martin Schabet, Dr., Neurologische Universitätsklinik, Hoppe-Seyler-Straße 3, 72076 Tübingen, FRG

Table 1. Diagnosis and differential diagnosis of brachial plexopathy

	Type of plexopathy[a]	
	Radiation-induced	Neoplastic
Symptoms		
Pain	++	+++
Paresthesia/hypesthesia	+++	+++
Weakness	+++	+++
Horner's syndrome	(+)	+
Lymphedema	+	+
Electrophysiological studies		
Myokymic discharges on EMG	++	(+)
Nerve conduction abnormalities	++	++
Abnormal imaging studies		
Computed tomography of plexus		
Loss of tissue planes	++	+
Demonstration of masses	(+)	++
Chest roentgenogram	(+)	++
Bone scan	(+)	++
Cervical spine roentgenogram	(+)	+
Myelography	(+)	+

EMG, electromyography.
[a]Estimated incidence: (+): <10%, +: 10–40%, ++: 40–80%, +++: >80%.

A wide range of latency periods, lasting several months or years after the end of radiotherapy, has been reported for both types of injury. Thus, the delay between irradiation and the onset of peripheral nerve injury is of no use in the differentiation of RPN and NPN (Bagley et al. 1978; Kori et al. 1981).

2.1 Signs and Symptoms

Progressive paresthesia or hypesthesia were shown to be the first symptoms in most patients with RPN (Table 1). In the study reported by Harper et al. (1989) patients with brachial RPN complained of pain, sensory dysfunction, and weakness when they sought medical attention. During the subsequent course of disease, the cumulative frequency of weakness exceeded 90%. Kori et al. (1981) suggested that upper brachial plexus lesions with lymphedema indicate radiation injury; however, this is not a consistent finding (Hildebrand 1992). In contrast, most authors agree that painful brachial plexopathy with Horner's syndrom implies tumor infiltration (Harper et al. 1989; Hildebrand 1992; Kori et al. 1981) (Table 1). Similarly, Thomas et al. (1985) found that the most reliable feature favoring a diagnosis of lumbosacral NPN was the presence of (mostly unilateral) nerve pain (Salner et al. 1981). In this study all patients with RPN presented with indolent mostly serious leg weakness which was bilateral in most cases and painless in half of them.

Lumbosacral neuropathy was found in 16 out of 50 patients treated with IORT for pelvic malignancies and consisted of pain in all 16 patients, numbness and tingling in 11, and weakness in eight (Shaw et al. 1990). The pain, numbness and tingling resolved in about 40% of patients, while weakness resolved in only one of eight. Similarly, irreversible mixed motor-sensory deficits were found in dogs treated in experimental studies of IORT-related neuropathy (Kinsella et al. 1988; Le Couteur et al. 1989).

2.2 Electrophysiological and Imaging Studies

Since it may be difficult to discriminate between RPN and NPN clinically (Cooke et al. 1988b; Hildebrand 1992), electrophysiological and imaging studies have been increasingly used for differential diagnosis (Cascino et al. 1983; Cooke et al. 1988a,b; Harper et al. 1989; Lederman and Wilbourn 1984). Harper et al. (1989) found myokymic discharges on electromyography (EMG) to be highly suggestive of RPN and no discriminative capacity of nerve conduction studies (Table 1). Lederman and Wilbourn (1984), however, reported that abnormal sensory but normal motor conduction of the affected nerves was more frequent in patients with RPN than in patients with NPN. They also found myokymia on EMG to be characteristic for RPN.

More recently, cross-sectional imaging techniques such as computed tomography (CT) were used in differential diagnosis of brachial plexopathy (CASCINO et al. 1983; COOKE et al. 1988a, b). In 51 patients with clinically diagnosed brachial plexopathy, CT revealed metastatic tumor in 46 and radiation fibrosis in five patients. In four patients with radiation fibrosis, CT showed distortion of normal tissue planes without a discrete mass, which did not exclude diffuse tumor infiltration (CASCINO et al. 1983). In a study by COOKE et al. (1988b) CT was able to identify varying grades of abnormality that were ascribed to radiation fibrosis. However, the changes on CT did not relate to the different radiotherapy techniques. In some patients with plexopathy neither clinical data nor electrophysiological nor imaging studies may be able to discriminate RPN from NPN. In these cases surgical exploration of the affected plexus may be indicated to prompt adequate treatment (BAGLEY et al. 1978).

3 Radiation Dose and Fractionation

3.1 Fractionated Radiotherapy

A number of previous studies have shown that the incidence of radiation-induced damage of peripheral nerves is related to both total dose and fractionation (Table 2). STOLL and ANDREWS (1966) reported on a series of patients treated with a high total dose (56.7 Gy) in large fractions (4.6 Gy) and detected brachial plexus injury in 73% of cases. When 54 Gy was given in 3 Gy fractions the incidence of brachial plexus lesions was 60%, but 45 Gy in 3 Gy fractions resulted in a 6% incidence (WESTLING et al. 1972).

PIERCE et al. (1992) reported on 1117 patients who received a median dose of 46 Gy to the supraclavicular lymph nodes with or without axillary irradiation, with 95% of patients receiving total doses of 44–45 Gy given in fractions of 1.8–2 Gy. With this schedule, only 20 patients (1.8%) developed a brachial plexopathy. The incidence was 1.3% (13/991) for axillary doses of less than 50 Gy and 5.6% (7/126) for doses greater than 50 Gy (Table 2). This difference was found to be statistically significant. Similarly, FOWBLE et al. (1991) found an overall incidence of radiation-induced brachial plexopathy of less than 1% if the regional lymph nodes received 46–50 Gy over a period of 4.5–5 weeks.

Recently, POWELL et al. (1990) compared two different fraction schedules supposed to be equivalent when using the Nominal standard dose formula. In this study the calculated doses administered to the brachial plexus were 45 Gy in 15 fractions and 54 Gy in 30 fractions. The incidence of radiation-induced brachial plexus injury at 5.9 years was significantly affected by fraction sizes, being 5.9% for the large fraction size group and 1.0% for the small fraction size group (Table 2). Applying the linear quadratic model to their own data and to comparable data of the literature POWELL et al. (1990) suggested that the α/β ratio for brachial plexus injury is approximately 2 Gy and thus similar to that of the central nervous system. However, there are insufficient data available to comment on the dependence upon overall treatment time (COHEN and SVENSSON 1978; POWELL et al. 1990).

3.2 Single Dose Radiotherapy

Recent experiences with single dose IORT strongly suggest that the size of the fraction doses is related to the risk of RPN (KINSELLA et al. 1988a,b; LE COUTEUR et al. 1989; SHAW et al. 1990). In an animal study LE COUTEUR et al. (1989) examined peripheral nerve lesions in the lumbar paraaortic region following fractionated external beam radiotherapy (EBRT), IORT, or a combination of both. The combination showed a similar incidence and latency of RPN as IORT alone. The incidence of RPN increased with increasing IORT doses beginning at 15 Gy, with an incidence of 100% for IORT doses of 25 Gy or more. Interestingly, RPN was not seen with EBRT alone at doses between 50 Gy and 80 Gy. Another animal study on IORT-related RPN (KINSELLA et al. 1988b) showed an inverse relation- ship between IORT dose (27–75 Gy) and the time to onset of hind limb paresis (1–12 months following IORT). Unilateral hind limb paresis occurred 8–9 months after IORT in all four dogs receiving 20 Gy and in none of the animals receiving IORT doses of 10 Gy or 15 Gy.

These experimental findings have been supported by preliminary results of human studies (KINSELLA et al. 1988a; SHAW et al. 1990). In a recent report (SHAW et al. 1990), RPN was seen in one of four patients receiving an IORT dose of 10 Gy compared to 14 of 28 patients receiving IORT doses of 15 Gy

Table 2. Incidenceof radiation-induced injury (RPN) of the brachial plexus for different radiation doses and fractionation schedules

Incidence of RPN			Radiation dose and fractionation			
Total group (%)	With chemotherapy (%)	Without chemotherapy (%)	Total dose (Gy)	Fraction dose (Gy)	Number of fractions	Reference
73			57	~4.6	12	Stoll and Andrews 1966
60[a]			54	3	18	Westling et al. 1972
35[b]	42	26	40–50	~4	10–12	Olsen et al. 1990
15			51	4.6	11	Stoll and Andrews 1966
6			45	3	15	Westling et al. 1972
5.9			45	3	15	Powell et al. 1990
5.6	7.9	3.2	50–55	1.8–2.0	25–28	Pierce et al. 1992
3.3			60	2.0	30	Basso-Ricci et al. 1980
1.3	3.7	0.4	45–50	1.8–2.0	23–28	Pierce et al. 1992
1.0			46–50	1.8–2.0	23–28	Fowble et al. 1991
1.0			54	1.8	30	Powell et al. 1990

[a] A 15% incidence for irradiation of supraclavicular region only.
[b] 48% incidence after more extended axillary surgery (> six lymph nodes removed) and 26% after less extended surgery (⩽six lymph nodes removed).

or more. Again, there was no relationship between the likelihood of developing complications and the total external beam dose.

4 Histopathological Features

In humans, histological evaluation of RPN revealed thickening of the epineurium and endoneurium and evidence of demyelination and endarteriitis in some cases (COOKE et al. 1988b; HILDEBRAND 1992). LE COUTEUR et al. (1989) performed histological studies of nerves in their beagle dogs 2 years following either IORT alone or IORT combined with EBRT. They found loss of axons and myelin and an increase of endoneurial, perineurial, and epineurial connective tissue as compared to untreated nerves. The number of axons and the amount of myelin decreased by 40% at 15 Gy IORT and to an even greater extent at higher doses. EBRT alone resulted in an insignificant decrease of axons and myelin. With most IORT doses, necrosis and hyalinization of the media of small arteries and arterioles within and around nerves were important findings. Severe vessel lesions occurred with a probability of 50% after 19.5 Gy IORT alone and after 18.7 Gy when IORT was combined with EBRT. Similar blood vessel lesions were not seen with any EBRT alone dose.

From these data it is concluded that RPN results from direct effects of irradiation on nerves and from secondary effects on the regional vasculature. The principal histological lesion observed by KINSELLA et al. (1988b) in IORT of nerves in dogs was loss of large nerve fibers without significant vascular injury. Similarly, histological alterations observed by SHAW et al. (1990) in autopsied IORT patients included perineurial fibrosis in the absence of radiation-related changes in major blood vessels.

5 Additional Effects of Chemotherapy and Surgery

Several authors have suggested that additional chemotherapy might enhance the radiation-induced effect on the brachial plexus (BAMBERG 1987; HILDEBRAND 1992; OLSEN et al. 1990; PIERCE et al. 1992; SALNER et al. 1981) (Table 2). OLSEN et al. (1990) found RPN in 26% of patients treated exclusively with postoperative irradiation for breast cancer and in 42% of patients additionally treated with two cycles of CMF chemotherapy. In both groups 40–50 Gy was administered to the axilla with 3 Gy fractions. Additional chemotherapy also resulted in diminishing the latency period. PIERCE et al. (1992) reported a significant increase of RPN by additional chemotherapy, from 0.4% to 3.7%, if a total dose of less than 50 Gy was given to the axilla in 1.8–2.0 Gy fractions. For patients receiving more than 50 Gy, incidences were 3.2% and 7.9% for patients treated without and with chemotherapy, respectively. However, this latter difference was not statistically significant. The majority of plexopathies found in this study was completely reversible. Similar findings have been reported by SALNER et al. (1981).

In addition, it has been suggested that the extent of surgery may contribute to the development of RPN (HILDEBRAND 1992; SAUER 1985). However, reliable data about this topic are still scarce. OLSEN et al. (1990) related the number of removed lymph nodes to the incidence of brachial plexopathy and found a significant increase, from 25% to 48%, if more than six lymph nodes had been removed during prior axillary surgery (Table 2).

6 Treatment of Radiation-Induced Peripheral Neuropathy

In the majority of patients, RPN has been reported to be an irreversible condition. The administration of steroids or actihaemyl has been reported to arrest RPN in some cases, but practically these drugs seem to be of limited benefit. Symptomatic relief of pain, however, may be obtained by tricyclic antidepressants (BAMBERG 1987; HILDEBRAND 1992; SAUER 1985).

Although some reports have suggested an improvement with decompressive surgery, these improvements are also limited to relief of pain without improvement in disability (HILDEBRAND 1992). BRUNELLI and BRUNELLI (1985), for instance, operated on 39 out of 67 patients with actinic brachial plexus lesions, including 31 cases by means of a free microvascular transfer of the greater omentum following neurolysis. The authors suggested that this technique is currently the best method for relieving pain. However, a good recovery was obtained only in patients with early neurological symptoms. As surgery may even lead to a worsening of symptoms in some patients, it should have a minor role in the treatment of RPN (HILDEBRAND 1992; SAUER 1985). Furthermore, in many patients, even symptomatic therapy of pain in RPN remains largely ineffective.

Management is therefore prevention and to devise safe but effective treatment strategies. In particular, restricted use of radiotherapy, safe total and fraction doses, and adequate radiation techniques avoiding local overdosage are warranted, particularly when administered concomitantly with cytotoxic therapy or after extensive surgery (Bamberg 1987; Hildebrand 1992; Pierce et al. 1992; Salner et al. 1981).

7 Summary and Therapeutic Recommendations

In recent years, radiation tolerance of peripheral nervous tissue has been addressed in a number of studies. Difficulties in interpreting and comparing the presented data are manyfold. They include different extent and time of neurological follow-up examinations, different methods of electrophysiological and imaging studies, differences in radiation techniques and dosage, in the extent of surgery and in the use of additional chemotherapy and the paucity of therapeutic data of RPN. Despite all these problems the following conclusions can be drawn from the available literature.

First of all, it should be kept in mind that peripheral neuropathy in cancer patients is considerably more likely to be caused by tumor infiltration than by prior radiation therapy. This is particularly true in patients with known metastatic disease elsewhere and in patients who have been irradiated with contemporary radiation techniques.

Second, although it may be difficult to discriminate between RPN and NPN, the presence of pain, the absence of myokymic discharges on EMG, and demonstration of metastases on CT are typical features in favor of a diagnosis of neoplastic neuropathy. The incidence of RPN is strongly related to the total dose and particularly to the size of fraction doses. With fraction doses of 1.8–2.0 Gy and total doses of less than 50 Gy RPN may occur in about 1% of patients. There is evidence that this risk is significantly increased if additional chemotherapy is administered or in the case of prior extended surgery in the irradiated volume. The peripheral nerve may become the principal dose-limiting normal tissue in single dose radiotherapy regimens. In IORT, for example, the incidence of RPN increases considerably if single doses in excess of 15–20 Gy are given.

The histological alterations in RPN include direct effects, such as loss of nerve fibers and fibrosis, and, less frequently, vascular injury. Usually, RPN is an irreversible condition, and the administration of drugs and the use of decompressive surgery are of limited benefit. Therefore, prevention is of utmost importance including careful indications for radiotherapy and concomitant chemotherapy, appropriate selection of radiation techniques and – most importantly – of safe and effective total and fraction doses.

References

Aho K, Sainio K (1983) Late irradiation-induced lesions of the lumbosacral plexus. Neurology 33: 953–955

Bagley FH, Walsh JW, Cady B et al. (1978) Carcinamotous versus radiation-induced brachial plexus neuropathy in breast cancer. Cancer 41: 2154–2157

Bamberg M (1987) Tumoren der peripheren Nerven. In: Scherer E (ed) Strahlentherapie. Springer, Berlin Heidelberg New York, p 1058

Basso-Ricci S, della Costa C, Viganotti G, Ventafridda V, Zanolla R (1980) Report on 42 cases of post irradiation lesions of the brachial plexus and their treatment. Tumori 66: 117–122

Brunelli G, Brunelli F (1985) Surgical treatment of actinic brachial plexus lesions: free microvascular transfer of the greater omentum. J Reconstr Microsurg 1: 197–200

Cascino TL, Kori S, Krol G, Foley KM (1983) CT of the brachial plexus in patients with cancer. Neurology 33: 1553–1557

Cherubino P, Berzero GF (1983) Post irradiation lesions of the brachial plexus. Ital J Orthop Traumatol 9: 357–363

Cohen L, Svensson H (1978) Cell population kinetics and dose-time relationships for post-irradiation injury of the brachial plexus in man. Acta Radiol Oncol 17: 161–166

Cooke J, Cooke D, Parsons C (1988a) The anatomy and pathology of the brachial plexus as demonstrated by computed tomography. Clin Radiol 39: 595–601

Cooke J, Powell S, Parsons C (1988b) The diagnosis by computed tomography of brachial plexus lesions following radiotherapy for carcinoma of the breast. Clin Radiol 39: 602–606

Fowble BL, Solin LJ, Schultz DJ, Goodman RL (1991) Ten year results of conservative surgery and irradiation for stage I and II breast cancer. Int J Radiat Oncol Biol Phys 21: 269–277

Harper CM, Thomas JE, Cascino TL, Litchy WJ (1989) Distinction between neoplastic and radiation-induced brachial plexopathy, with emphasis on the role of EMG. Neurology 39: 502–506

Hildebrand J (1992) Lesions of the peripheral nervous systems. In: Hildebrand J (ed) Management in neurooncology. Springer, Berlin Heidelberg New York, pp 75–87

Kinsella TJ, Sindelair WF, Lack E, Glatstein E, Rosenberg SA (1988a) Preliminary results of a randomized study of adjuvant radiation therapy in resectable adult retroperitoneal soft tissue sarcomas. J Clin Oncol 6: 10–25

Kinsella TJ, Sindelair WF, DeLuca (1988b) Threshold dose for peripheral nerve injury following intraoperative radiotherapy in a large animal model. Int J Radiat Oncol Biol Phys 15 [Suppl 1]: 205

Kori SH, Foley KM, Posner JB (1981) Brachial plexus

lesions in patients with cancer: 100 cances. Neurology 31: 45–50
Le Couteur RA, Gillette EL, Powers BE et al. (1989) Peripheral neuropathies following experimental intraoperative radiation therapy (IORT). Int J Radiat Oncol Biol Phys 17: 583–590
Lederman RJ, Wilbourn AJ (1984) Brachial plexopathy: recurrent cancer or radiation? Neurology 34: 1331–1335
Olsen NK, Pfeiffer P, Mondrup K, Rose C (1990) Radiation-induced brachial plexus neuropathy in breast cancer patients. Acta Oncol 29: 885–889
Pierce SM, Recht A, Lingos TI et al. (1992) Long-term radiation complications following conservatice surgery and radiation therapy in patients with early stage breast cancer. Int J Radiat Oncol Biol Phys 23: 915–923
Powell S, Cooke J, Parsons C (1990) Radiation-induced brachial plexus injury: follow-up of two different fraction- ation schedules. Radiother Oncol 18: 213–220
Salner AL, Botnick LE, Herzog et al. (1981) Reversible brachial plexopathy following primary radiation therapy for breast cancer. Cancer Treat Rep 65: 797–802
Sauer R (1985) Klinik der Strahlenfolgen an Hirn- und Nervengewebe. In: Diethelm L, Heuck F, Olsson O et al. (eds) Strahlengefährdung und Strahlenschutz. Springer, Berlin Heidelberg New York, pp 317–339 (Handbuch der medizinischen Radiologie, vol 20)
Shaw EG, Gunderson LL, Martin JK et al. (1990) Peripheral nerve and ureteral tolerance to intraoperative radiation therapy: clinical and dose-response analysis. Radiother Oncol 18: 247–255
Stoll BA, Andrews JT (1966) Radiation-induced peripheral neuropathy. Br Med J 1: 834–837
Thomas JE, Cascino TL, Earle JD (1985) Differential diagnosis between radiation and tumor plexopathy of the pelvis. Neurology 35: 1–7
Westling P, Svensson H, Hele P (1972) Cervical plexus lesions following post-operative radiation therapy of mammary carcinoma. Acta Radiol Ther Phys Biol 11: 209–216

2.5 Acute and Late Toxicity on Peripheral Nerves After Chemotherapy – A Review

CARSTEN BOKEMEYER, BERND FRANK, and HANS-JOACHIM SCHMOLL

CONTENTS

1 Introduction 51
2 Patients and Methods 52
2.1 Hodgkin's Disease 52
2.2 Testicular Cancer 52
3 Results 53
3.1 Hodgkin's Disease 53
3.2 Testicular Cancer 53
4 Discussion 54
5 Summary and Therapeutic Implications 56
References 57

1 Introduction

Peripheral neuropathy has long been recognized as a problem in cancer patients. The diagnosis of cancer itself is associated with peripherial neuropathy of different degrees in approximately 20%–40% of patients (PAUL et al. 1978). Furthermore, damage to the nervous system occurs as a common complication of antineoplastic therapy. Neurotoxicity may follow treatment with radiation therapy, chemotherapy, biological response modifiers, or combined modality therapy, with no portion of the nervous system being immune from potential damage. The peripheral nervous system represents a comment target for the toxic effects of many chemotherapeutic agents. For drugs like cisplatin and vincristine peripheral neurological toxicity may be the dose-limiting factor that prevents a more intensive use of these agents. A number of different cytotoxic drugs have been identified as a cause of peripheral neuropathy, out of which cisplatin and the vinca alkaloids are the most frequent (FORMAN 1990a, b; CASEY et al. 1973; ROELOFS et al. 1984). Table 1 summarizes chemotherapeutic agents which have been associated with toxic effects on the peripheral nervous system (MACDONALD 1992).

The pathological classification of peripheral neuropathies distinguishes between neuronopathies (loss of the anterior horn, dorsal root ganglion and autonomic ganglion cells), axonopathies, disorders of the Schwann cells and myelin and disorders of the supporting tissue affecting the vessels or the neural connective tissue (Table 2) (THOMAS 1984). For most chemotherapeutic agents the pathophysiological mechanisms causing neuropathy are not fully understood. After the use of vinca alkaloids, particularly vincristine and vindesine, damage is often found in the distal axonal part of the nerve (XU et al. 1989). The postulated underlying mechanism is interference of the drug with the axoplasmic transport of the neuron (FORMAN 1990b; MOLLMANN 1990).

While vincristine neuropathy affects large and small motor and sensory axons, the neuropathy following administration of cisplatin is rather specific to large sensory nerves. The pathological findings after the administration of cisplatin are consistent with an axonal neuropathy; however, segmental demyelination has also been described (THOMPSON et al. 1984; VON HOFF et al. 1979; MARIN and RIERSON 1979). Vinca alkaloids have been used in oncology for some time, and the neurotoxic effects of vinblastine and vincristine were recognized as early as 1962, while the first report of peripheral neuropathy following cisplatin appeared in 1978, approximately 5 years after its introduction into clinical oncology (KEDAR et al. 1978). Both cisplatin and the vinca alkaloids play a substantial role in modern combination chemotherapy, particularly for the treatment of curative neoplasms, such as malignant germ cell tumors of the testis and high grade lymphomas. In patients with Non-Hodgkin's and Hodgkin's lymphoma, the vinca alkaloids are an essential part of combination treatment regimens such as MOPP, COPP, CHOP or ABVD (Table 3). Cisplatin is the major component of those combination regimens which have brought

CARSTEN BOKEMEYER, Dr., H.-J. SCHMOLL, Prof., Dr., Zentrum für Innere Medizin und Dermatologie, Abteilung Hämatologie/Onkologie, Medizinische Hochschule, Konstanty-Gutschow-Strasse 8, 30623 Hannover, FRG
BERND FRANK, Dr., Universitätsklinikum Magdeburg, LeipzigerStrasse 44, 39120 Magdeburg, FRG

Table 1. Chemotherapeutic agents possibly associated with toxic effects on the peripheral nervous system

Agent	Comment
Amsacrine	Rare cases
Carboplatin	Only doses >1 g/m^2
Cisplatin	Frequently reported; dose-limiting
Etoposide	Rare cases; enhances neurotoxicity of other agents
Hexamethylmelamine	Frequency 10%–15%
Ifosfamide	Rare cases; central nervous system toxicity more common
Misonidazole	Sensory polyneuropathy
Procarbazine	10%–20% with myalgias
Taxol	20%–30% peripheral neurological symptoms
Vinca alkaloids	Frequency: vincristine > vindesine > vinblastine

Table 2. Pathological classification of peripheral neuropathies (according to THOMAS PK, 1984)

Neuronopathies: loss of the anterior horn, dorsal root ganglion and autonomic ganglion cells
Axonopathies: distal and proximal axonopathies; focal axonal interruption
Disorders of Schwann cells and myelin sheets
Disorders of the supporting tissues: vascular disorders; disorders of neural connective tissues

great progress in recent years in the treatment of patients with malignant germ cell tumors. Patients with either Hodgkin's disease or germ cell tumors will be cured in the majority of cases (EINHORN 1990; URBA and LONGO 1992). Therefore, the question of the frequency and severity of long-term neurological side effects is of particular concern.

This report describes an analysis of the incidence of late neurological side effects and their association with the therapy regimens used in two large patient groups treated for Hodgkin's disease or for testicular germ cell tumor at Hannover University Medical School over the last 15 years.

2 Patients and Methods

2.1 Hodgkin's Disease

A total of 76 patients (41 women and 35 men) who were treated between 1965 and 1988 at Hannover Medical University School were included into the current investigation. The mean age was 37 years (18–74) at the time of evaluation and 27.5 years (15–64) at the time of first diagnosis. All patients had been in complete remission for more than 2 years (median 72 months (27–234)). The median follow-up was 96 months. The patients' characteristics are summarized in Table 4. There were 12 patients (16%) who had received chemotherapy alone, 21 patients (28%) who had radiotherapy alone and 43 patients (56%) who were treated by combined chemo- and radiotherapy.

All patients were evaluated by a questionnaire in which they were able to subjectively grade the severity of their neurological complaints such as muscle cramps, muscle weakness and paresthesias. All patients were also examined by a skilled neurologist. Furthermore, electrophysiological measurements were performed in all patients, including determination of the orthodromic sensitive nerve conduction velocity of the sural nerve and the motor nerve conduction velocity of the peroneal nerve. Electrophysiological determinations were carried out at a standardized skin temperature (35 °C). Patients were also examined by electromyography (EMG) of the first interosseous dorsalis muscle. The following EMG criteria were analyzed: appearance of pathological spontaneous activity and the configurations of the motor potentials (polyphasia rate, mean duration and mean and maximal amplitude of the signal).

2.2 Testicular Cancer

A total of 115 patients with disseminated testicular cancer receiving standard induction or salvage

Table 3. Chemotherapeutic regimens used for the treatment of patients with Hodgkin's and Non Hodgkin's lymphomus

MOPP: mechlorethamine, Oncovin (vincristine), procarbazine, predinsone	ABVD: adriamycin, bleomycin, vinblastine, dacarbazine	CHOP: cyclophosphamide, hydroxydaunomycin (doxorubicin), Oncovin (vincristine), prednisone
COPP: cyclophosphamide, Oncovin (vincristine), procarbazine, prednisone		

Table 4. Characteristics of 76 patients treated for Hodgkin's disease at Hannover University Medical School[a]

Mean age	37 years (range: 18–74 years)	
Mean duration of follow-up	8 years (range: 27–234 months)	
Sex		
Female	54%	
Male	46%	
Stage (Ann Arbor)		
I	16%	
II	49%	
III	21%	
IV	14%	
Therapy		
Radiotherapy	28%	
Chemotherapy[b]	16%	
COPP		9%
COPP/ABVD		7%
Combined modality	57%	
COPP + radiotherapy		20%
COPP/ABVD/ IMEP + radiotherapy		24%
COP/ABV/IMEP + radiotherapy		10%
Others + radiotherapy		3%

[a]The patients were evaluated for long-term neurological side effects by subjective grading of symptoms, neurological examination and electrophysiological examinations.
[b]For definitions, see Table 3.

chemotherapy with cisplatin-containing combinations were included. The median age was 29.8 years (17–51) and the median time interval since chemotherapy was 58.1 months (14–149). All patients were in complete remission (CR) or had stable marker-negative unresectable disease for at least 1 year at the time of the neurological examination. There were 20 patients (17.4%) who had been treated by combination regimens with high dose cisplatin (> 150 mg/m^2 per chemotherapy cycle) and 95 patients (82.6%) who received standard dose cisplatin-containing regimens (100–120 mg/m^2 per cycle). Most patients had received either PEB (platinum/etoposide/bleomycin) or PVB (platinum/vinblastine/bleomycin) therapy. Eleven of these patients additionally received vincristine.

All patients were personally interviewed for subjective symptoms and complaints of peripheral neuropathy and received a careful neurological examination.

3 Results

3.1 *Hodgkin's Disease*

Some 27 (37%) of 73 evaluable patients complained of subjective neurological symptoms (muscle cramps, 18 patients; paresthesias, 11 patients; and sensory deficits, 13 patients). According to the neurophysiological examination 19 patients (26%) showed a distal symmetrical motor and sensory polyneuropathy. Of these, 13 patients (68%) were classified as having axonal polyneuropathy, five patients (26%) had a combined defect of the axonal and myelin structures and one patient showed affection of the myelin sheets alone.

Table 5. Correlation of subjective complaints and objective electrophysiological findings in 76 patients treated for Hodgkin's disease

Subjective neurological symptoms	Electrophysiological examination	
	Normal (%)	Abnormal (%)
None	37/54 (69)	9/19 (47)
Present	17/54 (31)	10/19 (53)

Only ten of 27 patients (37%) with subjective complaints of peripheral neuropathy also showed neurophysiological abnormalities. The other 17 patients (63%) had normal electrophysiological findings. In contrast to these, nine of 19 patients (47%) with electrophysiological findings indicating neuropathy were clinically free from subjective complaints. The latter findings were interpreted as "subclinical polyneuropathy." A comparison of electrophysiological and subjective findings in patients with Hodgkin's disease is shown in Table 5.

For all patients the median cumulative dose of vinca alkaloids (vincristine and/or vinblastine) received was evaluated. For those patients receiving vincristine, a median dose of 20 mg (4–84 mg) and for those receiving vinblastine a median cumulative dose of 80 mg (18–560) was determined. Of those 19 patients with abnormal findings in the electrophysiological examination 14 patients had received a cumulative dose of vinca alkaloids above the median dose of the total group and only five patients had received a cumulative dose below the median dose of vinca alkaloids in the study population ($p < 0.05$).

3.2 *Testicular Cancer*

In 65 patients (57%) no signs or symptoms of peripheral neuropathy were found. There were 36 patients (31%) who reported symptoms only during chemotherapy; these completely resolved by the follow-up examination. In 14 additional patients

Table 6. Neurological side effects in 115 patients treated for metastatic testicular cancer in relation to the administered doses of cytostatic agents

	No neurotoxicity	Neurotoxicity only during therapy	Late neurotoxicity
Percentage of patients	57%	31%	12%
Median dose (mg)			
Cisplatin	370	410	640 ($p < 0.05$)
Etoposide	1850	1950	2500 ($p = 0.07$)
Vinblastine	45	42	42 (n.s.)
Bleomycin	150	180	160 (n.s.)

n.s., not statistically significant.

(12%), the symptoms of peripheral neuropathy persisted after chemotherapy. The median cumulative dose of cisplatin in patients with the neurological toxicity was considerably higher (650 mg/m^2) than in patients reporting no neurotoxic effects (370 mg/m^2) ($p < 0.05$). In general, patients with persistent neurotoxic effects had also received a higher total dose of etoposide. Table 6 summarizes the median cumulative doses of cisplatin, bleomycin, etoposide and vinblastine received by our patients.

Of 20 patients (75%) receiving cisplatin doses >150 mg/m^2 per cycle, 15 reported symptoms of neurotoxicity, which appeared to be persistent in seven patients (35%). In comparison, patients receiving standard dose cisplatin regimens (100–120 mg/m^2 per cycle) reported neurological symptoms in 45% and persistent symptoms were present in only 16% of patients at the long-term follow-up evaluation.

Of 11 patients additionally receiving vincristine as part of their therapy regimen, eight reported reversible and one irreversible neurotoxicity. Overall, neurological symptoms were reversible within 1–36 months after the end of chemotherapy.

No risk factors for the development of neurological toxicity, apart from the total dose of cisplatin received, were found in these patients. There was no influence of age, renal function, smoking history or total dose of furosemide received during therapy.

4 Discussion

Peripheral neuropathy is a common side effect of cancer chemotherapy. However, the frequency of this toxicity depends largely on the type of regimen used and the total cumulative dose of the neurotoxic agent given to the patient (Vogelzang 1991).

Neurotoxic side effects of vinca alkaloids, particularly vincristine and vindesine, seem to be related to the patient's age and the cumulative dose of the drugs. However, peripheral neuropathy has also been described after administration of the first dose of vincristine (Sandler et al. 1969; Casey et al. 1973). Vincristine peripheral neuropathy involves both motor and sensory neurons. The decrease of the ankle reflexes is one of the first signs which may be followed by distal paresthesias during the following weeks. Myopathies are also rather common (MacDonald 1992). Damage to the autonomic nervous system has also been described and may lead to constipation, bladder atony and hypotension in some cases (Lahtinen et al. 1989; Raphaelson et al. 1983; Roca et al. 1985). Sometimes muscle cramps can be the first symptom of vincristine neurotoxicity and may start within the first days of chemotherapy (Haims et al. 1991). The use of etoposide or teniposide in combination regimens has been shown to increase the neurotoxic effects of vinca alkaloids (Griffiths et al. 1986).

Vinca alkaloids are part of almost all combination regimens for the treatment of patients with Hodgkin's disease. In our study population, 37% of patients with Hodgkin's disease reported subjective symptoms of peripheral neuropathy. However, in only half of these patients neurophysiological abnormalities could be detected, and most of these were consistent with axonal neuropathy. The frequency of peripheral neuropathies was related to the total cumulative dose of vinca alkaloids used. The use of more differentiated methods of examination, such as vibration threshold measurement or single fiber electromyography for the evaluation of additional nerve fibers, would probably increase the reported number of patients with objective neurophysiological abnormalities (Forman 1990a). In nine of 73 patients (12%) treated for Hodgkin's disease a "subclinical neuropathy" with electrophysiological abnormalities but without clinical signs was found. The meaning of this finding remains unclear, but it may be possible that additional toxic effects throughout the further life of these patients may enhance the generation of clinical symptoms.

Clinical studies have demonstrated that the neurotoxicity following vincristine treatment can be ameliorated by simultaneous administration of glutamic acid (JACKSON et al. 1988). The corticotropin-(4–9)-analogue Org 2766 has also been used to reduce the neurotoxic effects of vincristine in patients with Hodgkin's and Non-Hodgkin's lymphoma (VAN KOOTEN et al. 1992). The postulated mechanism of action of Org 2766 is based on the evidence that melanocortins, which are closely related to the family of corticotropins, enhance peripheral nerve repair mechanisms. They have, for example, been shown to increase the number of cross-sectioned axonal microtubules in an animal model (MÜLLER et al. 1991). However, these substances are not routinely used in patients with lymphomas receiving chemotherapy.

As demonstrated in our patients with Hodgkin's disease the incidence of chemotherapy-induced polyneuropathy is in the order of 20%–30% (BOKEMEYER et al. 1993). Although no severe neurotoxic effects were seen, even a mild neuropathy can be bothersome and sometimes disabling. Careful evaluation of patients during their treatment is important to identify neurotoxic side effects early. However, for the long-term follow-up of patients with Hodgkin's disease the incidence and severity of peripheral neuropathies does not support the routine use of neurophysiological examinations in these patients.

Cisplatin neuropathy is a common side effect in the treatment of patients with ovarian cancer and germ cell tumors. It can be particularly bothersome for patients for the latter group, since most of these will be cured even in cases of disseminated disease and may therefore be affected by long-term cisplatin side effects. The neuropathy of cisplatin is primarily sensory, affecting the long fibers of the neuron. Initial symptoms are often paresthesias in the feet. Mild motor involvement seems to be present in some cases (MACDONALD 1992). The occurrence of Lhermitte's sign has also been reported (LIST and KUMMET 1990). In one report, the use of high doses of cisplatin had also been associated with demyelination of central nerve structures (DAUGAARD et al. 1987).

Electrophysiological examinations in patients treated with cisplatin showed a decrease in sensory conduction velocity while motor nerve conductions remained normal (DAUGAARD et al. 1987; LIST and KUMMET 1990). Examinations of peripheral nerves by electron microscopy mainly showed axonal degeneration and secondary myelin breakdown. The highest tissue platinum levels were found in the dorsal ganglia, the dorsal root and in peripheral nerves, and a linear relationship between these tissue platinum levels and the cumulative dose of cisplatin given was found (GREGG et al. 1992). Although cisplatin neuropathy has been shown to resolve within months after treatment in a considerable number of patients, the platinum tissue levels in the neural structures did not dicrease with time.

Long-term symptoms of neuropathy following chemotherapy for testicular cancer have been reported in 18%–68% of patients (AASS et al. 1990; BOYER et al. 1990; FOSSA et al. 1991; ROTH et al. 1988; STOTER et al. 1989). In a careful examination using the determination of the vibration threshold, even an incidence of 80% was found up to 10 years after cisplatin-containing treatment in patients with testicular cancer (HANSEN et al. 1989). Reports of long-term neurological toxicity in the literature are summarized in Table 7. The use of the PVB (platinum/vinblastine/bleomycin), CisCA (cisplatin/cyclophosphamide/adriamycin plus vinblastine/bleomycin) or the VAB6 (ciplatin/actinomycin

Table 7. Reported long-term neurological side effects after cisplatin-containing chemotherapy in patients with testicular cancer

Reference	Symptoms	Comments
AASS et al. 1990	18% peripheral sensory neuropathy	30% symptoms in patients after PVB chemotherapy
BOYER et al. 1990	26% subjective symptoms	More than 3 years after treatment
FOSSA et al. 1991	40% mild peripheral neuropathy	
HANSEN et al. 1989	50% paresthesias	6 years after treatment
	80$ vibration threshold elevated	
ROTH et al. 1988	43% paresthesias	7 years after treatment
STOTER et al. 1989	68% subjective symptoms	10 years after treatment (with weekly cisplatin for 1 year)

PVB, cisplatin, vinblastine, bleomycin.

D/vinblastine/bleomycin) regimen seems to be more often associated with neurological side effects than the use of a standard PEB (platinum/etoposide/bleomycin) regimen (VOGELZANG 1991). In our study cohort 50 patients (43%) reported neurological symptoms during or after chemotherapy. In 14 patients (12%) the symptoms of neuropathy persisted. The use of high dose cisplatin with cumulative doses $>150\,mg/m^2$ per cycle was associated with a higher incidence of acute and long-term neurological toxicity than was found using a standard dose ($<150\,mg/m^2$ per cycle) of cisplatin-containing regimens. No influence of the patients age or renal function was found. Patients additionally receiving vincristine during their treatment were at higher risk for the development of reversible neuropathy but not for the development of persisting neuropathy.

In a randomized prospective trial in patients with ovarian cancer the development of cisplatin neuropathy was significantly delayed by the use of the corticotropin analogue Org 2766 (VAN DER HOOP et al. 1990). Both objective measurable neurological signs and subjective symptoms were reduced in patients receiving this drug. The radioprotective agent S-2-(3-aminopropylamino)-ethylphosphorotoic acid (WR 2721) has also been shown to significantly lower the incidence of neuropathy following cisplatin chemotherapy (MOLLMANN et al. 1988). The mean dose of cisplatin at the onset of clinical neurological symptoms was significantly higher for patients receiving WR 2721 than for historical controls. A lower incidence of long-term symptoms of neuropathy was also suggested.

The substitution of cisplatin by its analogue carboplatin in treatment protocols for patients with testicular cancer may be another option to dramatically reduce the incidence of neurological side effects, since these have only been reported after the use of very high doses of carboplatin ($>1000\,mg/m^2$ per cycle MACDONALD 1992). No neurotoxicity in patients receiving conventional doses of carboplatin has been reported (VOGELZANG 1991). However, the safety of this substitution in patients with "low risk" testicular germ cell tumors has so far not been proven in prospective randomized trials.

Peripheral, neurological, late-occurring toxicity following chemotherapy with cisplatin in patients with curable malignant diseases, such as testicular cancer, is a rather common side effect. However, very severe and disabling side effects occur with a frequency below 5%. With the development of definite indications for the use of prophylactic agents for neurotoxicity and with the definition of indications for a safe substitution of cisplatin by carboplatin, the incidence and severity of neurological side effects may hopefully be further reduced. Overcoming the dose-limiting neurotoxicity of cisplatin will help in the administration of full doses on schedule and may thereby possibly improve the outcome of cancer chemotherapy.

5 Summary and Therapeutic Implications

Neurological side effects are common complications of cancer chemotherapy. In particular, cisplatin and the vinca alkaloids have been shown to cause peripheral neuropathy at a notable frequency. Although their mechanisms of neurotoxicity are not fully understood, both drugs seem to cause damage to the axonal part of the nerve. Following vincristine or vindesine therapy, sensory and motor symptoms and symptoms of autonomic polyneuropathy with constipation, bladder atony and hypotension have been reported. The symptoms of cisplatin neuropathy are mainly sensory deficits and paresthesias. The development of acute and long-term neurological side effects of vinca alkaloids was ameliorated by the prophylactic administration of glutamic acid or Org 2766, a corticotropin analogue. Org 2766 and WR 2721, a radioprotective agent, have also been shown to significantly reduce neurological signs and symptoms of cisplatin-induced peripheral neuropathy.

Long-term neurological side effects in patients with curable malignancies, such as Hodgkin's disease and testicular cancer, may be particularly bothersome and disabling. In 76 patients treated for Hodgkin's disease at Hannover University Medical School, with a median follow-up of 8 years after therapy, an incidence of 37% of long-term neurological side-effects was found. However, in only ten of 27 patients (37%) with subjective complaints, the peripheral neuropathy was confirmed by electrophysiological abnormalities. Patients receiving a median cumulative dose of >20 mg of vincristine had a significantly elevated risk for the development of long-term side effects ($p<0.05$).

A second investigation included 115 patients treated for testicular cancer by cisplatin-based combination chemotherapy, who were also evaluated for late-occurring neurological toxicity after a median follow-up of 58 months. Of these patients 53% reported neurological symptoms during chemotherapy; 14 patients (12%) suffered from persistent symptoms of peripheral neuropathy. These latter patients had received a significantly higher median dose of cisplatin during chemotherapy. Furthermore, the use of high dose cisplatin regimens (doses > 150 mg/m²) was significantly more often followed by neurological side effects. No risk factors for the development of peripheral neurotoxicity apart from the cumulative dose of cisplatin administered were identified in these patients.

In patients with curable malignant diseases different clinical studies are currently investigating options to reduce treatment-associated long-term side effects without compromising the excellent chance of cure for these patients.

References

Aass N, Kaasa S, Lund E, Heier MS, Fossa SD (1990) Long-term somatic side-effects and morbidity in testicular cancer patients. Br J Cancer 61: 151–155

Bokemeyer C, Frank B, van Rhee J, Schrader A, Schmoll HJ, Poliwoda H (1993) Untersuchungen zur neurologischen Spättoxizität nach Therapie bei Patienten mit Morbus Hodgkin. In: Lang N, Jäger W (eds) Zytostatikabedingte Nebenwirkungen. Zuckschwerdt, Munich, pp 64–68 (Aktuelle Onkologie, vol 68)

Boyer M, Raghaven D, Harris PJ, Lietch J et al. (1990) Lack of late toxicity in patients treated with cisplatin-containing combination chemotherapy for metastatic testicular cancer. J Clin Oncol 8: 21–26

Casey EB, Jellife Am, Le Quesne PM, Millett YL (1973) Vincristine neuropathy. Clinical and electrophysiological observations. Brain 96: 69–86

Daugaard GK, Petrera J, Trojaborg W (1987) Electrophysiological study of the peripheral and central neurotoxic effect of cis-platin. Acta Neurol Scand 76: 86–93

Einhorn LE (1990) Treatment of testicular cancer: a new and improved model. J Clin Oncol 8 (11): 1777–1781

Forman A (1990a) Peripheral Neuropathy in cancer patients: clinical types, etiology and presentation. Oncology (Willison Park) 4: 85–89

Forman A (1990b) Peripheral neuropathy in cancer patients: incidence, features and pathophysiology. Oncology (Willison Park) 4: 57–62

Fossa SD, Aass N, Ous S, Waehre H (1991) The long term toxicity of polychemotherapy in successfully treated testicular carcinoma. Scand J Urol Nephrol [Suppl] 138: 241–246

Gregg RW, Malepo JM, Monpetit VJA et al. (1992) Cisplatin neurotoxicity: the relationship between dosage, time and platinum concentration in neurologic tissues and morphologic evidence of toxicity. J Clin Oncol 10(5): 795–803

Griffiths JD, Stark RJ, Ding JC, Cooper IA (1986) Vincristine neurotoxicity enhanced in combination chemotherapy including both teniposide and vincristine. Cancer Treat Rep 70(4): 519–521

Haims N, Barron SA, Robinson E (1991) Muscle cramps associated with vincristine therapy. Acta Oncol 30(6): 707–711

Hansen St W, Helweg-Larsen S, Trojaborg W (1989) Long-term neurotoxicity in patients treated with cisplatin, vinblastine and bleomycin for metastatic germ cell cancer. J Clin Oncol 7(10): 1457–1461

Jackson DV, Wells HB, Atkins JN et al. (1988) Amelioration of vincristine neurotoxicity by glutamic acid. Am J Med 84: 1016–1022

Kedar A, Cohen ME, Freemann AI (1978) Peripheral neuropathy as a complication of cis-dichlorodiammine-platinum (II) treatment: a case report. Cancer Treat Rep 62: 819–821

Lahtinen R, Koponen A, Mustonen J et al. (1989) Discordance in the development of peripheral and autonomic neuropathy during vincristine therapy. Eur J Hematol 43: 357–358

List AF, Kummet TD (1990) Spinal cord toxicity complicating treatment with cisplatinum and etoposide. Am J Clin Oncol 13(3); 256–258

MacDonald DR (1992) Neurotoxicity of chemotherapeutic agents. In: Perry MC (ed) The chemotherapy source book. Williams and Wilkens, Baltimore, pp 666–678

Marin AC, Rierson B (1979) Peripheral neuropathy secondary to cis-dichlorodiammino-platinum (II) (platinol): treatment for advanced ovarian cancer. Ariz Med 36: 898–899

Mollmann JE (1990) Cisplatin neurotoxicity. N Engl J Med 11(2): 126–127

Mollmann JE, Glover DJ, Hogan WM, Furman RE (1988) Cisplatinumneuropathy. Risk factors, prognosis and protection by WR-2721. Cancer 61: 2192–2195

Müller LJ, Moorer van Delft CM, Roubos EW et al. (1991) Neurons of the snail Lymnaea stagnalis as a model to study the neurotoxic side-effects of cytostatic compounds and the protective properties of Org 2766, an ACTH-analogue. In: Kits K, Boer HH, Joosse J (eds) Molluscan neurobiology. Elsevier Science, New York, pp 227–234

Paul T, Katayar BC, Misra S, Pant GC (1978) Carcinomatous neuromuscular syndromes. A clinical and quantitative electrophysiological study. Brain 101: 53–63

Raphaelson MI, Stevens, JC, Newman RP (1983) Vincristine neuropathy with bowel and bladder atony, mimicking spinal cord compression. Cancer Treat Rep 69: 604–605

Roca E, Bruera E, Politi PM et al. (1985) Vinca alcaloid-induced cardiovascular autonomic neuropathy. Cancer Treat Rep 69: 149–151

Roelofs RI, Hrushesky W, Rogin J, Rosenberg L (1984) Peripheral sensory neuropathy and cisplatin chemotherapy. Neurology 34: 934–938

Roth BJ, Greist A, Kubilis PS, Williams SD, Einhron LH (1988) Cisplatin-based combination chemotherapy for disseminated germ cell-tumors: long-term follow-up. J Clin Oncol 6: 1239–1247

Sandler SG, Tobin W, Henderson ES (1969) Vincristine induced neuropathy. A clinical study of fifty leukemic patients. Neurology 19: 367–374

Stoter G, Koopmann A, Vendrik CP, Stuyvenberg A et al. (1989) Ten-year survival and late sequelae in testicular cancer patients treated with cisplatin, vinblastine and bleomycin. J Clin Oncol 7: 1099–1104

Thomas PK (1984) The peripheral nervous system as a target for toxic substances. Acta Neurol Scand 70 [Suppl 100]: 21–26

Thompson StW, Davis LE, Kornfeld M et al. (1984) Cisplatin neuropathy. Clinical, electrophysiologic, morphologic and toxicologic studies. Cancer 54: 1269–1275

Urba WJ, Longo DL (1992) Hodgkin's disease. N Engl J Med 326: 678–687 van der Hoop RG, Vecht ChJ, van der Burg MEL et al. (1990) Prevention of cisplatinumneurotoxicity with an ACTH(4–9) analogue in patients with ovarian cancer. N Engl J Med 322(2): 89–94

van Kooten B, Moorer van Delft HAM, Roubos EW et al. (1992) A pilot study on the influence of a corticotropin (4–9) analogue on vinca alkaloid-induced neuropathy. Arch Neurol 49: 1027–1031

Vogelzang NJ (1991) The acute and chronic toxicitics of chemotherapy for metastatic testicular cancer. In: Horwich A (ed) Testicular cancer: Investigation and management. Chapman and Hall Medical, London, pp 331–352

von Hoff DD, Reichert CM, Cunco R et al. (1979) Demyelination of peripheral sensory nerves associated with cis-diamminedichloroplatinum (II) (DDP) therapy. Proc Am Assoc Cancer Res (abstract) 20: 91

Xu T, Sladky JT, Brown MJ (1989) Dose-dependent expression of neuronopathy after experimental pyridoxine intoxication. Neurology 39: 1077–1083

2.6 Endocrine Dysfunction After Brain Tumor Therapy in Children

HELMUTH G. DÖRR, ANDREAS KOCH, THORSTEN SAUERWALD, and JÖRN D. BECK

CONTENTS

1 Introduction 59
2 Growth and Growth Hormone Deficiency 59
2.1 Spinal Growth 60
2.2 Growth Hormone Therapy 60
3 Puberty 61
4 Thyroid Gland 61
5 Gonadal Dysfunction 62
6 Adrenal Cortex 62
7 Diabetes Insipidus 62
8 Summary 62
References 62

1 Introduction

Primary brain tumors represent, at 18%, the largest group of malignant solid tumors in childhood; 250–300 new cases occur every year in Germany (HAAF et al. 1991). The overall prognosis of children with malignant brain tumors has improved in recent years, but is still very poor. (KUMAR et al. 1990). The German survival rate after 5 years is almost the same as the international rate of 50%. These survival rates are attained by using aggressive therapeutic treatments such as neurosurgery, craniospinal irradiation and chemotherapy (HEIDEMAN et al. 1989; MAPSTONE and WARF 1991). However, they are achieved at the expense of late occurring effects such as neurological and behavioural disturbances, hearing loss, secondary malignancies and hormonal deficiencies (AHMED et al. 1986; ALBERTSSON-WIKLAND et al. 1987; BLATT and BLEYEC 1989; DANOFF et al. 1982; DUFFNER et al. 1983a; RAPPAPORT and BRAUNER 1989; SHALET 1983; SHALET et al. 1988). Regarding the occurrence of hormonal deficiencies, the type and location of the tumor itself must also be taken into account. Intra- and parasellar tumors, particularly craniopharyngiomas, may cause multiple hormonal deficiencies. This study reports on endocrine disorders in children with cranial tumors distant from the pituitary-hypothalamic area.

HELMUTH G. DÖRR, PRIVAT DOZENT, Dr., ANDREAS KOCH, Dr., THORSTEN SAUERWALD, Dr., Klinik für Kinder und Jugendliche, Pädiatrische Endokrinologie, Universität Erlangen. Loschgestrasse 15, 91054 Erlangen, FRG

JÖRN D. BECK, Prof. Dr., Klinik für Kinder und Jugendliche, Pädiatrische Hämatologie und Onkologie, Universität Erlangen, Loschgestrasse 15, 91054 Erlangen, FRG

2 Growth and Growth Hormone Deficiency

The growth and attainable final height of children with brain tumors are affected by various factors, such as growth hormone deficiency, reduced spinal growth, premature or delayed puberty, inadequate nutrition and/or tumor recurrence (BROWN et al. 1983; DANOFF et al. 1982; DUFFNER et al. 1983), whereby adequate nutrition seems to play an important part in the first year of therapy (SHALET 1983). The effects of radiation are less in older children than in younger ones (ALBERTSSON-WIKLAND et al. 1987; SHALET et al. 1988).

Numerous studies have been done on growth hormone deficiency (AHMED et al. 1986; ALBERTSSON-WIKLAND et al. 1987; DARENDELILER et al. 1990; DUFFNER et al. 1983b; HERBER et al. 1985; KANEV et al. 1991; LANNERING et al. 1988; RAPPAPORT and BRAUNER 1989; SHALET 1983; WINTER and GREEN 1985). Irradiation with doses of up to 50 Gy leads unavoidably to growth hormone deficiency in most of the patients within 2 years (DUFFNER et al. 1983; RAPPAPORT 1989; SHALET et al. 1988). There is a correlation between the radiation dose given and the extent of the growth hormone deficiency (SHALET et al. 1976, 1988).

Up until now, however, it has not been possible to define the threshold at which a disorder of growth hormone secretion may occur. In a recent report, damage is already found after a radiation dose of 18 Gy (CROWNE et al. 1992). If higher doses are given, reduction of other pituitary hormones may also occur, for example, FSH, LH, TSH or ACTH (CONSTINE et al. 1993; DANOFF et al. 1982; RAPPAPORT 1989). It is supposed that the hypothalamus is more sensitive to radiation than the anterior pituitary lobe (AHMED and SHALET 1984; BLACKLAY et al. 1986; LANNERING et al. 1988). Reduced secretion of GHRH over a longer period of time causes secondary damage to the pituitary gland, since it is no longer adequately stimulated and therefore growth hormone secretion is reduced. Normally, spontaneous growth hormone secretion in children over a 24 h period is pulsatile, with higher values during the night and significantly higher levels during puberty (ALBERTSSON-WIKLAND and ROSBERG 1988; ZADIK et al. 1985). In brain tumor patients, this pulsatility is reduced or even completely absent, the amplitude of growth hormone secretion is reduced and no growth hormone increase occurs in puberty (ALBERTSSON-WIKLAND et al. 1987; LANNERING et al. 1988).

To determine growth hormone deficiency, the concentration of growth hormone is measured after various pharmacological stimulation tests, e.g., arginine, insulin tolerance test (ITT) or L-dopa, and continuously over a period of several hours (12 or 24 h BROOK and HINDMARSH 1991; RANKE and HABER 1993. Differentiation between a hypothalamic and a pituitary disorder may be made using the GHRH test (AHMED and SHALET 1984; OBERFIELD et al. 1987). It remains difficult, however, to definitively prove a growth hormone deficiency, as contradictory results often appear. For example, a provocation test with arginine may cause an increase in growth hormone, while an ITT results in only a subnormal increase (AHMED et al. 1986). Deficient growth hormone responses after L-dopa, arginine and ITT with a normal growth hormone increase in a GHRH test have also been reported (LUSTIG et al. 1985). A pathological growth hormone secretion during 12–24 h with normal growth hormone increases in stimulation tests is also possible (AHMED et al. 1986; LANNERING et al. 1988).

It is questionable how far pharmacological stimulation can, in fact, mirror physiological reality. One should not forget that children with reduced growth and normal growth hormone concentrations (ALBERTSSON-WIKLAND et al. 1987; OBERFIELD et al. 1986) and children with normal growth and pathological growth hormone levels in stimulation tests (OBERFIELD et al. 1987) have been identified. Direct influence of growth hormone secretion by chemotherapy is rather unlikely (SHALET 1983), although an effect on insulin-like growth factors cannot be ruled out (PRICE et al. 1981).

2.1 Spinal Growth

There have been reports in the literature on the effects of spinal irradiaton on spinal growth (CLAYTON et al. 1988b; SHALET et al. 1987, 1988). It could be demonstrated almost 20 years ago that with doses of more than 20 Gy the vertebrae exhibit changes visible in X-ray, such as subcortical osteoporosis, irregular ossification or scoliosis (PROBERT and PARKER 1975).

With doses of more than 35 Gy there was a reduction in sitting height due to reduced growth of the vertebrae. Children under 6 years of age and those in puberty were especially affected. This dose and age dependency was confirmed in later studies (CLAYTON et al. 1988b; SHALET et al. 1988; SPOUDEAS 1989). The younger the child at the time of irradiation, the greater the effect on spinal growth (CLAYTON et al. 1988b). Particularly for medulloblastoma and ependymoma, spinal irradiation is unavoidable because of metastases in the spinal fluid. Thus, the vertebrae may be damaged directly resulting in reduced growth and reduced sitting height.

In addition, craniospinally irradiated children were −0.7 SDS smaller than "only" cranially irradiated children. Adult sitting height was −3.3 SDS after craniospinal irradiation and −1.4 SDS after cranial irradiation. A reduced head growth has also been determined (CLAYTON et al. 1987a).

2.2 Growth Hormone Therapy

The use of growth hormone (hGH) in children with radiation induced growth hormone deficiency is now widely accepted. In the study by ARSLANIAN et al. (1985), 71% of the affected children were treated with hGH. Despite this therapy, the final heights were still under the expected target heights. In a further investigation of 27 patients, only 12 reached a final height above the third percentile (HERBER et al. 1985). The mean final height was −2.05 SDS below the norm.

The decision to use hGH therapy is influenced by many factors: age, pubertal development and height at the beginning of therapy, age at irradiation, radiation dose and spinal irradiation, nutritional status, extent of the growth hormone deficiency, additional hormone deficiency (e.g., hypothyroidism or gonadotrophin deficiency), and/or tumor recurrence.

Success of hGH therapy of cranially irradiated patients cannot easily be compared to that of craniospinally irradiated patients, as the therapy cannot usually compensate for the reduced growth of the vertebrae after spinal irradiation (DARENDELILER et al. 1990; Shalet et al. 1988). Even if the gGH therapy cannot attain catch-up growth, at least a further loss of growth can be prevented (Lannering et al. 1988; Clayton et al. 1988a, b) and the percentile reached can be retained. Many children, in fact, show a significant increase in growth rate and an improved physical condition (Clayton et al. 1988a, b; Darendeliler et al. 1990; Herber et al. 1985).

At present, there are no clear criteria which can predict which children will profit from hGH therapy and which will not (Romshe et al. 1984). Growth in brain tumor patients due to hGH is less impressive than in patients with idiopathic growth hormone deficiency (Shalet et al. 1988; Sulmont et al. 1990). After treatment for several years, as with for children with idiopathic growth hormone deficiency, there is a drop in the rate of growth (Winder and Green 1985).

The time available for hGH therapy is often limited by precocious puberty (Clayton et al. 1988a). Frequently, due to hypothalamic damage of inhibitor neurones, the GnRH pulse generator is activated and pubertal development begins too soon (see Sect. 3). The effect of concomitant use of GnRH analogues in those patients entering relatively early puberty should be explored in further studies.

At present, there is no indication that the risk of tumor recurrence is increased by hGH therapy, although this is a frequently used argument against hGH treatment (Winter and Green 1985). Comparisons show that recurrences occur equally frequently for hGH treated and non-hGH treated patients (Arslanian et al. 1985; Clayton et al. 1987b). Observation over 10 years of medulloblastoma patients showed a recurrence of 18% in both groups (Shalet et al. 1988). Ogilvy-Stuart et al. (1992) examined 207 patients with different brain tumors, of which 47 had been treated with hGH for a mean time of 3.2 years. While 11% of the hGH treated patients had a recurrence, of the non-treated patients the rate was 26%. Even in those patients in whom a residual tumor could be determined by computed tomography, no progression was observed during hGH therapy. However, research remains to be done to determine possible mitogenic activity of hGH or hGH-dependent factors.

The question whether hGH therapy should be initiated after irradiation cannot be definitively answered (Shalet et al. 1988). Occasionally, in the first year after radiotherapy, the children show a decrease in growth rate followed by an increase (Herber and Milner 1986). Growth hormone deficiency is usually manifest only after the second year. However, the statistical probability of a recurrence for most malignant tumors is highest within 2 years of radiotherapy. In the case of highly malignant tumors, therefore, hGH treatment should be started only after 2 years.

3 Puberty

The increase in growth hormone stimulated by the sex steroids is absent in brain tumor patients (Albertsson-Wickdand et al. 1987). It has been shown that those children irradiated before puberty have the greatest loss of growth. If the children have already started puberty at the time of irradiation, the loss of growth is less. This is not surprising since, at a bone age of 11 years, boys have reached about 80% of their final height and girls about 90%.

There have been repeated reports of precocious puberty in children who hve been cranially irradiated (Brauner et al. 1984; Clayton et al. 1988a, b; Spoudeas 1989). Puberty starts in boys at a mean chronological age of 10.4 years and in girls at 9.9 years (Clayton et al. 1988b). The normal difference in the beginning of puberty has not been annulled, just brought forward in time. A positive correlation can be drawn between the start of puberty and the age at irradiation, that is, the earlier the child is irradiated, the earlier is started. This happens although growth hormone deficiency usually results in a delayed puberty (Shalet et al. 1988).

4 Thyroid Gland

Cranial or craniospinal irradiation can cause primary hypothyroidism due to direct damage to the thyroid gland. Radiation effects on the hypothalamus or pituitary gland may cause a secondary or tertiary hypothyroidism. A disorder of the thyroid gland can be determined in up to one third of the children at the end of treatment (Duffner et al. 1983; Oberfield et al. 1986). If the tumor is a craniopharyngioma, the rate is doubled or tripled (Arslanian et al. 1985). The most comprehensive investigation on thyroid function after irradiation and chemotherapy was carried out by Livesey and Brook (1989) on a total of 119 patients. The prevalence of primary hypothyroidism was 7%, of secondary 3%. Thyroidal dysfunction, i.e., elevated TSH values, were observed in 28%. Surprisingly, this study also revealed a significant influence of chemotherapy. Of the children with craniospinal irradiation and without chemotherapy, 23% showed a thyroid defect; for the children with craniospinal irradiation plus chemotherapy, the rate was 69%.

5 Gonadal Dysfunction

Gonadal disorders with elevated FSH and LH values are a usual result of chemotherapy (Ahmed et al. 1983; Sardelli et al. 1986; Livesey and Brook 1988). The damage observed in about a third of the patients could be attributed in particular to chemotherapy with alkylating substances (Clayton et al. 1988b; Danoff et al. 1982; Duffner et al. 1983b; Herber et al. 1985). The rate of gonadal damage is doubled or tripled with tumors in the hypothalamic-pituitary region and with craniopharyngiomas. However, a hypogonadotropic hypogonadism with reduced FSH and LH values may occur after hypothalamic-pituitary irradiation or because of the position of the tumor in this region (Constine et al. 1993).

An irradiation induced hyperprolactinemia may also cause secondary hypogonadism (Shalet 1983). Children with glioma in the hypothalamic-chiasma region rarely show somatic or sexual retardation. These children are more likely to have precocious puberty induced by central activation, which responds well to treatment with GnRH agonists (Laue et al. 1985).

6 Adrenal Cortex

The effects of therapy on the hypothalamo-pituitary-adrenal feedback control mechanism are less than on the thyroidal and gonadal mechanisms. At the most, only 14% of the irradiated and chemotherapy treated children exhibit reduced cortisol production (Duffner et al. 1983b; Rappaport 1989). If an ITT is carried out to determine growth hormone deficiency, then ACTH and cortisol levels must also be measured. A correlation between pathological GH and pathological ACTH levels has been described for seven patients (Petersen 1984).

7 Diabetes Insipidus

Central diabetes insipidus is one of the most commonly occurring endocrinological symptoms with brain tumors (Greger et al. 1986). A vasopressin deficiency may already be apparent during the diagnostic clarification of a brain tumor (Arslanian et al. 1985). However, during a 4 year observation of children after irradiation for brain tumors, not one case of diabetes insipidus was recorded (Brauner and Rappaport 1989).

8 Summary

The prognosis for children with malignant brain tumors has greatly improved with intensive treatment regimens. Endocrine dysfunctions after brain tumor therapy are common and unavoidable. However, one must not forget that these are malignant tumors, and without the aggressive therapy these children would have no chance of survival. Therefore, everything possible must be done during the follow-up of these children to recognize and treat hormonal deficiencies sufficiently early and to improve the quality of their lives.

References

Ahmed SR, Shalet SM (1984) Hypothalamic GH releasing factor deficiency following cranial irradiation. Clin Endocrinol 21: 483–488

Ahmed SR, Shalet SM, Campbell RHA, Deakin DP (1983) Primary gonadal damage following treatment of brain tumors in childhood. J Pediatr 103: 562–565

Ahmed SR, Shalet SM, Beardwell CG (1986) The effects of cranial irradiation on GH secretion. Acta Paediatr Scand 75: 255–260

Albertsson-Wikland K, Rosberg S (1988) Analyses of 24-hour growth hormone profiles in children. J Clin Endocrinol Metab 67: 493–500

Albertsson-Wikland K, Lannering B, Marky I, Mellander L, Wannholt U (1987) A longitudinal study on growth and spontaneous GH secretion in children with irradiated brain tumors. Acta Paediator Scand 76: 966–973

Arslanian SA, Becker DJ, Lee PA, Drash AL, Foley TP (1985) GH therapy and tumor recurrence. Findings in children with brain neoplasms and hypopituitarism. Am J Dis Child 139: 347–350

Blacklay A, Grossman A, Ross RJ, Savage MO, Davies PS, Plowman PN, Coy DH, Besser GM (1986) Cranial irradiation for cerebral and nasopharyngeal tumors in children: evidence for the production of a hypothalamic defect in GH release. J Endocrinol 108: 25–29

Blatt J, Bleyer WA (1989) Late effects of childhood cancer and its treatment. In: Pizzo PA, Poplack DG (eds) Pediatric oncology, Lippincott, Philadelphia, pp 1003–1025

Brauner R, Rappaport R (1989) Pituitary hormone secretion and growth after cranial irradiation. In: Frisch H, Thorner MO (eds) Hormonal regulation of growth. Raven, New York, pp 245–253 (Serono symposium, vol 58)
Brauner R, Czernichow P, Rappaport R (1984) Precious puberty after hypothalamic and pituitary irradiation in young children. N Engl J Med 311: 920
Brook CGD, Hindmarsh PC (1991) Tests for growth hormone secretion. Arch Dis Child 66: 85–87
Brown IH, Lee TJ, Eden OB, Bullimore JA, Savage DCL (1983) Growth and endocrine function after treatment for medulloblastoma. Arch Dis Child 58: 722–727
Clayton PE, Shalet SM, Price DA, Surtees RA, Pearson D (1987a) The role of GH in stunted head growth after cranial irradiation. Pediatr Res 22: 402–404
Clayton PE, Shalet SM, Gattamaneni HR, Price DA (1987b) Does GH cause relapse of brain tumors? Lancet 1: 711–713
Clayton PE, Shalet SM, Price DA (1988a) Growth response to growth hormone therapy following cranial irradiation. Eur J Pediatr 147: 593–596
Clayton PE, Shalet SM, Price DA (1988b) Growth response to GH therapy following craniospinal irradiation. Eur J Pediatr 147: 597–601
Constine LS, Woolf PD, Cann D, Mick G, McCormick K, Raubertas RF, Rubin P (1993) Hypothalamic-pituitary dysfunction after radiation for brain tumors. N Engl J Med 328: 87–94
Crowne EC, Moore C, Wallace WHB, Olgilvy-Stuart AL, Addison GM, Morris PH, Shalet SM (1992) A novel variant of growth hormone (GH) insufficiency following low dose cranial irradiation. Clin Endocrinol 36: 59–68
Danoff BF, Cowchock FS, Marquette C, Mulgrew L, Kramer S (1982) Assessment of the long-term effects of primary radiation therapy for brain tumors in children. Cancer 49: 1580–1586
Darendeliler F, Livesey EA, Hindmarsh PC, Brook CGD (1990) Growth and Growth Hormone secretion in children following treatment of brain tumors with radiotherapy. Acta Pediatr Scand 79: 950–956
Duffner PK, Cohen ME, Thom-as P (1983a) Late effects of treatment on the intelligence of children with posterior fossa tumors. Cancer 51: 233–237
Duffner PK, Cohen ME, Anderson SW, Voorhess ML, MacGillivray MH, Panahon A, Brecher ML (1983b) Long-term effects of treatment on endocrine function in children with brain tumors. Ann Neurol 14: 528–532
Greger NG, Kirkland RT, Clayton GW, Kirkland JL (1986) Central diabetes insipidus: 22 years' experience. Am J Dis Child 140: 551–554
Haaf HG, Kaatsch P, Keller B, Michaelis J (1991) Jahresbericht 1990 des Kinderkrebsregisters Mainz. Instut für Medizinische Statistik und Dokumentation
Heideman RL, Packer RJ, Albright LA, Freeman CR, Rorke LB (1989) Tumors of the central nervous system. In: Pizzo PA, Poplack DG (eds) Pediatric oncology. Lippincott, Philadelphia, pp 505–553
Herber SM, Milner RDG (1986) When are we diagnosing growth hormone deficiency? Arch Dis Child 61: 110–112
Herber SM, Dunsmore IR, Milner RDG (1985) Final status in brain tumors other than craniopharyngeoma: effect of GH. Horm Res 22: 63–67
Kanev PM, Lefebvre JF, Mauseth RS, Berger MS (1991) Growth hormone deficiency following radiation therapy of primary brain tumors in children. J Neurosurg 74: 743–748
Kumar R, Jones RAC, Tekkök IH (1990) Has modern management improved the outcome of infants with intracranial tumors? Childs Nerv Syst 6: 327–330
Lannering B, Marky I, Mellander L, Albertsson-Wikland K (1988) Growth hormone secretion and response to growth hormone therapy after treatment for brain tumor. Acta Paediatr Scand [Suppl] 343: 146–151
Laue L, Comite F, Hench K, Loriaux DL, Cutler GB, Hirsch-Pescovitz O (1985) Precocious puberty associated with neurofibromatosis and optic gliomas. Treatment with LHRH-analogue. Am J Dis Child 139: 1097–1100
Livesey EA, Brook CGD (1988) Gonadal dysfunction after treatment of intracranial tumours. Arch Dis Child 63: 495–600
Livesey EA, Brook CGD (1989) Thyroid dysfunction after radiotherapy and chemotherapy of brain tumors. Arch Dis Child 64: 593–595
Lustig RH, Schriock EA, Kaplan SL Grumbach MM (1985) Effect of growth hormone-releasing factor on GH release in children with radiation-induced GH deficiency. Pediatrics 76: 274–279
Mapstone TB, Warf BC (1991) Intracranial tumors in infants: characteristics, management and outcome of a contemporary series. Neurosurgery 28: 343–348
Oberfield SE, Allen JC, Pollack J, New MI, Levine LS (1986) Long-term endorine sequelae after treatment of medulloplastoma: prospective study of growth and thyroid function. J Pediatr 108: 219–223
Oberfield SE, Kirkland JL, Frantz A, Allen JC, Levine LS (1987) GH response to GRF 1–44 in children following cranial irradiation for central nervous system tumors. Am J Ped Hematol Oncol 9: 233–238
Ogilvy-Stuart AL, Ryder WDJ, Gattamaneni HR, Clayton PE, Shalet SM (1992) Growth hormone and tumor recurrence. Br Med J 304: 1601–1605
Petersen KE (1984) ACTH in normal children and children with pituitary and adrenal diseases. II. Plasma ACTH (cortisol and GH) values during insulin hypoglycaemia. Patients with idiopathic hypopituitarism and intracranial tumor. Acta Paediatr Scand 73: 372–378
Price DA, Morris MJ, Rowsell KV, Jones PH (1981) The effects of anti-leukaemic drugs on somatomedin production and carilage responsiveness to somatomedin in vitro. Pediatr Res 15: 1553
Probert JC, Parker BR (1975) The effects of radiation on bone growth. Radiology 114: 155–162
Ranke MB, Haber P (1993) Wachstumshromonstimulations- tests. In: Ranke MB (ed) Endokrinologische Funktions- diagnonstik im Kindes- und Jugendalter. Lehmann, Mannheim, pp 70–86
Rappaport R (1989) Growth after cranial radiation and chemotherapy for tumors or leucemia. In: Bierich JR, Cacciari E, Raiti S (eds) Growth abnormalities. Raven, New York, pp 93–105
Rappaport R, Brauner R (1989) Growth and endocrine disorders secondary to cranial irradiation. Pediatr Res 25: 561–567
Romshe CA, Zipf WB, Miser A, Miser J, Sotos JF, Newton WA (1984) Evaluation of GH release and hGH treatment in children with cranial irradiation-associated short stature. J Pediatr 104: 177–181
Sardelli S, Petraglia F, Massolo F, Messori A, Santoro V, Facchinetti F, Genazzani AR (1986) Changes in immunoreactive beta-endorphin, methionin-enkephaline and ACTH in bone marrow cells and fluid from leukemic children. Clin Immunol Immunopathol 41: 247–253

Shalet SM (1983) Disorders of the endocrine system due to radiation and cytotoxic chemotherapy. Clin Endocrinol 18: 637–659

Shalet SM, Beardwell CG, Pearson D, Jones PH (1976) The effect of varying doses of cerebral irradiation on GH-production in childhood. Clin Endocrinol 5: 287–290

Shalet SM, Gibson B, Swindell R, Pearson D (1987) Effect of spinal irradiation on growth. Arch Dis Child 62: 461–464

Shalet SM, Clayton PE, Price DA (1988) Growth impairment following treatment for childhood brain tumors. Acta Paediatr Scand [Suppl] 343: 137–145

Spoudeas HA (1989) The endocrine consequences of irradiation in childhood. Growth Matters 1(2): 6–10

Sulmont V, Brauner R, Fontoura M, Rappaport R (1990) Response to growth hormone treatment and final height after cranial or craniospinal irradiation. Acta Paediatr Scand 79: 542–549

Winter RJ, Green OC (1985) Irradiation-induced GH deficiency: blunted growth response and accelerated skeletal maturation to GH therapy. J Pediatr 106: 609–612

Zadik Z, Chalew SA, McCarter RJ, Meistas M, Kowarski AA (1985) The influence of age on the 24-hours integrated concentration of growth hormone in normal individuals. J Clin Endocrinol Metab 60: 513–516

2.7 Endocrine Dysfunction in Adults After Radiotherapy for Pituitary Adenomas and Suprasellar Tumors

MICHAEL BUCHFELDER and GERHARD GRABENBAUER

CONTENTS

1 Introduction 65
2 Investigation of Endocrine Function 65
3 Effects of Radiation on the Normal Pituitary and Hypothalamus 66
4 Effects of External Radiotherapy in Pituitary Adenomas 67
5 Effects of Heavy Particle Therapy 69
6 Effects of Interstitial Irradiation 70
7 Summary and Therapeutic Recommendations . . . 70
References 70

1 Introduction

Very early in this century, radiation therapy was already available and employed in the management of pituitary adenomas. Several studies demonstrated its favorable effects on the space-occupying lesion and on hormonal oversecretion. In the premicrosurgical era, surgery alone frequently could not eradicate a tumor and thus failed to sufficiently control tumor growth. Thus, postoperative irradiation was routinely performed and this appeared to prolong the interval in which symptomatic recurrences occurred. External irradiation also proved to be a valuable adjunct in the treatment of other tumors in the sellar region, such as craniopharyngiomas, suprasellar germinomas, chordomas and gliomas of the optic chiasm. Adequate coverage of the tumor within the radiation field often necessitates inclusion of adjacent normal structures. Therefore the normal pituitary and the hypothalamus are likely to receive a significant portion of the tumor dose. Soon after its introduction as a medical therapy it was noted that some children and adults treated with cranial irradiation for suprasellar tumors subsequently developed deficits in neuroendocrine function. We herein review the extensive studies which have been carried out to assess hormonal deficits following radiotherapy for these lesions. Since pituitary adenomas and other intra- and suprasellar tumors may affect pituitary function by primary or recurrent growth, it is also appropriate in this review to incorporate studies on hormonal sequelae in patients irradiated for other cranial tumors distant from the sellar region.

MICHAEL BUCHFELDER, Privatdozent, Dr., Neurochirurgische Klinik, Universität Erlangen-Nürnberg, Schwabachanlage 6, 91054 Erlangen, FRG
GERHARD GRABENBAUER, Dr., Klinik und Poliklinik für Strahlentherapie, Universität Erlangen-Nürnberg, Universitätsstrasse 27, 91054 Erlangen, FRG

2 Investigation of Endocrine Function

It is difficult to compare data on hormonal deficiencies of several hypothalamo-pituitary axes from different medical centers since the criteria to judge dysfunction are inconsistent. Certainly the true incidence of endocrine deficiency is not defined by the number of patients taking hormone replacement therapy because of symptoms. Also, blood samples measuring serum concentrations of pituitary hormones at a single time point do not reflect the secretion capacity of the system. Most of the hormones are secreted episodically; consequently, serum concentrations of growth hormone, prolactin, ACTH, TSH and gonadotropins may vary significantly in the same individual within short time intervals. Thus, dynamic endocrine testing by stimulation tests must be employed. Several tests challenging the system at different levels are available (FAHLBUSCH and BUCHFELDER 1992). Of these, insulin-induced hypoglycemia is probably the most reliable test available to assess growth hormone and ACTH reserve. It reliably determines the integrity of both the whole somatotrophic and adrenocorticotrophic axes. Alternatively, determination of the pituitary hormones before and after administration of the releasing hormones GRH, GnRH, CRH and TRH in individual tests or in combination may be employed. These stimulation tests, however, primarily assess pituitary function. Therefore they are not an ideal tool to identify radiation damage of the hypothalamus. Furthermore the determination of the serum levels of thyroid hormones and sex-steroid hormones is crucial to determine whether a patient has developed hypothyroidism or hypogonadism, irrespective of a normal TSH or gonadotropin regulation. Since appearance of a defect in hypothalamic-pituitary function may be delayed for several years after radiotherapy for pituitary region tumors, repeat testing of the patients in regular intervals is mandatory during their follow-up (LAM et al. 1991; LITTLEY et al. 1989, 1991b; RICHARDS 1980; SAMAAN et al. 1982).

3 Effects of Radiation on the Normal Pituitary and Hypothalamus

Data concerning radiation effects on the normal pituitary gland have been obtained under a variety of circumstances. Experimental studies in animal models suggest a relative radioresistancy of the systems (RODRIGUEZ et al. 1991). In most clinical situations the gland receives a significant portion of the tumor dose during the course of radiotherapy for either tumors of the sella turcica region, such as pituitary adenomas, craniopharyngiomas, optic nerve gliomas and other comparable lesions, or for other brain or skull base tumors distant from the sellar region, such as medulloblastomas or nasopharyngeal carcinomas (CONSTINE et al. 1993; LAM et al. 1991; SAMAAN et al. 1982; WARA et al. 1977). In the latter instances deterioration of previously normal pituitary function is considered an unavoidable adverse side effect of cranial irradiation. A completely different provocative situation was generated when a conscious effort was made to destroy the pituitary gland in order to achieve functional hypophysectomy, when required for palliative measures in hormonally dependent malignant tumors and in the control of diabetic retinopathy. Observations from these earlier therapeutic effects led to the conclusion that normal pituitary gland tissue is relatively radioresistant and its destruction requires high doses of radiation.

Thus, an unfractionated dose of 200 Gy to a very small volume is needed to destroy the gland by using external megavoltage irradiation (DE SCHRYVER et al. 1973). Fractionated doses are even better tolerated. However, doses between 200 and 260 Gy cause significant damage to the pituitary although their effect on hormonal secretion may only become manifest after several months (LITTLEY et al. 1991b; RICHARDS 1980; SHELINE 1979). With such high doses to the pituitary adminstered by conventional external megavoltage radiation therapy, the surrounding normal brain tissue would be severely affected. RUBIN and CASARETT (1968) reported on an autopsy series of 53 patients who had received 140–300 Gy of fractionated protons or α particles to the pituitary for the palliative treatment of metastatic cancer. They did not find radiation-induced necrosis when the dose was less than 200 Gy, but, when larger doses were employed, necrosis of up to 90% was observed as early as 5 days after completion of radiation therapy in individual cases. Of those who survived long-term, in almost all the gland became necrotic. This progressive decay of glandular cells is presumably caused by increasing ischemia resulting from vascular damage (LAWRENCE et al. 1971) or by a sublethal damage of the cells which only becomes manifest when the cell undergoes mitosis. In the latter case, necrosis may not be manifest until some years have elapsed (FUKS et al. 1976). Regeneration of the gland was not observed. When radiation doses are high enough, the acute effect is due to coagulation necrosis (FAJARDO 1982). However, low to intermediate doses of radiation do not produce specific morphological changes. Nonspecific changes such as a degranulation of acidophilic cells may be observed (FUKS et al. 1976). The posterior lobe is even more radioresistant and thus diabetes insipidus as a sequel to pituitary irradiation is virtually unknown (LITTLEY et al. 1991b). Pituitary adenoma tissue exhibits similar changes as a result of external radiotherapy (ANNIKO and WERSALL 1982). In contrast, functional damage to the hypothalamus is much more commonly observed. SAMAAN et al. (1982) observed an incidence of 83% of new endocrine deficiencies after irradiation for carcinoma of the nasopharynx. The fact that the hypothalamus is much more radiosensitive may explain much of the neuroendocrine sequelae observed following external megavoltage radiotherapy of the head and neck (AHMED and SHALET 1984; PERRY-KEENE et al. 1976; LARKINS and MARTIN 1973). Once the pituitary gland and the hypothalamus are both included in the radiation field, hypothalamic dysregulation may mimic anterior pituitary failure and consequently lead to hypofunction of the peripheral glands. Only the more focused beams of heavy particles may produce isolated pituitary lesions. Since hypothalamic exposure to radiation is avoided, a somewhat lower incidence of hypopituitarism following the latter treatment techniques can be explained.

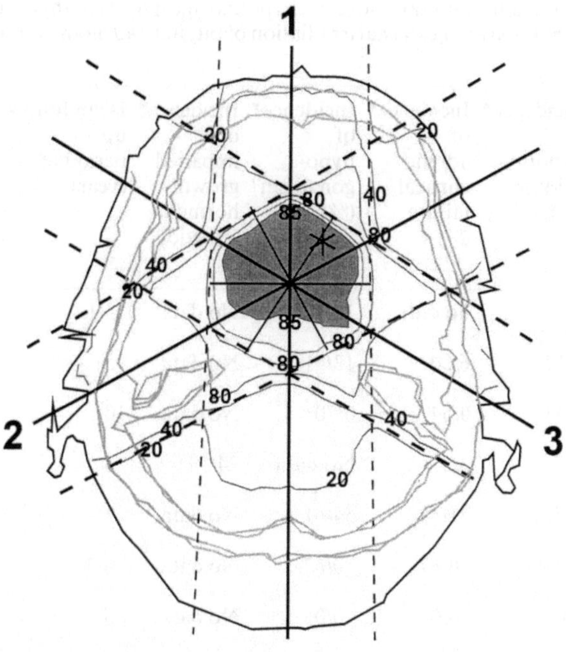

Fig. 1. Isodose curves for an irregularly shaped, 3.5 cm diameter tumor volume, using a 6 MeV linear accelerator and three fields

4 Effects of External Radiotherapy in Pituitary Adenomas

In the literature, there is considerable evidence of endocrine dysfunction as a sequel to pituitary irradiation. While early studies were largely based on circumstantial observations and thus could not clearly establish the exact incidence and etiology of any deficiency, more recent reports suggest that endocrine deficiencies may develop at any time after radiotherapy for tumors of the sellar region. The design of treatment fields for sellar or suprasellar tumors, either as primary therapy or after surgery, usually requires the inclusion of normal pituitary gland tissue and hypothalamus in the region that receives the tumor dose (Fig. 1), irrespective of whether external megavoltage radiotherapy or ^{60}Co irradiation is used (SHALET et al. 1979). Thus, the tumor, the pituitary gland and the hypothalamus all receive a similar dose of radiation. Growth hormone secretion is generally believed to be the most sensitive function to be affected by irradiation (LITTLEY et al. 1991b; SHELINE 1979). However, a clinical relevance of this type of deficiency in the adult has only recently been discussed and investigated (BENGTSSON 1993). CHROUSOS et al. (1982) have shown radiation-induced changes of the spontaneous pulsatile growth hormone secretion pattern which may occur even when dynamic endocrine testing does not reveal overt failure of growth hormone secretion after an iatrogenic stimulus. GROSSMAN et al. (1984) reported on an increase in the incidence of insufficient GH secretion from 24% before radiation therapy to 79% 3 years postradiation therapy in 36 women treated for prolactinoma by external megavoltage radiotherapy. Deficits in gonadotropin, ACTH and TSH secretion have also been documented following irradiation treatment of all types of pituitary tumors. The interest in these endocrine deficiencies has been greater because of their recognized clinical implications. The effect of external megavoltage radiotherapy on hypothalamic-pituitary function becomes manifest only with some delay. HALSE et al. (1981) did not observe an alteration in TRH-induced TSH secretion and in thyroid function 1 month after the completion of radiotherapy in their patients harboring pituitary adenomas. However, LAM et al. (1987) found an impairment of either gonadotropin, TSH or ACTH secretion when they tested patients with nasopharyngeal carcinomas who had received a higher dose to the putuitary region 1 year after irradiation. Table 1 summarizes the data from several studies. From the data available in the current literature it is clear that GH secretion is the most sensitive with respect to radiation injury, whereas TSH is the most resistant. Gonadotropin secretion seems to be slightly more sensitive than the corticotropic axis. Although in long-term follow-up studies deficiencies of ACTH and gonadotropin secretion develop with a similar incidence, an impaired LH and FSH secretion precedes the ACTH deficiency in most cases with the result that gonadotropin deficiency is more common in series with shorter follow-up periods. Although the sequence mentioned above is the most frequent, variations may occur. LITTLEY et al. (1991b) described a patient who developed ACTH deficiency before GH deficiency and the occurrence of TSH deficiency before ACTH deficiency in three others. Interestingly, they commonly observed the development of ACTH deficiency before gonadotropin secretion was affected. This sequence occurred in 39% of their patients who developed both abnormalities. In an attempt to characterize factors that might influence the development of endocrine disturbances after radiation therapy, these authors correlated hypothalamic-pituitary axis function against survival in subgroups of patients who had a normal hypothalamic-pituitary function before treatment. This analysis revealed that the rates at which pituitary deficiencies developed were not

Table 1. Incidence of radiation-induced disturbances of the hypothalamo-pituitary-adrenal, hypothalamo-pituitary-thyroid axes, hypothalamo-pituitary-gonadal axis and growth hormone secretion after external irradiation of pituitary adenomas and craniopharyngiomas

Reference	Patients (*n*)	Endocrinological classification	Total radiation dose (Gy)	Fractions/ duration of treatment (days)	Incidence* of hypothyroidism (%)	Incidence* of adrenocortical failure (%)	Incidence* of hypogonadism (%)	Incidence* of impaired growth-hormone secretion (%)	Heau follow-up period in (year)
Aloia et al. 1978	8	Acromegaly	55	28/	0/25 38–42	no data	17/100	No data	3.1
Eastman et al. 1979	47	Acromegaly	40–56	20–28/ 28–40	9/12	6/30	13/41	No data	5
Feek et al. 1984	46	Acromegaly	37.5	15/ ?	0/38	0/54	0/70	No data	10
Grossman et al. 1984	36	Prolactinoma	45	25/35	0–3	3/3	No data	24/79	3
Klijn et al. 1984	45	Acromegaly	46	23/35	11/24	21/59	54/61	No data	?
Snyder et al. 1986	35	Inactive adenomas	42.5	?/?	0/55	0/67	0/67	No data	4.2
Mehta et al. 1987	8	Prolactinomas	44–55	20–28/ 28–35	0/0	0/0	0/0	No data	15
Littley et al. 1991b	165	Pituitary adenomas and craniopharyngiomas	38–43	15–16/ 20–22	20/42	41/77	79/91	81/100	5
Littley et al. 1991b	59	Pituitary adenomas and craniopharyngiomas	20	8/9–11	20/26	42/64	59/77	No data	5

*(Incidences are provided in % before radiotherapy and at the end of the follow-up period).

related to the patient's age, gender, type of tumor, previous surgical intervention and the volume of brain tissue irradiated. However, the results of several other studies and the experience of the authors suggest that the volume of brain tissue irradiated has a significant effect on late sequelae (Sauer and Keilholz 1991; Sheline 1979).

In another report Littley et al. (1991a) studied the effect of external irradiation on serum prolactin levels in 58 patients. They found a continuous decrease of serum prolactin in all but three patients during observation periods of up to 12.8 years. However, the rate of fall of serum prolactin levels was greater in patients with true prolactin-secreting tumors than in those who only had functional, nontumorous hyperprolactinemia. The documentation of radiotherapy-induced hyperprolactinemia that has been repeatedly reported (Lam et al. 1991; Shalet et al. 1979; Samaan et al. 1982) accounts for a suprapituitary origin of disturbed function. It has virtually never been observed after interstitial irradiation or high energy particle beam therapy in intrasellar tumors in which the hypothalamus is not likewise exposed to radiation. Radiation-induced hyperprolactinemia has successfully been treated with dopamine agonists (Peterson et al. 1993).

The data on the incidence of radiation-induced hypopituitarism as a function of radiation dose are relatively meagre. Most such studies indicate that there is a latent period of several years and a dose-dependent relationship. High doses of radiation may cause radiation necrosis of the hypothalamus (Landolt 1980), particularly if the fractionation scheme leads to high radiation exposure in an individual fraction. The clinical picture here is mostly not dominated by the endocrine disturbances but by the space occupying effect causing visual impairment, deterioration of intellectual capability and dysregulations of vegetative functions. In these cases, the lesion may be depicted by CT, MR and PET scanning (Sauer and Keilholz 1991).

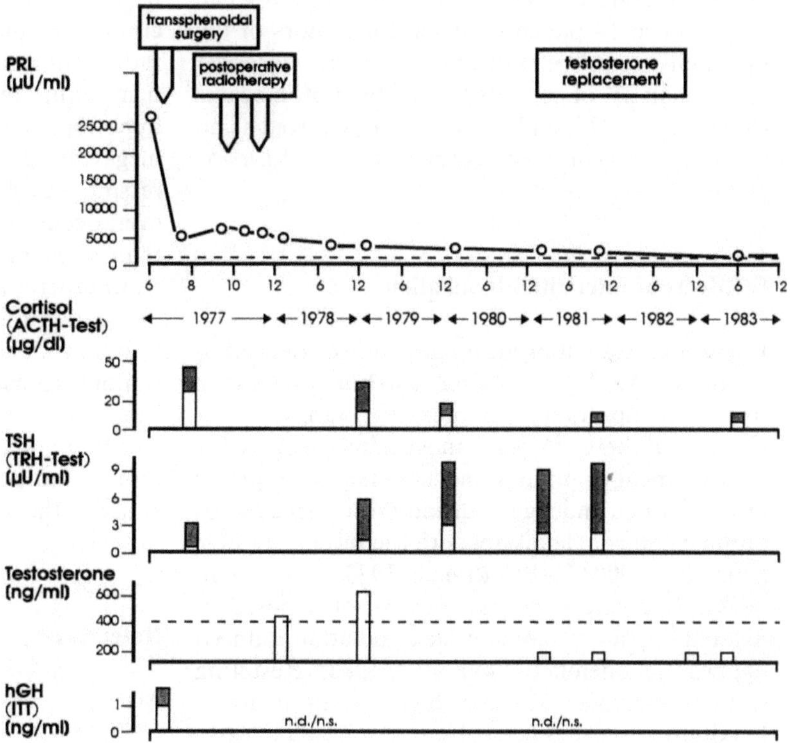

Fig. 2. Gradual development of hypopituitarism in a 41-year-old male patient who had surgery and external megavoltage radiotherapy (50 Gy in 25 fractions over 5 weeks) for a macroprolactinoma

The effect of external megavoltage radiotherapy on excessive autonomous oversecretion of pituitary hormones from functioning pituitary adenomas is similar to that on secretion from normal pituitary tissue. In both instances the effect is dose-dependent and increases with time. In individual cases the correction of hormonal oversecretion may be paralleled by the development of anterior pituitary failure requiring medical substitution therapy (Fig. 2). This has been documented for growth hormone- (FEEK et al. 1984; EASTMAN et al. 1979) and prolactin-secreting adenomas (GROSSMAN et al. 1984; LITTLEY et al. 1991b).

If one considers that most of the patients with pituitary adenomas have received radiotherapy after surgery and that there is a high prevalence of partial or total anterior pituitary failure, the incidence of clinically apparent pituitary deficiency following irradiation for pituitary adenomas is relatively low (BUCHFELDER 1984).

5 Effects of Heavy Particle Therapy

Although these techniques are now rarely used, a few data shall briefly be reviewed. By using proton (KJELLBERG 1975) or helium nuclei (LINFOOT 1980) very high radiation doses may be delivered to the pituitary region. With both high energy particles, accuracy of the beams requires the use of a stereotaxic frame. With these techniques the pituitary target dose may be 20–25 times greater than the beam dose. Thus, proton beams allow the administration of 60–100 Gy in order to achieve destruction of the pituitary or, alternatively, 20–40 Gy to a limited volume for the treatment of pituitary adenomas. Alpha particles, accelerated in a cyclotron, have been admistered to patients with acromegaly and Cushing's disease in treatments lasting for 5–12 days. Total doses ranged from 34 to 150 Gy. The damage to anterior pituitary function was much less than that expected after external magavoltage radiotherapy. However, similarly to the latter a delayed onset of hypopituitarism has been observed. Total pituitary insufficiency is expected to occur in approximately 15% of the patients 5 years after treatment. LINFOOT (1980) reports an incidence of 25%–28% of patients who developed radiation-induced hypoadrenalism, hypothyroidism or hypogonadism after α particle radiation therapy for acromegaly. SLATER et al. (1988) found that the endocrine abnormalities usually became manifest 2–5 years after irradiation when they studied 14 patients treated for tumors of the upper clivus. Diabetes insipidus has been observed in less than 2% of patients treated by proton beams (KJELLBERG 1975) and has not been reported as an adverse effect of proton radiosurgery (LINFOOT 1980).

6 Effects of Interstitial Irradiation

Interstitial irradiation using implants of the radioisotopes ^{198}Au, ^{32}P and ^{90}Y has also been used in the treatment of pituitary adenomas and craniopharyngiomas. Of these, ^{90}Y is the most suitable source for the treatment of pituitary adenomas. The implants are performed under general anesthesia using radiographic control. Total doses to the pituitary range from 100 to 500 Gy (BURKE et al. 1973; JOPLIN et al. 1979). Since the hypothalamus is not exposed to irradiation, these patients lack radiation-induced hyperprolactinemia (CLARK et al. 1983). Resulting from the exposure to very high radiation doses, hypopituitarism has been observed to occur as early as 1 month after implantation of ^{90}Y in some cases (SANDLER et al. 1987). However, many of the patients assessed after long-term follow-up did not require medical replacement therapy, which is further evidence for the relative radioresistancy of the normal pituitary gland. In patients in whom hypopituitarism occurred the sequence of sensitivity of the hypothalamopituitary-peripheral gland axes resembled those observed after external megavoltage radiotherapy. Diabetes insipidus has been reported to occur in about 14% of patients treated by internal irradiation (BURKE et al. 1973) but has been observed to improve spontaneously with time in many of the cases. It may in some instances have been due to the implantation procedure rather than to the radiation effect on the posterior lobe or on the pituitary stalk.

7 Summary and Therapeutic Recommendations

Patients with suprasellar tumors who underwent a course of external radiotherapy or had radioactive implants are at high risk of radiation-induced hypothalamic and pituitary injury. Several studies utilizing stimulation at various levels of neuroendocrine control suggest that hypothalamic dysfunction is more common than primary pituitary failure. Although growth hormone secretion was shown to be the most sensitive function to be affected by cranial irradiation; the clinical consequences of radiation-induced hypothyroidism and adrenocortical failure are more prominent. Deterioration of hypothalamic-pituitary function following external megavoltage radiotherapy usually is slowly progressing and delayed for a few years. It may, however, occur at any time between 1 month and more than 10 years after the completion of irradiation. It would therefore seem mandatory to repeatedly investigate patients who underwent radiation therapy, particularly those with intra- and perisellar tumors, to assess the neuroendocrine sequelae of irradiation. An adequate replacement therapy substituting gonadal, thyroid and adrenocortical hormones and possibly also growth hormone should enhance the quality of life in these patients.

References

Ahmed SR, Shalet S (1984) Hypothalamic growth hormone releasing factor deficiency following cranial irradiation. Clin Endocrinol (Oxf) 21: 483–488

Aloia JF, Archambean JO (1978) Hypopituitarism following pituitary irradiation for acromegaly. Heom Res 9: 201–207

Anniko M, Wersall J (1982) Morphological effects in pituitary tumors following radiotherpy. Virchows Arch 395: 45–58

Bengtsson BA (1993) The consequences of growth hormone deficiency in adults. Acta Endocrinol (Copenh) 128 [Suppl 2]: 2–5; Clin Endocrinol (Oxf) 21: 483–488

Buchfelder M (1984) Effekte der Radiotherapie supra- und parasellärer Hypophysenadenome. Inauguraldissertation, University of Erlangen-Nuremberg

Burke CW, Doyle FH, Joplin FG, Arnot RN, MacErlean DP, Fraser TR (1973) Cushing's disease: treatment by pituitary implantation of radioactive gold or yttrium seeds. Q J Med 42: 693–714

Chrousos GP, Poplack D, Brown T, O'Neill D, Schwade J, Bercu BB (1982) Effects of cranial radiation on hypothalamic-adenohypophyseal function: abnormal growth hormone secretory dynamics. J Clin Endocrinol Metab 54: 1135–1139

Clark AJL, Chahal P, Mashiter K, Joplin GF (1983) Lack or rise in serum prolactin following Yttrium-90 interstitial irradiation for acromegaly. Clin Endocrinol (Oxf) 19: 557–563

Constine LS, Woolf PD, Cann D, Mick G, McCormick K, Raubertas RF, Rubin P (1993) Hypothalamic-pituitary dysfunction after radiation for brain tumors. N Engl J Med 328: 87–94

De Schryver A, Ljunggren JG, Baaryd I (1973) Pituitary function in long-term survival after radiation therapy for nasopharyngeal tumors. Acta Radiol Ther Phys Biol 12: 497–508

Eastman RC, Gordon P, Roth J (1979) Conventional supervoltage irradiation is an effective treatment for acromegaly. J Clin Endocrinol Metab 48: 931–940

Fahlbusch R, Buchfelder M (1992) Tests of endocrine function for neurosurgical patients. In: Crockard A, Hayward R, Hoff JT (eds) Neurosurgery – the scientific basis of clinical practice. Blackwell, Oxford, pp 798–808

Fajardo LF (1982) Pathogenesis of radiation injury. In: Fajardo LF (ed) Pathology of radiation injury. Masson, New York

Feek C, McLelland J, Seth J, Toft AD, Irvine WJ, Padfield PL, Edwards CRW (1984) How effective is external pituitary irradiation for growth hormone-secreting pituitary tumours? Clin Endocrinol (Oxf) 20: 401–408

Fuks Z, Glatstein E, Marsa GW, Bagshaw MA, Kaplan HS (1976) Long-term effects of external radiation on the pituitary and thyroid glands. Cancer 37: 1152–1161

Grossman A, Cohen BL, Charlesworth M, Plowman PL, Rees LH, Wass JAH, Jones AE, Besser M (1984) Treatment of prolactinomas with megavoltage radiotherapy Brit Med J 288: 1105–1109

Halse J, Larsen IF, Rootwelt K (1981) Pituitary function during x-ray treatment of the hypothalamic-pituitary region as evaluated by the TRH test response. Acta Med Scand [Suppl] 645: 109–111

Joplin GF, Banks L, Casasar J, Doyle FH, Jadresic A, Kelly WF, Mashiter K (1979) Implantation of Yttrium-90 or Gold-198 seeds. In: Linfoot JA (ed) Recent advances in the diagnosis and treatment of pituitary tumors. Raven, New York, pp 331–335

Kjellberg RN (1975) A system of therapy of pituitary tumors-Bragg peak proton hypophysectomy. In: Seydel HG (ed) Tumors of the nervous system. Wiley, New York, pp 143–168

Klijn JGM, Lamberts SWJ, Van Woerkom-Eijkenboom WHM, Treurniet-Donker AD, Seeverens HJJ, de Lange SA, de Jong FH, Birkenhager JC (1984) Long-term follow up after external pituitary irradiation of pituitary adenomas. In: Lamberts SWJ, Tilders FJH, van der Veen EA, Assies J (eds) Trends in diagnosis and treatment of pituitary adenomas. Free University Press, Amsterdam, pp 359–372

Lam KSL, Tse VKC, Wang C, Yeung RTT, Ma JTC, Ho JHC (1987) Early effects of cranial irradiation on hypothalamic-pituitary function. J Clin Endocrinol Metab 64: 418–424

Lam KSL, Tse VKC, Wang C, Yeung RTT, Ho JHC (1991) Effects of cranial irradiation on hypothalamic-pituitary function – a 5-year longitudinal study in patients with nasopharyngeal carcinoma. Q J Med 78: 165–176

Landolt AM (1980) Hazards of Radiotherapy in patients with pituitary adenomas. In: Derome PJ, Peillon F, Jedynac GP (eds) 2nd European workshop on pituitary adenomas. Asclepios, France, Paris, pp 227–232

Larkins RG, Martins FIR (1973) Hypopituitarism after extracranial irradiation: evidence for hypothalamic origin. Br Med J 1: 152–153

Lawrence AM, Pinsky SM, Goldfine ID (1971) Conventional radiation therapy in acromegaly. Ann Intern Med 128: 369–377

Linfoot JA (1980) Alpha particles versus conventional radiotherapy to the pituitary region: a comparison of risk-benefit. Clin Neurosurg 27: 83–98

Littley MD, Shalet SM, Beardwell CG, Robinson EL, Sutton ML (1989) Radiation-induced hypopituitarism is dose-dependent. Clin Endocrinol (Oxf) 31: 363–373

Littley MD, Shalet SM, Reid H, Bearwell CG, Sutton ML (1991a) The effect of external pituitary irradiation on elevated serum prolactin levels in patients with pituitary macroadenomas. Q J Med 81: 985–998

Littley MD, Shalet SM, Beardwell CG (1991b) Radiation and the hypothalamo-pituitary axis. In: Gutin PH, Leibel SA, Sheline GE (eds) Radiation injury to the nervous system. Raven, New York, pp 303–324

Mehta AE, Reyes FI, Faiman C (1987) Primary radiotherapy of prolactinomas: 8–15 year follow-up. Am J Med 83: 49–58

Perry-Keene DA, Connelly JF, Young RA, Wettenhall HN, Martin FI (1976) Hypothalamic hypopituitarism following external radiotherapy for tumours distant from the adenohypophysis. Clin Endocrinol (Oxf) 5: 373–380

Petterson T, MacFarlane I, Foy PM, Hughes HJ, Jones B, Shaw D (1993) Hyperprolactinaemia and infertility following cranial irradiation for brain tumors: Successful treatment with bromocriptine. Br J Neurosurg 7: 571–574

Richards GE (1980) Effects of irradiation on the hypothalamic and pituitary regions. In: Gilbert HA, Kagan AR (eds) Radiation damage to the nervous system. Raven, New York, pp 175–180

Rodriguez A, Levy RP, Fabrikant JI: Experimental central nervous system injury after charged-particle irradiation. In: Gutin PH, Leibel SA, Sheline GE (eds) Radiation injury to the nervous system. Raven, New York, pp 149–182

Rubin P, Casarett GW (1968) Clinical radiation pathology, vol 2. Saunders, Philadelphia

Samaan NA, Vieto R, Schultz PN, Maor M, Meoz RT, Sampiere VA, Cangir A, Ried HL, Jesse RH (1982) Hypothalamic, pituitary and thyroid dysfunction after radiotherapy to the head and neck. Int J Radiat Oncol Biol Phys 8: 1857–1867

Sandler LM, Richards NT, Carr DH, Mashiter K, Joplin GF (1987) Long term follow-up of patients with Cushing's disease treated by interstitial irradiation. J Clin Endocrinol Metab 65: 441–447

Sauer R, Keilholz L (1991) The central nervous system: clinical aspects. In: Scherer E, Streffer C, Trott KR (eds) Medical radiology: radiopathology of organs an tissues. Springer, Berlin Heidelberg New York, pp 213–242

Shalet SM, MacFarlane IA, Beardwell CG (1979) Radiation-induced hyperprolactinaemia in a treated acromegalic. Clin Endocrinol (Oxf) 11: 169–171

Sheline GE (1979) Conventional radiation therapy in the treatment of pituitary tumors. In: Tindall GT, Collins WF (eds) Clinical management of pituitary disorders. Raven, New York, pp 287–314

Slater JD, Austin-Seymour M, Munzenrider J, Birnbaum S, Carroll R, Klibanski A, Riskind P, Urie M, Verhey L, Goitein M (1988) Endocrine function following high dose proton therapy for tumors of the upper clivus. Int J Radiat Oncol Biol Phys 15: 607–611

Snyder PS, Fowble BF, Schatz NJ, Savino PJ, Genarelli TA (1986) Hypopituitarism following radiation therapy of pituitary adenomas. Am J Med 81: 457–462

Wara WM, Richards GE, Grumbach MM, Kaplan SL, Sheline GE, Conte FA (1977) Hypopituitarism after irradiation in children. Int J Radiat Oncol Biol Phys 2: 549–552

2.8 Late Sequelae Affecting the Ear

STEFAN BIRKENHAKE

CONTENTS

1 Introduction 73
2 Middle Ear 73
3 Inner Ear 74
4 Bone 77
5 Summary and Therapeutic Recommendations 77
References 78

1 Introduction

Radiotherapy of cancer of the nasopharynx, maxilla, skull base, posterior fossa or brain stem causes significant X-ray exposure to the ear. Side effects on the stato-acoustical organ are probably of rare incidence and low severeness. Consequently the clinician may not pay regularly attention to them. In the past the prognosis of the above mentioned tumors was considered poor. In order to achieve the highest cure rates, injury of less important organs is often neglected. Nevertheless, over time the prognosis has become better and quality of life has an important influence on treatment planing. Though deafness or even less intense complaints will never be therapy limiting, these adverse effects of radiotherapy of the ear should be considered.

2 Middle Ear

It is a common observation that head and neck cancer patients undergoing radiotherapy regularly complain of suddenly appearing earache. This may be explained by serious effusion in the middle ear and disturbance of ventilation and drainage caused by edema of the mucous membrane in the pharynx, which leads to obstruction of the eustachian tubes (YAMAGUCHI et al. 1990).

Data from animal studies support this obvious theory: OHASHI et al. (1987, 1988) irradiated guinea pigs with a single dose of 30 Gy and killed the animals immediately afterwards. They found serious effusion in the tympanic cavity, degeneration of cilia or ciliated cells and capillary injury with increased permeability. These findings are comparable to those accompanying acute otitis media. BERG and LINDGREN (1961) analyzed morphology and lesion sites after irradiation to one half of the head of rabbits. They exposed the animals to single doses ranging from 21 Gy to 30 Gy or fractionated doses ranging from 54 Gy in 12 days to 105 Gy in 30 days; single doses thus varied from 2.2 Gy to 4.5 Gy. The animals were killed after 52 weeks. After high doses (e.g., 30 Gy single doses or a total of 105 Gy in doses of 3.5 Gy) fibrosis in the walls of the middle ear developed. The authors described a thickened and fibrotic mucous membrane. The ossicles were frequently involved and the epithelium was atrophic. In more severe cases the epithelium was often completely destroyed. However, no lesions were detected in the group which had been exposed to a 21 Gy single dose and no remarks we are made on alterations following conventional fractionation. The authors mentioned that only five of 30 animals which received fractionated doses did not have signs of otitis. BOHNE et al. (1985) exposed dogs to conventional fractionated doses of radiation for total doses ranging from 40 Gy to 90 Gy. The animals were killed 2 years after treatment and histopathological studies were performed. In contrast to the aforementioned investigations, no abnormalities in the middle ear were found. There was no evidence of previous or current infections when the animals had been killed. Neither mucosa nor tympanic membranes were found to have pathological alterations. Only in one dog, killed because of meningitis, serous effusion and purulent otitis media was described.

ELWANY (1985) carried out a study on six patients suffering from conductive hearing loss 6–11 months after they received doses of 65–85 Gy. In all patients a necrosis of the incus and in two patients necrosis of the stapes were found. The epithelium

STEFAN BIRKENHAKE, Dr., Klink und Poliklinik für Strahlentherapie, Universität Erlangen-Nürnberg, Universitätsstrasse 27, 91054 Erlangen, FRG

Table 1. Incidence of persistent otitis media following radiation of the mesopharynx

Authors	*n*	Incidence (%)
BAKER 1980	4/99	4
URDANETA et al. 1976	6/43	14
HUANG and CHU 1981	?/1032	44
LEE et al. 1992	11/4527	2

Data published by HUANG et al. include acute reactions described as "ear trouble due to eustachian tube."

showed variable degrees of ciliary loss and deterioration of ciliary motility. The cytoplasmic mass was diminished. Blood capillaries always had swollen endothelial cells, as is typical for radiation-induced injury. The connective tissue stroma was fibrotic.

Clinically, symptoms comparable to acute otitis media are found during radiatherapy. Persistent otitis media arises with a low but regular incidence varing between 2% and 14% (Table 1). HUANG and CHU (1981) reported on an incidence of 44% but acute otitis was included (HUANG 1980).

These chronic alterations may cause conductive loss, as has been described for chronic infections of other origin. Conductive hearing loss was reported by FROMM et al. (1980) who treated 19 children suffering from soft tissue sarcomas of the head and neck. In one patient, irradiated with 53 Gy, a thickened tympanic membrane was found. In the investigation of BAKER (1980) one of the four patients suffering from otitis media subsequently developed a cholesteatoma.

All in all, chronic alterations in the middle ear are of frequent occurrence; however, they seldom lead to serious complications but certainly reduce the quality of life. The clinician should nonetheless be aware of them because in rare cases they may even induce life threatening situations, for instance, when a meningitis arises.

3 Inner Ear

Concerning late sequelae on the ear, both experimental and clinical data exist. The former refer to the possible effects of ionizing radiation.

The animal study conducted by BERG and LINDGREN (1961) showed, apart from a high incidence of otitis, that marked vestibular lesions and changes of the nerves of the pons can occur both after a single dose and after a fractionated dose. In their investigation, the largest focal doses producing neither signs nor morphologic damage to the internal ear 1 year after treatment were 14 Gy single dose, 30 Gy à 2.5 Gy and 45 Gy à 1.5 Gy. Higher doses led to acute purulent otitis interna and lesions of pons nerves could be demonstrated. Furthermore, rarefaction of the cochlea and cochlear nerve were observed. The authors concluded that radiation induced vascular damage, which in turn led to infection thereby injuring structures important for hearing. They also pointed out that the radiosensitivity of the internal ear and the brain, at least in rabbits, seems to be in the same range.

After irradiation of dogs, BOHNE et al. (1985) identified degeneration of both sensory and supporting cells and a loss of the eighth nerve fibre. These effects depended on the amount of irradiated dose. Despite a considerable interanimal variability in the degree of cell loss, a linear regression between the percentage of missing hair cells and the radiation dose was calculated. The correlation coefficient amounted to 0.76 and was too low for a real linear dependency. Nevertheless, a trend for increasing loss of cells with higher doses of radiation was plainly recognizable. Eleven dogs had to be killed because of perioperative complications within the first month. The quantity of cell loss was significantly less than in those surviving 2 years. The authors concluded that radiation-induced cochlear destruction requires time to become manifest. Whereas cell loss showed a uniform distribution from apex to base of the cochlea, degeneration of nerve fiber was localized more often in the basal turn. Nerve fiber degeneration was also dose-dependent. In ears exposed to 50 Gy the incidence was 31%, while in the ears irradiated up to 90 Gy the incidence was 63%. The extent of damage was of sufficient magnitude to produce permanent sensorineural hearing loss. In contrast to the investigation of BERG and LINDGREN (1961) no inflammation was found. Consequently BOHNE et al. (1985) concluded that their results represent the primary effect of radiation on the cochlea.

LÖFFLER et al. (1988) treated children with medulloblastoma. The patients received postsurgical 100 mg/m^2 cisplatin every 3 weeks and 1.5 mg/m^2 vincristine once a week for a total of 9 weeks. For younger infants, monthly cycles of MOP were added until the second birthday. Afterwards radiotherapy was performed as follows: the whole brain received 30 Gy conventional fractionated and the spinal axis 25 Gy in doses of 1.5 Gy. The posterior fossa was irradiated up to 54 Gy. Three children developed clinically significant hearing loss at speech frequencies ($\leqslant$2000 Hz) after one, two or

Table 2. Severe hearing loss after treatment of brain tumors with and without chemotherapy/radiotherapy

Reference	RT (Gy)	Cisplatin	Ototoxicity	Incidence (%)
KRETSCHMAR et al. (1990)	50–60	+	Decrease at 2000 Hz	3/28(11)
	50–60	–	n.d.	0/19
LÖFFLER et al. (1988)	54	+	"Speech range"	0/15
ROZENTAL et al. (1989)	50	+	50 dB at 500–4000 Hz	3/31(10)
SCHELL et al. (1989)	—	+	50 dB at 500–4000 Hz	62/146 (42)
	29–83	+	50 dB at 500–4000 Hz	19/31(62)
	29–83	—		0/33

three cycles of cisplatin. Fifteen children were treated with radiation, all without any subjective hearing loss. Ten children underwent hearing evaluation without any deterioration compared to values before radiotherapy.

ROZENTAL et al. (1989) treated astrocytomas stages III and IV with ten courses of an "eight-drug-in-one-day" chemotherapy regimen, which included cisplatin. After two courses, radiotherapy was performed. The patients received brain irradiation up to 45 Gy to the involved area with a 3–4 cm margin and a 15 Gy boost. When the tumour was localized in the posterior fossa 50 Gy plus 10 Gy boost were given. Two weeks after radiotherapy chemotherapy was continued. Beside other severe complications ototoxicity was found in two patients before irradiation due to chemotherapy. Three further patients developed a decrease in auditory acuity over the speech range after the fourth cycle approximately 9 weeks after radiotherapy. One of them required a hearing aid and suffered from a 50 dB hearing loss. This was, of course, not necessarily due to radiotherapy; rather, the aggressive regimen gives rise to the suspicion that ear damage was caused by chemotherapy.

SCHELL et al. (1989) analyzed a group of 177 patients suffering from different cerebral neoplasms. Therapy consisted of repeated cisplatin infusions, radiotherapy alone or a combination of both in which radiation preceded. A relevant hearing loss was defined as a 50 dB decrease in the frequency of 500–4000 Hz, which was considered as the speech range. In this sense chemotherapy alone led to ototoxicity in 42% and the combined modality in 62%. Radiotherapy produced no relevant damage; however, minor hearing loss in the latter group was detected in 25%. The authors furthermore emphasized the importance of the cumulative cisplatin dose. Nonirradiated patiented with cisplatin up to 360 mg/m^2 had a negligible low risk of substantial deficits concerning speech frequency. As the dose increased to 720 mg/m^2 the risk increased to 25%. Another important observation was that, already after 270 mg/m^2 cisplatin, patients who had been irradiated had a risk of about 35% for a 50% decrease at 2000 Hz. Less severe loss at higher frequencies was found at 25% of the patients. The authors concluded that higher doses of cisplatin increase the risk of ototoxicity and that, at least in their investigation, cisplatin makes severe radiation-induced ototoxicity possible.

This is confirmed by several case reports. GRANOWETTER et al. (1983) noted a considerable increase in cisplatin-induced ototoxicity when it was administered after radiotherapy for brain tumors. Five children were as reported having significant audiographic changes after receiving only 120 mg/m^2 cisplatin. GOEBEL et al. (1983) confirmed this with two similar cases. WALKER et al. (1989) published three cases of sensorineural hearing loss after simultaneous radiochemotherapy and one case with cisplatin after radiation. It should be taken into consideration that in all cases radiotherapy preceded chemotherapy and no recovery was reported.

KRETSCHMAR et al. (1990) evaluated audiometric tests on 28 children with malignant brain tumors who had been treated with three courses of 100 mg/m^2 cisplatin each and vincristine 1.5 mg/m^2 weekly for a total of nine doses. MOP was added for infants until their second birthday. After chemotherapy radiotherapy was performed. Though the authors did not give explicitly the exact dose, one can conclude from the context that 50–60 Gy were applied. After 300 mg/m^2 cisplatin, in 11% significant hearing loss within speech frequencies, which were referred to as the interval between 1000 Hz and 2000 Hz, was noticed. In these frequencies, controls before and after radiotherapy of 19 patients failed to prove any deterioration. However, one patient with a former normal audiogram had loss at between 6000 Hz and 8000 Hz ascertained 12 months after radiation.

Several authors studied the question of late sequelae caused by radiotherapy of nasopharyngeal tumors (Table 3). BOHORQUEZ (1976) reported on

Table 3. Impairment of hearing following irradiation of nasaopharyngeal carcinoma

Reference	Radiotherapy (Gy)	*n* (%)	Hearing impairment
BOHORQUEZ (1976)	50–70	1/89(1)	Conductive hearing loss only
BORSANYI and BLANCHARD (1962)[a]	40–60	14/14(100)	Conductive type, no long-term follow up
GRAU et al. (1991)[a]	39–68	9/32(28)	Sensorineural hearing loss
LEE et al. (1992)	65	134/4527(3)	Bilateral deafness
		241/4527(5)	Impaired hearing
MESIC et al. (1981)	60–70	18/251(7)	Fluctuating hearing loss secondary to otitis
MORETTI (1976)[a]	20–203	7/13(54)	Sensorineural hearing loss

[a]Patients had both pre- and post-therapeutic examinations.

Table 4. Influence of radiotherapy for different tumors on the inner ear

Reference	Tumor	Radiotherapy (Gy)	*n* (%)	Remarks
EVANS et al. (1988)	Parotid cancer	55–60	0/18	Neither conductive nor sensorineural loss
FROMM et al. (1986)	Sarcomas of head and neck	7–60	1/25(4)	Mild sensorineural
GABRIELE et al. (1992)	Head and neck	25–51	11/25(44)	ENG abnormalities 3 and 6 months after radiotherapy
LEACH (1965)	Head and neck	30–120	20/56(36)	Impaired hearing
			2/56(4)	Complete deafness
SAKAI et al. (1988)	Maxillary	79	41/71(14)	Requiring hearing aid, postsurgical radiotherapy

152 patients treated in a three-field technique (two lateral and one nasal) with doses of 30–70 Gy. Some 89 people (60%) received more than 50 Gy. One patient developed conductive deafness due to fibrosis, which means an incidence of about 1%.

LEE et al. (1992) analyzed a cohort of 4527 patients irradiated for nasopharyngeal cancer. They applied a median dose of 65 Gy with a large portion of accelerated fractionation; 76% received 64–66 Gy. It is in the nature of such a retrospective analysis that treatment techniques and applied doses differ from each other. A decline of hearing was stated in 8% including 3% deafness. Interestingly enough, persistent otitis media was detected in only 2%, which is less than the described hearing loss. MESIC et al. (1981) discovered fluctuating hearing loss in 7.2% of 251 patients who underwent radiotherapy with 60 Gy at stage T1,2 and 70 Gy at stage T3,4 nasopharynx carcinoma. According to the authors themselves, this was secondary to acute and serous otitis media. GRAU et al. (1991) evaluated 35 ears before and after radiation for cancer of the nasopharynx. A sensorineural hearing loss of at least 10 dB was found in nine cases. The authors only evaluated frequencies up to 4000 Hz. Within this range hearing loss, was most pronounced in the higher frequencies. A latent period of 12 months or more was found. MORETTI (1976) examined 13 patients suffering from nasopharyngeal carcinoma before and after radiotherapy with doses ranging from 20 Gy to 203 Gy. Seven of these patients showed sustained senorineural deafness. BORSANYI and BLANCHARD (1962) analyzed a series of 14 patients with the same tumor. Doses to the cochlear region were 40–60 Gy. A deterioration of audiometric tests was found in all patients and was always of the conductive type. No long-term follow-up was made.

LEACH (1965) reviewed 56 cases of patients who underwent radiotherapy for different head and neck malignancies. Twenty of them complained of hearing loss and two patients developed complete deafness. This occurred in eight cases during radiotherapy. Leach reported two recoveries. He did not distinguish between conductive and sensorineural hearing loss. GABRIELE et al. (1992) treated 25 patients with head and neck cancer. The vestibular apparatus received 25–51 Gy. Electronystagmography (ENG) showed abnormalities in 11 patients cases 3 and 6 months after radiotherapy. Three patients complained of dizziness and two had balance disturbances. No correlation was found between the clinically described symptoms and the ENG abnormalities. SAKAI et al. (1988) reported on 171 patients with maxillary cancer who were postoperatively irradiated with 70 Gy in 7 weeks: 45

Table 5. Incidence of osteonecrosis following irradiation of the mastoid bone

Reference	n	Radiotherapy (Gy) Median dose/single dose
BIRZGALIS et al. (1992)	1/53	44–55/2.0–2.5
HANSEN and THOMSEN (1988)	0/57	50–54/2.0
KORZENIOWSKY and PSZON (1990)	1/29	60/2.5–3.0
PAASKE et al. (1987)	0/31	41–68/2
SAUERWEIN and FELDMAN (1988)	1/12	50–70/2.0

patients (26%) had tympanic effusion and 25% suffered from severe hearing loss requiring a hearing aid. FROMM et al. (1986) treated soft-tissue sarcomas of the head and neck. Middle and inner ear doses varied between 7 Gy and 60 Gy. Beside one case of conductivity hearing loss, there was mild sensorineural loss. Some 25 patients with a follow-up of 6 years had no alterations. EVANS et al. (1988) examined 18 patients who had received unilateral radical megavoltage therapy to the temporal bone because of unilateral parotid tumors. Doses between 55 Gy and 60 Gy in conventional fractionation had been applied to the involved side, whilst the dose of the contralateral ear was negligible. Examination took place between 2 and 16 years after radiotherapy. The results showed neither conductive nor sensorineural deficits. Table 4 summarizes the studies discussed here.

4 Bone

The only relevant side effect concerning bone is necrosis. A tolerance dose ($TD_{5/5}$) of 70 Gy in conventional fractionation is assumed. BERG and LINDGREN (1961) showed bone changes, mostly marked around the auditory canal and the middle ear of rabbits, after high dose irradiation, even in the absence of skin damage. A lower but from the clinical point of view still elevated dose (21 Gy single fraction) produced only slight lacunar absorption and sclerosis of bone. A focal dose of 71 Gy in 31 days was found to produce pure radionecrosis in the internal ear in 50% of the rabbits. This is still a considerable dose and it should be mentioned that the dose at the bone itself in practice rarely reaches this amount. BOHNE et al. (1985) irradiated dogs with up to 90 Gy in 2 Gy fractions and noticed no osteonecrosis (see Sect. 2).

Clinical data hint at the relative insensitivity of bone towards X-rays. PAASKE et al. (1987) for instance, applied a median dose of 55 Gy in single doses of 2 Gy to patients with cancer of the auditory canal (OHASHI et al. 1987). Like HANSEN and THOMSEN (1988), who treated glomus tumors, they saw no necrosis. Both KORZENIOWSKI and PSZON (1990) and BIRZGALIS et al. (1992) noticed one case of bone necrosis after treatment of cancer of the middle ear with doses varying from 45 Gy to 60 Gy in fractions ranging from 2 Gy to 3 Gy daily. Both groups treated postoperative patients, at least a biopsy had been performed before radiotherapy. SAUERWEIN and FELDMAN (1988) found one case of necrosis accompanying a relapse.

In summary, ostenonecrosis is a rare complication with an incidence of about 1%–2%. Conventional fractionation and healthy bone, i.e., not injured by cancer or surgery, prevent necrosis.

5 Summary and Therapeutic Recommendations

Persistent otitis media due to radiotherapy occurs in 2%–4% of patients. Taking the most comprehensive investigation of LEE et al. (1992) into account, a probably lower incidence of below 5% can be assumed. However, this was a retrospective study and therapy-related toxicity may be underestimated. The significance of otitis is that it may play a role in pathogenesis of conductive hearing loss. Animal data prove that acute reactions in the middle ear comparable to acute otitis can occur immediately after irradiation and can remain for months. Loss of ciliary cells and ciliary motility is found. This does not necessarily lead to chronic inflammation. But in connection with occluded eustachian tubes it may produce a thickened tympanic membrane and necrosis of ossicles, causing conductive hearing loss in return.

An effect of radiation on the inner ear resulting in sensorineural hearing loss is found in several studies and many case reports. The higher frequencies seem to be most often affected. Results are contradictory, with an incidence between 0% and 28% for realistic doses of maximum 70 Gy. LEE et al. (1992) analyzed more than 4500 patients and found bilateral deafness in 3% and in an additional 5% impairment of hearing. Unfortunately the authors did not distinguish between conductive and sensorineural hearing loss. Discussing these data it must again be taken into account that most investigations are retrospective and occurrences of side effects are underestimated.

Sensorineural deafness is caused by direct toxic effects both on sensory cells and the eighth nerve fiber, which is mostly affected in the basal turn of the cochlea. BOHNE et al. (1985) showed that these effects are dose-dependent. A latent period of several months can be assumed.

There is no doubt that the ototoxicity of cisplatin is increased by radiotherapy. Thus, for protection, it is recommended to use conventional fractionation, especially in connection with chemotherapy (KIRKBRIDE and PLOWMAN 1989). Though the skull base must be generously encompassed for the above discussed tumors, usually causing significant doses at the middle and inner ear when using standard field techniques, modern treatment planning should avoid unnecessary radiation to these obviously radiosensitive organs, for instance using multiple field techniques. Furthermore, it would be useful to obtain pre- and posttreatment audiograms, especially in children (TALMI et al. 1989). With regard to the relative-late onset, follow-up should be continued for several years.

References

Baker SR (1980) Nasopharyngeal carcinoma: clincal course and results of therapy. Head Neck Surg 3: 8–14

Berg NO, Lindgren M (1961) Dose factors and morphology of delayed radiation lesions of the internal and middle ear of rabbits. Acta Radiol 56: 305–315

Birzgalis AR, Keith AO, Farrington WT (1992) Radiotherapy in the treatment of middle ear and mastoid carcinoma. Clin Otolaryngeol 17: 113–116

Bohne BA, Marks JE, Glasgow GP (1985) Delayed effects of ionizing radiation of the ear. Laryngoscope 95: 818–828

Bohorquez J (1976) Factors that modify the radio response of cancer of the nasopharynx. AJR 126: 863–876

Borsanyi SJ, Blanchard CL (1962) Ionizing radiation and the ear. JAMA 181: 958–961

Dias A (1968) Effects on the hearing of patients treated by irradiation in the head and neck. J Laryngeol 80: 276–287

Elwany S (1985) Delayed ultrastructural radiation induced changes in the human mesotympanic middle ear mucosa. J Laryngeol Otol 99: 343–345

Evans RA, Liu KC, Azhar T, Symonds RP (1988) Assessment of permanent hearing impairment following radical megavoltage radiotherapy. J Laryngeol Otol 102: 588–589

Fromm M, Littman P, Raney RB, Nelson L, Handler S, Diamond G, Stanley C (1986) Late effects after treatment of twenty children with soft tissue sarcomas of the head and neck. Cancer 57: 2070–2076

Gabriele P, Orechchia R, Magnano M, Albera R, Sannazari GL (1992) Vestibular apparatus disorders after external radiation therapy for head and neck cancers. Radiother Oncol 25: 25–30

Gamble JE, Peterson EA, Chandler JR (1968) Radiation effects on the inner ear. Arch Otolaryngeol 88: 156–161

Goebel U, Lamprecht A, Beron B (1983) Akuter Hörverlust bei Kindern mit vorbestrahlten intrakraniellen Tumoren nach einmaliger hochdosierter Cis-Platinum-Gabe. Klin Padiatr 198: 277–280

Granowetter L, Rosenstock JG, Packer RJ (1983) Enhanced cis-platinum neurotoxicity in pediatric patients with brain tumors. J Neuro Oncol 1: 293–297

Grau C, Moller K, Overgaard M, Overgaard JH, Elbround O (1991) Sensori-neural hearing loss in patients treated with irradiation for nasopharyngeal carcinoma. Int J Radiat Oncol Biol Phys 21: 723–728

Hansen HS, Thomsen KA (1988) Radiotherapy in glomus tumors (paragangliomas). A 25 year-review. Acta Otolaryngeol Suppl (Stockh) 449: 151–154

Huang SC (1980) Nasopharyngeal cancer: a review of 1606 patients treated radically with cobald 60. Int J Radiat Oncol Biol Phys 6: 401–407

Huang SC (1981) Nasopharyngeal cancer: study II. Int J Radiat Oncol Biol Phys 7: 713–716

Kirkbride P, Plowman PN (1989) Platinum chemotherapy, radiotherapy and the inner ear: implications for standard radiation portals. Br Radiol 62: 457–462

Korzeniowski S, Pszon J (1990) The results of radiotherapy of cancer of the middle ear. Int J Radiat Oncol Biol Phys 18: 631–633

Kretschmar CS, Warren MP, Lavally BL, Dyer S, Tarbell NJ (1990) Ototoxicity of preradiation cisplatin for children with central nerbous system rumors. J Clin Oncol 8: 1191–1198

Leach W (1965) Irradiation of the ear. J Laryngeol 97: 870–880

Lee AWM, Law SCK, Chan DKK, Poon YF, Foo W, Tung SY, Cheung FK, Ho JHC (1992) Retrospective analysis of nasopharyngeal carcinoma treated during 1976–1985: late complications following megavoltage irradiation. Br Radiol 65: 918–928

Löffler JS, Kretschmar CS, Sallan SE, LaVally BL, Winston KR, Fischer EG, Tarbell NJ (1988) Pre-radiation chemotherapy for infants and poor prognosis children with medulloblastoma. Int J Radiat Oncol Biol Phys 15(1): 177–181

Mesic JB, Fletcher GH, Goepfert H (1981) Megavoltage irradiation of epithelial tumors of the nasopharynx. Int J Radiat Oncol Biol Phys 7: 447–453

Moretti JA (1976) Sensori-neural hearing loss following radiotherapy to the nasopharynx. Laryngoscope 86: 598–602

Ohashi Y, Nakai Y, Ikeoka H, Esaki Y, Koshimo H, Onoyama Y (1987) Mucosal pathology of an experimental otitis media with effusion after x-ray irradiation. Am J Otolaryngeol 8: 223–235

Ohashi Y, Nakai Y, Esaki Y, Ikeoka H, Koshimo H, Onoyama Y (1988) Acute effects of irradiation on middle ear mucosa. Ann Oto. Rhinol Laryngeol 97: 173–178

Paaske PB, Witten J, Schwer S, Hansen HS (1987) Results in treatment of carcinoma of the external auditory canal and middle ear. Cancer 59: 156–160

Rozental JM, Robins HI, Finlay J, Healey B, Levin AB, Steeves RA, Kohler PC, Schutta HS, Trump DL (1989) "Eight-drugs-in-one-day" chemotherapy administered before and after radiotherapy to adult patients with malignant gliomas. Cancer 63: 2475–2481

Sakai S, Kubo T, Mori N, Itoh M, Miyaguchi M, Kitaoku S, Sakata Y, Fuchihata H (1988) A study of the late effects of

the radiotherapy and operation on patients with maxillary cancer. Cancer 62: 2114–2117
Sauerwein W, Feldmann HJ (1988) Beitrag zur Strahlentherapie der Gehörgangskarzinome. Strahlenther Onkol 164: 567–573
Savic DL, Djeric DR (1991) Malignant tumors of the middle ear. Clin Otolaryngeol 16: 87–89
Schell MJ, McHaney VA, Green AA, Kun LE, Hayes FA, Horowitz M, Meyer WH (1989) Hearing loss in children and yound adults receiving cisplatin with or without prior cranial irradiation. J Clin Oncol 7: 754–760
Talmi YP, Finktelstein Y, Zohar Y (1989) Postirradiation hearing loss. Audiology 28: 121–126
Urdaneta N, Fischer JJ, Vera R, Gutierrez E (1976) Cancer of the nasopharynx: a review of 43 cases treated with supervoltage radiation therapy. Cancer 37: 1707–1712
Walker D, Pillow J, Waters K, Keir E (1989) Enhanced cis-platinum ototoxicity in children with brain tumors who have received simultaneous or prior cranial irradiation. Med Pediatr Oncol 17: 48–52
Yamaguchi N, Sando I, Hashida Y, Takahashi H, Myers EN (1990) Histopathologic study of otitis media in individuals with head and neck tumors. Ann Otol Rhinol Laryngeol 99: 827–823

2.9 Ototoxicity in Pediatric Oncology

SABINE HARTMANN

Since the 1960s, notions of how sound is processed in the inner ear have been dominated by van Bekesey's moving wave theory (VAN BEKESEY 1960) and the descriptions from electron microscope investigations of the inner and outer hair cells, which differ from each other especially in their ultrastructure and innervation pattern (HUDSPETH 1985; SPOENDLIN 1960; SPOENDLIN 1969; ZENNER et al. 1985). The outer hair cells contain contractile elements such as actin and myosin and can be made to produce longitudinal contractions or tilting movements of the cuticular plate by electrical, chemical and acoustic stimuli (ARNOLD et al. 1990; DRENCKHAHN et al. 1985; ZENNER 1986). They have predominantly efferent innervation via the neurotransmitters acetylcholine (ACh) and gamma-aminobutyricacid (GABA) which result in opposing functions (PLINKERT and ZENNER 1992; SPOENDLIN 1969).

The stimulus which produces contraction is the moving wave that occurs in the endolymphatic tube under acoustic exposure and which, depending on the frequency, reaches its maximum amplitude at a certain point on the basilar membrane. Through avulsion of the stereocilia, this results in the opening of ion canals in the apical hair cell region and leads to a positively charged inflow (KIM 1986). Depolarization is followed by release of the afferent neurotransmitter glutamate from the inner hair cells (ZENNER and GITTER 1987). Glutamate transmits the sound transduction to the acoustic nerve. In the region of the outer hair cells, a contraction is triggered by an energy-consuming inflow of potassium ions, i.e., ATP, and is bound to second messengers such as calcium, magnesium and inositol triphosphate (ZENNER and PLINKERT 1992).

According to numerous observations, a signal transfer takes place from the outer hair cell movements to inner hair cells, but whether this is generated by increased rigidity of the tectorial membrane or by a change of the moving wave, or by chemical effects through ion flows along the tectorial membrane or via nerve connections is still under discussion (KIM 1986; LIM 1986; MARK and RATTAY 1991; PLINKERT and LENARZ 1992; SPOENDLIN 1969; ZENNER 1986). Ultrastructurally, the outer hair cells, which are responsible for the active motile amplification mechanism, contain, in addition to actin and myosin, conspicuously large quantities of mitochondria and a clearly discernible endoplasmatic reticulum for protein and enzyme synthesis and for provision of energy (LIM 1986).

The motile properties of the outer hair cells can be measured in the external auditory canal as so-called otoacoustic emissions in a retrograde direction to the physiological sound movement (KEMP 1978; PROBST et al. 1987). According to a large number of studies, not only morphologically visible changes to the outer hair cells result in sound emission disturbances, but also functional deficiencies (PLINKERT and KRÖBER 1991; PROBST 1990). Therefore, early detection before the occurrence of manifest damage under ototoxic therapy may be possible.

Regarding ototoxicity, inorganic platinum compounds, especially cisplatin but also carboplatin, play a major role as cytostatic agents in pediatric oncology. They are believed to inhibit cell devision (ROSENBERG et al. 1965), bind DNA bases intracellularly and link complementary DNA strings via guanine molecules (EASTMAN 1986). As the correctibility of neoplastic cells is reduced, a certain tumor selectivity manifests itself in this way (ZWELLING and KOHN 1979). Cisplatin is mainly excreted renally (DE SIMONE et al. 1979), so that the tissue concentration depends on the renal flow, which in view of the substantial nephrotoxicity must be taken into account (FLEISCHMANN et al. 1975). In addition to other side effects, serum electrolyte losses such as calcium and magnesium deficiency have also been described (Table 1, Fig. 1).

SABINE HARTMANN, Dr., Klinik für Phoniatrie und Pädiatrische Audiologie, Universität Münster, Kardinal-von-Galen-Ring 10, 48129 Münster, FRG

Table 1. Morphological and pathophysiological side effects in the cochlea after cisplatin

Damage of OHC beginning in the first row	From basal coil up to the upper coil of the cochlea	Atrophy of stria vascularis after higher dose	Decrease of second messenger function	Decrease of plasma membrane enzymes	Decrease of EP	Chemical changes	Increase after furosemide or aminoglycosides	References (animal studies)
					×			LAURELL and ENGSTRÖM 1989
	×							KURT et al. 1992
	×							FEDERSPIL et al. 1992
×								FLEISCHMANN et al. 1975
×		×						ANNIKO and SOBIN 1986
			×					KOCH and GLODDEK 1991
×	×						×	MARCO-ALGARRA et al. 1985
×	×	×			×			KOMMUNE et al. 1979
×	×			×		×		SPIRO et al. 1986
×	×							FERNÁNDEZ-CERVILLA et al. 1993

OHC, outer hair cells; EP, endocochlear potential.

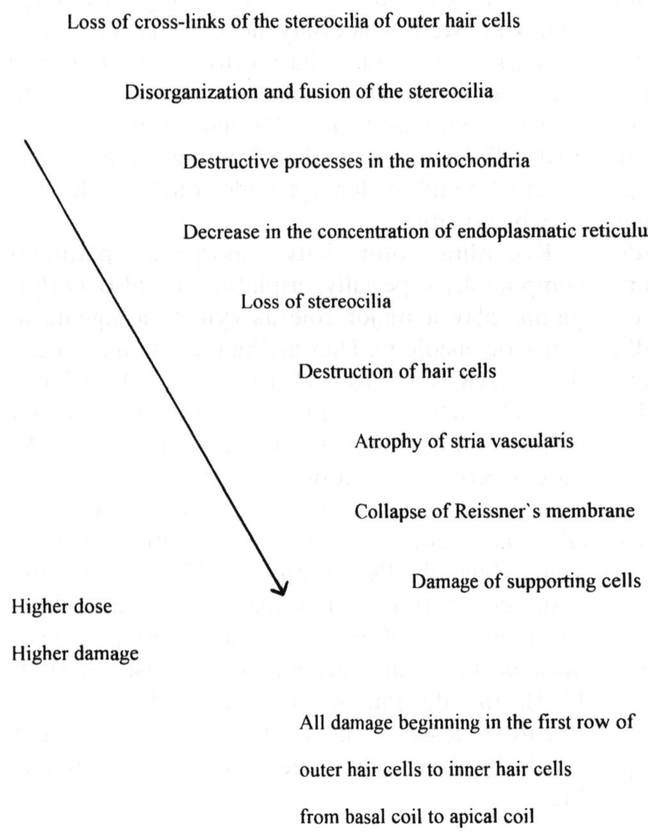

Fig. 1. Histopathological changes in the inner ear after cisplatin (see KOMMUNE et al. 1981; MARCO-ALGARRA et al. 1985; SPIRO et al. 1986; FERNÁNDEZ-CERVILLA et al. 1993)

Table 2. Ototoxicity of cisplatin and carboplatin in clinical studies

Hearing loss after CP	Hearing loss after CaP	CaP less ototoxic than CP	Ototoxicity in relation to age	Remissions	Ototoxicity in relation to mode of administration	References
48%			No		×	SCHRÖDER et al. 1986
34%				×		PLINKERT and KRÖBER 1991
		×				KEHRL et al. 1992
	32% >10 dB		No			BAUER et al. 1992
		×				FEDERSPIL et al. 1992
43% >20 dB						DELB et al. 1992
50% Related to dose 27%–69%						LENARZ et al. 1992
			Yes		×	BECK et al. 1992
Related to dose 35% >10 dB 35%	37% >10 dB					WELKOBORSKY et al. 1992
High frequency			No			BROCK et al. 1992

CP, cisplatin; CaP, carboplatin.

Following administration of cisplatin, ultrastructural damage to the organ of hearing may be observed, depending on the dosage and form of administration. Initially, a decrease in the number of cross-links of the stereocilia of outer hair cells is seen, which may progress to produce clumping and loss of the sensory hairs (SPIRO et al. 1986). The morphological damage begins in the most peripheral row of the outer hair cells, until all rows of hair cells are affected, and progresses from basal to apical until ultimately also the inner hair cells and sustentacular cells show structural changes (MACRO-ALGARRA et al. 1985). The mitochondria become conspicuously swollen at a relatively early stage, and a reduction in the endolymphatic reticulum can also be seen. In other stages, atrophic changes to the stria vascularis, which in conjunction with other factors is responsible for maintaining the endolymphatic ion environment, and defects in Reissner's membrane can be found (KOMMUNE et al. 1981).

Pathophysiological investigations suggest that cisplatin attacks functional processes, controlled by second messengers, of the outer hair cells and of the stria vascularis and also has an inhibiting effect on adenyl cyclase, i.e., there is an effect on the energy metabolism followed by a reduction in contractility (KOCH and GLODDECK 1991). A further indication of this is a fall of the endocochlea potential (LAURELL and ENGSTRÖM 1989). The electrolyte losses caused by cisplatin and its nephrotoxicity indicate the same point of attack. Earlier studies describe protein synthesis disturbance and losses of activity of various plasma membrane enzymes, i.e., alkaline phosphatase, 5-nucleotidase, calcium-, sodium- and potassium-ATPase (MARCO-ALGARRA et al. 1985; SPIRO et al. 1986; Table 2).

The studies of the last few years have given a frequency of auditory defects due to cisplatin ranging between 5% and 91%, depending on the different dosages, forms and points of administration and on differing concepts of auditory damage

(BAUER et al. 1992; BECK et al. 1992; PLINKERT and KRÖBER 1991; SCHRÖDER et al. 1986). To summarize, with a medium total cisplatin dose of 600 mg per m^2 body surface area, high-frequency auditory defects occur in approximately 50% of the cases, while the hearing loss rises in line with the dose and also extends into the middle frequency range. The greatest ototoxic effects are caused by bolus injections. Already existing damage to the organs of hearing and increasing age appear to intensify the hearing loss. Reports of sudden deafness are extremely rare, and where it does occur, it is after rapid highdose infusion (150–200 mg/m^2 body surface area). A rise in ototoxicity through certain diuretics like furosemide and ethacrynic acid was demonstrated in animal experiments (KOCH and GLODDEK 1991; RYBAK 1982), and a decrease was seen in the use of osmotic diuretics, e.g., mannitol (MAROSO and BLAIR 1983). If an additional aminoglycoside therapy is necessary or if cranial radiation takes place prior to cytostasis, a significant increase in auditory damage must be considered (GÖBEL et al. 1986; KAUS 1992).

For some time now, carboplatin, a substance developed from cisplatin, has been available, and is reported to have higher myelotoxicity, lower nephrotoxicity and, in general, a lower rate of side effects. According to the few studies available, the ototoxicity appears to be smaller, though not with statistical significance (BAUER et al. 1992; DELB et al. 1993; WELKOBORSKY et al. 1992).

The changes in cell morphology due to administration of cisplatin appear to be preceded by a loss of function of the outer hair cells, as measured by the otoacoustic emissions. At our disposal a specific method of measurement is available which permits an assessment of the function of the outer hair cells. KUMPF and HOKE (1970) succeeded in measuring spontaneous sound emissions of the inner ear in the external auditory canal. KEMP (1978) gave a description of evoked otoacoustic emissions (OAE). Click-evoked OAE can be observed in over 95% of all ears with normal hearing, though it should be pointed out that for registering click-evoked OAE above all a preserved hearing ability between 1 and 2 KHz is of importance (PROBST 1990).

According to all available studies and our own results, OAE cannot be demonstrated in persons with a hearing loss greater than 25–30 dB, at above 90% sensitivity and specificity (KEMP 1978; PROBST 1990). The amplitude of sound emissions is regularly reduced under hypoxia, exposure to noise and ototoxic medication such as cisplatin without a loss of hearing being initially discernible in the sound threshold audiogram (BECK et al. 1992; PLINKERT and KRÖBER 1991; PROBST 1990; SPOENDLIN 1969). A recovery of the amplitude has not been observed so far. Distortion product OAE (DP OAE) are responses of the cochlea to intermodulation products or combination tones occurring after stimulation with two sinus tones of defined frequency and volume, whose frequency can be described mathematically and whose amplitude depends on the volume of the primary tones (PROBST 1990). Thus, it appears possible in many cases to perform frequency-specific measurements, whereby the amplitude often seems to follow the structure of the hearing curve in the sound audiogram (HAUSER et al. 1991; Table 3).

Table 3. Hearing defects after cisplatin therapy: sound audiogram vs EOAE

Sound audiogram	EOAE	References
5%	57%	LENARZ 1992
R > 20 dB	RA: 20%	
48%	86%	BECK et al. 1992
R > 10 dB	RA: 13.3%–37.9%	
7%	34%	PLINKERT and KRÖBER 1991
R > 10 dB	RA: 30%	

EOAE, evoked otoacoustic emissions; R, reduction; RA, reduction of amplitude.

In approximately 30% of cases, cochlear damage can already be diagnosed before clinical symptoms under cisplatin therapy occur (PLINKERT and KRÖBER 1991). The increasing loss of function of the outer hair cells apparently leads to a reduction in emission response before the emergency of major morphological damage.

Regular controls of hearing ability using OAE should be performed before and after each administration of cisplatin, as the method is quick (approximately 1–2 min per ear), independent of the subjective statements of the patient and is not excessively distressing for the patient.

References

Anniko M, Sobin A (1986) Cisplatin: evaluation of its ototoxic potential. Am J Otolaryngol 7: 276–293

Arnold W, Anniko M, Pfaltz CR (1990) Funktionelle Morphologie der äußeren Haarzellen des Menschen. Laryngorhinootologie 69: 177–186

Bauer FP, Westhofen M, Kehrl W (1992) Zur Ototoxizität des Zytostatikums Carboplatin bei Patienten mit Kopf-Hals Tumoren. Laryngorhinootologie 71: 412–415

Beck A, Maurer J, Welkoborsky HJ et al (1992) Veränderungen transitorisch evozierter otoakustischer Emissionen unter Chemotherapie mit Cisplatin und 5FU. HNO 40: 123–127

Brock PR, Yeomans EC, Bellmann SC et al (1992) Cisplatin therapy in infants: Short and long-term morbidity British Journal of Lancer 66 Suppl 18: 36–40

Delb W, Koch A, Kurt P et al (1992) Klinische Untersuchungen zur Ototoxizität des Cisplatin bei pädiatrischen Patienten. In: Lang N, Jäger W (eds) Aktuelle Onkologie 68, Zytostatika bedingte Nebenwirkungen. Zuckerschwerdt, Munich

Delb W, Feilen S, Koch A et al (1993) Vergleichende Untersuchungen zur Ototoxizität des Cisplatin und des Carboplatin. Laryngorhinootologie 72: 24–27

De Simone PA, Yancey RS, Coupal JJ et al. (1979) Effect of a forced diuresis on the distribution and excretion of ^{195m}platinum when given as ^{195m}platinum. Cancer Treat Rep 63: 2023–2025

Drenckhahn D, Schäfer T, Prinz M (1985) Actin myosin and associated proteins in the vertebrate auditory and vestibular organs. In: Drescher DG (ed) Auditory biochemistry. Thomas, Springfield, pp 317–335

Eastman A (1986) Reevaluation of interaction of cisdichloro (ethylendiammine) platinum(2) with DNA. Biochemistry 25: 3912–3915

Federspil P et al (1992) Vergleichende Untersuchungen zur Ototoxizität von Cisplatin und Carboplatin. In: Lang N, Jäger W (eds) Aktuelle Onkologie 68, Zytostatika bedingte Nebenwirkungen. Zuckerschwerdt, Munich

Fernández-Cervilla F, Crespo PV, Ciges M et al (1993) Early morphofunctional alterations induced by cisplatin in the cochlea. Oto Rhino Laryngol 55: 337–340

Fleischmann RW, Stadnicki SW, Ethien MF et al (1975) Ototoxicity of cis-dichlorodiammineplatinum (2) in the guinea pig. Toxicol Appl Pharmacol 33: 320–332

Göbel U, Lamprecht A, Beron B (1986) Akuter Hörverlust bei Kindern mit vorbestrahlten intrakraniellen Tumoren nach einmaliger hochdosierter Cis-Platin-Gabe. Klin Padiatr 198: 277–280

Hauser R, Probst R, Harris FP et al (1991) Die klinische Anwendung otoakustischer kochleärer Distorsionsprodukte. Laryngorhinootologie 70: 123–131

Hudspeth AJ (1985) The cellular basis of hearing: the biophysics of hair cells. Science 230: 745–752

Kaus S (1992) The influence of calcium on the ototoxicity of aminoglycosides. Acta Otolaryngol (Stockh) 112: 83–87

Kehrl W, Flöttmann T, Bauer FP et al (1992) Vergleichende Untersuchungen zur Toxizität von Cisplatin und Carboplatin bei der Kombinationstherapie mit 5-FU. In: Lang N, Jäger W (eds) Aktuelle Onkologie 68, Zytostatika bedingte Nebenwirkungen. Zuckerschwerdt, Munich

Kemp DT (1978) Stimulated acoustic emissions from within the human auditory system. J Acoust Soc Am 64(5): 1386–1391

Kim DO (1986) Active and nonlinear cochlear biomechanics and the role of outer-hair cell subsystem in the mammalian auditory system. Hear Res 22: 105–114

Koch T, Gloddek B (1991) Inhibition of the adenylate cyclase-coupled G protein complex by ototoxic diuretics and cis-platinum in the inner ear of the guinea pig. Arch Otorhinolaryngol 248: 459–464

Kommune S, Asakuma S, Snow JB (1981) Pathophysiology of the ototoxicity of cis-diamine dichloroplatinum. Otolaryngol Head Neck Surg 89: 275–282

Kumpf W, Hoke M (1970) Ein konstantes Ohrgeräusch bei 4000 Hz. Arch Klin Exp Ohr Nase Kehlkopfheilkd 196: 243–247

Kurt P, Loew M, Federspil A et al (1992) Die Cisplatin-Ototoxizität-Einfluß von Dosisaufteilung und Furosemidgaben. In: Lang N, Jäger W (eds) Aktuelle Onkologie 68, Zytostatika bedingte Nebenwirkungen. Zuckerschwerdt, Munich

Laurell G, Engström B (1989) The ototoxic effect of cisplatin on guinea pigs in relation to dosage. Hear Res 38: 27–34

Lenarz T (1992) Neue Verfahren zur Erfassung der Ototoxizität von Zytostatika. In: Lang N, Jäger W (eds) Aktuelle Onkologie 68, Zytostatika bedingte Nebenwirkungen. Zuckerschwerdt, Munich

Lim DJ (1986) Cochlear micromechanics in understanding otoacoustic emission. Scand Audiol Suppl 25: 17–25

Macro-Algarra J, Basterra J, Macro J (1985) Cis-diamine-dichloro platinum ototoxicity. Acta Otolaryngol (Stockh) 99: 343–347

Mark HE, Rattay F (1991) Das Innenohr als elektrosensorisches Sinnesorgan. Laryngorhinootologie 70: 340–349

Moroso MJ, Blair RL (1983) A review of cis-platinum ototoxicity. J Otolaryngol 12: 365–369

Plinkert PK, Kröber S (1991) Früherkennung einer Cisplatin-Ototoxizität durch evozierte otoakustische Emissionen. Laryngorhinootologie 70: 457–462

Plinkert PK, Lenarz T (1992) Evozierte otoakustische Emissionen und ihre Beeinflussung durch kontralaterale akustische Stimulation. Laryngorhinootologie 71: 74–78

Plinkert PK, Zenner HP (1992) Sprachverständnis und otoakustische Emissionen durch Vorverarbeitung des Schalls im Innenohr. HNO 40: 111–122

Probst R, Lonsbury-Martin L, Martin GK et al (1987) Otoacoustic emissions in ears with hearing loss. Am J Otolaryngol 8: 73–81

Probst R (1990) Otoacoustic emissions: an overview. In: Pfaltz CR (ed) New aspects of cochlear mechanics and inner ear pathophysiology. Adv Otorhinolaryngol 44: 1–91

Rosenberg B, Van Camp L, Krigas T (1965) Inhibition of cell devision in Escherichia coli by electrolysis products from a platinum electode. Nature 205: 698–699

Rybak LP (1982) Pathophysiology of furosemide ototoxicity J Otolaryngol 11: 127–133

Schröder M, Laskawi R, Stennert E et al (1986) Cis-Platin Ototoxizität. Laryngorhinootologie 65: 86–89

Spiro DC, Rhys-Evans PH, Osborne MP et al (1986) Early morphological and chemical changes induced by cisplatin in the guinea pig organ of corti. Laryngol Otol 100: 1375–1383

Spoendlin HH (1960) Submikroskopische Strukturen im Cortischen Organ der Katze. Acta Otolaryngol (Stockh) 52: 11

Spoendlin HH (1969) Innervation patterns in the organ of corti of the cat. Acta Otolaryngol (Stockh) 67: 239–254

Van Bekesey G (1960) Experiments in hearing. Mc Graw-Hill, New York

Welkoborsky HJ, Bleier R, Wissen-Siegert I (1992) Antineoplastische Wirksamkeit und underwünschte Nebenwirkungen der Polychemotherapie ausgedehnter Oro- und Hypopharyngxkarzinome. Laryngorhinootologie 71: 261–266

Zenner HP, Gitter A, Zimmermann U et al. (1985) Die isolierte, lebende Haarzelle. Laryngorhinootologie 64: 642

Zenner HP (1986) Aktive Bewegungen von Haarzellen: ein neuer Mechanismus beim Hörvorgang HNO 34: 133–138

Zenner HP, Gitter AH (1987) Die Schallverarbeitung des Ohres. Physik Unserer Zeit 18: 97–105

Zenner HP, Plinkert PK (1994) Aspekte der Physiologie und Pathophysiologie der Schallverarbeitung im Innenohr bei Lärmexposition. In: Dieroff HG (ed) Lärmschwerhörigkeit. Fischer, Jena

Zwelling LA, Kohn KW (1979) Machanism of action of cis-dischlorodiammineplatinum (2). Cancer Treat Rep 63: 1439–1444

3 Skin and Mucosal Toxicity

3.1 Biological Basis for Skin and Mucosal Toxicity

KLAUS-RÜDIGER TROTT

CONTENTS

1 Introduction 89
2 The Pathogenesis of Acute Mucositis 89
3 Mechanisms of the Regenerative Response of the Irradiated Mucosa 90
4 The Pathogenesis of Chronic Epithelial Atrophy . . 90
5 Conclusions 90
References 91

1 Introduction

Both the epidermis, which is a keratinizing squamous epithelium, and the oral mucosa, which is a nonkeratinizing squamous epithelium, are characterized by rapid cell turnover. In normal squamous epithelium, cell production and cell differentiation are well organized in separate cell layers with unidirectional flow of cells from the suprabasal to the superficial cell layers. The life span of a newly formed cell in the germinative layer of the human oral mucosa until its sequestration from the mucosal surface is about 5 days; i.e. about once per week the mucosa is completely replaced by a new mucosal membrane through cell production by the stem cells and the transit cells in the germinative layer. Irradiation causes mucositis (and, in an analogous way, dermatitis) by inhibiting the cell production which is needed for this continuous replacement. For this reason, after high single doses or very accelerated irradiation, the latency to the characteristic signs of acute radiation injury is similar or only a little longer than the normal epithelial turnover time, i.e. about 1 week in oral mucosa and 2 weeks in skin. The radiation-induced inhibition of cell production causes an acute hypoplasia in the epithelium. The symptoms of acute radiation injury such as erythema and pain, however, do not arise in the hypoplastic epithelium itself but in the supporting vascular connective tissue, i.e. the submucosa and dermis, respectively, probably in response to the functional insufficiency of the hypoplastic epithelium.

KLAUS-RÜDIGER TROTT, Prof. Dr., Department of Radiation Biology, St. Bartholomew's Medical College, Charterhouse Square, London EC1M 6BQ, UK

2 The Pathogenesis of Acute Mucositis

This simple pathogenetic model of acute epidermal and mucosal radiation injury (POTTEN 1985) becomes much more complicated if radiation is not given as single or concentrated irradiation but in daily fractions of about 2 ($\pm$0.5) Gy. Signs and symptoms of mucositis do not appear before the third radiotherapy week, i.e. after an accumulated radiation dose of about 25 Gy. As treatment continues, the severity of mucositis increases to patchy erosions, often reaching a plateau during the last 2 weeks of radiotherapy and occasionally even improving despite further accumulation of dose (FLETCHER et al. 1962).

This typical pattern of oral mucositis demonstrates that even during an ongoing course of radiotherapy compensatory processes are initiated which in most patients effectively counteract any further increase in radiation injury. Their cellular basis is accelerated repopulation which, during the last week of radiotherapy, is capable of compensating the cytotoxic effect of nearly 2 Gy per day (THAMES et al. 1990).

During daily irradiation with 2 Gy, epithelial cell density in pig skin decreases linearly over time but much slower than predicted by the normal epithelial cell turnover rate (MORRIS and HOPEWELL 1986). A similar effect is seen in mouse oral mucosa (KUMMERMEHR et al. 1992). The increased regeneration rate is well regulated and exactly balances the rate of radiation-induced cell killing. In this way a new steady state of cell production and cell killing is established on a reduced level of epithelial cellularity (KUMMERMEHR et al. 1992).

Detailed studies on the proliferation kinetics of the epidermis and of the mucosal epithelium during this new steady state identified profound changes in the pattern of cell proliferation and cell differentiation (TROTT and KUMMERMEHR 1993). Most important is a shift from the asymmetrical stem cell divisions which are characteristic for unperturbed continually renewing tissues such as the epidermis, to symmetrical divisions only: Whereas in normal mucosa, 50% of the newly born stem cells leave the stem cell compartment to enter the transit compartment, during the new steady state all newly born stem cells remain stem cells. In addition, the cell cycle time of stem cells and transit cells may be reduced and the pool of transit cells may be enlarged (TROTT and KUMMERMEHR 1993). It is tempting to speculate that this adaptive mechanism is regulated by changes in the expression of some cytokines both in the epithelium and in the supportive connective tissue. Yet little is known so far on the cytokine network which regulates proliferation and differentiation in oral mucosa and in skin. Even less is known about the signals which trigger those changes of proliferation and differentiation at a well defined level of radiation-induced cell depletion. Histologically, the mucosal epithelium, although reduced with regard to cell numbers, looks remarkable intact (KUMMERMEHR et al. 1992).

3 Mechanisms of the Regenerative Response of the Irradiated Mucosa

Since accelerated repopulation starts at about the same time as radiation-induced erythema, a causal relation between inflammatory and regenerative response of the oral mucosa and the skin to the radiation injury appears a plausible hypothesis.

The observation of FLETCHER et al. (1962) that frequently signs and symptoms of oral mucositis plateau or even improve during the last week of a 6–7 weeks course of radiotherapy, indicates that the mucosa should be able, in principle, to compensate completely the daily dose by accelerated regeneration. Yet nearly all patients treated for head and neck cancer by curative radiotherapy develop painful acute oropharyngeal mucositis. Obviously, the mucosa does not register the ongoing radiation damage during the first few weeks and therefore does not call in the reserves of its regenerative potential until too late, i.e. until too much dose has been accumulated and too many mucosal stem cells have been sterilized. The clinical problem of acute mucositis despite the pronounced regenerative capacity of the mucosa is caused by the delay between induction of radiation injury and manifestation of radiation damage. It is only the latter which is registered by the tissue and which triggers the regenerative response.

Experimental studies (DÖRR and KUMMEMEHR 1992) and clinical experiments (MACIEJEWSKI et al. 1991) demonstrate that acute radiation tolerance of the oral mucosa can be improved if the manifestation of radiation injury is made to occur earlier or by unspecific stimulation of cell turnover. These preliminary data suggest principles of potential therapeutic strategies to improve acute radiation tolerance by manipulating the molecular and cellular regulation of cell proliferation and differentiation in irradiated epithelia.

4 The Pathogenesis of Chronic Epithelial Atrophy

Whereas acute radiation damage of oral mucosa and skin may be described as inflammatory reaction of the supportive vascular-connective tissue to the radiation-induced epithelial hypoplasia, chronic radiation damage such as epithelial atrophy is due to direct radiation injury to the vascular- connective tissue with secondary effects on the epithelium. The primary target appears to be the capillary endothelial cell which may suffer functional radiation damage (see chapter by SCHULTZ-HECTOR, this volume). By yet undisclosed mechanisms, the radiation damage of individual endothelial cells results in the loss of entire capillaries causing ischaemia and further leading to tissue fibrosis and sclerosis and, in dependent parenchyma such as epithelium, to atrophy. There is some evidence that these processes, too, do not progress in a deterministic way but are subject to various regulatory processes. Cytokines may play a role here, too. Transforming growth factor-ß mRNA is increased in irradiated pig skin during the erythema stage to remain there for the entire process of dermal fibrosis (MARTIN et al. 1993). The continuous production of this cytokine may be an important signal causing increased fibroblast proliferation and differentiation.

5 Conclusions

No tissue has been studied more extensively with regard to the pathogenesis and biology of acute and chronic radiation damage than skin and oral mucosa. Yet new radiobiological and molecular research has opened a different appreciation of these presumedly well understood radiation effects. The most important new message is that both acute and chronic radiation injury should no longer be regarded as a deterministic progression defined by radiation dose and cell inactivation alone but as a process which is subject to complex regulations and, therefore, potentially subject to therapeutic interference.

References

Dörr W, Kummermehr J (1992) Increased radiation tolerance of mouse tongue epithelium after local conditioning. Int J Radiat Biol 61: 369–379

Fletcher GH, MacComb WS, Shalek RJ (1962) Radiation therapy in the management of cancer of the oral cavity and oropharyngx. Thomas, Springfield, Illinois

Kummermehr J, Dörr W, Trott KR (1992) Kinetics of accelerated repopulation in normal and malignant squamous epithelia during fractionated radiotherapy. Br J Radiol Suppl 24: 193–199

Maciejewski B, Zajusz A, Pilecki B, Swiatnicka J, Skladowski K, Dörr W, Kummermehr J, Trott KR (1991) Acute mucositis in the stimulated oral mucosa of patients during radiotherapy for head and and neck cancer. Radiother Oncol 22: 7–11

Martin M, Lefaix JL, Pinton P, Crechet F, Daburon F (1993) Temporal modulation of TGFß1 and ß-actin gene expression in pig skin and muscular fibrosis after ionizing radiation. Radiat Res 134: 63–70

Morris GM, Hopewell JW (1986) Changes in the cell kinetics of pig epidermis after repeated daily doses of X-rays. Br J Radiol Suppl 19: 34–38

Potten CS (1985) Radiation and skin. Taylor and Francis, London

Thames HD, Benzen SM, Turesson I, Overgaard M, van den Bogaert W (1990) Time-dose factors in radiotherapy: a review of the human data. Radiother Oncol 19: 219–235

Trott KR, Kummermehr J (1993) The time factor and repopulation in tumors and normal tissues. Semin Radiat Oncol 3: 115–125

3.2 Radiation-Induced Fibrosis: Experimental Studies

H. Peter Rodemann, Anke Binder, and Michael Bamberg

CONTENTS

1 Introduction . . . 93
2 Materials and Methods . . . 94
3 Results . . . 94
3.1 Radiation-Induced Terminal Differentiation . . . 94
3.2 Transforming Growth Factor-ß-Induced Terminal Differentiation . . . 94
3.3 Radiation-Induced Growth and Differentiation Promoting Factors . . . 95
4 Discussion . . . 95
References . . . 97

1 Introduction

Fibrosis is a common sequela of both cancer treatment by radiotherapy and accidental irradiation and has been described in many tissues, including skin (Brocherion et al. 1986), lung (Bentzen et al. 1989), heart (Lopez Cardoso et al. 1985) and liver (Fajardo and Stewart 1973). Fibrotic lesions contain infiltrating inflammatory cells, fibroblasts and large amounts of various extracellular matrix components. In fibrotic tissues an enhanced synthesis and deposition of the interstitial collagens fibronectin and proteoglycans have been described (Althan and Gerber 1983). At the cellular level the histologically observed abnormal proliferation of fibroblasts is considered to be a major event occurring during the onset and progression of the fibrotic reaction in vivo. However, the mechanisms triggering normal fibroblasts to undergo fibrotic changes have not been identified.

Using cytomorphological, biochemical and molecular biological markers, the fibroblast cell system of the connective tissues of skin, lung, and kidney of various mammalian species, including humans, has been shown to be comprised of three mitotically active progenitor fibroblast cell types, MFI, MFII, MFIII, and three postmitotic fibrocytes, PMFIV, PMFV, PMFVI) (Bayreuther et al. 1989; Rodemann et al. 1989a, 1993). The postmitotic fibrocyte PMFVI represents the terminally differentiated cell of the fibroblast system, with specific functions in the synthesis and deposition of extracellular matrix components and other factors interacting with neighboring cell systems (Bayreuther et al. 1986; Rodemann et al. 1989a, b, 1993). In vivo there is probably a well balanced, cellular steady state ratio between progenitor fibroblasts and postmitotic fibrocytes that maintains tissue function. Since the lifespan of the postmitotic fibrocytes is limited, these cells have to be renewed from the mitotically active progenitor fibroblasts via induction of differentiation divisions (Rodemann 1993). Thus, disturbances in the differentiation processes of fibroblasts due to exogenous factors, e.g., radiation, could be a basis for connective or interstitial tissue alterations.

Based on recent in vitro data analyzing the effect of cytokines on fibroblast proliferation and collagen synthesis, it can be speculated that cytokines, e.g., transforming growth factor-ß (TGF-ß), which control the growth, differentiation and function of mesenchymal cells might be involved in the induction of fibrosis. TGF-ß is known to activate gene transcription and to increase the synthesis and secretion of matrix proteins such as type I and III collagens or fibronectin. Furthermore, TGF-ß reduces the synthesis of matrix degrading proteolytic enzymes and enhances the production of certain protease inhibitors (Varga et al. 1987). Thus, TGF-ß resembles a good candidate for one of the key cytokines which may be involved in the cascade of events resulting in fibrosis.

In the present study we have analyzed how radiation affects the differentiation pattern of lung fibroblasts and how these processes are influenced by TGF-ß. We will provide evidence that radiation-induced and/or TGF-ß-dependent changes in the differentiation pattern of human lung fibroblasts that are observable in vitro could be relevant for

H. Peter Rodemann, Prof. Dr., Anke Binder, Dr., Michael Bamberg, Prof. Dr., Abteilung Strahlenbiologie, Universität Tübingen Röntgenweg 11, 72076 Tübingen, FRG

understanding the mechanisms resulting in the onset and progression of the fibrotic reaction in vivo.

2 Materials and Methods

Normal human lung fibroblast cultures from fetal (cell line Wi 38) or adult (CCD14) lung were routinely cultured in Dulbecco's modification of Eagle's medium (DMEM) supplemented with pretested 10% fetal calf serum (Fcs) and standard amounts of antibiotics. Cells were passaged once weekly with constant seeding density of 1×10^6 cells per 50 cm^2 dish. Cultures used for the various experiments were at identical passage levels (P12–15).

Cells to be irradiated were seeded at a density of 250 cells per 9 cm^2 multiwell dishes and incubated with DMEM and 20% FCS. Some 24 h after seeding, cells were irradiated with varying radiation doses (0–12 Gy) generated by a linear accelerator (2 Gy/min) and incubated thereafter for an additional 14 days. Both colony formation and the differentiation states of the surviving colonies were determined after fixing and staining the cells according to standard procedures (Bayreuther et al. 1988a; Rodemann et al. 1989a).

For coculture experiments, cells to be irradiated were seeded at a density of 10 000 cells per cm^2 on Cyclopore coculture inserts (Becton Dickinson) precoated with serum to increase cell attachment. After 24 h, cells were irradiated with a single dose of 5 Gy. Directly after irradiation coculture inserts were placed over test fibroblast cultures either prepared for colony formation or for analysis of DNA synthesis.

Using the colony formation assay the effect of TGF-ß on the differentiation pattern of human lung fibroblasts was analyzed. Therefore, cells were treated permanently with varying doses of TGF-ß (0, 0.2, 1.0, and 10 ng/ml) added to the culture medium. After 14 days the differentiation pattern of the cultures were analyzed according to standard procedures (Bayreuther et al. 1988a; Rodemann et al. 1989a).

In order to determine the fraction of proliferating cells after the various treatment procedures (radiation, TGF-ß, cocultures) cells were incubated with 5-bromodeoxyuridine (BUdr) for 17 h. The incorporation of BUdr in the fraction of growing cells was demonstrated by a BUdr-specific antibody staining procedure.

3 Results

3.1 Radiation-Induced Terminal Differentiation

Fibroblast cultures predominantly composed of MFII-type cells (MFII 80%, MFIII 17%, PMF 3%) showed an accelerated terminal differentiation within 15 days of postirradiation culture. The cell composition of control populations showed no change during the incubation time, while in cultures irradiated with either 1 or 7 Gy significant changes in the cell type frequencies occurred. After approximately 3 days, the amounts of cell type MFII decreased while cell type MFIII increased until day 7–8. Thereafter, MFIII cells disappeared resulting in increasing amounts of postmitotic fibrocytes up to day 15. At day 15 approximately 70% (1 Gy) or 93% (7 Gy) of all cells present were of the postmitotic differentiation state (Rodemann et al. 1991).

As demonstrated by the method of high resolution 2-dimensional gel electrophoresis the radiation-induced postmitotic fibrocytes expressed the same marker proteins described earlier for spontaneously arisen PMF-type cells (Bayreuther et al. 1988a; Rodemann et al. 1989a; data not shown). Likewise, radiation-induced PMF-type cells showed approximately the same changes in collagen synthesis (enhancement of total collagen synthesis by a factor of 4–5, with specific alterations in the relative amounts of the interstitial collagens) as described for PMF type cells resulting from spontaneous terminal differentiation (Rodemann et al. 1991).

3.2 Transforming Growth Factor-ß-Induced Terminal Differentiation

In order to elucidate whether TGF-ß might act as a modulator of fibroblast differentiation, cells were treated with varying doses of TGF-ß. As shown in Table 1, TGF-ß induced within 14 days of culture a significant shift towards postmitotic cell types, as analyzed in a colony formation assay. When untreated control cultures were compared to cultures treated with 0.1, 1.0 or 10 ng/ml TGF-ß the amount of PMF-type cells increased concentration dependently by a factor of 4–14 above controls (Table 1). Likewise, within 14 days of TGF-ß treatment the amount of growing cells decreased from about 30% to 3%–5% (data not shown) indicating an increase in the fraction of noncycling postmitotic cells (data

Table 1. Effect of TGF-ß on fibroblast differentiation in vitro: relative amounts (%) MFII, MFIII, and PMF after 14 days of culture

	Starting population	TGF-ß (ng/ml) 0	0.1	1.0	10.0
MFII	38	36	32	13	12
MFIII	59	61	56	50	48
PMF	3	3	12	37	40

TGF-ß, transforming growth factor-ß; MFII, MFIII, mitotically active progenitor fibroblasts; PMF, postmitotic fibrocytes.

not shown). However, during the first 3–5 days there was a slight increase in the number of proliferating cells.

3.3 *Radiation-Induced Growth and Differentiation Promoting Factors*

Coculture experiments of irradiated and nonirradiated cells were performed in order to analyze whether irradiated cells produce factors which are able to modulate the proliferation and differentiation potential of nonirradiated cocultured cells. As demonstrated in Fig. 1, colony formation of nonirradiated fibroblasts was significantly affected when these cells were cocultured with irradiated fibroblasts. The cloning efficiency of the nonirradiated fibroblasts was stimulated by about 40% above the control values of fibroblasts cocultured with nonirradiated cells. Furthermore, when the colonies formed were analyzed for the differentiation states a strong stimulation (of about 100%) of colonies of cell type MFI could be observed, while colony formation of the cell type MFII was decreased by approximately 30%. No change was observable with cell type MFIII; however, the amount of postmitotic cells increased by about 40% above control level. These data, proliferation and differentiation induction caused by the irradiated coculture cell system are further supported by the result of the BUdr incorporation measurements. The growth fraction of the test lung fibroblast culture could be stimulated by about 30%–35% after 24 h of coculture with 5 Gy irradiated fibroblasts as compared to the nonirradiated controls.

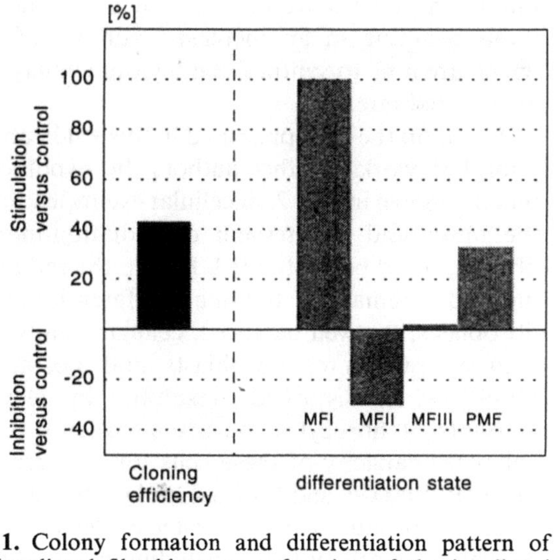

Fig. 1. Colony formation and differentiation pattern of nonirradiated fibroblasts as a function of the irradiated cocultured cells. Fibroblasts irradiated with a single dose of 5 Gy were cocultured immediately after irradiation with test fibroblast cultures of defined differentiation state. After 14 days, colony formation and differentiation pattern of the test cultures were analyzed. *MFI, MFII, MFIII,* progenitor fibroblasts: *PMF,* postmitotic fibrocytes

4 Discussion

The cellular mechanism(s) triggering the fibrotic reaction in response to irradiation have not yet been resolved. It has long been held that chronic fibrosis may be caused by some mechanisms of cell activation and it has been suggested that an abnormal production of growth factors in irradiated tissues may play a role in the activation of certain cells, e.g., fibroblasts (Martin et al. 1993).

In the present study we have shown that irradiated fibroblast cultures undergo a premature and accelerated terminal differentiation process, from mitotically active progenitor cells to irreversible postmitotic mature fibrocytes. In the context of the organization of the fibroblast cell system terminally differentiated fibrocytes have been described to be the major cell type being responsible for the synthesis of the specific extracellular matrix components, e.g., interstitial collagens type I, III, and V (Rodemann et al. 1992). Ex vivo-in vitro experiments using primary cell cultures of human skin revealed that the connective tissue of skin in vivo contains a constant ratio of potentially mitotic progenitor fibroblasts and postmitotic mature fibrocytes (Bayreuther et al. 1988b). Thus, this cellular homeostasis could be essential for the function of the connective tissue. As demonstrated in long-term cultures of postmitotic human fibrocytes, these cells have a genetically determined life span of

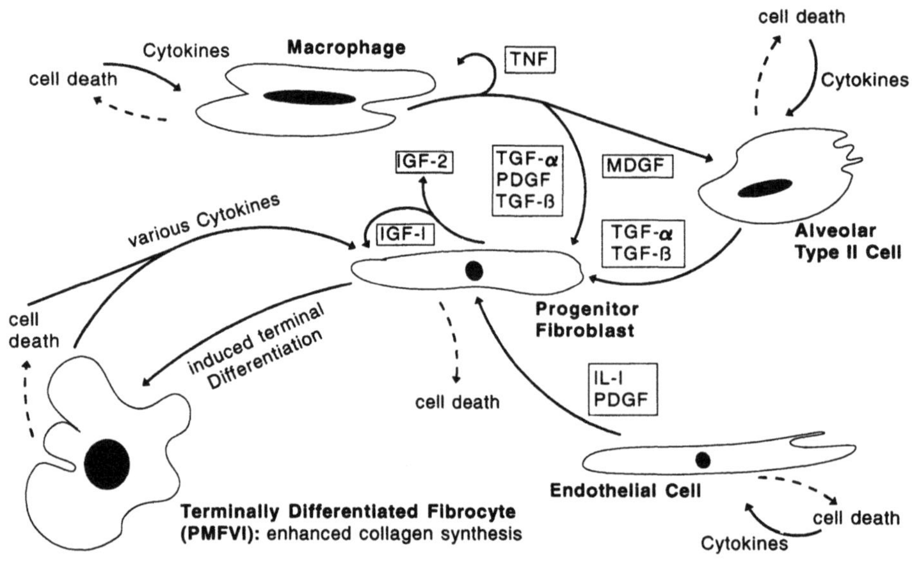

Fig. 2. Possible cellular communication pathways and events after irradiation injury in lung tissue. *TNF*, tumor necrosis factor, *IGF*, insoluble growth factor; *PDGF*, platelet-derived growth factor; *TGF*, transforming growth factor; *MDGF*, macrophage-derived growth factor; *IL*, interleukin

about 15 weeks in culture (BAYREUTHER et al. 1993). Thereafter, they undergo spontaneous degeneration presumably by the induction of apoptotic processes (BAYREUTHER et al. 1993). In order to maintain the cellular tissue homeostasis a loss of functioning mature fibrocytes in connective tissues due to the genetically determined lifespan most likely results in the induction of differentiation divisions of the progenitor fibroblasts into mature fibrocytes. A disturbance of this well coordinated, cellular tissue steady state ratio by factors affecting the differentiation process of progenitor fibroblasts into mature postmitotic fibrocytes could, thus, cause severe tissue alterations.

As demonstrated by the use of coculture systems irradiated cells produce some factor(s) which is (are) able to promote growth of nonirradiated cells, most likely by the induction of proliferation and differentiation divisions. It is well known that certain cell systems produce signals, such as cytokines or growth factors, in response to irradiation (MARTIN et al. 1993). The involvement of TGF-ß in particular has recently been suggested in the occurrence of radiation-induced fibrotic alterations in liver (ANSCHER et al. 1990) and colon (CANNEY and DEAN 1990). Furthermore, in various models of fibrosis, e.g. bleomycin-induced fibrosis of the lung (RAGHOW et al. 1989) or carbon tetrachloride-induced fibrosis of the liver (NAKATSUKASA et al. 1990), the involvement of TGF-ß has been demonstrated. Our results of a TGF-ß-induced premature terminal differentiation into postmitotic fibrocytes support the assumption that TGF-ß may act as a fibrogenic modulator. On the basis of our data it could be speculated that TGF-ß exhibits its fibrogenic action via the induction of differentiation divisions from mitotically active progenitor fibroblasts to postmitotic fibrocytes (RODEMANN and MÜLLER 1991). Thus, the amount of postmitotic fibrocytes would increase above normal levels resulting in an increased number of cells which are able to synthesise interstitial collagen at an elevated rate.

Based on the data presented in this study and on published work of other authors the hypothetical scheme shown in Fig. 2, of cellular events leading to the onset and progression of radiation-induced fibrosis, could be postulated. Due to the radiation-induced premature terminal differentiation of fibroblasts, the well balanced, cellular steady state between progenitor fibroblasts and postmitotic fibrocytes is disturbed, resulting in elevated amounts of fibrocytes. As a consequence of the enhanced capacity of these cells for collagen synthesis (RODEMANN and MÜLLER 1991), interstitial collagens are produced and deposited at elevated rates. Neighboring cell systems, including macrophages, alveolar type II pneumocytes and endothelial cells, may produce specific factors/ cytokines (e.g., TGF-ß) in response to irradiation which in turn react with the progenitor fibroblasts. Due to the action of these cytokines progenitor fibroblasts might be induced to differentiate into postmitotic fibrocytes. Based on this cytokine-induced disturbancy of the well balanced cellular homeostasis of progenitor fibroblasts and postmitotic fibrocytes, collagen synthesis and deposition in the irradiated tissue would be affected resulting in the fibrotic lesion. As demonstrated in this study and by others, TGF-ß could be one of the key cytokines involved in the onset of fibrosis. Thus, using well defined fibroblast cell systems for the analysis of biochemical and molecular biological events triggered by TGF-ß and other cytokines, it should be possible to elucidate the molecular mechanism(s) of radiation-induced fibrosis.

Acknowledgments. The authors are very grateful to Heidi Löffler for excellent technical assistance. This work was supported by a grant from the Deutsche Forschungsgemeinschaft, SFB 120, project B11.

References

Altman KI, Gerber GB (1983) The effect of ionizing radiations on connective tissue. In: Lett JT, Adler H (eds) Advances in radiation biology, vol. 10. Academic Press, New York, pp 237–304

Anscher MS, Crocker IR, Jirtle RL (1990) Transforming growth factor-ß1 expression in irradiation liver. Radiat Res 122: 77–85

Bayreuther K, Rodemann HP, Hommel R, Dittmann K, Albiez M, Francz PI (1988) Human skin fibroblasts in vitro differentiate along a terminal cell lineage. Proc Natl Acad Sci USA 85: 5112–5116

Bayreuther K, Rodemann HP, Francz PI, Maier K (1988) Differentiation of fibroblast stem cells. J Cell Sci 10: 115–130

Bayreuther K, Francz PI, Rodemann HP (1993) Fibroblasts in normal and pathological terminal differentiation, ageing, apoptosis and transformation. Arch Gerontal Geriatr Suppl 3: 47–74

Bentzen SM, Thames HD, Overgaard M (1989) Latent-time estimation for late cutaneous and subcutaneous radiation reactions in a single follow-up clinical study. Radiother Oncol 15: 267–274

Brocheriou C, Verola O, Lefaix J-L, Daburon F (1986) Pathology of high dose radiation-induced lesions. Br J Radiol Suppl 19: 101–108

Canney PA, Dean S (1990) Transforming growth factor beta: a promotor of late connective tissue injury following radiotherapy? Br J Radiol 63: 620–623

Fajardo LF, Stewart JR (1973) Pathogenesis of radiation-induced myocardinal fibrosis. Lab Invest 29: 244–257

Lopez-Cardozo BL, Zoctelief H, van Bekkum DW, Zurcher G, Hagenbeck A (1985) Lung damage following bone marrow transplantation. The contribution of irradiation. Int J Radiat Oncol Biol Phys 11: 907–914

Martin M, Lefaix JL, Pinton Ph, Crechet F, Daburon F (1993) Temporal modulation of TGF-ß and ß-actin gene expression in pig skin, muscular fibrosis after ionizing radiation. Radiat Res 134: 63–70

Nakatsukasa H, Nagy P, Evarts RP, Hsia CC, Marsden E, Thorgeirsson S (1990) Cellular distribution of transforming growth factor-ß1 and procollagen types I, III and IV in carbon tetrachloride-induced rat liver fibrosis. J Clin Invest 85: 1833–1843

Raghow R, Irish P, Kang AH (1989) Coordinate regulation of transforming growth factor ß, gene expression and cell proliferation in hamster lungs and undergoing bleomycin-induced pulmonary fibrosis. J Clin Invest 84: 1836–1843

Rodemann HP, Bayreuther K, Francz PI, Dittmann K, Albiez M (1989a) Selective enrichment and biochemical characterization of seven human skin fibroblast cell types in vitro. Exp Cell Res 180: 84–93

Rodemann HP (1989b) Differential degradation of intracellular proteins in human skin fibroblasts of mitotic and mitomycin-C-induced postmitotic differentiation states in vitro. Differentiation 42: 37–43

Rodemann HP, Peterson HP, Schwenke K, von Wangenheim K-H (1991) Terminal differentiation of human fibroblasts is induced by radiation. Scann Microsc 5: 1135–1143

Rodemann HP, Müller GA (1991) Characterization of human renal fibroblasts in health and disease: II. In vitro growth, differentiation and collagen synthesis of fibroblasts from kidneys with interstitial fibrosis. Am J Kidney Dis 17: 684–686

Rodemann HP, Wecke P, Jaeschke M (1992) Low-frequency electromagnetic fields induce premature terminal differentiation of in vitro cultured human skin and lung fibroblasts. Bioelectrochem Bioenerg 27: 269–280

Rodemann HP (1993) Differential gene expression, protein synthesis and degradation in ageing fibroblasts. In: Bernd A (ed) Cell and tissue culture models for dermatological research. Springer, Berlin Heidelberg New York, pp 272–278

Varga J, Rosenbloom J, Jimenez S (1987) TGF-ß causes a persistent increase in the steady-state amounts of type I and type III collagen and fibronectin mRNAs in normal dermal fibroblasts. Biochem J 247: 597–604

3.3 Lymphedema of the Arm After Treatment of Breast Cancer

HEINRICH SCHÜNEMANN and NORMAN WILLICH

CONTENTS

1 Introduction 99
2 Patients and Methods 99
3 Results 100
4 Discussion 101
References 103

1 Introduction

Lymphedema arises if the lymph load exceeds the transport capacity due to blockage of the lymph vessel. This may be caused by mechanical strangulation of the lymph vessel or after partial destruction and scarring following surgery and radiotherapy. Since alternative drainage routes, including lymphatic bypasses, do not have the capacity to drain the lymph fluid completely, edema results (FÖLDI and FÖLDI 1993; INGIANNI and HOLZMANN 1985; LOTZE and RICHTER 1989; RÜNZI and HÜBNER 1985). Secondary lymphedema of the arm is frequently seen after primary treatment of a breast cancer (BATES 1988; BRISMAR and LJUNGDAHL 1983; RAY et al. 1983; WILLICH et al. 1989; YEO et al. 1986). However, the literature reveals significant differences in the reported lymphedema rate after similar treatment modalities (GÖLTNER et al. 1985; HUGHES and PATEL 1966; KINDLER 1984; LOBB and HARKINS 1949; RYTTOV et al. 1983). This can be explained by the lack of a well established definition of significant lymphedema and by the use of a variety of methods to measure the degree of lymphedema. While some investigators measure the circumference of the middle of the upper arm or the middle of the forearm, others determine the circumference at up to ten levels of the whole arm (BRISMAR and LJUNGDAHL 1983; GREGL et al. 1978; KINDLER 1984; LOBB and HARKINS 1949). Another method is volumetry by water plethysmometry, in which the extremity is dipped into water, but again either completely or incompletely (FÖLDI and FÖLDI 1993; LARSON et al. 1986; SWEDBORG and WALLGREN 1981; TRACY et al. 1961). Optoelectronical measurement by a commercially available volumeter (Volometer, Bösl Medizintechnik, Aachen, FRG) seems to be the most reliable method (FISCHBACH et al. 1986; GÖLTNER et al. 1985). The contralateral arm serves as the standard.

An accurate posttherapeutic assessment is only possible when a preoperative measurement of both arms has been done. Additionally, not only postoperative muscle atrophy, caused by adopting a compensating posture, may distort measurement of the affected arm, but also the physiologically large circumference of the normally preferred arm compared to the contralateral arm.

2 Patients and Methods

Since 1972, at the Bad Trissl hospital, the circumferences of the right and left upper arms and forearms have been recorded in centimeters, 10 cm above and below the olecranon. In this retrospective study the only patients analyzed were those with an increased circumference of at least 2 cm and for whom the histology of the tumor, the type of surgery and the technique of radiation were documented. Discrete lymphedemas measuring up to 1.9 cm in circumference were not included in this study to avoid methodological errors.

The primary treatment of the analyzed patients had already been partly carried out in the 1950s. In some cases the date of origin of the edema was not known due to a lack of documentation, but the frequency of the edema could be established. All cases were classified according to the UICC classification of 1987, which required a reclassification of

HEINRICH SCHÜNEMANN, Dr., Abteilung für Gynäkologie I und Lymphtherapie, Onkologische Klinik Bad Trissl, Bad Trissl-Straße 73, 83080 Oberaudorf, FRG
NORMAN WILLICH, Prof. Dr., Klinik und Poliklinik für Strahlentherapie – Radioonkologie, Westfälische Wilhelms-Universität Münster, Albert-Schweitzer-Straße 33, 48129 Münster, FRG

all cases up to 1987. In those cases in which the size of the primary tumor was not described quantitatively, but rather qualitatively and the number of removed axillary lymph nodes was not given by the pathologists, the stage was estimated as TX (size of primary tumor unknown) or as NO (no axillary lymph nodes involved) or as N+ (axillary lymph nodes involved).

3 Results

Between 1972 and 1989 a total of 4011 female patients with breast carcinoma were analyzed at the Bad Trissl hospital. There were 90 (2.2%) who had bilateral breast cancer. The total number of breast cancers therefore was 4101 (100%). Some 2009 tumors were located in the right breast (49.0%) and 2092 in the left breast (51.0%) (Table 1).

Secondary lymphedema of the arm was detected in 1107 (27%) breast cancers, 526 (47.5%) involved the right arm and 581 (52.5%) the left arm (Table 1).

Lymphedemas were found which had existed preoperatively due to axillary lymph node metastases or else occurred either immediately following surgery or only many years after primary treatment. In one patient lymphedema of the arm occurred 13 years after mastectomy and irradiation and without evidence of disease. On the average, for all 1107 lymphedemas, the increase of circumference was 4.2 cm with a maximum of 14 cm for the right arm and 24 cm for the left arm. The swelling of the right arm was on the average 4.6 cm and of the left arm 3.7 cm.

A total of 1630 breast cancers were treated by surgery alone, an incidence of subsequent edema of 20.3%. The rate of edema following combined surgery and irradiation of 2471 carcinomas was 31.4% (Table 2).

After radical mastectomy (Rotter-Halsted) for 731 breast cancers, after modified radical mastectomy for 3149 cancers and after breast conserving surgery for 221 cancers the lymphedema rates were 39.8%, 25.2% and 9.5%, respectively (Table 3).

The significance of irradiation for the development of lymphedema is evident: lymphedema rates were increased by radiotherapy after radical mastectomy (alone 22.7%) to 44.7%, after modified radical mastectomy (alone 19.9%) to 29.3% and after breast conserving surgery (6.9%) to 10.4% (Table 4).

Primary treatment before 1971 resulted in an edema rate of 37.6%, up to 1981 of 25.3% and up to 1989 of 18.1% (Fig. 1). This reduction of the lymphedema rate reflects the change in treatment modalities, from radical mastectomy with conventional X-ray irradiation in the early years to modified radical mastectomy with or without

Table 1. Breast cancer and secondary lymphedema 1972–1989

	n(%)
Breast cancer	4101 (100)
Unilateral	4011 (97.8)
Bilateral	90 (2.2)
Right side	2009 (49.0)
Left side	2092 (51.0)
Lymphedema of arm	1107 (27)
Right	526 (47.5)
Left	581 (52.5)

Table 2. Primary treatment ($n = 4101$): rate of edema

Procedure	Number of cases of edema	(%)
Surgery alone[a]	1630	(20.3)
Surgery + irradiation[b]	2471	(32.4)

[a]10% radical mastectomy, 86% modified radical mastectomy, 4% breast conserving surgery.
[b]23% radical mastectomy, 71% modified radical mastectomy, 7% breast conserving surgery.

Table 3. Rate of edema according to different surgical methods

Procedure	Number of cases of edema	(%)
Radical mastectomy[a]	731	(39.8)
Modified radical mastectomy[b]	3149	(25.2)
Breast conserving surgery[c]	221	(9.5)

[a]21% surgery alone, 79% surgery and irradiation.
[b]44% surgery alone, 56% surgery and irradiation.
[c]28% surgery alone, 72% surgery and irradiation.

Table 4. Rate of edema according to different surgical methods with and without radiotherapy

Procedure	Number of cases of edema	(%)
Radical mastectomy	163	(22.7)
With radiotherapy	568	(44.7)
Modified radical mastectomy	1381	(19.9)
With radiotherapy	1768	(29.3)
Breast conserving surgery	58	(6.9)
With radiotherapy	163	(10.4)

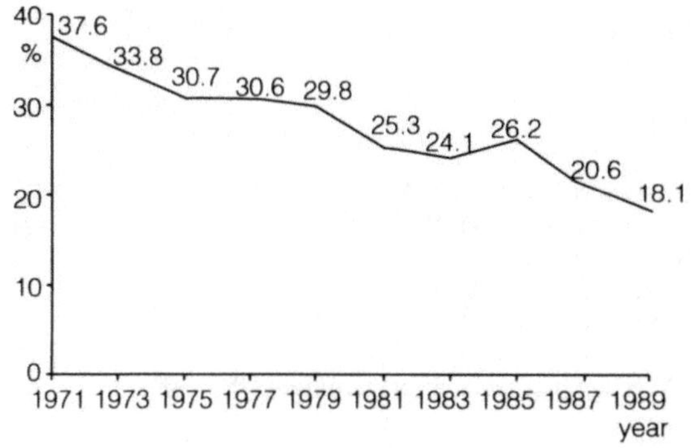

Fig. 1. Reduction of edema rate following changes in treatment modalities ($n = 4101$)

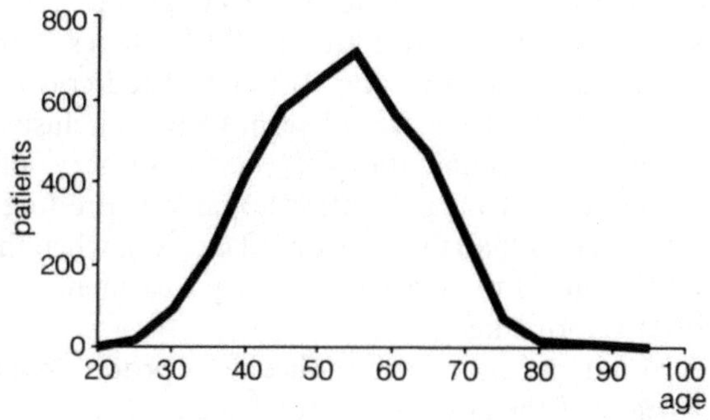

Fig. 3. Age distribution of breast cancer patients ($n = 4011$)

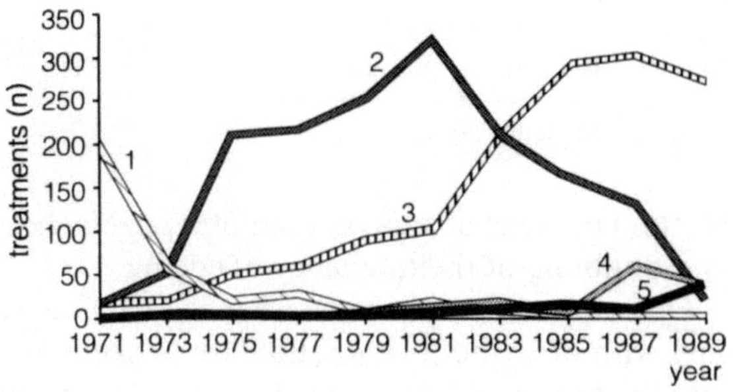

Fig. 2. Treatment schedule ($n = 4101$ treatments): *1*, radical mastectomy + conventional X-ray irradiation; *2*, modified radical mastectomy + megavoltage irradiation; *3*, modified radical mastectomy alone; *4*, breast conserving surgery + megavoltage irradiation; *5*, breast conserving surgery alone

Table 5. Stage distribution of tumors

n	(%)	pTN	Number of cases of edema	(%)
411	(10.8)	pTX	179	(43.6)
45	(1.1)	pTis	3	(6.7)
1496	(36.5)	pT1	277	(18.5)
1774	(43.5)	pT2	495	(27.9)
219	(5.3)	pT3	75	(34.6)
158	(3.9)	pT4	78	(49.4)
2026	(49.4)	pNO	428	(21.1)
436	(10.6)	pN+	168	(38.5)
1160	(28.3)	pN1	316	(27.2)
435	(10.6)	pN2	176	(40.5)
44	(1.1)	pN3	19	(43.2)

megavoltage irradiation in the 1970s and breast conserving treatments with or without modern radiotherapy in the 1980s (Fig. 2).

The relation between pathological stage and the incidence of lymphedema is shown in Table 5. Only 37.6% of the primary tumors were under 2 cm (Tis and T1), the majority of tumors were advanced. The axilla was not involved (NO) in 50%. The frequency of occurrence of edema increased with the size of the primary tumor and with the degree of axillary involvement.

The age distribution of the patients at the time of the primary therapy is shown in Fig. 3. Some 61% of the patients were between 45 and 65 years old, with a peak between the 55th and 60th year of life. The youngest patient was 22 years, the oldest 91 years of age.

4 Discussion

To our knowledge our patients represent the largest group ($n = 4101$) which has been analyzed; the next largest group, followed by Gregl et al. (1978), consisted of 1203 patients.

The patients came from all over Bavaria and only a small percentage (6.5%) were from other states in Germany. This means that the edema frequency found is not the result of selection of only a few hospitals which prefer more radical or more moderate treatment modalities, but is based on an average from all over Bavaria. The age distribution and the tumor stages are typical for breast cancer (Leonhardt 1988).

Most of the edemas developed in the first 2–5 years after primary therapy (Földi and Földi 1993; Göltner et al. 1985; Gregl et al. 1978; Hughes and Patel 1966; Schünemann and Willich 1990), but some occurred even after 10 years; others occurred without any signs of tumor progression (Gregl et al. 1978), though these events were rare.

Table 5 demonstrates a close correlation between increasing edema frequency, increasing tumor size and extent of the involvement of the axilla. The TX/N+ stages, however, do not correlate, probably because it is a heterogeneous group (T1-4, N1-3). However, since the TX/N+ stages were mostly recruited from the Rotter-Halsted era, the frequency of edema would seem to be conclusive, because the combination of radical surgery and conventional X-ray irradiation apparently produced more edemas than those recorded later on, when the patients generally received primary treatment with lower tumor stages.

In our patients, the lymphedemas produced expansion of the circumference of the arm to 4.2 cm (2.0 cm–24.0 cm). The edemas of the right arm were larger than those of the left arm (4.6 cm vs 3.7 cm). It should be noted that about 90% of the German population are right-handed, with a physiological increase of circumference of the working arm up to 1.9 cm. For this reason, in this analysis, differences between the two arms of less than 2 cm were not considered significant; otherwise an artifactually higher number of edemas would result for the right arm. In contrast there was a slightly higher number of edemas of the left arm (52.5%). Other authors have found twice the number of edemas for the right arm as for the left (GREGL et al. 1978; TRACY et al. 1961). In our opinion this can only be explained by methodological errors or selection.

There was a distinct difference between the patients complaints and the objectively recorded findings (ENGEL et al. 1988); but there was no doubt that early treatment of the secondary edema, for example the complex physical lymph therapy of (FÖLDI 1989; HEYTMANEK and KUBISTA 1988; RÜNZI and HÜBNER 1985), is required and effective. This has been used successfully by us for many years (SCHÜNEMANN 1993).

The above mentioned problems with respect to the comparability of the different methods to measure the extent of lymphedemas of the arm are documented in Table 6. After radical mastectomy without postoperative irradiation, LOBB and HARKINS (1949) reported a lymphedema rate of 6.7%–62.5% in a review of several collected series. KINDLER (1984) reported 12.7%. Both SAY and DONEGAN (1974) and HUGHES and PATEL (1966) reported a 30% lymphedema rate. Including some other publications (FLETCHER et al. 1980) the average is about 20%–30%. In our group the lymphedema rate was 22.7%.

After radical mastectomy combined with postoperative irradiation (Table 7) the lymphedema rates reported in the literature are in the range of 45%–52% (GREGL et al. 1978; TRACY et al. 1961; ZESCHICK 1987). In our patients we found a rate of 45.7%. The effect of adjuvant radiotherapy is shown by a doubling of the frequency of edema.

Table 6. Edema of the arm after radical mastectomy

Reference	Incidence (%)[a]
LOBB and HARKINS 1949	6.7–62.5
HUGHES and PATEL 1966	30
SAY and DONEGAN 1974	31
FLETCHER et al. 1980	20
KINDLER 1984	12.7

[a] Average incidence approximately 20%–30%.

Table 7. Edema of the arm after radical mastectomy plus irradiation

Reference	Incidence (%)[a]
TRACY et al. 1961	47
GREGL et al. 1978	45
ZESCHICK 1987	52

[a] Average incidence 50%.

Our data on lymphedema after radical mastectomy with or without irradiation are in accordance with the reported data in the literature. This proves to be different after modified radical mastectomy without irradiation. For this situation RYTTOV et al. (1983) found an incidence of edema of only 4% and LEIS (1978) 15.4%. We had a rate of edema of 19.9%, although we did not consider an increase of circumference of the arm below 2 cm to be edematous. Due to our large number of breast cancer patients in this group ($n = 1381$), we suspect that these differences can possibly be explained by too few cases in other authors' reports. The fact that the radical operation, according to Rotter-Halsted, without irradiation yielded only a slight elevation of the edema rate, in comparison to modified radical mastectomy (22.7% vs 19.9%), might be explained by the hypothesis that the modalities of surgery of the thoracic wall are only of minor value with respect to edemas if the differences between these modalities consist in the removal or nonremoval of the pectoral muscles. The completeness of the axillary dissection cannot be evaluated reliably in the Rotter-Halsted era data because in general the pathologist did not mention the number of lymph nodes removed. However, our rate of edema of 29.3% after modified radical mastectomy with postoperative irradiation is in good agreement with the literature, in which an average of 30% is reported (GÖLTNER et al. 1985; RYTTOV et al. 1983; ZESCHICK 1987).

After breast conserving surgery the lymphedema rates of the arms, as derived from the literature, are in the range of about 7%, (Adamczyk 1989, Browse 1987; Danoff et al. 1985; Kissin et al. 1986; Ryttov et al. 1983), which agrees with our 6.9% after breast conserving therapy without postoperative irradiation. After additional radiotherapy, the edema rate in 163 breast cancers was 10.4%.

There are several reasons for the insignificant incidence of edema after breast conserving therapy despite obligatory axillary dissection:

1. A breast conserving operation will only be carried out if the axilla is clinically negative.
2. Only small primary tumors up to 2–3 cm in size are operated on.
3. If the axilla is also histologically negative only the breast and not the axilla is postoperatively irradiated. This also applies to nodal positive patients after complete axillary disection without tumor remnants.
4. As a consequence of the above, the lymph vessels connecting the breast and the axilla remain to a great extent intact, and the axillary lymph nodes are only slightly affected by lymphonodectomy, because radical cleaning of the axilla is nowadays considered to be overtreatment in clinically nodal negative patients. Indeed at least ten lymph nodes should be removed from levels 1 and 2.

The radical mastectomy with radical cleaning of the axilla and curative intention, as it was introduced by Halsted in 1894, resulted from Virchow's theory on lymphatic tumor cell drainage and the hypothesis of the lymphatic node barrier. After the end of the second World War, in response to the development of radiotherapy and other related disciplines, attempts were made to reduce the aggressiveness of the standard operation and to complement surgery by modern adjuvant radiotherapy. In Germany radical mastectomy, according to Rotter-Halsted, was replaced by the modified radical mastectomy, which became the standard modality in the early 1970s (Günther 1989).

As it had been proven that the survival rate of breast cancer patients is not reduced by the more limited surgical methods (Eiermann and Hepp 1989; Fisher et al. 1985), it is not surprising that breast conserving treatment modalities have become increasingly popular in Germany since the early 1980s. However, it has now taken more than 20 years for the French approach to breast conserving therapy irradiation alone of breast cancer to be accepted here (Günther 1989).

Our results demonstrate that the lymphedema rate has clearly decreased with the introduction of the modified radical mastectomy plus megavoltage irradiation instead of Halsted's classical radical operation and conventional X-ray treatment (Bates 1988). After 1983, the radical mastectomy was largely replaced by the modified radical mastectomy without radiotherapy the use of which reached a maximum in 1987. This modality of treatment has been partly substituted by breast conserving therapy combined with megavoltage irradiation (Bertelli et al. 1991). As a result the frequency of edema has decreased from an initial nearly 38% down to 18%.

Breast conserving surgery has shown that the reduction of aggressiveness of treatment yields not only no disadvantage with respect to survival of the patient but the quality of life is significantly improved by a clear reduction of the rate of edema, down to about 10%. A further reduction in the incidence of secondary lymph edema should be strived for.

References

Adamczyk M (1989) Ergebnisse brusterhaltender Therapie bei Mammakarzinon 1984–1987. Inaugural dissertation, Medizinische Fakultät, LMU Munich

Bates TD (1988) The 10-year results of a prospective trial of postoperative radiotherapy delivered in 3 fractions per week versus 2 fractions per week in breast carcinoma. Radiol 61: 625–630

Bertelli G, Venturini M, Forno G, Macchiavello F, Dini D (1991) Conservative treatment of postmastectomy lymphedema. A controlled, randomized trial. Ann Oncol 2: 575–578

Brismar B, Ljungdahl I (1983) Postoperative lymphoedema after treatment of breast cancer. Acta Chir Scand 149: 687–689

Browse NL (1987) Lymphoedema of the arm. Br Med J 295: 3–4

Danoff BF, Pajak TF, Solin LJ, Goodman RL (1985) Excisional biopsy, axillary node dissection and definitive radiotherapy for stage I and II breast cancer. Int J Radiat Oncol Biol Phys 11: 479–483

Eiermann W, Hepp H (1989) Brusterhaltende Therapie. Indikation und Grenzen. Krebsmedizin 10: 35–38

Engel K, Müller A, Kaufmann M, Fournier von D, Schmidt W (1988) Zur Frage der Lebensqualität nach brusterhaltender Therapie des Mamma-Carcinoms. Frauenarzt 6: 697–703

Fischbach JU, Mönter B, Göltner E (1986) Messungen von Armödemen durch optoelektronische Volumetrie. Phlebol Proktol 4: 3–15

Fisher B, Wolmark N, Fisher ER, Deutsch M (1985) Lumpectomy and axillary dissection for breast cancer: surgical, pathological and radiation considerations. World J Surg 9: 692–698

Fletcher GH, Montague ED, du V Tapley N, Barker JL (1980) Radiotherapy in the management of nondisseminated breast cancer. In: Fletcher GH (ed) Textbook of radiotherapy. Leau u. Febiger, Philadelphia, pp 527–579

Földi M (1989) Die komplexe physikalische ('2-Phasen") Entstauungstherapie des Lymphödems. Vasomed Aktuell 3: 40–44

Földi M, Földi E (1993) Das Lymphödem. Fischer, Stuttgart

Göltner E, Fischbach U, Mönter B, Kreus A, Vorherr H (1985) Objektivierung des Lymphödems nach Mastektomie. Dtsch med Wochenschr 110: 949–952

Gregl A, Heitmann D, Krack U (1978) Häufigkeit, klinische und radiologische Symptomatik sowie Therapie des Armödems beim Mammakarzinom. Strahlentherapie 154: 482–488

Günther B (1989) Operative Onkologie, Krebsmedizin 10: 22–25

Halsted W (1894) The results of operations for the cure of cancer of the breast performed of the Johns Hopkins Hospital from June 1889 to January 1894. Ann Surg 20: 497–555

Heytmanek G, Kubista E (1988) Therapie des postoperativen Lymphödems beim Mammakarzinom: die Lymphdrainage. Geburtsh Frauenheilkd 48: 433–435

Hughes JH, Patel AR (1966) Swelling of the arm following mastectomy. Br J Surg 53: 4–15

Ingianni G, Holzmann T (1985) Klinische Erfahrungen in der Anwendung von lympho-venösen Anastomosen beim sekundären Lymphödem. Handchir Microchir Plast Chir 17: 43

Kindler M (1984) Lymphödem des Arms nach Mastektomie – Symptom eines Rezidivs? Zentralbl Chir 109: 479–482

Kissin MW, Querci della Rovere G, Easton D, Westbury G (1986) Risk of lymphoedema following the treatment of breast cancer. Br J Surg 73: 580–584

Larson D, Weinstein M, Goldberg I, Silver B, Recht A, Cady B et al. (1986) Edema of the arm as a function of the extent of axillary surgery in patients with stage I–II carcinoma of the breast treated with primary radiotherapy. Int J Radiat Oncol Biol Phys 12: 1575–1582

Leis HP (1978) Selective moderate surgical approach for potentially curable breast cancer. In: Gallagher HS, Leis HP, Snydermann RK, Urban JR (eds) The breast, Ist edn Mosby, St Louis, pp 232–247

Leonhardt, A (1988) Die klinische Erkennung von 2511 Mammakarziomen der Jahre 1977 bis 1986. Geburtsh Frauenheilkd 48: 92–98

Lobb AW, Harkins HN (1949) Postmastectomy swelling of the arm with note on effect of segmental resection of axillary rein at time of radical mastectomy. West J Surg 57: 550–557

Lotze W, Richter P (1989) Sekundäre Lymphödeme bei gynäkologischen Malignomen. Zentralbl Gynaekol 111: 92–98

Ray GR, Fish VJ, Lee, RH, Marzoni FA Jr, Trollope ML et al. (1983) Biopsy and definitive radiation therapy in stage I and II carcinoma of the female breast. Int J Radiat Oncol Biol Phys 9: 23–28

Rünzi M, Hübner K (1985) Das Lymphödem, eine vergessene Erkrankung. Therapiewoche 35: 4226–4233

Ryttov N, Blichert-Toft M, Madsen EL, Weber J (1983) Influence of adjuvant irradiation on shoulder joint after mastectomy for breast cancer. Acta Radiol Oncol 22: 29–33

Say CC, Donegan W (1974) A biostatistical evaluation of complications from mastectomy. Surg Gynecol Obstet 138: 370–376

Schünemann H, Willich N (1990) Das sekundäre Lymphödem beim Mammakarzinom. Eine Studie über 3067 Fälle. Krebsmedizin 11: 19–25

Schünemann H (1993) Sekundäres Lymphödem. In: Schünemann H, Beaufort F, Scheidel P, Willich N (eds) Gynäkologische Malignome. Zuckschwerdt, Munich

Swedborg I, Wallgren A (1981) The effect of pre- and postmastectomy radiotherapy on the degree of edema, shoulder-joint mobility, and gripping force. Cancer 47: 877–881

Tracy GD, Reeve TS, Simons Fitz E, Rundle FF (1961) Observation on the swollen arm after radical mastectomy. Aust NZJ Surg 30: 204

Willich N, Zeschick A, Zeschick L, Wendt T (1989) Ergebnisse der Bestrahlung nach Mastektomie. In: Sauer H (ed): Mammakarzinom. Zuckschwerdt, Munich, pp 56–63

Yeo EK, Denham JW, Davies SA, Spittle MF (1986) Primary breast cancer. Complications of axillary management. Acta Radiol Oncol 25: 105–108

Zeschick A (1987) Lokoregionäre Rezidive und Fernmetastasen nach postoperativer Strahlentherapie des Mammakarzinoms. Inaugural dissertation, Medizinische Fakultät, LMU Munich

3.4 Skin and Mucosal Damage After Radiotherapy for Head and Neck Tumors

Marcus Niewald, Werner Berberich, Christoph Schlichting, Michael Engel, Armand Koch, and Klaus Schnabel

CONTENTS

1	Introduction	105
2	Patients and Methods	105
2.1	Patients	105
2.2	Radiotherapy	105
2.3	Assessment of Side Effects	106
3	Results	106
3.1	Acute Side Effects	106
3.1.1	Dermatitis	106
3.1.2	Mucositis	106
3.2	Late Side Effects	106
3.2.1	Skin Fibrosis	106
3.2.2	Mucosal and Bone Necroses	107
4	Discussion	107
4.1	Critical Evaluation of the Results	107
4.2	Critical Evaluation of the Literature	109
5	Summary and Therapeutic Recommendations	109
	References	110

1 Introduction

Acute and long-term side effects on the skin and mucous membranes are very frequent after definitive radiotherapy of tumors in the head and neck region and may severely alter the general status of the patient. An interruption of the radiotherapy can become necessary because of intolerable damage especially to the mucous membranes.

In a retrospective study prognostic factors for the occurrence or the degree of acute and late side effects in the skin and the mucosa of the head and neck region were looked for.

Marcus Niewald, Dr., Klaus Schnabel, Prof. Dr., Abteilung für Strahlentherapie, Radiologische Universitätsklinik, 66421 Homburg/Saar, FRG

Werner Berberich, Privatdozent, Dr., Institut fur Strahlentherapie, Strädtisches Klinikum St. Marien, 92224 Amberg, FRG

Michael Engel, Dr. Dr., Abteilung für Mund-, Kiefer- und Gesichtschirurgie der Universitäts-Zahn-, Mund- und Kieferklinik, 66421 Homburg/Saar, FRG

Armand Koch, Privatdozent, Dr., Universitäts-HNO-Klinik und Poliklinik, 66421 Hamburg, FRG

2 Patients and Methods

2.1 Patients

In the period October 1983 to April 1993 375 patients were irradiated for cancer in the oral cavity (49.9%) or in the oropharynx (50.1%). The mean age at the beginning of therapy was 55.9 years (30.4–84.1 years), the mean Karnofsky performance status was 7.45 (5–10). Nearly all patients were heavy drinkers and smokers. There were 245 patients (65.3%) who had been operated on before radiotherapy; the remaining 130 (34.7%) had no pretreatment. Patients having received chemotherapy were excluded from the analysis due to the heterogeneity of chemotherapy schedules. The T classification was: T1: 14%, T2: 35%, T3 24%, T4 27%. The N classification was: N0: 33%, N1: 23%, N2: 26%, N3: 18%. Distant metastases were diagnosed in 4% of the patients. The UICC stage distribution was: I: 7%, II: 13%, III: 23%, IV: 57%.

2.2 Radiotherapy

All patients received a careful dental examination and therapy (mostly extraction of several teeth) first. Radiotherapy was then performed by irregular, lateral, parallel opposing portals using 60 Co γ-rays (up to 1988) or 4 or 6 MV photons from a linear accelator. A total of 247 patients (65.9%) received a conventionally fractionated therapy with a single dose administered once daily five times a week up to a total dose mostly in the range of 60–70 Gy. Another 118 patients (31.5%) were treated with hyperfractionation with single doses of 1.2 Gy administered twice daily (time interval at least 6 h) five days a week up to a total dose mostly in the range of 80.4–85.2 Gy. The remaining ten patients were treated using several fractionation schedules. In 13% radiotherapy could not be completed due to deterioriation of the patient's status. Treatment of 32% of the patients was subject to minor interruptions, up to 5 days duration, due to holidays and machine defects; 19% of the patients experienced major interruptions (more than 5 days). The mean follow-up was 748 days (0–3133 days).

2.3 Assessment of Side Effects

Acute dermatitis and mucositis were recorded immediately after the conclusion of radiotherapy and graded according to the World Health Organization (WHO) classification. The intensity of skin fibrosis and the occurrence of mucosal or bone ulcers were recorded during every follow-up examination. Skin fibrosis was graded according to the EORTC-RTOG classification. Prognostic factors for the side effects mentioned above were computed using the Cox regression hazard test. Variables tested were age, KARNOFSKY performance status, pretreatment, TNM classification, UICC stage, delay between diagnosis and beginning of therapy, single dose, total dose, duration of therapy, and local and regional tumor control. Furthermore, dose-effect curves were constructed, and failure curves using the KAPLAN-MEIER estimate were computed.

3 Results

3.1 Acute Side Effects

The frequency and grade of acute side effects are depicted in Fig. 1.

3.1.1 Dermatitis

The multivariate analysis of possible prognostic factors for the occurrence of radiogenic dermatitis showed a statistical significance of the total dose, the single dose (hyperfractionated vs conventionally fractionated treatment), the pretreatment and the UICC stage of the primary tumor. Assuming the total dose as the only influencing factor, a correlation with the frequency of acute skin reactions could be seen (Fig. 2), but not with the grade of dermatitis (Fig. 3). There might be more intense dermatitis using low single doses (1.2 Gy twice a day).

3.1.2 Mucositis

For the occurrence and degree of acute mucositis, single dose (hyperfractionated vs conventionally fractionated treatment) and total dose were prognostically significant. The univariate dependence on total dose is depicted in Fig. 4. Higher amounts of mucositis were seen in the group which was treated hyperfractionally.

3.2 Late Side Effects

3.2.1 Skin Fibrosis

The frequency and grade of skin fibrosis are shown in Fig. 5. Using multivariate analysis a prognositic significance of T classification, pretreatment and regional tumor control for the degree of skin

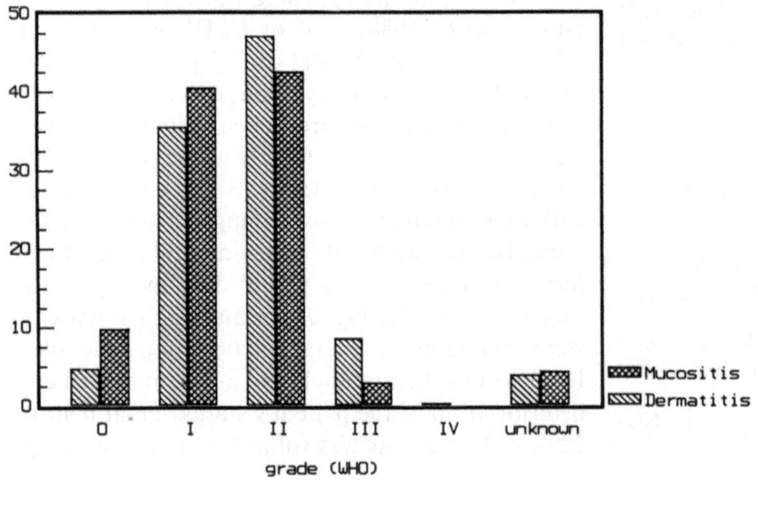

Fig. 1. Distribution of acute side effects

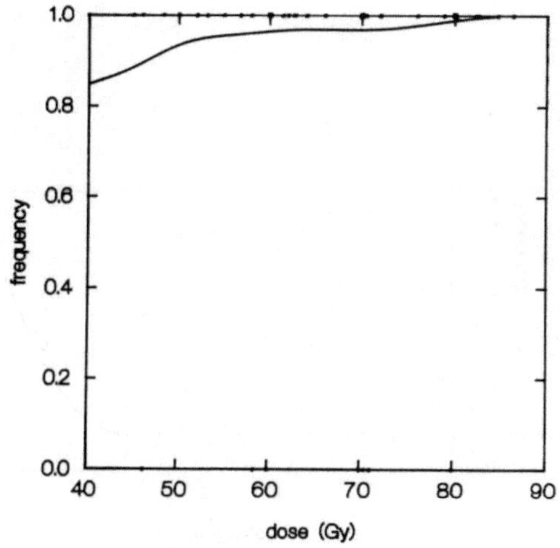

Fig. 2. Dose-effect relationship (frequency of dermatitis)

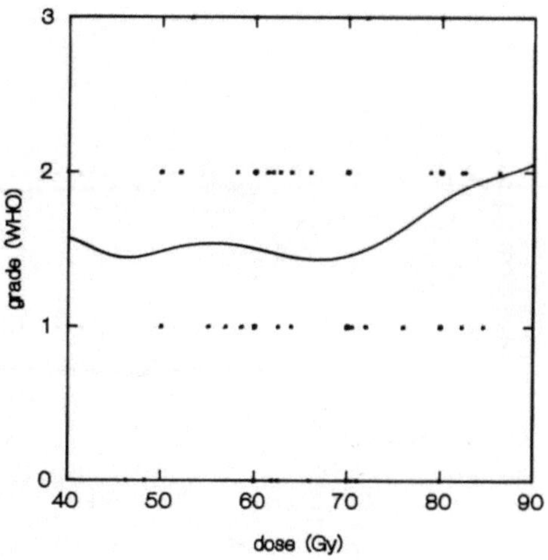

Fig. 4. Dose-effect relationship (grade of mucositis)

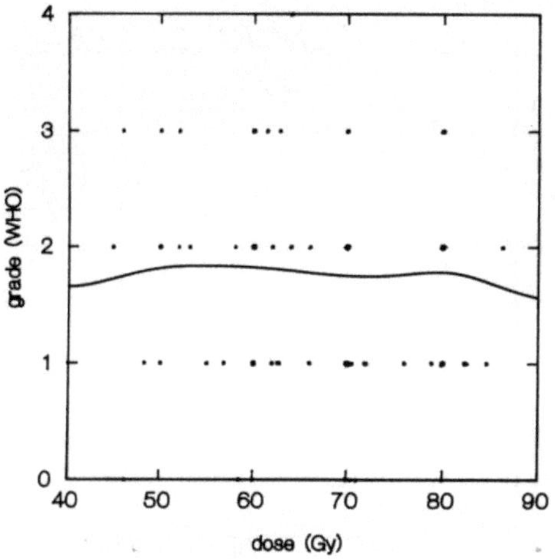

Fig. 3. Dose-effect relationship (grade of dermatitis)

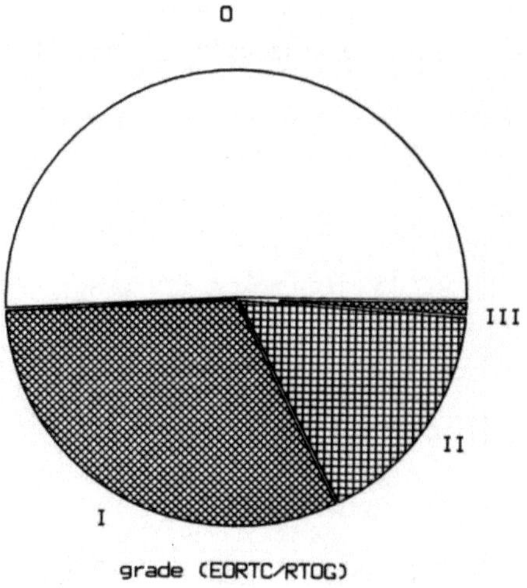

Fig. 5. Distribution of skin fibrosis

fibrosis could be computed. No dependency on dose was seen univariately (Fig. 6) or multivariately for total doses above 60 Gy. Using the KAPLAN-MEIER estimate it can be shown that the risk of skin fibrosis grade II EORTC/RTOG or higher steadily rose during follow-up and had not yet reached a peak (Fig. 7).

3.2.2 Mucosal and Bone Necroses

The occurrence of fatal late effects of the mucous membranes such as ulcers or necroses was analysed. The overall frequency in our collective is 5.3% at the present time, in 2.7% an osteoradionecrosis has also been observed. The only significant prognostic factor is the total dose. Since there is a strong dependency of total dose on single dose a correlation with single dose must be assumed as well. The univariate analysis of the dose-effect dependency resulted in a risk of necrosis rising steeply with doses above 70 Gy (Fig. 8). The failure curve (KAPLAN-MEIER estimate) shows an ascending risk during follow-up and that a plateau might be reached in 4 years after completion of radiotherapy (Fig. 9).

4 Discussion

4.1 Critical Evaluation of the Results

The correlation of the frequency of acute dermatitis with the total dose is well known. The correlation with the single dose was negative, that means that

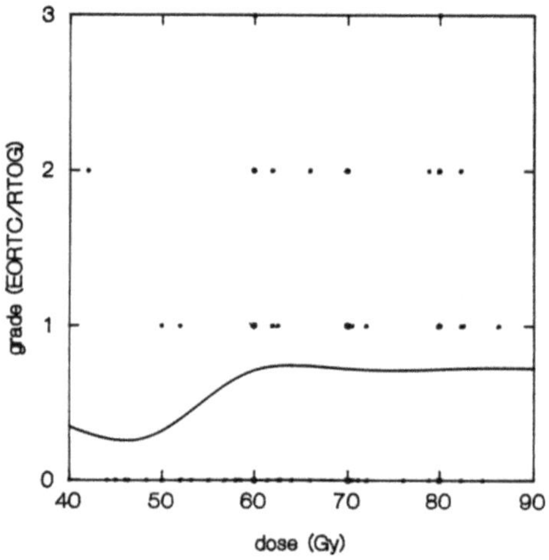

Fig. 6. Dose-effect relationship (grade of skin fibrosis)

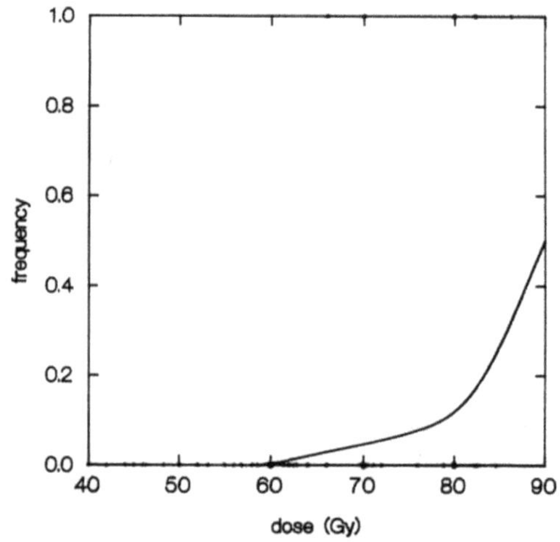

Fig. 8. Dose-effect relationship (frequency of mucosal necroses)

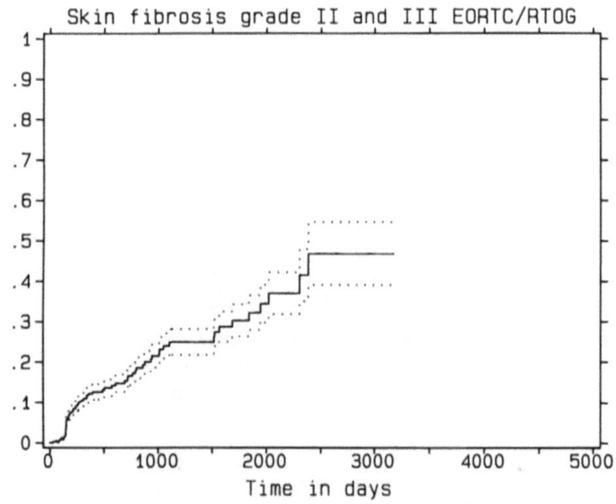

Fig. 7. Dependency of the probability of skin fibrosis on time

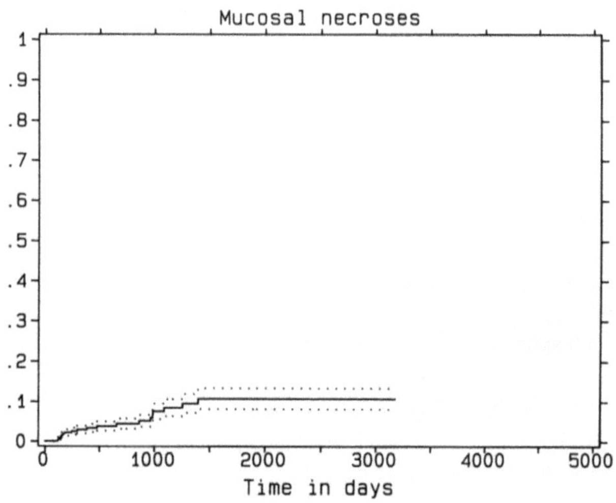

Fig. 9. Dependency of the probability of mucosal necroses on time

patients with the smallest single doses (hyperfractionated treatment twice a day) experienced the greatest amount of dermatitis. This can be explained easily by considering that patients who were irradiated hyperfractionally received a single dose of 1.2 Gy twice a day, resulting in a daily dose of 2.4 Gy compared to 2.0 Gy administered once a day. The dependency on the pretreatment may be explained by assuming that surgery can irritate the skin. An explanation for the dependency on UICC stage might be that the bigger target volume in patients with advanced tumor stages had an influence on the grade of side effects. In addition, there was more intense mucositis after hyperfractionated radiotherapy, which is a generally well known experience. The explanation might be the same as for dermatitis.

The nondependency of the grade of skin fibrosis on dose was unexpected. Statistical analysis indicates that pretreatment (surgery or not) played a major role in producing fibrosis. It may be that local tumor recurrence causes additional irritation of the tissues, thereby enhancing skin fibrosis. The dependency on T classification might be explained by an influence of the bigger target volumes in patients with advanced T stage tumors.

The statistical analysis of the dose-effect relationship for mucosal and bone ulcers showed that patients with the highest total doses had the most

Table 1. Total effect (TE) values

Radiotherapy schedule	TE value
30 × 2.0 Gy in 42 days	360
35 × 2.0 Gy in 49 days	420
69 × 1.2 Gy in 49 days	437
41 × 2.0 Gy in 57 days	492

TE = $(\alpha/\beta + d)D$ for d = single dose and D = total dose.

necroses. These were also the patients irradiated hyperfractionally.

Using the LQ model (assumptions: a/ß for bone: 4.0 Gy, *hm* = 0.0625) we computed the total effect (TE) values for the various fractionation schedules used. These are listed in Table 1. One can see that the TE value of our hyperfractionated radiotherapy regimen (82.8 Gy total dose, 1.2 Gy twice a day single dose) is in fact somewhat higher than that for a 70 Gy total dose administered conventionally, in contrast to the equivalence assumed in the beginning of the study. That means that the unexpected high incidence of fatal side effects in the hyperfractionated group may be due to a relative overdosage; the additional influence of surgery cannot be assessed statistically. Comparing the hyperfractionated regimen (82.8 Gy) to a hypothetical conventionally fractionated schedule (single dose 2.0 Gy, total dose 82 Gy), however, there is an important sparing of side effects, as demonstrated by the TE values. This has been predicted and shown by numerous radiobiological and clinical trials.

4.2 Critical Evaluation of the Literature

WANG et al. (1985) and VAN DER SCHUEREN et al. (1990) state that, in general, mucositis begins 2 weeks after the start of therapy, the accumulated dose at this time being nearly 20 Gy. The intensity progresses rapidly if radiation is continued. Complete healing can be expected in 2–3 weeks after the end of therapy. Acute dermatitis starts later and progresses far less rapidly than mucositis. The time needed for complete healing a much longer. Some side effects were recorded, especially after the use of unconventional fractionation schedules. WANG et al. (1985) noted only insignificant side effects after hyperfractionated radiotherapy (2 × 1.6 Gy daily up to 38.4 Gy, 2 week interval, than 1.8 Gy daily up to 65 Gy). SHUKOVSKY and FLETCHER (1973) recorded 27% mucosal ulcers after total doses of 70–75 Gy fractionated conventionally; a dependency on field size was stated. NGUYEN et al. (1988) reported 33% cervical fibroses and 24% mucosal necroses after a hyperfractionated schedule (0.9 Gy eight times daily up to 36 Gy, 2 weeks interval, then repeated). The authors conclude that the short time intervals between the fractions were responsible for the high incidence of side effects.

There are several risk factor analyses for side effects. MACIEJEWSKI et al. (1990) computed a dependency of the intensity of acute mucositis on single dose, total dose, and duration of therapy. There was no correlation with field size. Late effects were correlated with the dose per fraction, the overall treatment time, and the amount of acute reactions, but not with the field size. KALZ et al. (1990) recorded a dependency of the occurrence of mucosal necroses only on the pretreatment but not on the dose or field size. LARTIGAU et al. (1991) stated that the intensity of late reactions of skin and mucosa depended on the dose per fraction and the total dose, the interval between the fractions (CHART radiotherapy) also being very important. According to TURESSON and NOTTER (1984a, b) the amount of late-occurring effects strongly depends on the dose per fraction. The frequency of skin fibroses was found to rise over a long time (several years) reaching a plateau.

5 Summary and Therapeutic Recommendations

Using a total dose of 70 Gy in 49 days with conventional fractionation there are tolerable acute and late side effects. Higher doses with conventional fractionation should be avoided because of the rapidly rising risk of mucosal necroses.

Unconventional fractionation schedules should be biologically planned as carefully as possible using the LQ model with the different α/β values known for the organs at risk (mucous membranes, bone, spinal cord) especially when total doses exceeding 76 Gy are intended and patients already operated on are to be irradiated. Our experience is that a total dose of 82.8 Gy (single dose 1.2 Gy twice a day) certainly is too high and causes intolerable side effects.

The incidence of late reactions is significantly influenced by the length of follow-up (or survival). Finally patients should generally be included in a dental prophylaxis program prior to radiotherapy.

References

Kalz W, Dallüge P, Marquardt P, Marquardt S (1990) Klinische Studie zu oralen radiogenen Komplikationen bei der Tumortherapie im Kopf-Hals-Bereich. Zahn Mund Kieferheilkd 78: 521–523

Lartigau E, Saunders MI, Dishe S, Warburton MF, Rochers CD (1991) A comparison of later radiation changes after three schedules of radiotherapy. Radiother Oncol 20: 139–148

Maciejewski B, Withers HR, Taylor JMG, Hliniak A (1990) Dose fractionation and regeneration in radiotherapy for cancer of the oral cavity and oropharynx, part 2. Normal tissue responses: acute and late effects. Int J Radiat Oncol Biol Phys 18: 101–111

Nguyen TD, Panis X, Froissart D, Legros M, Coninx P, Loirdtte M (1988) Analysis of late complications after rapid hyperfractionated radiotherapy of advanced head and neck cancers. Int J Radiat Oncol Biol Phys 14: 23–25

Shukovsky LJ, Fletcher GH (1973) Time-dose and tumor volume relationships in the irradiation of squamous cell carcinoma of the tonsillar fossa. Radiology 107: 621–626

Turesson I, Notter G (1984a) The influence of fraction size in radiotherapy on the later normal tissue reaction – I: comparison of the effects of daily and once-a-week fractionation on human skin. Int J Radiat Oncol Biol Phys 10: 393–398

Turesson I, Notter G (1984b) The influence of fraction size in radiotherapy on the late normal tissue reaction – II: comparison of the effects of daily and twise-a-week fractionation on human skin. Int J Radiat Oncol Biol Phys 10: 599–606

Van der Schueren E, Van den Bogaert W, Vanuytsel L, Van Limbergen E (1990) Radiotherapy by multiple fractions per day (MFG) in head and neck cancer: acute reactions of skin and mucosa. Int J Radiat Oncol Biol Phys 19: 301–311

Wang CC, Blitzer PH, Suit HD (1985) Twice-a-day radiation therapy for cancer of the head and neck. Cancer 55: 2100–2104

3.5 Mucosal Toxicity After Radiochemotherapy

LUDWIG PLASSWILM and VRATISLAV STRNAD

CONTENTS

1	Introduction	111
2	Mucosal Toxicity	111
2.1	Radiation-Induced	111
2.2	Chemotherapy-Induced	112
2.2.1	5-Fluorouracil and Cisplatin	112
2.2.2	Folinic Acid and Interferon	113
2.2.3	Other Drugs	113
3	Radiochemotherapy-Induced Mucosal Toxicity in the Oral Cavity	113
3.1	Platinum Analogues and 5-Fluorouracil	113
3.2	Mitomycin C	114
3.3	Therapeutic Recommendation	114
4	Radiochemotherapy-Induced Mucosal Toxicity in the Gastrointestinal System	114
4.1	5-Fluorouracil and Radiation	114
4.2	5-Fluorouracil and Folinic Acid	114
4.3	Doxorubicin	115
4.4	Other Drugs	115
4.5	Therapeutic Recommendation	115
5	Prevention and Treatment of Therapy-Associated Mucosal Toxicity	115
5.1	Head and Neck Cancer Patients	115
5.1.1	Dental Care and Oral Hygiene	115
5.1.2	Pharmacological Agents	115
5.1.3	Physical Therapy	116
5.2	Colorectal Cancer Patients	116
5.2.1	Pentoxifylline	116
5.2.2	Octreotide and Loperamide	116
5.3	Therapeutic Recommendation	117
6	Summary	117
	References	117

1 Introduction

Combined modality therapy for tumors is based on the failure of surgery, radiotherapy or chemotherapy alone to produce cures. Laboratory and clinical research has been performed to identify the mechanisms of interaction and possible side effects between radio- and chemotherapy and to optimize their clinical applications. Today, when recent improvements in supportive care sometimes allow intensification of treatment with equal-acute toxicity, e.g., stomatitis, the chronic side effects and late organ damage such as ulcers or fistulas may be considered as therapy limiting. Oral and gastrointestinal sequelae resulting from radiochemotherapy have a tremendous effect on the patient's quality of life. Pretherapeutic existing parameters, including performance status, age, and renal and liver function, may always influence the severity of possible side effects.

This chapter is a summary of theoretical considerations, laboratory findings and clinical data regarding the interaction of radiotherapy with some frequently used chemotherapeutic agents at the mucosa.

LUDWIG PLASSWILM, Dr., VRATISLAV STRNAD, Dr., Strahlentherapeutische Klinik und Poliklinik, Universität Erlangen-Nürnberg, Universitätsstraße 27, 91054 Erlangen, FRG

2 Mucosal Toxicity

2.1 *Radiation-Induced*

It should be remembered that there are no pathognomic features of radiation injury (FAJARDO 1989). Mucous membranes are rapidly proliferating tissues and therefore it is not suprising that radiation injury occurs early. Shortly after irradiation, cells of the squamous epithelium undergo degeneration, atrophy, dysplasia, atypia and necrosis. The submucosa becomes edematous, capillaries are dilated, and the endothelium is swollen. Depression of cell proliferation and continuing loss of postmitotic mucosal cells lead to desquamation of mucosal epithelium. Clinical signs and symptoms develop after the postmitotic differentiated cells have exhausted their physiological life span. In the oral mucosa this causes an erythema. After approximately 2–4 weeks erosion and desquamation of the mucosa will occur. The denuded surface becomes covered with a pseudomembrane of fibrin, cell debris and leukocytes. Later, atrophy, fibrosis or necrosis can occur.

When analyzing the changes in the gastro-intestinal renewal system, one must bear in mind that the most important changes after irradiation occur in the small intestine. Irradiation results in cell depletion in the intestinal villi and crypts due to the killing of proliferating cells and the sterilization of stem cells (HENDRY et al. 1983). The most typical sign of acute intestinal injury is the development of diarrhea due to acute mucosal hypoplasia with decreased intestinal surface area; mucosal denudation is not required. In the submucosa edema and eosinophilic infiltration can be seen (BERTHRONG and FAJARDO 1981). In the chronic phase, the mucosa is usually atrophic, and finally, hyalinic fibrosis and telangiectasia can occur, sometimes terminating with intestinal obstruction.

Fistulas and perforation, representing segmental geographic loss of mucosa and its smooth musculature, cannot possibly be explained as a simultaneous cellular hypoplasia of two differnt cell types, i.e., mucosa and smooth muscle. The association of obliterative endoarteritis in zones of necrosis and perforation indicate infarction and necrosis of supplying vessels as the essential mechanism (RUBIN and CASARETT 1968).

2.2 *Chemotherapy-Induced*

Many drugs cause toxicity because of their preferential activity against rapidly proliferating cells. Tissues that maintain a high rate of cellular proliferation include the bone marrow, hair follicles, gonads, and the mucosa.

Ulceration of the intestinal mucosa is a common and sometimes dose limiting toxicity that occurs in treatment with several anticancer agents (Table 1). Mucosal damage, usually beginning a few days after drug administration, or in the case of continuous infusion also sometimes during treatment, is due to interruption of the production of new cells that normally replace the mature cells that are continuously sloughed into the lumen. Full recovery is possible with repopulation from slowly proliferating stem cells that are situated in the base of the intestinal crypts. Early signs of mucositis and stomatitis, as an inflammatory response of the mucosa following administration of cytotoxic drugs, include mild erythema and edema. This generalized reaction can be drug-, dose- and schedule-related. The inflammation may progress to enteritis, painful ulcerations, and secondary infections and lead to complications such as malnutrition, diarrhea, dehydration, and bleeding with interruption of therapy.

Table 1. Several chemotherapeutic drugs that might lead to mucosal injury

Alkylating agents	Antimetabolites	Natural products
Cyclophosphamide	Methotrexate	Doxorubicin
Ifosfamide	5-Fluorouracil	4-Epi-doxorubicin
Methyl-CCNU	Cytosine arabinoside	Actinomycin D
	Piritrexim	Bleomycin
	10-EDAM	Mitomycin C
	Methotrexate	Vinca alkaloids
		VP-16
		Paclitaxel
		Taxotere

Some drugs, e.g., cyclophosphamide or 5-fluorouracil, seem to act only on proliferating cells in the crypts of the intestinal mucosa, whereas other agents, e.g., doxorubicin or radiation alone, also appear to damage stem cells near the base of the crypts (IJIRI and POTTEN 1987).

The progressive component of the possible late effects of radiation is arteriocapillary fibrosis and alteration of fibroconnective tissues. The late effects of chemotherapy are postulated to be predominantly a result of parenchymal cell depletion, but with sparing of the microcirculation and fibroconnective tissue. (RUBIN 1984).

2.2.1 5-Fluorouracil and Cisplatin

A drug which is often used in chemotherapy and radiochemotherapy, especially in treatment of head and neck tumors and colorectal cancer, is 5-fluorouracil (5-FU). When used as a continuous infusion (e.g. 1000 mg/m^2/24 h through 96 or 120 h) the predominant toxicity is mucositis (TAPAZOGLU et al. 1986), while hematological toxicity is more frequently seen after 5-FU bolus administration.

5-FU, a halogenated pyrimidine that mimics uracil biochemically, is an effective inhibitor of RNA function and thymidilate synthesis. The drug requires enzymatic conversion to the nucleotide in order to exert its cytotoxic activity. The folate cofactor, N^{5-10}-methylenetetrahydrofolate, and 5-dUMP (active fluorinated nucleotide) form a covalently bound terenary complex with the enzyme (KEYOMARSI and MARON 1986). The dissociation rate of this complex is decreased in the presence of excess cofactor.

A randomized trial of three courses of cisplatin (100 mg/m^2, day 1) and 5-FU infusion (1000 mg/m^2, days 1–4) vs cisplatin (100 mg/m², day 1) and bolus 5-FU (600 mg/m², days 1 and 8) in head and neck cancer patients showed a statistically significant difference in response for the infusion arm. Stomatitis was more frequent in the 5-FU infusion arm (KISH et al. 1985).

2.2.2 Folinic Acid and Interferon

Biochemical modulation of 5-FU with folinic acid (Leucovorin) or biological response modifiers such as interferon have increased complete response rates without clearly improving survival, but severe mucositis and diarrhea continue to be the dose limiting side effects (DIMERY and HONG 1993; TAYLOR et al. 1992).

2.2.3 Other Drugs

Some other frequently used or newly discussed anticancer drugs with mild to significant mucosal injury are adriamycin (ROSENTHAL and ROTMAN 1991), mitoxantrone (DOBROWSKY et al. 1992), ifosfamide (MARTIN et al. 1993), 10-EDAM (GREEN et al. 1992), piritrexim (UEN et al. 1992), paclitoxel (SPRIGGS and TONDINI 1992) and taxotere (PAZDUR et al. 1992).

3 Radiochemotherapy-Induced Mucosal Toxicity in the Oral Cavity

Though the mechanisms underlying the interaction between most of the cytotoxic agents and radiation still remain largely undefined, a fundamtental concept of combined modality treatment is to administer each modality, i.e., irradiation and chemotherapy, in an effective dosage. Therefore we recommend using drugs with the highest efficacy in effective dosages even in combination with radiotherapy, e.g., cisplatin and 5-FU in head and neck cancer or 5-FU in rectal cancer. The full doses of 5-FU may increase the radiation induced mucosal reaction. Some clinical data give an idea about the possible mucosal injury in radiochemotherapy of head and neck cancer.

3.1 Platinum Analogues and 5-Fluorouracil

Cis- or carboplatin are well documented drugs that do not lead to remarkable mucosal toxicity when used in a single agent treatment with doses of about 100 mg/m² (once every 3–4 weeks) or 25 mg/m² (on 5 consecutive days, every 3–4 weeks). Even when a platinum analogue is given simultaneously with conventional doses of radiotherapy it does not increase mucosal toxicity. Mucositis is seen in 80% of the patients but it is not more severe than that observed with radiation alone (JACOBS et al. 1989).

The experimental data of BOTNIK et al. (1979) in a variety of tissues show that, after chemotherapy, regenerated cells and tissues, despite their normal appearance, may have lost some of their proliferative reserve capacity. Nevertheless, clinical investigations of an adjuvant chemotherapy vs sequential chemo- and radiotherapy for resectable head and neck carcinomas showed no significant difference in acute and late toxicity for patients treated postoperatively by radiotherapy alone or by chemotherapy followed by radiation (LARAMORE et al. 1992).

A prospectively randomized trial of concurrent vs sequential radiochemotherapy (ADELSTEIN et al. 1990) with a 5-FU infusion and cisplatin bolus showed a significantly better relapse-free survival on the simultaneous arm. Mucosistis and the resultant weight loss were more severe on the simultaneous arm.

Particularly in treatment protocols with hyperfractionated irradiation plus chemotherapy (Table 2), increased mucosal damage has been observed (WENDT et al. 1987, 1990; WENDT 1993; GLANZMANN et al. 1990; VOLLING et al. 1991).

Table 2. Acute mucosal toxicity after hyperfractionated radio- and radiochemotherapy (from WENDT 1993)

	Regimen A[a] (*n*)	(%)	Regimen B[b] (*n*)	(%)
WHO grade				
No data	3	2.5	2	1.9
0	2	1.7	2	1.9
1–2	94	79.0	60	57.7
3–4	20	16.8	40	38.5
Total	119	100.0	104	100.0

Data of 223 patients from a randomized German multicenter trial for locally advanced head and neck cancer (ARO 89–1).
[a] Regimen A: hyperfractionated radiotherapy up to 70,20 Gy.
[b] Regimen B: hyperfractionated radiotherapy up to 70,20 Gy plus concomitant chemotherapy with cisplatin, 5-fluorouracil and Leucovorin.

3.2 Mitomycin C

Mitomycin C, also associated with some mild mucosal toxicity and commonly used in the treatment of head and neck cancers, does not seem to lead to a dose limiting increase of the mucosal reaction in radiochemotherapy (DOBROWSKY et al. 1992).

3.3 Therapeutic Recommendation

Summarizing these data, at the present time our standard treatment regimen in Erlangen for head and neck cancer patients is concurrent radiochemotherapy with 5-FU and cisplatin. We know that this therapy leads to a higher risk of mucositis than sequential chemo- and radiotherapy or irradiation alone; however, the increased mucosal damage is usually reversible. Weight loss is not a remarkable problem since we use a percutaneous endoscopic gastrostomy for almost all head and neck patients at the beginning of treatment. The grade of weight loss seems to have no impact on mucosal toxicity (SENFT 1993).

4 Radiochemotherapy-Induced Mucosal Toxicity in the Gastrointestinal System

Acute and late radiation-induced gastrointestinal toxicity is well documented, but chemotherapy-induced mucosal damage has only been described as an acute toxicity, e.g., for 5-FU and methyl-CCNU (DANJOUX and CATTON 1979; RUBIN et al. 1992). Late chemotherapy-induced gastrointestinal injury can be found only in combination with radiation (DETHLEFSEN 1979; SCHENKEN et al. 1979).

Early mucosal damage due to radiochemotherapy does not always predict the severity of the late effects of the intestine. This was seen in the ECOG study using split course irradiation (60 Gy in 10 weeks) and maintenance chemotherapy (5-FU and methyl-CCNU) for 1 year (DANJOUX and CATTON 1979). Although no undue acute toxicity occurred, catastrophic late complications such as fistulization and necrosis in 29% of patients 6 months to 2 years after therapy were registered. This high incidence of severe side effects is possibly explained by the following: With fractionated radiation the microcirculation is altered, but no late effects occur until another challenge is made to the organ system. Concomitant or maintenance chemotherapy uses up crypt stem cell reserve and the "recall" or surfacing of a radiation syndrome may occur. Chemotherapy can accelerate and deplete crypt stem cells in zones of focal radiation ischemia and then despite a different mechanism of action, an unexplained or enhanced effect is encountered (RUBIN 1984).

4.1 5-Fluorouracil and Radiation

For many years 5-FU has been the mainstay of chemotherapy for patients with gastrointestinal adenocarcinoma. Some laboratory findings (BYFIELD et al. 1982; VIETTI et al. 1971) showed radiation enhancement depending on the duration of exposure to 5-FU, especially in a colon cancer cell line (SMALLEY et al. 1991). These data have not been confirmed uniformly (WEINBERG and RAUTH 1987; NAKAJIMA et al. 1979; STEPHENS et al. 1977) The main determinants of the amount of additive toxicity, e.g., nausea and diarrhea, are the degree of cytotoxicity achieved with 5-FU infusion and the radiation dose. The often required 5-FU dose (1000 mg/m^2/24 h over a period of 4–5 days) and the radiation dose (50–60 Gy) produce a markable mucosal toxicity each on its own (CHU and TAKIMOTO 1993; GUNDERSON and MARTERSON 1989; RUBIN and CASARETT 1992). Therefore it is not suprising that an increased mucosal toxicity can be observed when these modalities are combined as a concurrent radiochemotherapy (PHILLIPS 1980; DANJOUX and CATTON 1979; GRIGSBY and PEREZ 1991).

Usually the symptoms may be well controlled with analgesics, antiemetics or anticholinergics. In our experience cessation of chemotherapy or radiotherapy is normally not required in patients without pretreatment, e.g., patients undergoing preoperative radiochemotherapy for rectal cancer. After exensive surgery however, the tolerance seems to be reduced.

4.2 5-Fluorouracil and Folinic Acid

The results o some clinical trials seem to confirm that the addition of the prodrug 5-formyltetrahydrofolate (Leucovorin) increases the cytotoxicity and efficacy of 5-FU (KEYOMARSI and MORA 1986). However, gastrointestinal toxicity is also increased.

A principle directive of the US National Cancer Institute is that patients with resected colon cancer (UICC stage III, Dukes C) unable to enter a clinical trial should reveive an adjuvant therapy with 5-FU and levamisole.

4.3 *Doxorubicin*

An additive mucosal toxicity of adriamycin and irradiation has been reported (ROSENTHAL and ROTMAN 1991). Mucosal injury strongly depends on the dose of adriamycin and radiation dose per fraction. If adriamycin is escalated to more than 12 mg/m^2 per day × 5 (by continuous infusion), mucositis increases exponentially. If adriamycin is administered as a concomitant continuous infusion regimen with 12 mg/m^2 per days × 5, a remarkable increasing mucosal injury develops only with 2.0 Gy per fraction compared to 1.0 or 1.5 Gy (ROSENTHAL and ROTMAN 1991).

4.4 *Other Drugs*

Concerning other chemotherapeutic agents, such as cisplatin or mitomycin C, which are also used frequently in radiochemotherapy of abdominal tumors, no remarkable increase of mucosal toxicity has been reported (SAUER et al. 1990; DEWIT et al. 1987).

4.5 *Therapeutic Recommendation*

Our routine treatment in high risk, lower gastroinestinal cancer is concomitant radiotherapy with 5-FU infusion. We avoid combinations with biomodulating agents (folinic acid or interferon) because of their possibly increased acute and late side effects.

5 Prevention and Treatment of Therapy-Associated Mucosal Toxicity

5.1 *Head and Neck Cancer Patients*

Most prevention and treatment procedures described in the literature are based on clinical experience and show great diversity. There are only a few clinical and experimental findings attempting to identify possible agents that may ameliorate radiation- and chemotherapy-induced inflammation.

5.1.1 Dental Care and Oral Hygiene

All head and neck patients must receive a comprehensive dental evaluation before they enter into therapy. After extraction or other surgical intervention a rest period of at least 2 weeks until the onset of therapy is necessary.

During therapy smoking is strongly discouraged because it contributes to mucosal irritation (RUGG et al. 1990) as does the use of alcohol. The radiation therapist should inspect the oral mucosa weekly.

A daily review of a symptom survey by a radiation nurse combined with well defined analgetic use and careful oral hygiene may result in improved management of radiation- and radiochemotherapy-induced oropharyngeal mucosits (JANJAN et al. 1992a, b).

5.1.2 Pharmacological Agents

It appears that resolution of mucositis is accelerated by using Kamillosan Liquidum as an oral rinse (CARL and EMRICH 1991).

The local application of prostaglandin E_2 tablets (0.5 mg four times a day) has a potent effect on the therapy of mucositis without a significant amount of the substance entering the circulation (MATEJKA et al. 1990).

The use of sucralfate as an effective drug in the therapy and prevention of therapy-related stomatitis or diarrhea remains controversial (HENRIKSSON et al. 1992; PFEIFFER et al. 1990; SHENEP et al. 1988).

Allopurinol may protect against mucositis; however, the precise biochemical mechanism for its effect on 5-FU-metabolism has not been clearly defined. CLARK and SLEVIN (1985) found that an allopurinol mouthwash substantially decreased the incidence and severity of stomatitis in patients after exposure to 5-FU. In contrast, LOPRINZI et al. (1990) demonstrated that an allopurinol mouthwash regimen does not offer any protective effect against 5-FU-induced mucositis.

MACIEJEWSKI et al. (1991) reported that an acute reaction is significantly decreased in the mucosa when it has been repeatedly painted with a 2% silver nitrate solution for several days before radiotherapy. Another conditioning procedure which might increase the tolerance of the oral mucosa is the local application of biological substances, e.g., tannin. Polyphenols (tannins) are effective as medical agents due to their astringent action. They produce an impervious layer (polyphenol-protein and/or polysaccharide complex) under which the natural healing process can occur (HASLAM et al. 1989; OKUDA et al. 1988).

Successful prevention of mucositis has been reported by eradication of gram-negative bacilli in patients receiving irradiation because of head and neck cancer (SPIJKERVET et al. 1991) These bacilli could play a role in irradiation mucositis (VAN SAENE and MARTIN 1990). In a prospective, double-blind randomized trial some increase in gram-negative bacilli was noted in patients treated with a 0.12% chlorhexidine digluconate mouth rinse. In patients undergoing high dose radiotherapy no differences were observed in oral mucositis between chlorhexidine-treated patients and a control group. Yet chlorhexidine mouth rinse significantly reduced the incidence of oral mucositis in chemotherapy patients (FERRETI et al. 1990).

SEITER et al. (1993) reported that intravenous uridine administration allows dose escalation of 5-FU when used in combination with methotrexate and *N*-phosphon-acetyl-*L*-asparate. The investigators showed significant vascular toxic effects associated with intravenous uridine. Whether the oral use of uridine leads to better 5-FU tolerance in chemo- or radiochemotherapy is still unknown.

Pilocarpine, a parasympathomimetic agonist, has been shown to be effective in the treatment of salivary gland hypofunction after radiation therapy (GREENSPAN and DANIELS 1987). In a double-blind, placebo-controlled trial VALDEZ et al. (1993) showed that pilocarpine stimulates the salivary tissue outside the field of radiation therapy. So, if the portal arrangement allows some gland tissue to be spared, the use of pilocarpine during radiation may lead to a lower frequency of xerostomia and dysphagia. Carbacholine, another cholinergic drug, also seems to be useful in the treatment of radiation-induced xerostomia (JOENSUU et al. 1993).

5.1.3 Physical Therapy

DOSE et al. (1990) reported that oral cryotherapy decreases the incidence and severity of stomatitis associated with bolus 5-FU/Leucovorin treatment. Cryotherapy consisted of having patients retain crushed ice in their mouth for 30 min.

5.2 Colorectal Cancer Patients

During radiochemotherapy of colorectal cancer, mucositis with diarrhea is the most burdensome side effect. Drug management of these side effects are discussed below.

5.2.1 Pentoxifylline

Pentoxifylline (PTX) is a xanthine derivative which down-regulates tumor necrosis factor-α (TNF-α) in patients with hematologic malignancies. Bone marrow transplantation patients receiving PTX at doses in excess of 1200 mg/day, from day -10 through day 100 posttransplant, experienced less mucositis and fewer other side effects than a good risk control group (BIANCO et al. 1991). PTX has been shown to have a marked effect on cellular mediators of inflammation and tissue injury (SULLIVAN et al. 1988; HAN et al. 1990). Methylxanthine derivatives have immunodepressive properties (which may explain their effect on the incidence of graft-vs-host disease in human bone marrow transplant) by direct depression of T cell activation (SINGER et al. 1992). We could not find any reports describing the use of PTX in radiochemotherapy regimens.

5.2.2 Octreotide and Loperamide

Due to the efficacy of the somatostatin analogue octreotide in the treatment of secretory diarrhea, e.g., in Zollinger-Ellison syndrome and the carcinoid syndrome, KENNEDY et al. (1990) used this drug to treat 5-FU Leucovorin-related diarrhea. CASCINU et al. (1993) performed a randomized trial that compared octreotide with loperamide in patients with grade 2 or 3 diarrhea after 5-FU containing chemotherapy. Octreotide, at a dosage of 0.1 mg subcutaneously twice per day for 3 days, was more effective than loperamide, 4.0 mg orally initially and then 2.0 mg every 6 h for 3 days, in the control of diarrhea. The cost of octreotide is extremely high compared to that of loperamide.

In our department we investigated somatostatin analogues (Sandostatin, 3×0.1 mg/day) in three patients with rectal cancer and treatment-related diarrhea after administration of concurrent radiochemotherapy with 5-FU-infusion and irradiation of the pelvis. The effect was not better than our routine administration of loperamide (Imodium, Janssen Gmbh, Germany) in a dosage of 4.0 mg

Table 3. Basic measures in prevention and treatment of mucosal toxicity of head and neck cancer patients

Careful dental evaluation before therapy
A 2 week rest period until the onset of therapy after oral surgical intervention
No smoking or drinking of alcohol
Weekly to daily inspection of the oral mucosa by the radiation therapist
Daily dexpanthenol mouthwash
Sufficient local prevention of candida infection
Nutritional support care to hold performance status without weight loss
Local (e.g., viscous xylocaine) or systemic analgestics
Interruption of therapy in case of mucosal toxicity grade 4 (WHO)
Drug therapy with pilocarpine if some salivary gland tissue can be spared of radiation

Table 4. Clinical options in case of unexpected gastrointestinal toxicity

Loperamide administration in case of diarrhea
Intravenous fluid and electrolyte substitution
Sufficient analgetic medication
Reduction of 5-fluorouracil dose
Interruption of therapy if symptoms are not reversed 2 days after the onset of supportive therapy

initially and than 2.0 mg after every stool up to 12.0 mg/day.

5.3 Therapeutic Recommendation

Table 3 summarizes our routine prevention and treatment procedures of mucosal toxicity in head and neck cancer. Table 4 shows the clinical options in case of unexpected gastrointestinal side effects.

6 Summary

Radiation-induced mucosal toxicity is a well known phenomen. Acute toxicity can usually be managed with standard medication. Late toxicity should be avoided by careful radiation treatment planning (e.g., dose per fraction, fractionation and the total dose).

Chemotherapy-induced acute mucosal toxicity is also well-known. Late mucosal injury can be seen only in combination with irradiation. Toxicity depends upon the type of chemotherapeutic drugs, the doses and the manner of administration – bolus or continuous infusion.

Individual patient data such as performance status, age, and renal and liver function also have a strong influence on the degree of mucosal toxicity.

References

Adelstein DJ, Saharan VM, Earle AS, Shah AC, Vlastou C, Haria CD, Damm C, Carter S, Hines JD (1990) Simultaneous versus sequential combined technique therapy for squamous cell head and neck cancer. Cancer 65: 1685–1690

Berthrong M, Fajardo LF (1981) Radiation injury in surgical pathology. II. Alimentary Tract Am J Surg Pathol 5: 153–178

Bianco JA, Appelbaum FR, Nemunaitis J, Almgren J, Andrews F, Kettner P, Shields A, Singer JW (1991) Phase I–II trial of pentoxifylline of transplant-related toxicities following bone marrow transplantation. Blood 78: 1205–1211

Botnik LE, Hannon ECM, Hellman S (1979) Late effects of cytotoxic agents on the normal tissue of mice. Front Radiat Ther Oncol 13: 36–47

Byfield JE, Calabro-Jones P, Klisak I (1982) Pharmacologic requirements for obtaining sensitization of human tumor cells in vitro to combined 5-fluorouracil or ftorafur and x-rays. Int J Radiat Oncol Biol Phys 8: 1923–1933

Carl W, Emrich LS (1991) Management of oral mucositis during local radiation and systemic chemotherapy: a study of 98 patients. J Prosthet Dent 66: 361–369

Cascinu S, Fedeli A, Fedeli SL, Catalano G (1993) Octreotide versus loperamide in the treatment of fluorouracil-induced diarrhea: a randomized trial. J Clin Oncol 11: 148–151

Choi KN, Rotman M, Aziz H, Potters L, Stark R, Rosenthal J (1991) Locally advanced paranasal sinus and nasopharynx tumors treated with hyperfractionated radiation and concomitant infusion cisplatin. Cancer 67: 2748–2752

Chu E, Takimoto CH (1993) Antimetabolites. In: DeVita, VT, Hellman S, Rosenberg SA (eds) Cancer, principles and practice of oncology, 4th edn. Lippincott, Philadelphia, pp 358–374

Clark PI, Slevin ML (1985) Allopurinol mouthwash and 5-fluorouracil induced oral toxicity. Eur J Surg Oncol 11: 267–268

Danjoux CE, Catton GE (1979) Delayed complications in colorectal carcinoma treated by combination radiotherapy and 5-fluorouracil – Eastern Cooperative Oncology Group (ECOG) Pilot Study. Int J Radiat Oncol Biol Phys 5: 311–316

Dethlefsen LA (1979) Cellular recovery kinetic studies relevant to combined modality research and therapy. Int J Radiat Oncol Biol Phys 5: 1175–1184

Dewit L, Oussoren Y, Bartelink H (1987) Early and late damage in the mouse rectum after irradiation and cisdiamminedichloroplatinum. Radiother Oncol 8: 57–70

Dimery IW, Hong WK (1993) Overview of combined modality therapies for head and neck cancer. J Natl Cancer Inst 85: 95–111

Dobrowsky W, Neude J, Millesi W, Grasl M, Kohler W, Kautzky M, Pavelka R, Toth M, Dobrowsky E (1992) Atypical fractionation in advanced squamous-cell carcinomas of the head-neck area. Strahlenther Onkol 168: 686–691

Dose AM, Mahood D, Loprinzi CL, Gainey D, Sorensen JM, Therneau T, Veeder M, Althman L, Mailliard J, Gusa N (1990) A controlled trial of oral cryotherapy for preventing stomatitis in patients receiving 5-Fluorouracil (5-FU) plus leucovorin (LV). North Central Cancer Treatment Group and Mayo Clinc Study. Proc ASCO 9: 321

Fajardo LF (1989) Morphologic patterns of radiation injury. In: Vaeth JM, Meyer JL (eds) Radiation Tolerance of Normal Tissues. Karger, Basel, pp 75–84

Ferretti GA, Raybould TP, Brown AT, Maxdonald JS, Greenwood M, Maruyama Y, Geil J, Lillich TT, Ash RS (1990) Chlorhexidine prophylaxis for chemotherapy- and radiotherapy-induced stomatitis: a randomized double-blind trial. Oral Surg Oral Med Pathol 69: 331–338

Glanzmann C, Sartorelli B, Thum P, Lütolf UM (1990) Hyperfraktionierte Bestrahlung und simultane Chemotherapie mit Cisplatin bei Patienten mit fortgeschrittenen Karzinomen der Kopf-Hals-Region. Strahlenther Onkol 166: 397–401

Green MD, Sherman P, Zalcberg J (1992) Phase II study of 10-EdAM in patients with squamous cell carcinoma of the head and neck previously untreated with chemotherapy. Invest New Drugs 10: 31–34

Greenspan D, Daniels TE (1987) Effectiveness of pilocarpine in postradiation xerostomia. Cancer 59: 1123–1125

Grigsby PW, Perez CA (1991) Efficacy of 5-fluorouracil by continuous infusion and other agents as radiopotentiators for gynecological malignancies. In: Rotman M, Rosenthal CJ (eds) Concomitant continuous infusion chemotherapy and radiation, Springer, Berlin Heidelberg New York, pp 259–267

Gunderson LL, Marterson JA (1989) Gastrointestinal Tract Radiation Tolerance. In: Vaeth JM, Meyer JL (eds) Radiation tolerance of normal tissues. Karger, Basel, pp 277–298

Han J, Thompson P, Beutler B (1990) Dexamethasone and pentoxifylline inhibit endotoxin-induced cachectin/tumor necrosis synthesis at separate points in the signaling pathway. J Exp Med 172: 391

Haslam E, Lilley TH, Cai Y, Marin R, Magnolato D (1989) Traditional herbal medicines – the role of polyphenols. Planta Med 55: 1–8

Hendry JH, Potten CS, Roberts NP (1983) The gastrointestinal syndrome and mucosal clonogenic cells; relationship between target cell sensitivities, LD50 and cell survival and their modification by antibiotics. Radiat Res 96: 100–112

Henrikson R, Franzen L, Littbrand B (1992) Effects of sucralfate on acute and late bowel discomfort following radiotherapy of pelvic cancer. J Clin Oncol 10: 969–975

Ijiri K, Potten CS (1987) Further studies on the response of intestinal crypt cells of different hierarchical status to eighteen different cytotoxic agents. Br J Cancer 55: 113–123

Jacobs MC, Eisenberger M, OH MC, Sinibaldi V, Gray W, Elias G, Salazar OM (1989) Carboplatin and radiotherapy for stage IV carcinoma of the head and neck: a phase I–II study. Int J Radiat Oncol Biol Phys 17: 361–363

Janjan NA, Weissman DE, Pahule A (1992a) Improved pain management with daily nursing intervention during radiation therapy for head and neck carcinoma. Int J Radiat Oncol Biol Phys 23: 647–652

Jansma J, Vissink A, Spijkervet FK, Roodenburg JL, Panders AK, Vermey A, Szabo BG, 's-Gravenmade EJ (1992b). Protocol for the prevention and treatment of oral sequelae resulting from head and neck radiation therapy. Cancer 70: 2171–2180

Jansma J, Vissink A, Bouma J, Vermey A, Panders AK, 's-Gravenmade EJ (1992c) A survey of prevention and treatment regimens for oral sequelae resulting from head and neck radiotherapy used in dutch radiotherapy institutes. Int J Radiat Oncol Biol Phys 24: 359–367

Joensuu H, Bosttröm P, Makkonen T (1993) Pilocarpine and carbacholine in treatment of radiation-induced xerostomia. Radiother Oncol 26: 33–37

Kemeny N, Younes A, Seiter K (1990) Interferon alpha 2a and 5-fluorouracil for advanced colorectal carcinoma. Cancer 66: 2470–2475

Kennedy P, Presant CA, Blaynei D (1990) Sandostatin therapy for chemotherapy and radiotherapy related diarrhea. Proc ASCO 9: 324

Keyomarsi K, Moran RG (1986) Folinic acid augmentation of the effects of fluoropyrimidines on murine and human leukemic cells. Cancer Res 46: 5229–5235

Kish JA, Ensley JF, Jacobs J, Weaver A, Cummings G, Al-Sarraf M (1985) A randomized trial of cisplatin (CACP) + 5-fluorouracil (5-FU) infusion and CACP + 5-FU bolus for recurrent and advanced squamous cell carcinoma of head and neck. Cancer 56: 2740–2744

Laramore GE, Scott CB, AL-Sarraf M, Haselow RE, Ervin TJ, Wheeler R, Jacobs JR, Schuller DE, Gahbauer RA, Schwade JG, Campbell BH (1992) Adjuvant chemotherapy for resectable squamous cell carcinomas of the head and neck: report on intergroup study 0034. Int J Radiat Oncol Biol Phys 23: 705–713

Loprinzi C, Cianeflone SG, Dose AM, Etzel PS, Burnham NL, Therneau TM, Hagen LR, Gainey DK, Cross M, Athmann LM, Fischer T, O'Connel MJ (1990) A controlled evaluation of an allopurinol mouthwash as prophylaxis against 5-fluorouracil-induced stomatitis. Cancer 65: 1879–1882

Maciejewski B, Zajusz A, Pilecki B, Swiatnicka J, Skladowski K, Dorr W, Kummermehr J, Trott KR (1991) Acute mucositis in the stimulated oral mucosa of patients during radiotherapy for head and neck cancer. Radiother Oncol 22: 7–11

Martin M, Diaz-Rubio E, Gonzales-Larriba JL, Casado A, Sastre J, Lopez-Vega JM, Almenarez J, Domingues S (1993) Ifosfamide in advanced epidermoid head and neck cancer. Cancer Chemother Pharmacol 31: 340–342

Matejka M, Nell A, Kment G, Schein A, Leukauf M, Porteder H, Mailath G, Sinzinger H (1990) Local benefit of prostaglandin E2 in radiochemotherapy-induced oral mucositis. Br J Oncol Maxillofac Surg 28: 89–91

Moertel CG, Flemming TR, MacDonald JS (1990) Levamisole and fluorouracil for adjuvant therapy of resected colon carcinoma. N Engl J Med 322: 352–358

Nakajima Y, Miyomoto T, Tanabe M (1979) Enhancement of mammalian cell killing by 5-fluorouracil in combination with X-rays. Cancer Res 39: 3763–3767

National Institute of Health Consensus Development Conference Statement (1990): Adjuvant therapy for patients with colon and rectum cancer. 16–18 April, Office of Medical Applications of Research. JAMA 1990

Okuda T, Yoshida T, Hatano T (1988) Ellagitannins as active constitutents of medical plants. Planta Med 55: 117–122

Pazdur R, Newman FA, Newman BM, Fuentes A, Benvenuto J, Bready B, Moore D jr, Jaiyesimi I, Vreeland F, Bayssass MM (1992) Phase I trial of taxotere: five-day schedule. J Natl Cancer Inst 84: 1781–1788

Piedbois P, Buyse M, Rustum Y (1992) Modulation of flourouracil by leucovorin in patients with advanced colorectal cancer: evidence in terms of response rate. J Clin Oncol 10: 896–903

Phillips TL (1980) Tissue toxicity of radiation-drug interactions. In: Sokol GH, Maickel RP (eds) Radiation-drug interactions in the treatment of cancer, Wiley, New York

Pfeiffer P, Madsen EL, Hansen O, May O (1990) Effect of sucralfate suspension on stomatitis induced by cancer chemotherapy. Acta Oncol 29: 29–30

Rosenthal CJ, Rotman M (1991) Concomitant continuous infusion adriamycin and radiation: evidence of synergistic effects in soft tissue sarcomas. In: Rotman M, Rosenthal CJ (eds) Concomitant continuous infusion chemotherapy and radiation. Springer, Berlin Heidelberg New York, pp 272–280

Rubin P (1984) The Franz Buschke Lecture: late effects of chemotherapy and radiation therapy: a new hypothesis. Int J Radiat Oncol Biol Phys 10: 5–34

Rubin P, Casarett GW (1968) Clinical radiation pathology, vols I and II. Saunders, Philadelphia

Rubin P, Casarett G (1972) A direction for clinical radiation pathology – the tolerance dose. In: Vaeth JM (ed) Frontiers of radiation therapy and oncology, vol. 6. University Park Press, Baltimore, pp 1–16

Rubin P, Coustine LS, Nelson DE (1992) Late effects of cancer treatment: radiation and drug toxicity. In: Perez CA, Brady LW (eds) Principles and practice of radiation oncology. Lippincott, Philadelphia, pp 124–161

Rugg T, Saunders MI, Dische S (1990) Smoking and mucosal reactions to radiotherapy. Br J Radiol 63: 554–556

Sauer R, Dunst J, Altendorf-Hofmann A, Fischer H, Bornhof C, Schrott KM (1990) Radiotherapy with and without cisplatin in bladder cancer. Int J Radiat Oncol Biol Phys 19: 687–691

Schenken LL, Burdolt DR, Kovacs J (1979) Adriamycin radiation induced combinations: drug-induced delayed gastrointestinal radiosensitivity. Int J Radiat Oncol Biol Phys 5: 1265–1270

Seiter K, Kemeny N, Martin D, Schneider A, Williams L, Colofiore J, Sawyer R (1993) Uridine allows dose escalatian of 5-fluorouracil when given with N- phosphonacetyl-L-asparate, methotrexate, and leucovorin. Cancer 71: 1875–1881

Senft M (1993) Lebensqualität und Ernährungstherapie bei Patienten mit Tumoren im Kopf-Hals-Bereich. Thesis, Medical faculty, University of Erlangen

Shenep JL, Kalwinsky DK, Hutson PR, George SL, Dodge RK, Blankenship KR, Thornton D (1988) Efficacy of oral sucralfate suspension in prevention and treatment of chemotherapy-induced mucositis. J Pediat 113: 758–763

Singer JW, Bianco JA, Takahashi G, Simrell C, Petersen J, Andrews DF (1992) Effect of methyxanthine derivates on T cell activation. Bone Marrow Transplant 10: 19–25

Smalley SR, Kimler BF, Evans RG (1991) 5-fluorouracil modulation of radiosensitivity in cultured human carcinoma cells. Int J Radiat Oncol Biol Phys 20: 207–211

Spijkervet FK, van Saene HK, van Saene JJ, Panders AK, Vermey A, Mehta DM, Fidler V (1991) Effect of selective elimination of the oral flora on mucositis in irradiated head and neck cancer patients. J Surg Oncol 46: 167–173

Spriggs DR, Tondini C (1992) Toxol administered as a 120 hour infusion. Invest New Drugs 10: 175–278

Stephens JC, Peacock SH, Steel GG (1977) Cell survival in B16 melanoma after treatment with combination of cytotoxic agents: lack of potentiation. Br J Cancer 36: 84–93

Sullivan GW, Carper HT, Novick WJ, Mandell GL (1988) Inhibition of the inflammatory action of interleukin-1 and tumor necrosis factor alpha on neutrophil function by pentoxifylline. Infect Immunol 56: 1722

Tapazoglou E, Kish J, Ensley J, Al-Sarraf M (1986) The activity of a single-agent 5-fluorouracil infusion in advanced and recurrent head and neck cancer. Cancer 57: 1105–1109

Taylor CW, Modiano MR, Woodson ME, Marcus SG, Alberts DS, Hersh EM (1992) A phase I trial of fluorouracil, leucovorin, and recombinant interferon alpha-2b in patients with advanced malignancy. Semin Oncol 19: 185–190

Uen WC, Huang AT, Mennel R, Jones SE, Spaulding MB, Killion K, Havlin K, Keegan P, Clendeninn NJ (1992) A phase II study of piritrexim in patients with advanced squamous head and neck cancer. Cancer 69: 1008–1011

Veldez IH, Wolff A, Atkinson JC, Macynskii AA, Fox PC (1993) Use of pilocarpine during head and neck radiation therapy to reduce xerostomia and salivary dysfunction. Cancer 71: 1848–1851

van Saene HK, Martin MV (1990) Do microorganisms play a role in irradiation mucositis? Eur J Microbiol Infect Dis 9: 861–863

Vietti T, Eggerding F, Valeriote F (1971) Combined effect of X radiation and 5-fluorouracil on survival of transplanted leukemic cells. J Natl Cancer Inst 47: 865–870

Vokes EE (1993) Interactions of chemotherapy and radiation. Sem Oncol 20: 70–79

Volling P, Staar S, Achterrath W, Müller RP (1991) Carboplatin plus radiation therapy in head and neck cancer. Semin Oncol 18 [Suppl 2]: 17–22

Weinberg MJ, Rauth AM (1987) 5-fluorouracil infusions and fractionated doses of radiation: studies with a murine squamous cell carcinoma. Int J Radiat Oncol Biol Phys 13: 1691–1699

Wendt TG (1993) Kombinierte Radio-Chemotherapie I. Neue Aspekte zum Einsatz von Strahlen- und Chemotherapie bei der Behandlung von Mundhöhlen- und Pharynxkarzinomen. 1st Cologne workshop, 17–19 Nov 1993

Wendt TG, Wustrow TPU, Hartenstein RC, Rohloff R, Trott KR (1987) Accelerated split-course radiotherapy and simultaneous cis-dischlorodiammine-platinum and 5-fluorouracil chemotherapy with folinic acid enhancement for unresectable carcinoma of the head and neck. Radiother Oncol 10: 277–284

Wendt TG, Wustrow TP, Schalhorn A (1990) Ergebnisse der simultanen Radio-Chemotherapie bei fortgeschrittenen Kopf-Hals-Tumoren. Strahlenther Onkol 166: 569–579

Zaniboni A, Ehrlichman C, Seitz J (1993) FUFA increases disease free survival in resected B2C colon cancer: results of a prospective pooled analysis of 3 randomized trials. Proc Am Soc Clin Oncol 12: 191

3.6 Complications of the Small Intestine and the Pancreas After Intraoperative Radiotherapy

CHRISTIAN RÜBE, HANS-JÖRG KRÄMLING, NORMAN WILLICH, JOACHIM GRAB, and RALF WILKOWSKI

CONTENTS

1 Introduction 121
2 Materials and Methods 121
3 Results 122
4 Discussion 124
5 Summary and Therapeutic Recommendations . . 125
References 126

1 Introduction

Intraoperative radiotherapy (IORT) has been used as an additional approach to improve local control of cancer, in the abdomen the largest experience exists for pancreatic and for gastric cancer. Other applications in the abdomen are the local treatment of cancer of the gallbladder, the bile ducts and advanced rectal carcinoma. There is some experience in the treatment of gynecological cancers, mainly in recurrences.

Most of the clinical studies (ABE and TAKAHASHI 1981; CALVO et al. 1992; FROMMHOLD et al. 1991; GUNDERSON et al. 1984, 1987; RICH 1985; TEPPER et al. 1991) have showed a significant improvement in local control of the tumor; nevertheless, a prolongation of overall survival was only rarely seen, due to hematogeneous dissemination of the disease. Our own results, for patients with inoperable carcinoma of the pancreas treated with palliative surgery such as biliodigestive anastomosis, IORT and external beam irradiation with 50 or 34 Gy for cases without distant metastases, showed very good pain reduction resulting from good local control; because of the high incidence of distant metastases, no benefit regarding survival could be achieved (KRÄMLING et al. 1992; RÜBE et al. 1992; WILLICH et al. 1988, 1989).

Patients with resectable pancreatic cancer treated with 20 Gy IORT survived longer than a historical group of patients treated without IORT; the difference was not statistically significant (GRAB et al. 1992). In an ongoing randomized trial for IORT of gastric cancer, no definitive results on the clinical outcome are yet available.

The therapeutic value of any new treatment modality has to be measured by comparing unwanted side effects with the advantages of the treatment. In this chapter we report our experience concerning side effects of IORT of pancreatic and gastric cancer and summarize data from the literature. Potentially occurring side effects and complications are malabsorption, disturbance of small and large bowel peristaltis, and ulcers and other lesions of the mucosa. Furthermore, stenoses, bleedings and necroses of parts of the bowel may appear. Perforation, anastomotic leakage and the development of fistula and local or generalized peritonitis with abscess are also described in the literature.

The analysis of clinical data is limited by the fact that, in many cases, it is difficult to differentiate complications caused by IORT from those which result from the surgical procedures or the tumor itself.

2 Materials and Methods

From 1986 to 1992, 101 patients underwent IORT of the upper abdomen at the University Hospital of Munich. Of the 74 patients who suffered from pancreatic cancer, 44 were inoperable and 30 were treated surgically. There were 27 patients who had operable gastric cancer.

In the group of patients with inoperable pancreatic cancer, 32 had a palliative operation (biliodigestive anastomosis or gastroenteroanastomosis). IORT was performed with round tubes

CHRISTIAN RÜBE, Dr., RALF WILKOWSKI, Dr., Radiologische Klinik Grosshadern, Abteilung Strahlentherapie, Marchioninistraße 15, 81377 Munich, FRG
HANS-JÖRG KRÄMLING, Privatdozent, Dr., JOACHIM GRAB, Dr., Chirurgische Klinik Grosshadern, Marchioninistrasse 15, 81377 Munich, FRG
NORMAN WILLICH, Prof. Dr., Klinik und Poliklinik für Strahlentherapie/Radioonkologie, Westfälische Wilhelms-Universität Münster, Albert Schweitzer-Straße 33, 48129 Münster, FRG

5–8 cm in diameter, including the macroscopically determined tumor extension. The applied dose was 20 Gy ($n = 30$) or 30 Gy ($n = 14$) with fast electrons; the electron energy varied according to the tumor size, between 9 and 19 MeV.

There were 22 patients who additional percutaneous radiation, ten patients with 50 Gy (5 × 1.8 Gy/week), as recommended by Abe and coworkers (ABE and TAKAHASHI 1981). Twelve patients received a reduced percutaneous dose of 34 Gy (5 × 1.8 Gy/week). These patients were simultaneously treated with 5-FU chemotherapy (1000 mg/m^2/per 24 h) for 96 h with a continuous infusion. Of the 30 patients with operable pancreatic cancer, 26 had Whipple's operation and four had a left-sided hemipancreatectomy. All patients were treated with IORT of 20 Gy using 9 MeV electrons and tube sizes between 5 and 8 cm. The irradiated volume included the tumor bed (Fig. 1). Except for the area of the celiac trunk, irradiation of the locoregional lymphnodes was not routinely performed.

The third group of patients represented one arm of a randomized trial for gastric cancers. At the time of the analysis, 60 patients were included in the trial; all had a total or subtotal gastrectomy, 27 received IORT with 28 Gy using 9 MeV electrons and mostly pentangular tubes (Fig. 2); 33 patients were treated with surgery only.

All patients were closely followed by clinical examination, CT of the abdomen and X-ray examination of the upper gastrointestinal tract with oral contrast media, in most cases every 3–4 months.

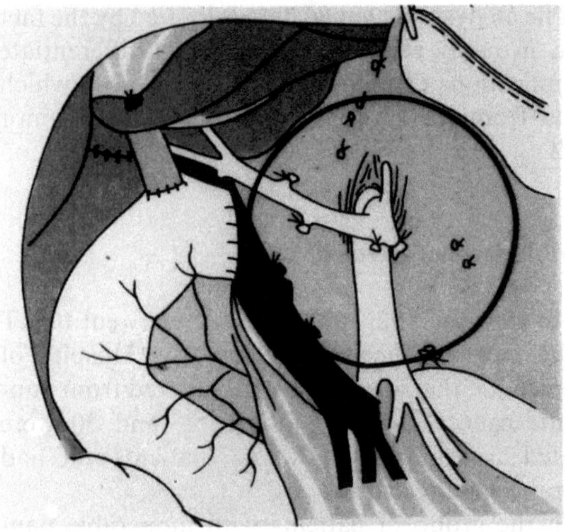

Fig. 1. Round-shaped irradiation field for intraoperative radiotherapy (IORT) after Whipple's operation including the tumor bed. (From SCHILDBERG et al. 1992)

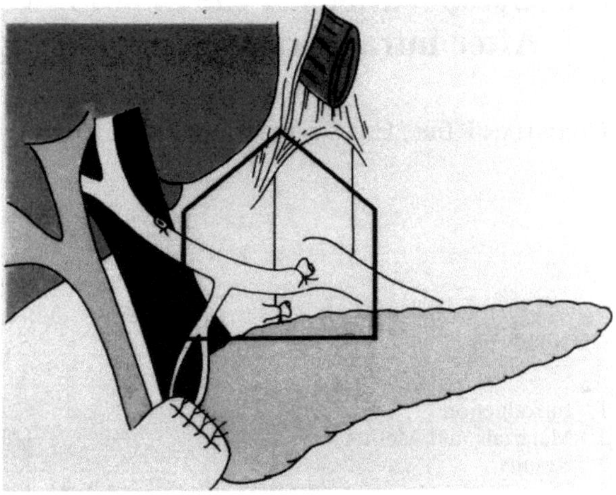

Fig. 2. Pentangular-shaped irradiation field for intraoperative radiotherapy (IORT) after gastrectomy including the tumor bed and the upper edge of the pancreas. (From SCHILDBERG et al. 1992)

This chapter deals only with those complications of the bowel and the pancreas. The complications may have been due to surgery, intraoperative and/or external beam irradiation or the tumor growth itself. In many cases it was difficult to discriminate between the different possibilities and their interactions.

3 Results

Of the patients treated for operable and inoperable pancreatic cancer, there were two who had anastomotic leakage after hemipancreatectomy, none in the group of palliative operations. There were three patients with bowel stenosis, two of these cases concerning the duodenum. In two of 74 patients, a generalized peritonitis took place (Table 1). None of these complications had a lethal outcome.

The most frequent complication in the group of pancreatic cancer patients was bleeding, which occurred 12 times (Table 1). There was only one bleeding in the group of resected patients, who were irradiated only intraoperatively. There were 11 patients with inoperable tumors, who were treated both intraoperatively and with external beam radiotherapy (Table 2). The bleedings occurred 2–9 months after irradiation (mean: 5.6 months). Seven of these bleedings were lethal. Further detailed analysis of the bleedings showed that, except for one intraoperative surgical bleeding, all occurred in those patients who had IORT plus external

Table 1. Complications of the bowel and pancreas after intraoperative radiotherapy ($n = 101$)

Complication	Unresectable pancreatic cancer ($n = 44$)	Resectable pancreatic cancer ($n = 30$)	Gastric cancer ($n = 27$)
Pancreatic fistula/necrosis	0	0	4
Gastrointestinal obstruction	2	1	0
Anastomotic leakage	0	2	1
Hemorrhage	11	1	1
Abscess	1	1	2
Total number	14	5	8

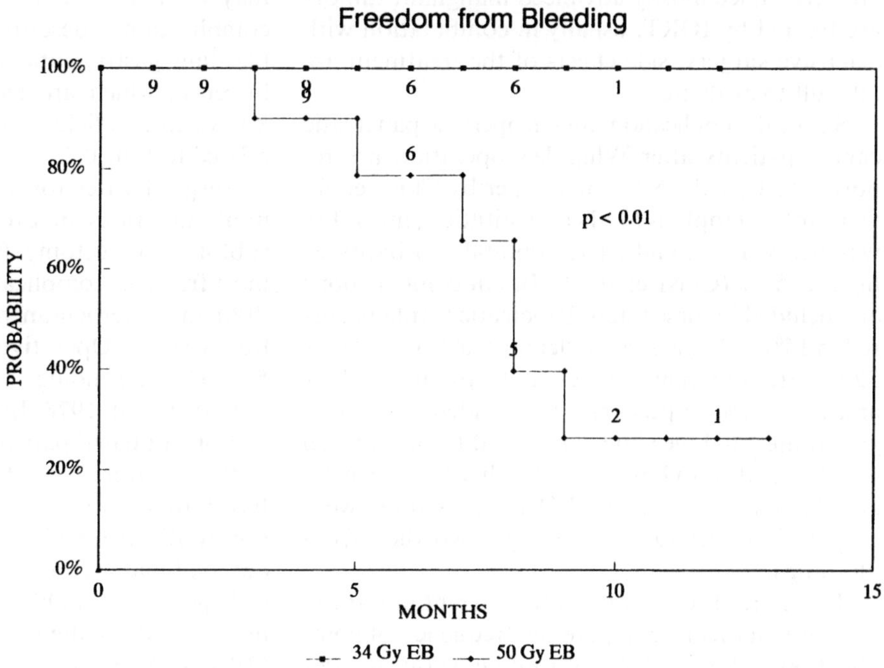

Fig. 3. Probability of a bleeding event after 20 Gy intraoperative radiotherapy (IORT) for patients with unresectable pancreatic cancer; there was a significant reduction of bleedings after reducing the external beam (*EB*) dose from 50 Gy to 34 Gy

beam irradiation (Fig. 3.) In the 22 patients in whom only IORT with 20 Gy ($n = 8$) or 30 Gy ($n = 14$) was performed, only one surgical bleeding was seen (Table 2).

In the early days of IORT, parts of the duodenum were included into the IORT field. If those cases are excluded from the analysis the bleeding events are seen only in the group of patients who had 20 Gy IORT *plus* 50 Gy external beam radiotherapy. After the reduction of the external dose from 50 to 34 Gy (both fractionated 5 × 1.8 Gy/week), no more bleedings occurred. The difference is statistically significant (Fig. 3).

Table 1, shows the incidence of complications in patients with gastric cancer and IORT. A total of eight events occurred (one bleeding without clinical relevance, one pancreatic necrosis and three pancreatic fistulas, one anastomotic leakage and two cases of peritonitis with abscess). Two patients died from

Table 2. Inoperable pancreatic cancer: bleedings according to therapy with and without external beam irradiation

IORT (Gy)	EB (Gy)	Bleedings	Corrected[a]
20	50	7/10	6/9*,*
20	34	3/12	0/8*
20	–	1[b]/8	1[b]/8**
30	–	0/14	0/14

IORT, intraoperative radiotherapy; EB, external beam; * and **, statistically significant comparisons.
[a]Corrected: patent with bowel inside IORT field eliminated.
[b]Surgical bleeding.

complications. Compared to the unirradiated arm of the trial, only the pancreatic complications seemed to be more frequent. Compared to the literature, the overal incidence of complications in both groups was not elevated concerning lethal and other events.

4 Discussion

Published data regarding complications of IORT are rare. Since mostly advanced malignant tumors are treated by IORT, usually in combination with extensive surgery, side effects of the treatment are difficult to evaluate.

Surgical complication rates in operable pancreatic cancer patients after Whipple's operation are reported to be 12%–52%. In a paper by CRIST et al., from Johns Hopkins Medical Institution, mortality was between 2% and 24%, nonfatal morbidity as high as 52% (CRIST et al. 1987). All complications are included in these totals. Pancreatic fistula occurred in 14%–22%, gastric outlet obstruction in 24%–32%, intra-abdominal abscess and sepsis in 4%–17% and 11%–29%, respectively. The incidence of upper gastrointestinal bleeding is reported to be between 6%–15%, intra-abdominal hemorrhage between 2% and 12%. Six out of 88 (7%) patients underwent reoperation because of bleedings; two died from bleedings.

There are three reports in the current literature, that systematically compare the frequency of complications after IORT to routine surgical procedures (CROMACK et al. 1989; AVIZONIS et al. 1989; NOYES et al. 1992). For pancreatic cancer, Avizonis et al. reported a morbidity rate of 19% for their patients (both resected and unresected) treated with IORT ($n = 26$) compared to 32% with surgery alone ($n = 28$) in a nonrandomized trial; mortality was 8% (IORT) vs 18% (surgery alone). CROMACK et al. published data from two randomized trials treating pancreatic cancer with and without IORT. Intra-abdominal abscess, pancreatic fistula and hemorrhage were the most frequent complications both for resected and unresected tumors. Mortality and morbidity did not differ significantly in the treatment groups (Tables 3, 4). In the analysis of NOYES et al., 13 of the 59 patients who received IORT (22%) developed complications compared to only three of 26 (12%) in the non-IORT group. Even though the difference is not statistically significant, this suggests that IORT to the pancreatic region may be associated with a higher morbidity. The complications described included anastomotic bleeding, gastric outlet obstruction and wound dehiscence, which are technical complications well known in this field of surgery and not necessarily related to IORT.

Surgical series for gastric cancer report overall morbidity rates in excess of 50% after total or subtotal gastrectomy (DUPONT et al. 1978). The most frequent complications were wound infection (9%) and enterocutaneous fistula and anastomotic leakage (4%). Operative mortality is reported to be 5%–16% depending on the surgical procedure (DUPONT et al. 1978; BONENKAMP et al. 1992).

For irradiated patients, in the series of Avizonis et al. the overall morbidity in patients receiving IORT ($n = 14$) was 35% compared to 25% in the non-IORT group (Table 5). Nevertheless, the incidence of major complications such as anastomotic leakage or intra-abdominal abscess was slightly higher in the patients who received surgery only (25% vs 18%). The mortality rate was 5% in both groups. The report of CROMACK et al. showed a higher incidence of fistulas in the IORT (five of 12) than in the control group (four of 21). This finding correlates with our own experience and may be due to the compression of the upper edge of the pancreas by the irradiation tube (see Fig. 2). Other complications e.g. hemorrhage or abscess, showed no difference in occurrence in both groups, except

Table 3. Unresectable pancreatic cancer

	NOYES et al.		CROMACK et al.		Our results
Complication	IORT ($n = 59$)	Control ($n = 26$)	IORT ($n = 16$)	Control ($n = 13$)	IORT ($n = 44$)
Fistula	1	0	0	1	0
Hemorrhage	2	1	6	3	11
Obstruction	1	0	4	2	2
Intra-abdominal abscess	0	0	2	1	1

IORT, intraoperative radiotherapy.

Table 4. Resectable pancreatic cancer

Complication	CROMACK et al. 1989 IORT (n = 10)	CROMACK et al. 1989 Control (n = 12)	AVIZONIS et al. 1989 IORT (n = 16)	Our results IORT (n = 30)
Fistula	1	0	0	0
Hemorrhage (gastro-intestinal and intra-abdominal	3	2	0	1
Obstruction	0	2	0	1
Intra-abdominal abscess	4	4	1	1
Anastomotic leak	n.r.	n.r.	2	2

n.r., not reported.

Table 5. Reports of complications in gastric cancer

Complication	CROMACK et al. 1989 IORT (n=12)	CROMACK et al. 1989 Control (n=21)	NOYES et al. 1992 IORT (n=31)	NOYES et al. 1992 Control (n=22)	AVIZONIS et al. 1989 IORT (n=14)	SINDELAR et al. 1993 IORT (n=16)	SINDELAR et al. 1993 Control (n=25)	Own results IORT (n=27)	Own results Control (n=33)
Pancreatic fistula	5	4	1	0	0	0	1	3	0
Hemorrhage	2	1	0	0	0	2	1	1	1
Gastrointes-tinal obstruction/ stricture	1	0	0	0	0	4	3	0	0
Abscess	5	5	0	0	2	4	8	2	3
Anastomotic leak	n.r.	n.r.	1	2 (1[a])	3	2	3	1	0
Pancreatitis	n.r.	n.r.	2[a]	0	n.r.	n.r.	n.r.	1	0

n.r. = not reported.
[a]Fatal
IORT, intraoperative radiotherapy.

for enteritis-obstruction which was increased in the surgery group only. The RTOG data from the protocol 85–04, which combined gastrectomy with IORT and postoperative external beam radiotherapy (40–50 Gy) (NOYES et al. 1992) showed that only the incidence of pancreatic complications was higher in the IORT group (three of 31) than in the group that received surgery and external beam irradiation (none of 22). This again indicates that IORT to open pancreatic surfaces may increase the risk of pancreatitis or pancreatic fistula.

Our own data concerning complications of IORT are in accordance with the reports from the literature, except for the fact that we saw a higher incidence of lethal bleedings in the patient group treated with palliative surgery, IORT (20 Gy) and postoperative external beam irradiation with 50 Gy. Other investigators who used the same treatment schedule reported no complications at all (ABE and TAKAHASHI 1981) or only minor bleedings (RICH 1985; TEPPER et al. 1984). The reason for the high incidence of bleedings in our patients is unclear. As there is a statistically significant reduction of bleedings after reducing the external beam dose to 34 Gy without a worsening of the results, a dose of 20 Gy intraoperatively plus 50 Gy external beam seems to be too high.

5 Summary and Therapeutic Recommendations

According to the literature and our own experience, IORT in the upper abdomen causes no increase of the known surgical complications such as anastomotic leak, abscess and gastrointestinal obstruction. There may be a tendency towards a higher rate of pancreatic complications after irradiation of the tumor bed after gastrectomy for gastric cancer. This complication may be due to the compression of the IORT tube to the upper part of the pancreas; thus, great caution is recommended while positioning the tube in this area.

As we saw a high incidence of bleedings in our patients with unresectable pancreatic cancer treated with 20 Gy IORT plus 50 Gy external beam irradiation, we recommend a reduction of the external beam dose to 34 Gy. This is possible without compromising the good results on local control.

References

Abe M, Takahashi M (1981) Intraoperative radiotherapy: the Japanese Experience. Int J Radiat Oncol Biol Phys 7: 863–868

Avizonis VN, Sause WT, Noyes RD (1989) Morbidity and Mortality Associated with Intraoperative Radiotherapy. J Surg Oncol 41: 240–245

Bonenkamp JJ, Van de Velde CJH, Sasako M, Hermans J (1992) R2 Compared with R1 Resection for gastric cancer: morbidity and mortality in a prospective, randomized trial. Eur J Surg 158: 413–418

Calvo FA, Azinovic I, Zornoza G, Voltas J, Pardo F, Alvarez-Cienfuegos J (1992) Pancreatic cancer intraoperative radiotherapy. Springer, Berlin Heidelberg New York, pp 57–64

Crist DW, Sitzmann JV, Cameron JL (1987) Improved hospital morbidity, mortality, and survival after the whippel procedure. Ann Surg 206(3): 358–365

Cromack DT, Maher MM, Hoekstra H, Kinsella TJ, Sindelar WF (1989) Are complications in intraoperative radiation therapy more frequent than in conventional treatment? Arch Surg 124: 229–234

Dupont JB, Lee JR, Burton GR, Cohn I (1978) Adenocarcinoma of the stomach: review of 1497 Cases. Cancer 41: 941–947

Frommhold H, Albrecht T, Glaser K, Nilles A (1991) Individualisierte Intraoperative Radiotherapie des Pancreaskarzinoms. Radiologe 31: 147–152

Gunderson LL, Martin JK, Earle JD, Byer De, Voss M, Fieck JM, Kvols LK, Rorie DK, Martinez A, Nargoney DM, O'Connell MJ, Weber FC (1984) Intraoperative and external beam irradiation with or without resection: Mayo pilot experience. Mayo Clin Proc 59: 691–699

Gunderson LL, Martin JK, Kvols LK, Nargoney DM, Fieck JM, Wieland HS, Martinez A, O'Connell MJ, Earle JD, McIlrath DC (1987) Intraoperative and external beam irradiation ±5 FU for locally advanced pancreatic cancer. Int J Radiat Oncol Biol Phys 13: 319–329

Krämling HJ, Willich N, Schildberg FW (1992) Intraoperative Radiotherapie (IORT) in der onkologischen Chirurgie. Jahr Chir 117–129

Noyes D, Weiss SM, Krall JM, Sause WT, Ovens JR, Wolkov HB, Lanciano R, Hanks GE, Hoffmann J (1992) Surgical complications of intraoperative radiation therapy: the radiation therapy oncology group experience. J Surg Oncol 50: 209–215

Rich TA (1985) Radiation therapy for pancreatic cancer: eleven year experience at the JCRT. Int J Radiat Oncol Biol Phys 11: 759–763

Rübe C, Wilkowski R, Krämling HJ, Grab J, Willich N, Lissner J (1992) Acute, subacute and late effects of IORT in the upper abdomen. Strahlenther 168(8): 463–464

Rübe C, Willich N, Wendt T, Grab J, Pratschke E, Kiszel Z (1992) Intraoperative Bestrahlung (IORT) des Pancreaskarzinoms: das Großhaderner Patientenkollektiv (1986–1991). Zentralbl Radiol 146 (1–2): 76–77

Schildberg FW, Willich N, Krämling HJ (1992) Intraoperative Strahlentherapie bei malignen Tumoren des Gastrointestinaltrakts. Chirurg 63(4): 251–259

Sindelar WF, Kinsella TJ, Tepper JE, DeLaney TF, Maher MM, Smith R, Rosenberg SA, Glatstein E (1993) Randomized trial of intraoperative radiotherapy in carcinoma of the stomach. Am J Surg 165: 178

Tepper JE, Gunderson LL, Orlow E, Cohen AM, Hedberg SE, Shipley WU, Blitzer PH, Rich T (1984) Complications of intraoperative radiation therapy. Int J Radiat Oncol Biol Phys 10: 1831–1839

Tepper JE, Noyes D, Krall JM, Sause WT, Wolkov HB, Dobelbower RR, Thomson J, Owens J, Hanks GE (1991) Intraoperative radiation therapy of pancreatic carcinoma: a report of RTOG-8505 Int J Radiat Oncol Biol Phys 21: 1145–1149

Willich N, Teichmann R, Krimmel K, Naujokat B, Denecke H, Wendt T, Rohloff R (1988) Intraoperative Elektronenbestrahlung (IORT) maligner Pankreastumoren-erste Großhaderner Erfahrung. Strahlenther Oncol 164(4): 187–194

Willich N, Denecke H, Krimmel K, Grab J (1989) The Munich experience in intraoperative irradiation therapy of pancreatic cancer. Ann Radiol 32(6): 484–486

3.7 Skin Toxicity

MICHAEL LANDTHALER

CONTENTS

1 Introduction 127
2 Toxic Reactions 127
2.1 Alopecia 127
2.2 Stomatitis 127
2.3 Hyperpigmentation 127
2.4 Nail Disorders 128
2.5 Photosensitivity Reactions 128
2.6 Extravasation 128
2.7 Acral Erythema 128
2.8 Radiation Reactions 128
3 Allergic Reactions 128
4 Pseudoallergies 129
5 Assignment of Skin Changes to Various Anticancer Drugs 129
6 Various Skin Reactions 129
References 130

1 Introduction

Skin lesions in cancer patients may be caused by many reasons (Table 1). They may vary dramatically in clinical presentation and their classification is often difficult (CHREN et al. 1993). A major cause is chemotherapeutic agents, the side effects of which can be divided into toxic reactions, allergies, and pseudoallergies. It is also possible to assign various other skin reactions to certain chemotherapeutic agents.

2 Toxic Reactions

Patterns of cutaneous toxicity include alopecia, stomatitis, hyperpigmentations, nail disorders, photosensitivity, extravasation injury, radiation reactions, and acral erythema (DESPAIN 1991; REST and HORN 1992).

MICHAEL LANDTHALER, Prof. Dr., Dermatologische Klinik und Poliklinik, Universität Regensburg, Franz-Josef-Strasse-Allee 11, 93053 Regensburg, FRG

Table 1. Skin lesions in tumor patients

Toxic drug reactions
Allergies
Pseudoallergies
Secondary tumors
Skin metastases
Radiation effects
Paraneoplastic syndromes
Infections (fungi, bacteria, viruses)
Graft vs host reaction

2.1 Alopecia

Toxic hair loss caused by cytostatics is often observed. Depending on the dose given and the length of time, either alopecia of the immediate type, with a dystrophic hair root pattern, or alopecia of the late type, with a telogen hair root pattern (BRAUN-FALCO et al. 1984), develops.

2.2 Stomatitis

This is a well known side effect of chemotherapy. Drugs often causing stomatitis include 5-fluorouracil, methotrexate, dactinomycin, doxorubicin, daunorubicin, bleomcin, cytarabine, and less frequently cyclophosphamide. Symptoms usually begin within 1 week of therapy with exanthema and may progress rapidly to confluent ulceration. Complications through secondary infection by bacteria, viruses, or *Candida* species are common (REST and HORN 1992).

2.3 Hyperpigmentation

Hyperpigmentations of skin, mucous membranes, and nails are often caused by alkylating agents and antibiotics, which may have a direct stimulating effect on melanocytes or lead to toxic postinflammatory hyperpigmentation.

Clinically, different types of hyperpigmentations can be distinguished (DeSpain 1991; Rest and Horn 1992; Tsuij and Sawabe 1993):

1. Diffuse cutaneous hyperpigmentation mimicking Addison's disease by busulfan, cyclophosphamide, methotrexate, 5-fluorouracil, dactinomycin, and hydroxyurea.
2. Serpignous hyperpigmented streaks overlying veins after infusion of 5-fluorouracil.
3. Flagellate pigmentations in patients receiving bleomycin.
4. Darkened horizontal bands within hair (flag sign) following high dose methotrexate.
5. Nail hyperpigmentations after cyclophosphamide, 5-fluorouracil, daunorubicin, doxorubicin, and bleomycin.
6. Generalized hyperpigmentations following ifosfamide.
7. Oral mucous membrane hyperpigmentations with doxorubicin and 5-fluorouracil.

2.4 Nail Disorders

The cytotoxic effects of chemotherapy on the nail matrix are reflected by Beau's lines occurring weeks after therapy, transverse white bands, hyperpigmentations, toxic onycholysis, and true leukonychia. (DeSpain 1991; Rest and Horn 1992; Unammo et al. 1992).

2.5 Photosensitivity Reactions

These reactions are rarely caused by chemotherapeutic agents. Clinically, sunburn-like reactions are typical. Triggering drugs include dacarbazine, 5-fluorouracil, vinblastine, and mitomycin (DeSpain 1991).

2.6 Extravasation

Many drugs can cause extravasation injury leading to skin necrosis and ulceration (Table 2). Dacarbazine, dactinomycin, daunorubicin, doxorubicin, and vinblastine may result in phlebitis; bleomycin, cisplatin, and dacarbazine induce chemical cellulitis (Breathnach and Hinter 1992).

2.7 Acral Erythema

Clinically, acral erythema (palmar-plantar erythrodysaesthesia) is characterized by palmar-plantar erythema and swelling, and in severe cases by blister formation and disabling pain (4). There seem to be different types of reactions. Type A has been observed during long-term continuous infusion of doxorubicin or 5-fluorouracil. In this type, severity of skin alterations increases and remission only occurs when treatment is discontinued or the responsible agent is changed. Type B develops a few days after a short-term chemotherapy including cytarabine or methotrexate. It is a self-limited condition that can be treated symptomatically. In some patients oral corticosteroids may be effective. Typically, chemotherapeutic treatment need not to be discontinued (Wiedemann et al. 1992). A similar reaction of erythema and ear swelling was described after cytarabine treatment for leukemia (Kruldner et al. 1990).

Table 2. Agents causing type I reactions, e.g., urticaria and angioedema

L-Asparaginase	
Busulfan	
Chlorambucil	Thio-TEPA
Cisplatin	Methotrexate
Cyclophosphamide	Etoposide
Daunorubicin	Mitotane
Doxorubicin	Procarbazine
Melfalan	

From Peters et al. (1986); Rest and Horn (1992).

2.8 Radiation Reactions

Radiation reactions are caused by the combined effects of radiation and chemotherapeutic drugs including radiation enhancement and radiation recall phenomenon. The latter is an inflammatory reaction in tissues previously irradiated, following administration of chemotherapeutic agents. Dactinomycin and doxorubicin are the drugs most frequently causing this phenomenon. Clinically, this reaction is characterized as erythema, edema, vesiculation, and desquamation (DeSpain 1991). Recently, radiation recall toxicity was observed in a patient with AIDS-related Kaposi's sarcoma and bleomycin therapy (Stelzer et al. 1993).

3 Allergic Reactions

According to Coombs and Gell (1963) hypersensitivity reactions can be classified into four groups.

Type I reactions are mediated by specific IgE antibodies and clinically manifest as urticaria, angioedema or anaphylactic shock. Most commonly, L-asparaginase causes this type of reaction and about 10% of patients suffering from urticarial reaction to L-asparaginase may progress to life-threatening anaphylaxis (DeSpain 1991). Other agents which also may cause type I reactions are listed in Table 2.

Type II reactions are mediated by complement activating IgG antibodies which are fixed on target cells such as erythrocytes, leukocytes or platelets. Clinically, these reactions present as hemolytic anemia, thrombocytopenia, and agranulocytosis. Primary skin lesions have not been described.

Type II reactions are caused by circulating immune complexes and the skin may react in two different patterns: (1) as cutaneous allergic leukocytoclastic vasculitis or (2) skin involvement in serum sickness, characterized by urticaria, vasculitis, arthritis, and lymphadenophathy. Drugs known to cause type III reactions are listed in Table 3.

Type IV reactions are cell-mediated allergic reactions of the delayed type, i.e., eczema tuberculin type reactions. In about 50% of mycosis fungoides patients treated with topical aqueous mechlorethamine an allergic contact dermatitis develops (DeSpain 1991). Other drugs which can lead to contact dermatitis after skin contact are daunorubicin, doxorubicin and 5-fluorouracil (Peters et al. 1986). Exanthematous allergic drug reactions are also considered to be a tuberculin type IV reaction. Clinical manifestations include morbilliform, scarlatiniform, or rubeoliform drug eruptions. Erythema multiforme may be caused by type III and IV reactions (Braun-Facco et al. 1984). Exanthematous drug eruptions can follow therapy with high dose thio-TEPA, methrotrexate, triazinate, and long-term high dose hydroxyurea (DeSpain 1991). Additionally, these eruptions can be caused by supportive drugs such as antibiotics or analgesics.

Table 3. Agents causing type III reactions

L-Asparaginase
Busulfan
Chlorambucil
Cyclophosphamide
Hydroxyurea
Mechlorethamine
Procarbazine
Thio-TEPA
Cytarabine

From Peters et al. (1986); Rest and Horn (1992).

4 Pseudoallergies

Pseudoallergy reactions may clinically imitate true allergies but they are *not* mediated by antibodies or antigen-specific lymphocytes (Brain-Falco et al. 1984). Anaphylactoid reactions resemble an anaphylaxis and clinical signs, e.g., erythema and urticaria are mediated by histamine. They often result from direct action of drugs on mast cells, platelets or other immune competent cells. Anticancer drugs that may initiate pseudoallergies are listed in Table 4.

5 Assignment of Skin Changes to Various Anticancer Drugs

Besides the classification of skin reactions as toxic, allergic, and pseudoallergic, it is possible to assign various other skin reactions to alkylating agents, antibiotics, and antimetabolites (Table 5–8) (Breathnach and Hinter 1992).

6 Various Skin Reactions

Multiple reactions to anticancer drugs, which cannot be classified as toxic or allergic reactions, have been observed. Neutrophilic eccrine hidradenitis presents as a papular rash without a characteristic distribution. Recently, it has been observed in patients with acute mylogenous leukemia receiving induction chemotherapy. It may be caused by cytarabine and bleomycin. The lesions usually resolve spontaneously. Histologically one finds infiltration of eccrine coils with neutrophils and necrosis of secretory epithelium (Breathnach and Hinter 1992). A related skin lesion is syringosquamous

Table 4. Agents which may cause pseudoallergies

Chlorambucil
Melfalan
Thio-TEPA
Methotrexate
Bleomycin
Daunorubicin
Doxorubicin

Table 5. Skin reactions by alkylating agents

Busulfan	Bullous erythema multiforme
	Urticaria
	Hyperpigmentation (Addisonian-like)
	Porphyria cutanea tarda
	Allergic vasculitis
Chlorambucil	Morbilliform exanthema
	Urticaria, periorbital edema
Cyclophosphamide and mesna	Hair loss
	Hyperpigmentation (localized, widespread)
	Allergic reactions to mesna (urticaria, rashes)
Mechlorethamine	Angioedema, pruritus
	Contact dermatitis
Melfalan	Morbilliform rashes
	Anaphylactic shock (patients with IgA, κ myeloma)
	Urticaria
	Allergic vasculitis
	Melanonychia striata
Thio-TEPA	Pruritus, urticaria, angioedema (after intravesical installation)
	Patterned hyperpigmentation (after i.v. administration)
DTIC	Photosensitivity
Procarbazine	Urticaria, angioedema, arthralgia

From Breathnach and Hinter (1992).

Table 7. Skin reaction by antimetabolites

Aminoglutethimide	Systemic lupus erythematosus
Azathioprine	Exanthematous rashes
	Virus papillomas
	Skin tumors
Cytarabine	Acral erythema (type B)
5-fluorouracil	Photosensitivity
	Hyperpigmentations
	Acral erythema (type A)
	Anaphylaxis
Methotrexate	Acral erythema (type B)
	Urticaria
	Hair loss
	Photosensitivity
	Macular rash
	Anaphlyaxis

From Breathnach and Hinter (1992).

Table 8. Skin reactions to various drugs

Vinblastine	Light sensitivity
Cisplatin	Types I, III and IV allergies
DTIC	Light sensitivity
Interferon	Skin necrosis
Interleukin-2	Erythema, desquamation, local induration

From Breathnach and Hinter (1992).

metaplasia, which clinically presents as an erythematous and papular rash (Breathnach and Hinter 1992).

Inflammation of solar keratosis has been described after administration of fluorouracil or after combined therapies (DeSpain 1991).

Recently, patients with multiple skin tumors on light-exposed areas during long-term treatment with hydroxyurea have been observed (Papi et al. 1993). In 1984, multiple eruptive melanocytic naevi were described in a homozygotic twin after chemotherapy of acute leukemia with cortisone, 6-mercaptopurine, and methotrexate (Heyne et al.1984). Recently, it could be demonstrated that children receiving chemotherapy for hematologic malignancy have an excessive number of melanocytic naevi (Baird et al. 1992).

By the immune suppressive effects of anticancer therapy, infections of the skin with fungi, bacteria, and viruses are common (Rest and Horn 1992).

Subcutaneous injections of interferon-α may result in local necrosis of the skin (6).

A maculopapular eruption, which developed after an 8 day cycle of doxorubicin, 5-fluorouracil, and cyclophosphamide, was histologically characterized by a benign, multifocal, and spontaneously disappearing dermal invasion of atypical basal keratinocytes (Hann et al. 1993).

Table 6. Skin reaction by antibiotics

Bleomycin	Flagellate erythema and hyperpigmentations
	Alopecia
	Glossitis, buccal ulceration
	Drug fever
	Raynaud's phenomenon
	Systemic sclerosis-like changes
	Localized erythematous indurations
Dactinomycin	Acneiform rash
Daunorubicin	Angioedema, urticaria
	Hyperpigmentations
Doxorubicin	Erythema and urticaria along injected vein
	Angioedemia, urticaria
	Hyperpigmentations (skin, nails)
	Acral erythema (type A)
Mitomycin	Urticaria
	Dermatitis (face, palms, soles)

From Breathnach and Hinter (1992).

References

Baird EA, McHenry PM, MacKie RM (1992) Effect of maintenance chemotherapy in childhood on numbers of melanocytic naevi. Br Med J 305: 799–801

Braun-Falco O, Plewig G, Wolff HH, Winkelman RK (1984) Dermatology Springer, Berlin Heidelberg New York
Breathnach SM, Hinter H (1992) Adverse drug reactions and the skin. Blackwell, London, pp 281–304
Burgdorf WHC, Gilmore WA, Ganick RG (1982) Peculiar acral erythema secondary to high-dose chemotherapy for acute myelogenous leukemia. Ann Intern Med 97: 61–62
Chren MM, Lazarus HM, Bickers DR (1993) Rashes in immuno compromised cancer patients. Arch Dermatol 129: 175–181
Christian B, Derriennic X, Aymard JP (1993) Nécrose cutanée locale après injection d'interféron alpha. Presse Med 22: 783
Coombs RRA, Gell PGH (1963) The classification of allergic reactions underlying disease. In: Gell PGH, Coombs RRA (eds) Clinical aspects of immunology. Davis, Philadelphia, pp 317–330
DeSpain JD (1991) Dermatologic toxicity. In: Perry MC (ed) The chemotherapy source book. Williams and Wilkins, Baltimore, pp 531–547
Hann SK, Rhoe BS, Kang WH, Park YK (1993) Self limited dermal invasion of keratinocytes in maculopapular eruptions after systemic chemotherapy. J Dermatol 20: 94–101
Heyne K, Hof M, Hansen HG (1984) Pigmented naevi after therapy of leukemia in a monozygotic twin. Eur J Pediatr 142: 70
Krulder JWM, Vlasveld LT, Willemze R (1990) Erythema and swelling of ears after treatment with cytarabine for leukemia. Eur J Cancer 26: 649–650
Papi M, Didona B, DePità O, Abruzzese E, Stasi R, Papa G, Cavalieri (1993) Multiple skin tumors on light-exposed areas during long-term treatment with hydroxyurea. J Am Acad Dermatol 28: 485–486
Peters HD, Fink U, Schmoll HJ (1986) Dermatoxizität. In: Schmoll HJ, Peters HD, Fink U (eds) Kompendium Internistische Onkologie, part 1. Springer, Berlin Heidelberg New York, pp 239–248
Rest EB, Horn TD (1992) Dermatology. In: Armitage JO, Antman KH (eds) High dose cancer therapy. Pharmacology, hematopoietnis, stem cells. Williams and Wilkins, Baltimore, pp 518–546
Stelzer KJ, Griffin TW, Koh WJ (1993) Radiation recall skin toxicity with bleomycin in a patient with Kaposi sarcoma related to acquired immune deficiency syndrome. Cancer 71: 1322–1325
Tsuij T, Sawabe M (1993) Hyperpigmentation in striae distensae after bleomycin treatment, J Am Acad Dermatol 3: 503–505
Unammo P, Fernandez-Lopez E, Santos C (1992) Leukonychia due to cytostatic agents, Clin Exp Dermatol 17: 273–274
Wiedemann M, Meller-Henn M, Mahrle G (1992) Erythrodysaesthesia palmoplantaris – Vorkommen von zwei klinischen Erscheinungsbildern? Z Hautkr 67: 1070–1072

4 Lung Toxicity

4.1 Radiation Pneumopathy – Experimental and Clinical Data

THOMAS HERRMANN, JOHANNES SCHORCHT, and MICHAEL MOLLS

CONTENTS

1 Introduction 135
2 Animal Experiments 135
3 Clinical Data 136
4 Clinical Problems Associated with Lung Sparing . . 137
5 Summary and Practical Consequences 138
References 139

1 Introduction

Radiation-induced lung damage presents as a typical "black box" situation. The input, i.e., the dose dependence, and the output, i.e., the clinical, histological and radiographic (including CT) features of disease, are well known. However, the pathogenetic mechanisms which transform the lung tissue, normally filled with air, first into alveoli with thickened alveolar capillary membranes filled with exudate and finally into a fibrotic scar are largely unknown. Recent studies, moreover, demonstrate that interstitial pneumonia developing after total body irradiation and bone marrow transplantation is fundamentally different from radiation pneumonitis after fractionated localized radiotherapy with regard to mechanism and radiobiology. The development of interstitial pneumonia associated with bone marrow transplantation is influenced by a variety of factors which also target the lung, including chemotherapy, viremia and decreased immunological defenses (VAREKAMP 1990; MOLLS and VAN BEUNINGEN 1991). Yet the increasing therapeutic use of total body irradiation and bone marrow transplantation has highlighted the dose-limiting complications imposed by the lung. Increased research efforts into the radiobiology of radiation-induced pneumopathy has yielded some fundamental observations, which will be discussed here.

2 Animal Experiments

The dose-response relationship after irradiation of the lung is very steep, reflecting the narrow therapeutic response range of the lung (Fig. 1). Experiments by TRAVIS et al. (1985) demonstrated that lung tolerance increases considerably as dose rate decreases, with an optimum at about 0.01 Gy/min. This dose-rate effect is significant in animal experiments and has been confirmed by clinical reports from different bone marrow transplantation centers (WEINER et al. 1986).

Radiobiological experiments in different animal models (mice, rats) have been carried out to study

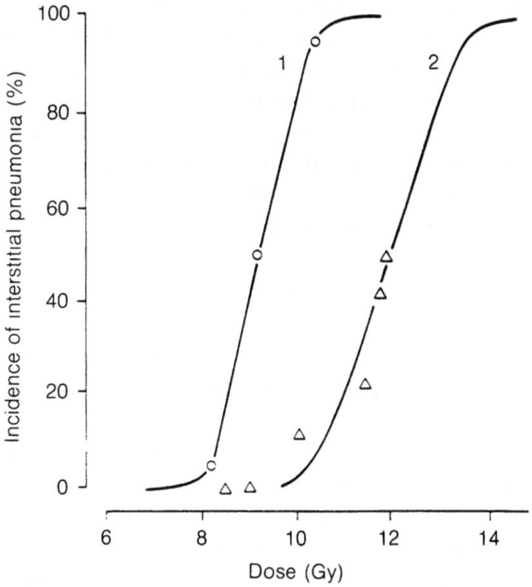

Fig. 1. Dose-effect curve of pneumonitis after single dose with higher dose rate (*curve 1*, 0.5–4.0 Gy/min) (VAN DYK et al. 1989) and lower dose rate (*curve 2*, 0.028–0.15 Gy/min) (KEANE et al. 1989). (From MOLLS et al. 1991)

THOMAS HERRMANN, Prof. Dr., JOHANNES SCHORCHT, Privatdozent, Dr., Medizinische Akademie Carl Gustav Carus, Abteilung Strahlentherapie, Fetscherstraße 74, 01307 Dresden, FRG
MICHAEL MOLLS, Prof. Dr., Klinik für Strahlentherapie, Technische Universität, Ismaninger Straße 15, 81675 Munich, FRG

Table 1. The α/β ratios and repair halftimes for lung damage (MOLLS et al. 1991)

	α/β	Repair halftime: $T^{1/2}$	Author
Mouse		0.76 h (trend toward shorter halftime with large fraction sizes)	TRAVIS et al. (1987a)
Mouse		0.8–1.2 h	PARKINS et al. 1988)
Mouse	3.74 Gy	0.84 h	DOWN et al. (1986)
Mouse	4.0 Gy	0.75 h	VEGESNA et al. (1989)
Mouse	3.7 Gy, analysis of data from TRAVIS et al. (1987a)		THAMES et al. (1989)
Mouse	3.7 Gy, analysis of data from VEGESNA et al. (1985)		THAMES et al. (1989)
Mouse	2.5–4.0 Gy, analysis of data from PARKINS et al. (1985)		TUCKER and TRAVIS (1990)
Mouse	5.5 Gy, analysis of data from FIELD et al. (1976)		TUCKER and TRAVIS (1990)
Mouse	3.7 Gy, analysis of data from WARA et al. (1973)		TUCKER and TRAVIS (1990)
Mouse	about 3.0 Gy (ignoring a time factor)		FOWLER (1990)
Rat	3.5 Gy (pneumonitis) 2.3 Gy (fibrosis)	0.95 h (pneumonitis) 1.13 h (fibrosis)	VAN RONGEN et al. (1990)
Rat	2.7 Gy (ignoring a time factor)		VAN DYK et al. (1990)
Pig	3.7 Gy		HERRMANN et al. (1986a, 1987)
Animals	5.0 ± 10 Gy (acute damage) 2.0 Gy (late damage)	Analysis of data from the literature, including a factor for overall treatment time	VAN DYK et al. (1989)
Human	3.3 ± 1.5 Gy		VAN DYK et al. (1989)
Beagle	3.4 Gy		GILETTE et al. (1992)

the influence of the most important variables of fractionated radiotherapy, e.g., dose per fraction or number of fractions, and overall treatment time. These experiments consistently showed the particular importance of the size of the dose per fraction (or the number of fractions) whereas overall treatment time was of considerably less importance, in accordance with its very small impact on tolerance dose. Obviously, the lung, or the target cells which are responsible for the development of radiation pneumopathy, have a pronounced capacity for sublethal damage repair. Nonetheless, the lack of any significant increase of radiation tolerance with increasing overall treatment time suggests little or no regeneration of target cells during the course of radiotherapy.

Experiments in adolescent pigs, whose lungs are structurally and functionally very similar to those of humans, confirmed the conclusions drawn from rodent experiments (HERRMANN et al. 1986). The equation $D \sim N^{0.32} \times T^{0.05}$ describes the fractionation response of pig lung well and the size of the respective exponents reflects the radiobiological mechanisms just described. From these data, an α/β value of 3.7 could be derived.

Other experiments and the reevaluation of some older data yielded α/β values for the lung of between 2 and 5 Gy (Table 1). Therefore, the lung fits into the group of late responding tissues which all are characterized by a pronounced repair capacity and a small or absent capacity for repopulation of the target cells (van RONGEN et al. 1990). Lung sparing in clinical practice, therefore, can only be achieved by reducing the dose per fraction as much as feasible. Prolongation of overall treatment time or split-course irradiation is not an effective method of lung sparing possibly actually favoring tumor growth. Either of these approaches would thus be deleterious to the overall results of radiotherapy (MACIEJEWSKI et al. 1983).

3 Clinical Data

Table 2 is a review of some older published data (HERRMANN et al. 1987) describing attempts made in the 1960s and 1970s to spare the lung from radiation injury by using the split course technique. These attempts all failed, in accordance with experimental data in animals. Yet reduction of the daily

Table 2. Effect of overall treatment time (split course technique vs continuous treatment) on pneumonitis and fibrosis (HERRMANN et al. 1987)

Author	Tumor	Number of patients	Fraction × dose (Gy) (rest period)	Time d	Pneumonitis (%)	Fibrosis (%)	Effect
EICHBORN 1963	Lung	73	20···45 × 2.0	61		42.5	None
		37	25···30 × 2.0 (6 weeks)	101		62	
			15 × 2.0				
HOLSTI 1967	Lung	33	25···30 × 2.0	40	75		None
		74	13···15 × 2.0 (3 weeks)	61	70		
			13···15 × 2.0				
LEVITT 1967	Lung	14	30 × 2.0	40		7	None
		15	3 × 6.0 (4 weeks)	70		33	
			3 × 6.0				
LANDBERG 1971	Hodgkin's lymphoma	3	20 × 1.6···2.0	38	100		Small
		8	20 × 1.6···2.0 (5 weeks)	75	75		
			10 × 1.6···2.0				
EICHHORN 1972	Lung	60	11 × 6.0	55		35	None
		30	16 × 2.5 (3 weeks)	65		37	
			16 × 2.0				
JOHNSON 1976	Hodgkin's lymphoma	82	20 × 2.0	26	13		Small
		54	10 × 2.0 (3 weeks)	47	3.7		
			10 × 2.0				
SALAZAR 1976	Lung	101	30 × 2.0	40	17		None
		59	12 × 2.5 (2 weeks)	46	17		
			12 × 2.5				
EMAMI 1979	Lung	76	30 × 2.0	40	No difference		
		24	10 × 2.5 (3 weeks)	47			
			10 × 2.5				
KATS 1980	Lung	47	26 × 2.0	36		47	None
		32	14 × 2.0 (3 weeks)	53		75	
			14 × 2.0				
SHAH 1981	Lung	56	25 × 2.0	33		18	None
		70	10 × 3.0 (3 weeks)	49		17	
			10 × 3.0				

dose was very effective. The problem may be better discussed in relation to dose distribution in the lung, since in clinical practice straightforward reduction of dose per fraction is limited by the required tumor control dose.

This is particularly obvious in postmastectomy radiotherapy of the chest wall (LINGOS et al. 1991). The shape and the thickness of the chest wall varies enormously between patients. The dose distribution was calculated using a computerized planning system based on a computed tomography (CT) image (Fig. 2). The 80% isodose transects the anterior part of the lung and it is exactly there where radiogenic lung reactions are found. Yet these changes are only seen in CT images and not in normal chest X-rays. Radiogenic lung reactions are almost always clinically asymptomatic. Table 3 shows the data obtained from many patients who were treated in Dresden and demonstrates the success achieved by reducing the dose per fraction in the irradiated lung (by improved treatment plans) from 2.0 Gy to 1.8 Gy, with a significant reduction both of radiation pneumonitis and fibrosis. This clinical example demonstrates that reduction of the dose per fraction is the crucial factor and, actually, the only factor which effectively reduces lung toxicity. Unfortunately, there are a few practical problems with the clinical application of this treatment strategy, and these are discussed below.

4 Clinical Problems Associated with Lung Sparing

Even modern treatment planning systems have some problems in dealing with the highly variable anatomy of the thorax and the different shapes of its cross-sections. It is desirable to plan for radiotherapy of many cross-sections. However, since radiotherapy involving the thorax is very common, with 50% of all indications for radiotherapy in or

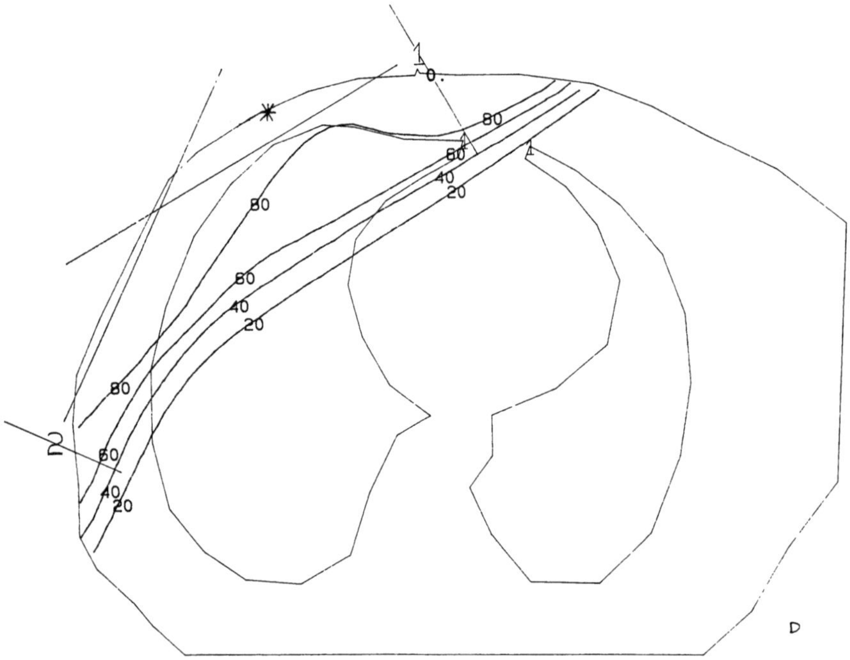

Fig. 2. Dose distribution in postmastectomy radiotherapy of the chest wall. The 80% isodose transects the anterior part of the left lung

Table 3. Pneumonitis and fibrosis in patients with postmastectomy radiotherapy of the chest wall: effects of dose per fraction

Dose per fraction	2.0 Gy	1.8 Gy
Number of patients	77	75
Fractions × dose	30 × 2 Gy	33 × 1.8 Gy
Pneumonitis	26 (34%)*	13 (17%)
Radiographic fibrosis	7 (9%)*	0 (0%)
	*$p < 0.05$	

near the thorax and including the lung, there remains a risk of producing hot spots in those lung regions which have not been planned. This is because lung density is very low and locally very heterogeneous (MAH and VAN DYK 1991). Therefore, even in properly planned radiotherapy in the thorax, increased fractional doses are likely to occur in partial volumes, which may not be well tolerated by the lung. A compromise has to be reached which is both feasible and safe.

While this problem may be of great practical importance, the as yet unresolved questions regarding the pathogenesis of radiation pneumonitis and the lack of clearly identifiable target structures (GRAHAM et al. 1990) still haunt the radiobiologist, whose interest is concentrated on type I and II pneumocytes and on capillary endothelial cells. These three cell types are among the approximately 40 separate ones known to exist in the lung. They have a very slow turnover rate, a limited capacity for repopulation, and are sensitive to damage by other cytotoxic agents, particularly to a number of anticancer drugs. Since injury may persist for quite some time, additive damage to lung tissue may occur even with sequential administration of radiotherapy and chemotherapy (YAN et al. 1991).

Progression from pneumonitis to fibrosis appears to be the natural course of events. It is, at present, an unresolved question whether each pneumonitis leads to fibrosis or whether limitation to very early types of injury may allow a reversion to normal (SLANINA et al. 1988). Clinical experience, however, demonstrates the difficulties in therapeutically influencing fibrotic lung disease in general and radiation induced lung fibrosis in particular. Yet there are some suggestions of potential therapeutic value which have come from experimental studies (WARD et al. 1990.)

5 Summary and Practical Consequences

The lung is the dose-limiting tissue in the thorax. A radiation dose of 40 Gy given in 20 daily fractions of 2 Gy leads to a 50% incidence of pneumonitis in the treated volume which will progress further to fibrosis. Smoking, drugs and preexisting lung disease all may increase the radiosensitivity of the lung. Therefore, it is imperative for the radiotherapist to assess, before the start of radiotherapy, the functional and radiographic status of the unirradiated lung. Only if the unirradiated lung is well enough to guarantee the essential breathing function and even if the entire irradiated lung volume fails, can radiotherapy with potentially curative doses be delivered even while deliberately running the risk of pneumopathy. If lung volume is already poor, or the unirradiated volume is small, or the entire lung is to be irradiated (e.g., in total body irradiation) everything has to be done to avoid radiation pneumonitis, as this would be lethal. A total dose of 20 Gy (with conventional fractionation) may not be exceeded.

Treatment planning has to be particularly careful if large lung volumes are to be included, taking into consideration the special physical problems associated with the air spaces to avoid excessive daily dose fractions.

Acknowledgment. The authors would like to thank Prof. K.-R. Trott/London for his critical comments and his help in preparing this manuscript.

References

Down JD, Easton DF, Steel GG (1986) Repair in the mouse lung during low dose rate irradiation. Radiother Oncol 6: 29–42

Eichhorn HJ, Lessel A, Rotte KH (1972) Einfluß verschiedener Bestrahlungsrhythmen auf Tumor- und Normalgewebe in vivo. Strahlentherapie 143: 614–629

Eichhorn HJ, Mateev B (1963) Über die Häufigkeit von Strahlenfibrosen im gesunden Lungengewebe nach intensiver Strahlentherapie beim Bronchialkarzinom. Strahlentherapie, Sonderband 52, 4: 149–155

Emami B, Munzenrider JE, Ding Jen Lee, Rene JB (1979) Radical radiation therapy of advanced lung cancer. Cancer 44: 446–456

Field, SB, Hornsey S, Kutsutani Y (1976) Effects of fractionated on mouse lung and a phenomenon of slow repair. Brit J Radiol 49: 700–707

Fowler JF (1990) Radiation-induced lung damage: dose-time fractionation considerations. Radiother Oncol 18: 184–187

Gillete SM, Gillete EL, Shida T, Boon J, Miller CW, Powers BE (1992) Late radiation response of canine mediastinal tissues. Radiother Oncol 23: 41–52

Graham MM, Margaret LE, Dahlen DD, Mahler PA, Rasey JS (1990) Pharmacological alteration of the lung vascular response to radiation. Int J Radiat Oncol Biol Phys 19: 329–339

Herrmann TH, Voigtmann L, Knorr A, Lorenz J (1987) Zum Reparaturverhalten der Lunge – experimentelle und klinische Ergebnisse. Strahlenther Onkol 163: 370–377

Herrmann TH, Voigtmann L, Knorr A, Lorenz J, Johannsen U (1986) Dose-time relationship of the radiogenic lung reaction in pigs. Radiother Oncol 5: 127–135

Holsti LB, Vuorinen P (1967) Radiation reaction in the lung after continuous and split-course megavoltage radiotherapy of bronchial-carcinoma. Brit J Radiol 40: 280–284

Johnson RE, Rühl U, Johnson SK, Glover M (1976) Splitcourse radiotherapy of Hodgkin's disease. Cancer 37: 1713–1717

Kats MS, Breuer DM, Zholkiver KI, Zevrieva IF (1980) Snatschenie welitschiny dosy i faktora wremeni w rasitii lutschewych pnewmosklerosow. Med radiol (Moskau) 25: 28–34

Kean TJ, van Dyk J (1989) TBI schedules prior to bone marrow transplantation: requirements for comparison (Letter to the editor). Radiother Oncol 15: 207–209

Landberg T, Svahn-Tapper G, Wintzell K (1971) Mantle treatment of Hodgkin's disease. Acta Radiol Ther Phys Biol 10: 174–186

Levitt SH, Bogardas CR, Ladd G (1967) Split-dose intensive radiation therapy in the treatment of advanced lung cancer: a randomized study. Radiology 88: 1159–1161

Lingos TI, Recht A, Vicini F, Abner A, Silver B, Harris JR (1991) Radiation pneumonitis in breast cancer patients treated with conservative surgery and radiation therapy. Int J Radiat Oncol Biol Phys 21: 355–360

Maciejewski B, Preuss-Bayer G, Trott KR (1983) The influence of the number of fractions and of overall treatment time on local control and late complication rate in squamous cell carcinoma of the larynx. Int J Radiat Oncol Biol Phys 9: 321–328

Mah K, van Dyk J (1991) On the impact of tissue inhomogeneity corrections in clinical thoracic radiation therapy. Int J Radiat Oncol Biol Phys 21: 1257–1267

Molls M, van Beuningen D (1991) Radiation injury of the lung: experimental studies, observations after radiotherapy and total body in adiation prior to bone marrow transplantation. In: Scherer E, Streffer C, Trott KR (eds) Medical radiology diagnostic imaging and radiation oncology (radiopathology of organs and tissues) Springer, Berlin Heidelberg New York

Parkins CS, Fowler JR, Maughan RL, Roper MJ (1985) Repair in mouse lung for up to 20 fractions. Brit J Radiol 58: 225–241

Parkins CS, Whitsed CA, Fowler JF (1988) Repair kinetics in mouse lung after multiple X-ray fractions per day. Int J Radiat Biol 54: 429–443

Salazar OM, Rubin P, Brown JC, Feldstein ML, Keller BE (1976) The assessment of tumor response to irradiation of lung cancer: continuous-vs-split course regimes. Int J Radiat Oncol Biol Phys 1: 1107–1118

Shah K, Olsen MH, Ray P (1981) Comparison of dose-time-fractionation schemes in non-oat-cell lung cancer. Cancer 48: 1127–1132

Slanina J, Sigmund G, Hinkelbein W, Wenz W, Wannenmacher M (1980) Die pulmonale Strahlenreaktion nach Mantelfeldbestrahlung Vergleich der Verlaufsstadien im konventionellen Röntgenbild und im Computertomogramm. Radiologie 28: 20–28

Thames HD, Hendry JH, Moore JV, Ang KK, Travis EL (1989) The high steepness of dose-response curves for late-responding normal tissues. Radiother Oncol 15: 49–53

Travis EL, Peters LJ, McNeill J, Thames HD, Karolis C (1985) Effect of dose-rate on total body irradiation: lethality and pathologic findings. Radiother Oncol 4: 341–351

Travis EL, Thames DL, Watkins TL, Kiss I (1987) The kinetics of repair in mouse lung after fractionated irradiation. Int J Radiat Biol 52: 903–919

Tucker SL, Travis EL (1990) Comments on a time-dependent version of the linear-quadratic model. Radiother Oncol 18: 155–163

van Dyk, Mah K, Keane TJ (1989) Radiation-induced lung damage: dose-time-fractionation considerations. Radioth Oncol 14: 55–69

van Dyk J, Mah K, Keane TJ (1990) Further comments on dose-time-fractionation considerations for lung damage, Letters to the editor. Radiother Oncol 18: 183–184

van Rongen E, Madhuizen HT, Tan CHT, Durham SK, Gijbels MJJ (1990) Early and late effects of fractionated irradiation and the kinetics of repair in rat lung. Radiother Oncol 17: 323–337

Varekamp AE (1990) Interstitial pneumonitis following bone marrow transplantation. Thesis, University of Leiden (also published by Institut of Applied Radiobiology and Immunology TNO, Rijswijk)

Vegesna SL, Withers HR, Thames HD, Mason KA (1985) Multifraction radiation response of mouse lung. Int J Radiat Biol 47: 413–422

Vegesna V, Withers HR, Taylor JMG (1989) Repair kinetics of mouse lung. Radiother Oncol 15: 115–123

Wara WM, Philips TL, Margolis LW, Smith V (1973) Radiation pneumonitis: a new approach to the deviation of time-dose factors. Cancer 32: 547–552

Ward WF, Molteni A, Ts'ao CH, Hinz JM (1990) Captopril reduces collagen and mast cell accumulation in irradiated rat lung. Int J Radiat Oncol Biol Phys 19: 1405–1409

Weiner RS, Bortin MM, Gale RP, Gluckman E, Kay HEM, Kolb HJ, Hartz AJ, Rimm AA (1986) Interstitial pneumonitis after bone marrow transplantation. Assessment of risk factors. Ann Intern Med 104: 168–175

Yan R, Peters LJ, Travis EL (1991) Cyclophosphamide 24 hours before total body irradiation: effects on lung and bone marrow. Radiother Oncol 21: 149–156

4.2 Lung Toxicity of Chemotherapeutic Agents

ULRICH GATZEMEIER

CONTENTS

1 Introduction 141
2 Experimental Data 141
3 Clinical Features 144
4 Laboratory Tests 144
5 Clinical Results 145
6 Summary and Therapeutic Recommendations . . . 147
References 149

1 Introduction

Many cytostatic drugs cause a significant incidence of clinically relevant pulmonary toxicity which influences therapeutic strategies (COLLIS 1980; COOPER et al. 1986; GINSBERG and COMIS 1982; MUGGIA 1983; SOSTMAN et al. 1977; WILLSON 1978). The most important drugs concerning these lung toxic effects are bleomycin and mitomycin C. Less frequent pulmonary toxicity is seen after cyclophosphamide, nitrosoureas and other (Table 1). The pathogenesis and morphological development of lung toxicity has been intensively examined (BEDROSSIAN 1982; COMIS 1992; FASSKE and MORGENROTH 1983; MARTIN and KACHEL 1987). Chemotherapeutic agents that are potentially lung toxic drugs play an important role in the combination chemotherapy of different solid tumors, for example, germ cell tumors. Due to the curative intent of the chemotherapy in these tumor types there is a need for both prevention and effective therapy of this specific side effect (MACKES et al. 1992).

The occurrence of free oxygen radicals (SINHA 1989; SLATER 1984) and dysfunction of the glutathione system are the most important factors (Table 2) (BEDROSSIAN 1982; BEREND 1985; COMIS 1992; FASSKE and MORGENROTH 1983; MARTIN and KACHEL 1987). Bleomycin induces a dose-related interstitial edema, proliferation of type II pneumocytes and activation of fibroblasts. The end point of this damage is an interstitial fibrosis similar to idiopathic diffuse interstitial fibrosis.

ULRICH GATZEMEIER, Dr., Lungenfachklinik, Onkologische Abteilung, Klinik Grosshansdorf, Woehrendamm 80, 22927 Grosshansdorf/Hamburg, FRG

Table 1. Drugs with potential pulmonary toxicity

Bleomycin	Melphalan
Mitomycin C	Azathioprine
BCNU	Methotrexate
Busulfan	Ara-C
Cyclophosphamide	Procarbazine
Chlorambucil	Teniposide
	Vinblastine

Table 2. Mechanisms of pulmonary toxicity

Bleomycin	Development of free radicals
Anthracyclines	Development of free radicals
Mitomycin C	Development of free radicals
Etoposide	Development of free radicals
Cyclophosphamide	Reduction of intracellular glutathione (liver and lungs)
BCNU	Inhibition of glutathione reductase

2 Experimental Data

We developed an animal model to examine the pathological and anatomic course of mitomycin C-induced pulmonary toxicity.

Table 3. Experimental data: Material and methods

Group	Weeks of administration	Total dose of mitomycin C (mg)
1	6	0.3
2	8	0.4–0.5
3	10	0.5–0.6
4	12	0.6–0.7
5	14	0.7–0.8
6	16	0.8–0.9
7	18	0.9–1.0

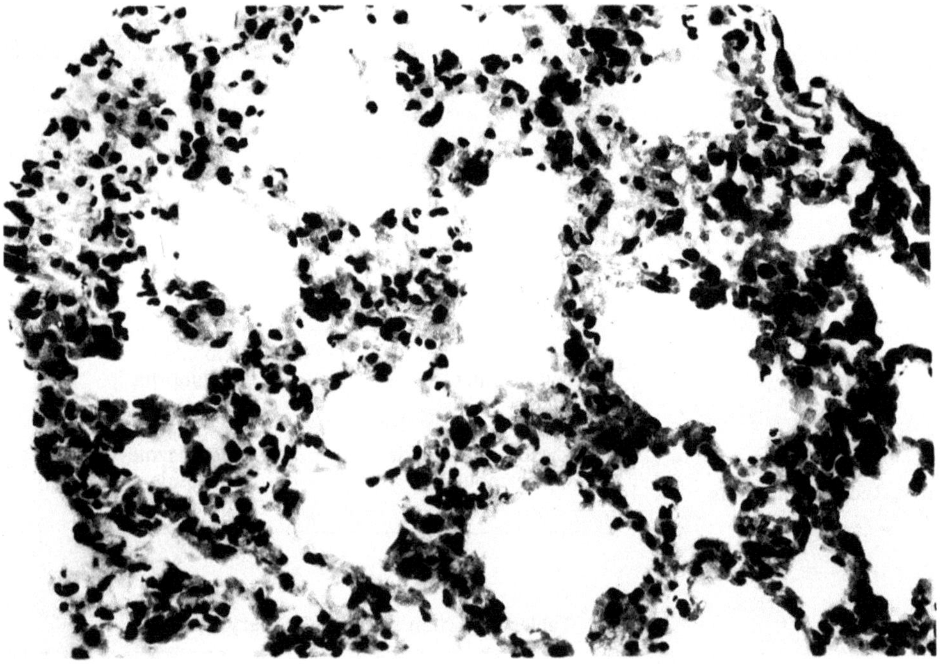

Fig. 1. Light microscopy photograph of lung tissue after 0.95 mg mitomycin C. Note swelling of type II pneumocytes and widening of the alveolar septal walls. × 360

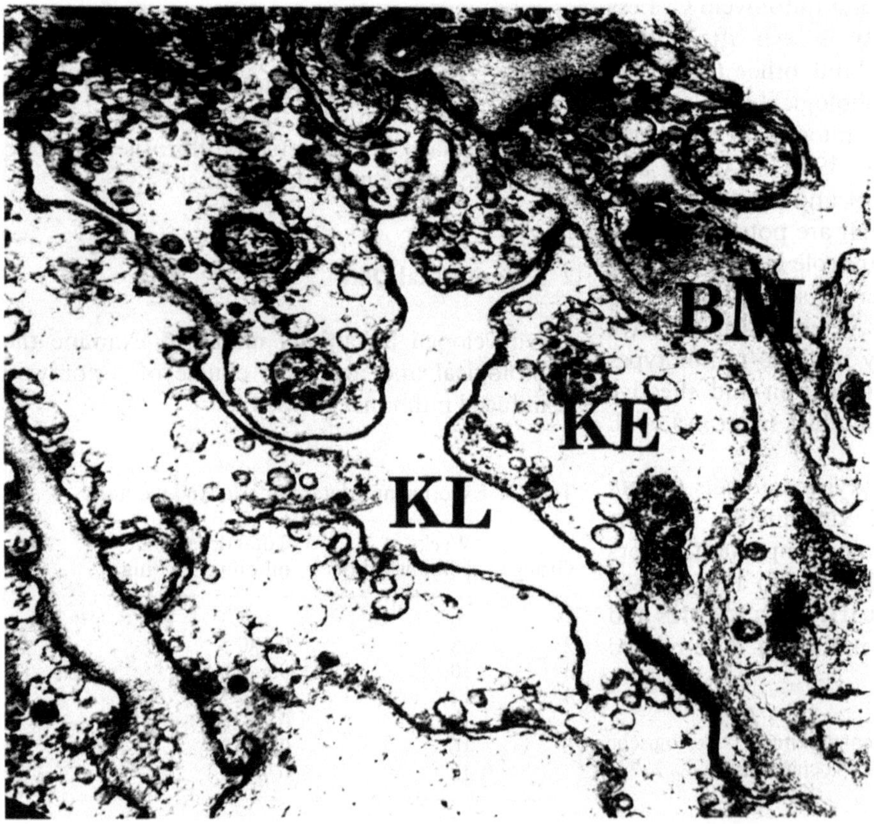

Fig. 2. Electron micrograph of a mouse lung capillary after 1.15 mg mitomycin C. Note remarkable swelling of the capillary endothelium, stenosis of the lumen, and thickening of the basement membrane. *KE*, endothelial cell; *KL*, lumen; *BM*, basement membrane. × 22000

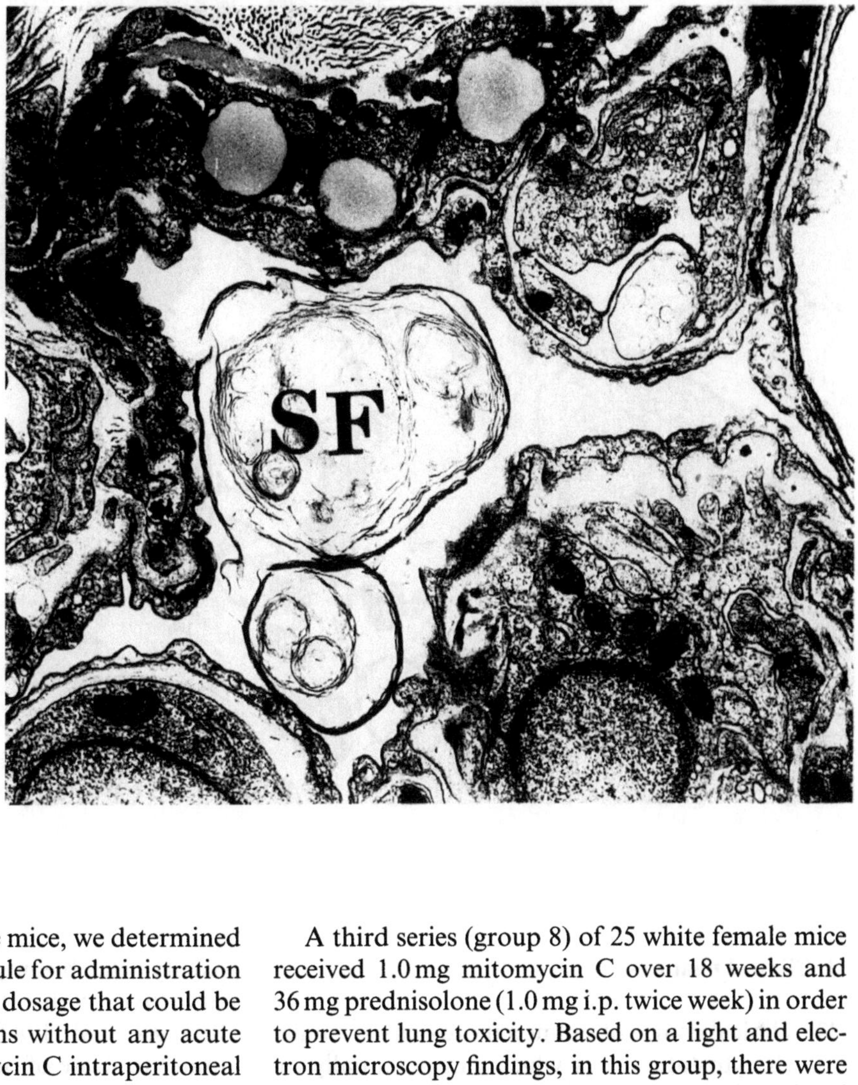

Fig. 3. Electron micrograph of mouse lung alveoli after 0.95 mg mitomycin C. *SF*, lamellar surfactant in the alveolar lumen. × 11000

In a first series of 250 white mice, we determined the optimal dosage and schedule for administration of mitomycin C. The optimal dosage that could be given over a period of months without any acute toxicity was 0.025 mg mitomycin C intraperitoneal twice a week. The second and main series included 90 female white mice. Seven groups of these animals received 0.025 mg mitomycin C twice a week up to 18 weeks (Table 3). The maximum dosage of mitomycin C given ranges from 0.3 mg after 6 weeks up to 1.0 mg after 18 weeks. The lung tissue was examined by light and electron microscopy. The pathological findings were dose- and time-related.

The earliest changes were swelling of type II pneumocytes and widening of the alveolar septal walls (Fig. 1). We observed a remarkable swelling of the capillary endothelium, with stenosis of the lumen and thickening of the basement membrane (Fig. 2).

Lambellar surfactant was expressed in the alveolar lumen (Fig. 3) and a large amount of surfactant was found in the alveoli (Fig. 4). The end point was a fibrosis with collagen and free surfactant (Fig. 5).

A third series (group 8) of 25 white female mice received 1.0 mg mitomycin C over 18 weeks and 36 mg prednisolone (1.0 mg i.p. twice week) in order to prevent lung toxicity. Based on a light and electron microscopy findings, in this group, there were no major pathological defects in the lung tissue in all animals. Only very early signs of swelling of the capillary endothelium were found. The conclusions from these experimental data are:

1. In the development of mitomycin C-induced interstitial fibrosis, the most important cells are type II pneumocytes and alveolar macrophages.
2. Damage of the capillary endothelium results in overproduction of surfactant by type II pneumocytes. Alveolar macrophages are activated and produce mediator substances, e.g., macrophage growth factor and macrophage-dependent fibroblast stimulating activity. Fibroblasts were stimulated to produce collagen.
3. There is a dose-time relationship in the development of interstitial fibrosis.
4. Steroids given simultaneously with mitomycin C can prevent interstitial fibrosis in mice.

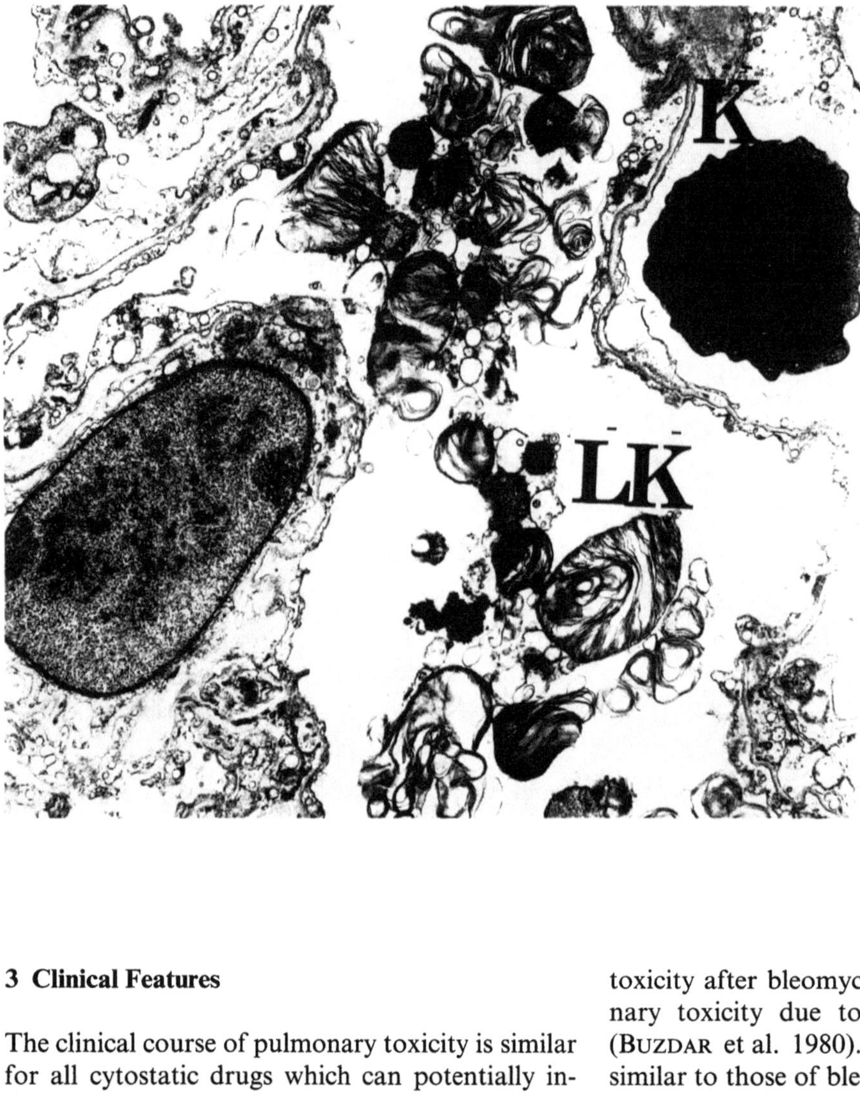

Fig. 4. Electron micrograph of mouse lung alveoli after 1.15 mg mitomycin C. Note the abundant surfactant material in the alveoli. *LK*, lamellar bodies; *K*, capillary. ×6000

3 Clinical Features

The clinical course of pulmonary toxicity is similar for all cytostatic drugs which can potentially induce lung injury. Development of a dry, hacking cough, progressive dyspnea at rest, tachypnea, fever and cyanosis are typical for fatal pulmonary toxicity. The earliest physical finding is fine crackling bibasilar rales involving the lower third of the lung fields. Methotrexate can also induce an acute toxicity like edema 6–12 h after the first and further doses. In 4%–8% of patients, an acute pleural pain is also reported after methotrexate. The late toxicity is similar to that of bleomycin. After bleomycin treatment, 1%–2% fatal toxicity is reported (Comis 1992; Ginsberg and Comis 1982).

The clinical incidence of fatal bleomycin toxicity is 3%–4%. Based on lung function measurements, the incidence of lung toxicity after bleomycin is 40%.

Age above 70 years and simultaneous radiotherapy are risk factors in developing pulmonary toxicity after bleomycin. The incidence of pulmonary toxicity due to mitomycin C is 3%–12% (Buzdar et al. 1980). The clinical symptoms are similar to those of bleomycin. Also, after busulfan therapy lung toxicity occurs with an incidence of 4%–12% (Ginsberg and Comis 1982).

BCNU induces lung injury in up to 30% of patients. There is a dose-dependent relationship, with a tremendous increase of pulmonary toxicity at >1000 mg/m2. Preexisting risk factors such as smoking can potentiate the development of lung toxicity. Finally, there is a probable synergy between cyclophosphamide and radiotherapy.

4 Laboratory Tests

The most sensitive way to detect lung toxicity is to measure lung function, especially the diffusion capacity (DLCO) (Collis 1980; Comis 1992; Ginsberg and Comis 1982). Abnormalities and a decrease in DLCO can also be found in asymptomatic patients (up to 40%–50%) Arterial blood

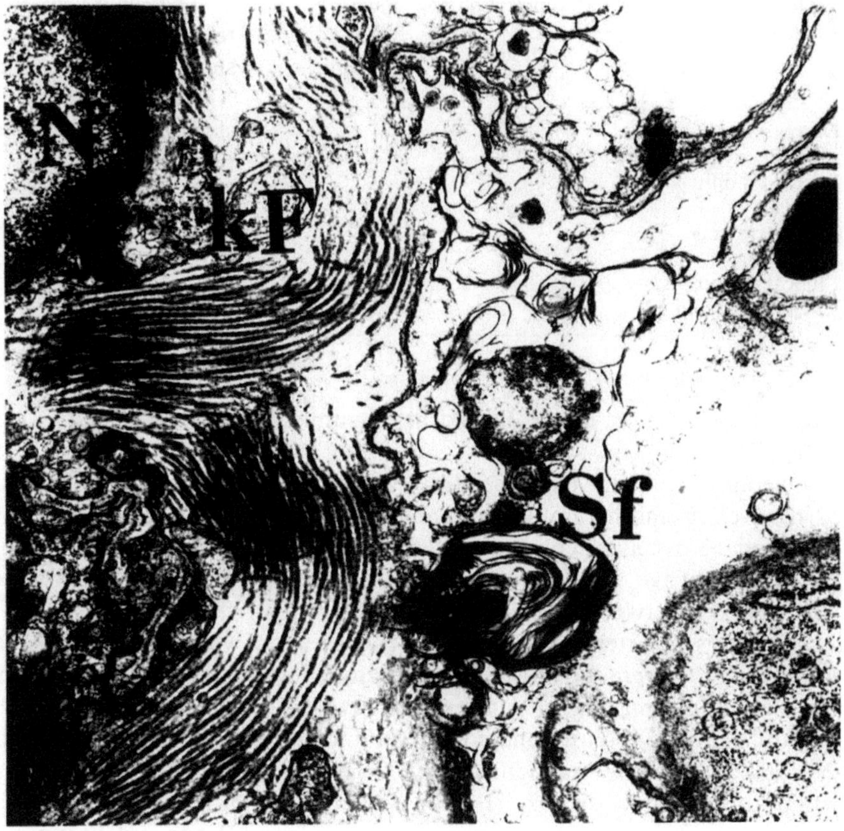

Fig. 5. Electron micrograph of mouse lung after 0.975 mg mitomycin C. Fibrosis with collagen (*KF*) and free surfactant (*SF*). *N*, nucleus. × 14000

gases indicate hypoxemia and hypocapnea when significant pulmonary toxicity develops. Blood gases under exercise are another sensitive parameter. Spirometric and body plethysmographic tests are less sensitive for detecting pulmonary toxicity.

In chest radiography, the earliest manifestation of lung toxicity is fine reticular bibasilar infiltrates that may progress to bibasilar alveolar and interstitial infiltrates. Computed tomographic scanning shows discrete nodular densities. A more aggressive, but also very sensitive, test is bronchoscopy with transbronchial biopsy and bronchoalveolar lavage (BAL). In the biopsy there are pathological changes including interstitial alveolitis or fibrosis. In the BAL there is mostly an increase in both the total number of cells and the percentage of lymphocytes as a sign of interstitial pneumonitis.

5 Clinical Results

Patients with inoperable non-small cell lung cancer (NSCLC) received combination chemotherapy either with mitomycin C/ifosfamide or mitomycin C/vindesine. Parameters measured before and after

Table 4. Clinical study: Patient characteristics

	Without steroids	With steroids
Number of patients	52	53
Age		
Median	60	55
Range	36–73	34–79
Sex		
Male	35	44
Female	17	9
Performance status		
ECOG 0–1	41	44
ECOG 2	11	9
Mitomycin C (mg)		
Mean	45	48
Range	15–80	17–80

chemotherapy were: (a) spirometric data; (b) DLCO; (c) arterial blood gas; (d) clinical symptoms; (e) chest X-ray; and (f) bronchoscopy with transbronchial biopsy and BAL.

Patients were randomized to receive either 250 mg prednisolone i.v. as a bolus injection 30 min before mitomycin C or no concomitant supportive therapy. The steroids were given to prevent the toxic

Table 5. Clinical study: Pathological parameters

	Without steroids (%)	With steroids (%)
Decreased arterial blood oxygen pressure	44.4	34.0
Decreased diffusion capacity	44.4	38.6
Restrictive lung disorder	28.6	37.8
Clinical symptoms	25.5	15.1
Radiological findings	10.4	13.2

lung reaction, as we demonstrated in our animal data.

Overall 105 patients have been treated (Table 4): 52 received chemotherapy without any supportive care and 53 received concomitant steroids. The distribution of age, sex and performance status, was well balanced between the two groups.

Decreases in arterial blood gases (Fig. 6) and DLCO (Fig. 7) were the most sensitive parameters for detecting lung toxicity after mitomycin C therapy (Table 5). With concomitant steroids the decrease in DLCO was significantly lower than without supportive therapy (Fig. 7). Other lung function parameters, e.g., vital capacity, are of less value for detecting pulmonary lung function changes due to drug-induced toxicity (Fig. 8).

The incidence of clinical symptoms due to lung toxicity was 25.5% without steroids and 15.1% with steroids (Fig. 9). Radiological findings in the chest X-ray were in the range of 10%–13% without a statistically significant difference between the two groups.

In the BAL there was significantly less frequent lymphocytosis in the steroid-treated patients (Table 6, Fig. 10), in accordance with a slightly lower total number of cells. Thus, these data show a preventive effect of steroids concerning lung toxicity of mitomycin C. Furthermore, by lung function criteria, especially DLCO and BAL, the pulmonary toxicity of mitomycin C can be detected before clinical symptoms occur.

Another clinical study of prevention of bleomycin-induced pulmonary toxicity has been carried out by Mackes et al. (1992) (Table 7). Patients with germ cell tumors received a combination chemotherapy consisting of bleomycin/ifosfamide/cisplatin/vinblastine with and without *N*-acetylcysteine (NAC). This drug has an antioxidative potential that can influence lung toxicity induced by free oxygen radicals, as occurs with bleomycin (Bernard 1992). There are some experimental data that show a pneumoprotective effect of NAC (Berend 1985; Blum and Fridovich 1985; Clemens and Schmid 1991; Cotgreave et al. 1987; Ward et al. 1986). Patients were intensively examined by lung function

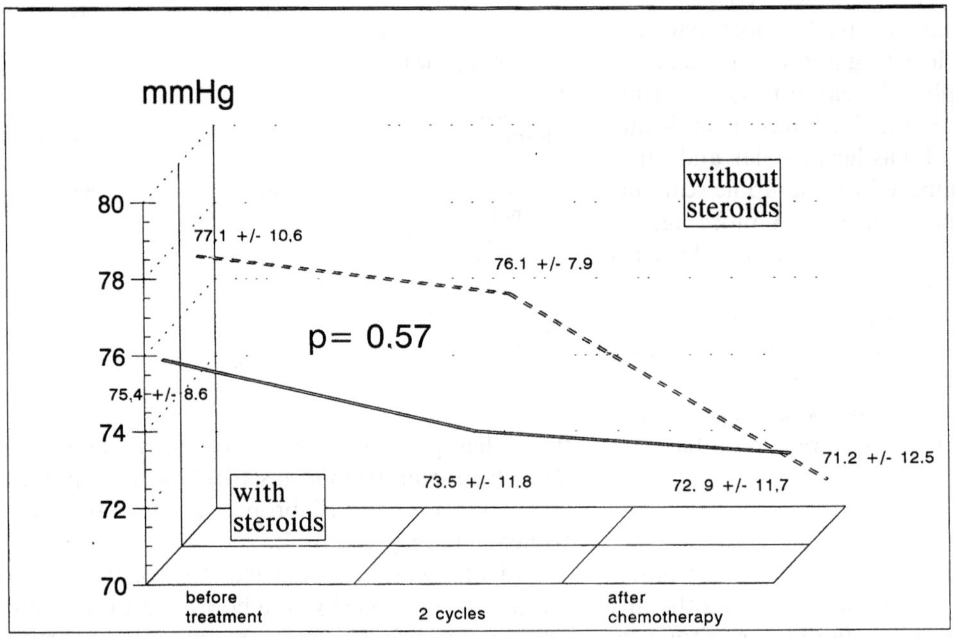

Fig. 6. Course of arterial blood gas

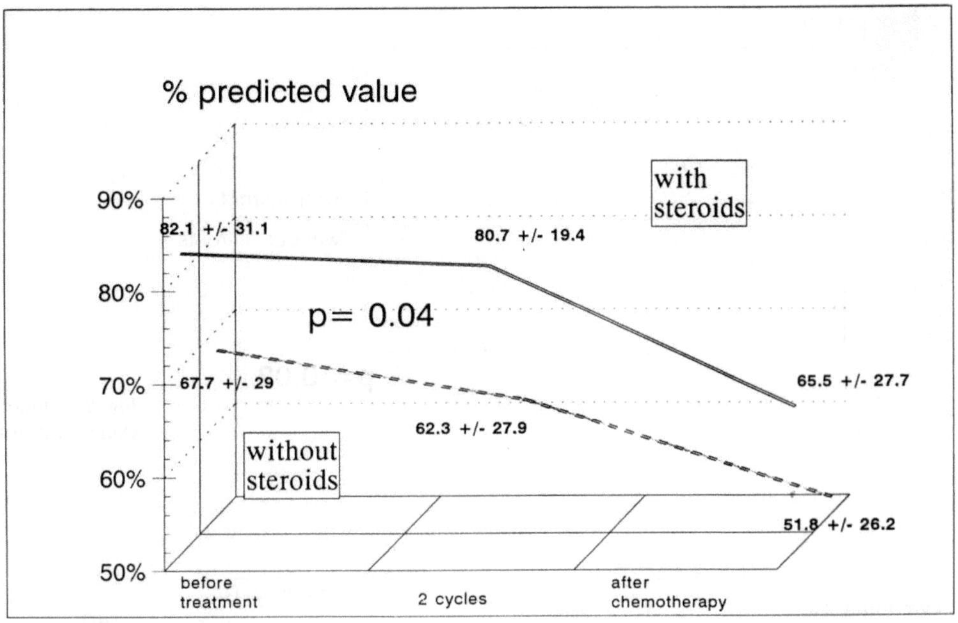

Fig. 7. Course of diffusion capacity (DLCO)

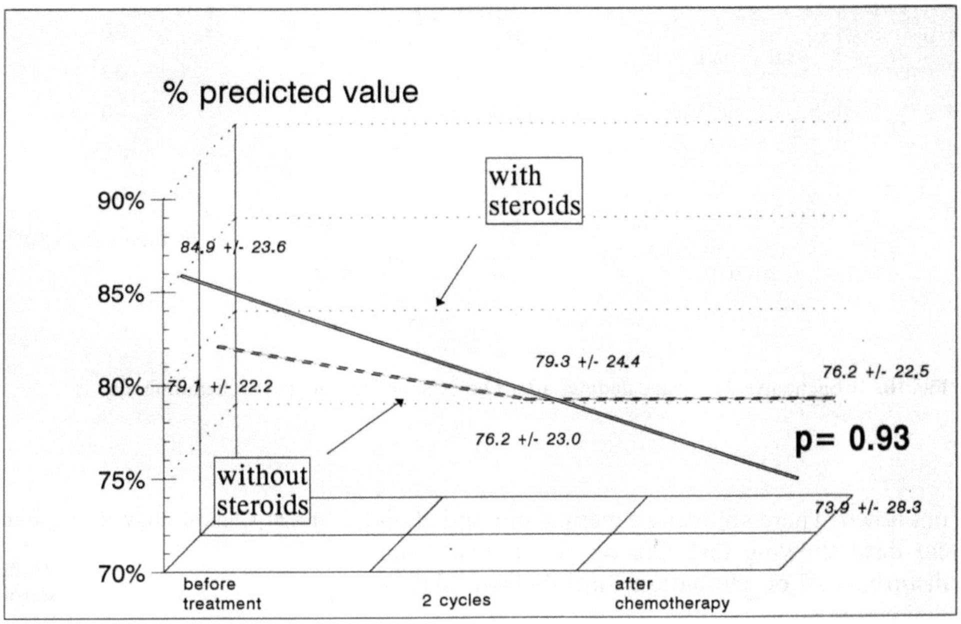

Fig. 8. Course of vital capacity

tests and right heart catheterization. The results are shown in Table 7. There were 14 patients who received chemotherapy without NAC and 16 patient who were treated with high dose NAC. Without NAC treatment the decrease in vital capacity and DLCO at rest and under exercise were significantly higher than with prophylactically given NAC. This study thus also demonstrates that prevention of the pulmonary toxicity of cytostatic agents is possible.

6 Summary and Therapeutic Recommendations

The complete mechanism of the pathogenesis of pulmonary toxicity of cytostatic drugs is still

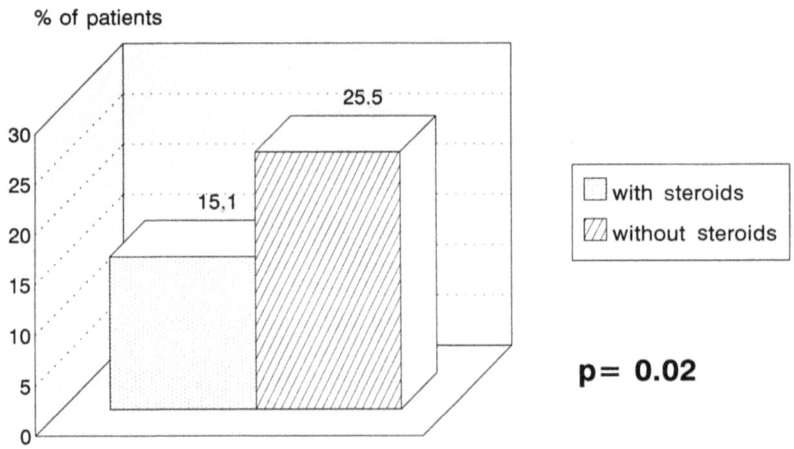

Fig. 9. Clinical symptoms after two cycles of mitomycin C chemotherapy

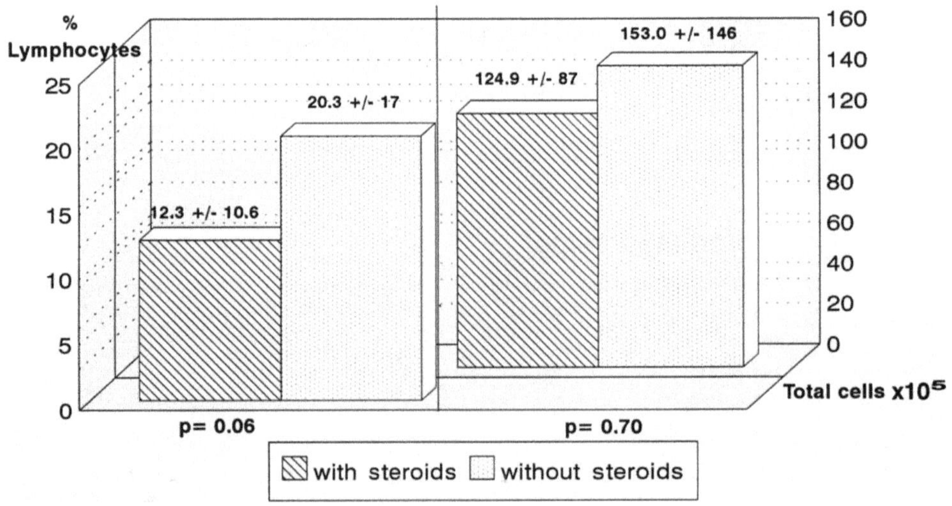

Fig. 10. Bronchoalveolar lavage findings after two cycles of mitomycin C chemotherapy

unknown. There are many experimental and clinical data showing that free oxygen radicals and disturbances of gluthatione metabolism play a major role.

Drugs that can influence these mechanisms for example, as "oxidant scavengers" (HEFFNER and REPINE 1989; SIES 1991), may be important for the prevention and therapy of pulmonary toxicity. Steroids and NAC have been shown to be effective in experimental and clinical studies (JENSEN et al. 1989; MACKES et al. 1992).

Another important aspect is the accurate diagnosis before and during chemotherapy with potentially lung toxic drugs. An exact lung function test, especially of DLCO, and, if necessary, bronchoscopy with BAL are important measurements to assess pulmonary toxicity before clinical symptoms occur. Risk factors for additional lung injury, e.g., radiotherapy or maximum dose should be considered.

Table 6. Clinical study: BAL parameters

BAL	Without steroids	With steroids
Lymphocytosis	20.3%	12.3%
Total cells ($\times 10^5$)	153.0	124.9

BAL, bronchoalveolar lavage.

Table 7. Prevention of bleomycin-induced lung toxicity with *N*-acetylcysteine (from MACKES et al. 1992)

Therapy[a]	Number of patients	Decrease in vital capacity (%)	Decrease in DLCO (%)	Decrease in DLCO under exercise (%)	Pulmonary capillary resistance (%)
Bleomycin (60 mg/m2) + Ifosfamide + cisplatin + vinblastine					
Without *N*-acetyl-cysteine	14	6.0*	7.8*	10.2*	5.0 (increased)
With *N*-acetyl-cysteine	16	21.0	2.9	1.8	2.0 (decreased)

DLCO, diffusion capacity; * significant.
[a] Two to three cycles.

References

Bedrossian CWM (1982) Pathology of drug-induced lung diseases. Semin Respin Med 4: 98–105

Berend N (1985) Inhibition of bleomycin lung toxicity by N-acetylcysteine in the rat. Pathology 17: 108

Bernard GR (1992) N-Acetylcystein bei akuter (eds) experimenteller und klinischer Lungenschädigung. In: Crystal RG, Nolte D (eds) Das Glutathionsystem und seine Bedeutung in der antoxidativen Abwehr. Excerpta Medica, Amsterdam, pp 70–82

Blum J, Fridovich I (1985) Inactivation of glutathione peroxidase by superoxide radical. Arch Biochem Biophys 240: 500–508

Buzdar AU, Legha SS, Luna MA, Tashima CK, Hortobagyi GN, Blumenschein GR (1980) Pulmonary toxicity of mitomycin. Cancer 45: 236–244

Clemens MR, Schmid B (1991) Freie Radikale und Antioxidantien in Hämatologie und Onkologie. Atemw Lungenkrh Jahrgang 17 [Suppl] S26–S34

Collis CH (1980) Lung damage from cytotoxic drugs. Cancer Chemother Pharmacol 4: 17–27

Comis RL (1992) Bleomycin pulmonary toxicity: current status and future directions. Semin Oncol 19(2, Suppl 5) 64–70

Cooper JAD, White DA, Matthay RA (1986) Drug-induced pulmonary disease. Am Rev Respir Dis 133: 321–340

Cotgreave IA, Eklund A, Larsson K, Moldeus P (1987) Oral N-acetylcysteine, how does it work? Eur J Respir Dis 70: 71–72

Fasske E, Morgenroth K (1983) Experimental Bleomycin-lung in mice. Lung 161: 133–146

Ginsberg SJ, Comis RL (1982) Pulmonary toxicity of antineoplastic agents. Semin Oncol 9 (1): 34–51

Heffner JE, Repine JE (1989) Pulmonary strategies of antioxidant defense. Am Rev Respr Dis 140: 531–554

Jensen IL, Goel R, Venner PM (1989) The effect of corticosteroid administration on bleomycin lung toxicity. Cancer 65: 1291–1297

Mackes KG, Müller T, Retter C, Harlapp J (1992) Pneumoprotektive Wirkung von N-Acetylcystein bei Bleomycinbehandlung von Patienten mit malignen Hodentumoren. In: Crystal RG, Nolte D (eds) Das Glutathionsystem und seine Bedeutung in der antoxidativen Abwehr. Excerpta Medica, Amsterdam, pp 187–198

Martin WJ II, Kachel DL (1987) Bleomycin-induced pulmonary endothelial cell injury: evidence for the role of iron-catalyzed toxic oxygen-derived species. Lab Clin Med 110: 153–158

Muggia FM (1983) Pulmonary toxicity of antitumor agents. Cancer Treat Rev 10: 221–243

Sies H (1991) Natürliche und synthetische Antioxidantien. Atemw Lungenkrkh 17 [Suppl 1]: S16–S25

Sinha B (1989) Free radicals in anticancer drug pharmacology. Chem Biol Interact 69: 293–317

Slater TF (1984) Free radical mechanisms of tissue injury. Biochem J 222: 1–15

Sostman HS, Matthay RA, Puman CE (1977) Cytotoxic drug- induced lung disease. Am J Med 62: 608–615

Ward HE, Nicholson A, Berend N (1986) Does systemic N-acetylcysteine protect against bleomycin induced lung injury? Am Rev Respin Dis 132 [Suppl 4]: part 2: 51

Willson JKV (1978) Pulmonary toxicity of antineoplastic drugs. Cancer Treat Rep 62: 2003–2008

4.3 Differential Diagnosis of Treatment Sequelae in the Lung

MICHAEL GALANSKI, REGINE RATHMANN, and CORNELIA SCHAEFER-PROKOP

CONTENTS

1 Introduction 151
2 Therapy Modalities 152
3 Underlying Disease and Tumor Activity 154
4 Onset of Manifestation and Course 155
5 Clinical Symptoms 157
6 Analysis and Interpretation of Radiographic Findings 157
6.1 Interstitial Opacities 157
6.2 Alveolar Opacities 157
6.3 Nodular Opacities 158
7 Summary 158
References 158

1 Introduction

With the advancement in tumor treatment and the increasing use of potent yet aggressive modalities of tumor therapy, the incidence of therapy-related side effects increases, e.g., drug-induced lung disease. This is especially true for patients treated with chemotherapy (with known lung toxicity) and resultant immunosuppressive effects and/or those treated with radiation of the lungs. Patients with malignant lymphoma, myeloproliferative disease, testicular tumors, chemotherapy-sensitive sarcomas (Ewing, neuroblastoma, rhabdomyosarcoma), HIV-associated tumors, breast cancer or gastrointestinal tumors all belong to this group. If these patients express symptoms such as fever, dyspnea and/or pulmonary infiltrates, it may be considerably difficult to differentiate the various potential causes. However, these difficulties must be overcome in order to induce the correct therapy. Depending on the diagnosis, different and even partially contradictory treatments are the necessary consequence.

The definition of diagnosis is impeded for two other reasons: First, the tumor itself may lead to immunodeficiency irrespective of treatment resulting in an increased disposition for infection. Second, due to better treatment modalities, more advanced tumor stages are seen, with unusual tumor manifestations and metastases, and a resultant higher rate of complete response and survival has been achieved. The etiologic spectrum of pulmonary disease has increased, while the morphologic response of lung parenchyma, however, is stereotypic, such that the clinical and radiographic appearance is rather nonspecific.

Table 1. Differential diagnosis of pulmonary changes observed in patients receiving cancer therapy

Toxic/allergic drug effects
Radiation-induced pneumonitis
Opportunistic infection
Intrapulmonary hemorrhage
Pulmonary edema
Tumor manifestation
Paraneoplastic syndrome

Pulmonary opacities and/or complications that appear in the context of oncologic treatment may be caused by direct therapy effects, i.e., either as drug-induced disease or as radiation effects, or by indirect therapy effects (Table 1). Therapy can: (1) induce immunosuppression and promote opportunistic infections, (2) cause interstitial or alveolar edema (by therapy-induced renal or cardiac damage or by infusion therapy), and (3) cause parenchymal bleeding (most likely due to thrombocytopenia). In addition, pulmonary opacification can be caused by metastases or manifestation of the tumor itself. A polythrombotic state may be due to tumor-related disease (ovarian carcinoma or oat cell carcinoma of the lung), or to hormonal therapy causing an increase in the production of coagulating substances.

With few exceptions, imaging modalities alone are insufficient in making a definitive diagnosis. Only in the context of clinical data pertaining to both history and previous experience can the radiological diagnosis exceed a pure definition of anatomical and pathological findings such that it

MICHAEL GALANSKI, Prof. Dr., REGINE RATHMANN, Dr., CORNELIA SCHAEFER-PROKOP, Dr., Diagnostische Radiologie I, Medizinische Hochschule Hannover, Konstanty Gutschow-Straße 8, 30625 Hannover, FRG

Table 2. Basic clinical information mandatory for correct diagnosis

Knowledge of primary malignancy and of therapeutic regimen
Tumor response to therapy
Time of manifestation
Clinical course
Symptomatology
Electrolyte and fluid balance

may be useful for diagnosis and differentiation of disease. The data should refer to tumor disease and staging, tumor activity, onset and course of pulmonary complication, and clinical symptoms, drug therapy and fluid balance (Table 2; REED 1984).

The following article will describe additional information necessary to correctly interpret the radiographic findings. Finally, analysis of the radiographic images will be discussed.

2 Therapy Modalities

Knowledge of the therapy, whether chemotherapy and/or radiation therapy are involved, is a necessary precondition for the evaluation of potential adverse side effects. The most important cytostatic agents that lead to pulmonary disease are the cytotoxic antibiotics bleomycin (15%–20%) and mitomycin, the alkylants busulfan (1%–12%) and cyclophosphamide, the nitrosamines BCNU and CCNU, and the antimetabolites methotrexate (15%–20%) and cytarabine (Table 3; COOPER et al. 1986; KREISMAN and WOLKOVE 1992; SCHAEFER et al. 1990).

For the various substances, data concerning type and frequency of pulmonary complications, latent period, risk factors and the predominant radiographic morphology are listed in Table 4. One should note that these data are only for orientation purposes. The broad range of variations is in part due to different dosage requirements, examination modalities and evaluation parameters (clinical parameters, pulmonary function parameters, chest X-ray or computed tomography) and to different combinations of therapy modalities (KREISMAN and WOLKOVE 1992). The combination of bleomycin and methotrexate may not lead to more frequent side effects, but instead to more severe ones. High dose chemotherapy is associated with a higher incidence of complications than standard dose therapy (PETERS et al. 1986). The majority of therapy-induced pulmonary disease is caused by dose-dependent toxic reactions that may be subacute or chronic.

Table 3. Chemotherapeutic agents causing pulmonary, cardiac, or renal toxicity

Pulmonary toxicity		
	Cytostatic antibiotics	
		Bleomycin and its derivatives
		Mitomycin
		Doxorubicin
	Alkylating agents	
		Busulfan
		Cyclophosphamide
	Nitrosoureas	
		BCNU
	Antimetabolites	
		Methotrexate
		Cytarabine
	Cytokines	
		Interleukin-2
Cardiac toxicity		
	Anthracyclines	
		Adriamycin
		Daunorubicin
		Mitoxantrone
Renal toxicity		
	Alkylating agents	
		Cisplatin
		Nitrosoureas
		Nitrogen mustard derivatives
	Antimetabolites	
		Methotrexate

A toxic drug reaction in the lung clinically presents as chronic pneumonitis, an acute allergic reaction, or a noncardiac edema. The symptoms range from a simple gas diffusion disturbance to cough, dyspnea, fever or to a severe respiratory insufficiency requiring artificial respiration. The Eastern Cooperative Oncology Group (ECOG) proposed a clinical grading scheme based on a five point scale ranging from a mild reduction in diffusion capacity to severe reactions with a fatal outcome (Table 5; OKEN et al. 1982).

The radiographic morphology is characterized by interstitial reticulonodular or mixed interstitial-alveolar opacities, which may vary considerably depending on severity and extent of disease, i.e., ranging from discrete interstitial disease to widespread airspace disease (Figs. 1, 2). Chronic pneumonitis-like reactions usually present as progressive fibrous disease while an acute hypersensitivity reaction will present as either edema, infiltration of the lung, or respiratory distress syndrome (RDS). RDS is described to occur after treatment with methotrexate, cyclophosphamide, cytarabine and interleukin. It is most likely caused by capillary leaking and presents as alveolar edema. Pleural effusion is rarely seen after treatment with

Table 4. Incidence, latent period, threshold dose, risk factors, and the common X-ray pattern associated with the various cytotoxic drugs

Cytostatic drug	Frequency	Latent period	Threshold dose	Risk factors	X-ray findings
Bleomycin	5%–10%	1–3 Months	>450 mg	Age > 70, radiation, O_2, combined therapy	Fine reticular, subpleural, basal, seldom nodular
Mitomycin	3%–12%	6–12 Months	–	O_2, combined therapy, radiation?	Reticulonodular (ARDS)
Busulfan	1%–12%	Months-years	>400 mg	Radiation	Basal reticular, also acinar
Melphalan	Rare	Weeks-months	–	–	Diffuse reticular
Chlorambucil	Rare	Months-years	–	–	Basal reticular
Cyclophosphamide	1%	Weeks-years	–	O_2, combined therapy	Basal reticulonodular
BCNU	1%–30%	Weeks-years	> 1 g/m³	O_2, combined therapy, concomitant disease	Basal reticulonodular
Methotrexate	7%	Immediate and delayed	–	Combined therapy	Edema/ARDS (immediate) reticulonodular (delayed)
Cytarabine	5%–15%		+	–	Edema/ARDS

ARDS, adult respiratory distress syndrome.

Table 5. ECOG grading of pulmonary toxicity

Grade I:	mild symptoms, 25%–50% reduced diffusion capacity
Grade II:	moderate symptoms, > 50% reduced diffusion capacity
Grade III:	severe symptoms, intermitt. O_2-therapy
Grade IV:	continuous O_2 therapy or assisted respiration
Grade V:	dead

mitomycin, bleomycin and busulfan; however, if present, it is usually small and always associated with pulmonary disease.

In some cases the radiographic image may be normal despite the manifestation of clinical symptoms. This discrepancy is the result of either a poor sensitivity of the chest X-ray or of bronchiolitis. In both instances, higher resolution computed tomography (HRCT) may be helpful. A bronchiolitis is described to occur with bleomycin, cyclophosphamide, methotrexate and procarbazine (PADLEY et al. 1992; ROSENOW 1972; ROSENOW et al. 1985).

The differentiation of infectious diseases, especially opportunistic infections, can be difficult or even impossible (McLEOD and MÜLLER 1990; MÜLLER and MILLER 1990; PENNINGTON 1983). Opacities with a nodular character that have the radiographic appearance of metastases or mycotic infection are rare and have been described for bleomycin in some cases. Allergic-toxic reactions that normally take an acute course appearing with alveolar edematous opacities or with RDS were described for cytarabine, procarbazine, and especially for combination therapies. Despite its undoubtedly higher sensitivity HRCT did not prove to be an aid for differentiation (specificity) (JANZEN et al. 1993).

Antineoplastic substances with cardiotoxic or nephrotoxic side effects can lead to an alveolar or interstitial edema and induce a radiographic image that cannot be differentiated from an opportunistic infection, a lymphatic spread of tumor or a simple fluid overload after infusion therapy. The most important substances with cardiotoxic effects are the anthracyclines adriamycin and daunorubicin and the synthetic substance mitoxantrone. The most important substances with nephrotoxic effects are the alkylant cisplatin and the antimetabolite methotrexate (Table 3; DRINGS 1988; PETERS et al. 1986). For example, the frequency of side effects is 10% with a dose threshold of 500 mg/m³. Risk factors for cardiotoxic effects are increased in patients greater than 70 years of age, especially if there has been preexisting coronary or myocardial damage, a history of hypertension, or radiation to the mediastinum. In addition, all cytotoxic substances can provoke a rapid tumor lysis syndrome of the kidneys due to extensive tumor necrosis.

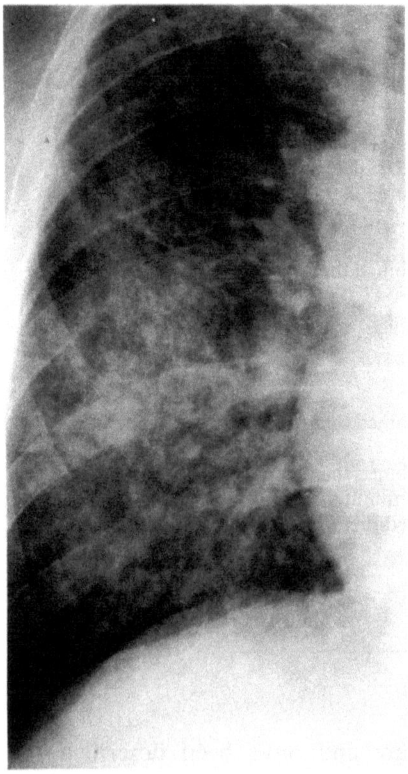

Fig. 1. Pulmonary changes induced by interferon therapy. A mixed interstitial and alveolar pattern in both lungs

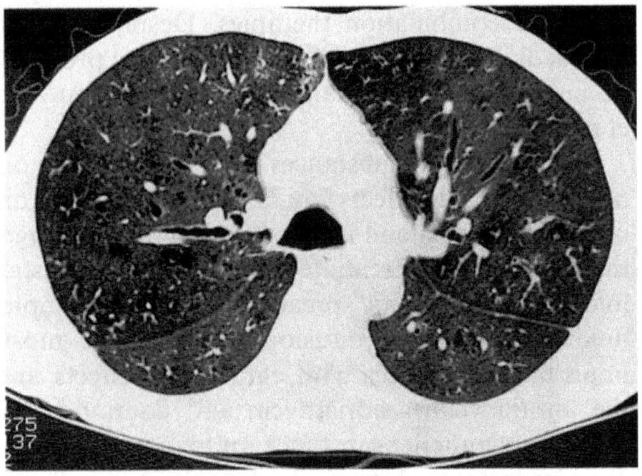

Fig. 2. Diffuse ground glass opacification affecting both lungs simulating alveolitis due to methotrexate therapy

3 Underlying Disease and Tumor Activity

Important factors influencing prognosis are the underlying disease itself, tumor stage, activity and course, and the occurrence of hematogenic or lymphogenic metastases or of direct tumor infiltration.

Lymphatic spread of the tumor, interstitial pneumonia, interstitial edema and a predominantly interstitial allergic-toxic drug-induced pulmonary reaction all demonstrate very similar radiographic morphologies. The chest X-ray can only be interpreted in conjunction with the clinical history.

In cases in which a rather uniform image and no or few clinical symptoms are present, interstitial edema would be the first diagnosis, especially if the patient was treated with infusion therapy or had a known electrolyte imbalance. When accompanied by fever and a nonproductive cough, diagnosis of opportunistic pulmonary infection is favored, e.g., pneumocystis carinii or viral pneumonia, both of which are indications for bronchoalveolar lavage (Reed 1984). A pneumonia due to legionella or mycoplasma can be more easily differentiated from other agents due to opacities which usually occur within the segmental or lobular distribution (Pennington 1983).

In patients with an advanced tumor stage and/or a very aggressive tumor, lymphatic spread should be considered quite early as part of the diagnosis (Fig. 3). This is especially true if tumors which have a preference for lymphatic spread are involved, i.e., breast, stomach, pancreas, and bronchial carcinomas. This is also the case if the interstitial changes in the chest X-ray are more localized and less uniform,

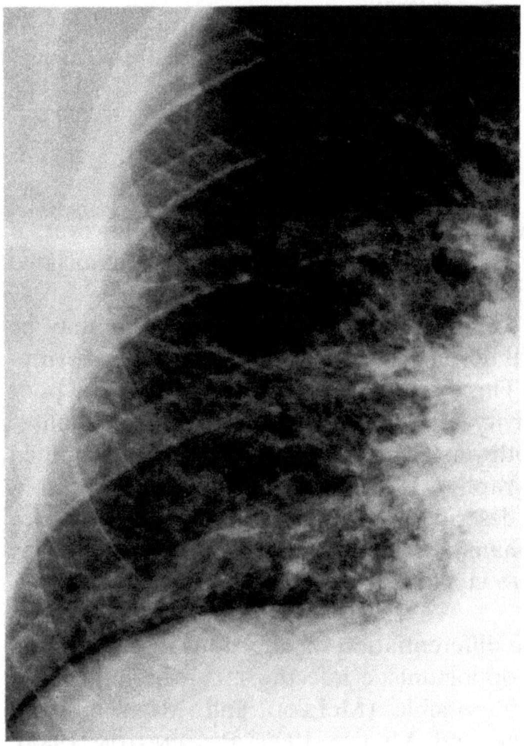

Fig. 3. Coarse reticulonodular pattern observed in a patient with lymphatic carcinomatosis

as seen in edema. For the early diagnosis of lymphatic spread of the tumor computed tomography has proven to be very sensitive. In contrast to the edema, findings include not only thickening of the interlobular septa and pleural structures but also consolidation of the central peribronchial and perivascular interstitial space. Thickening of the interstitial structures due to tumor infiltration is typically irregular and nodular (MUNK et al. 1988; MAIDICH et al. 1991; ZERHOUNI 1989).

4 Onset of Manifestation and Course

The onset of manifestation and the course of the pulmonary changes are important factors for the differential diagnosis (Table 6). The onset of a bacterial or a pneumocystis carinii infection follows an acute course, in contrast to an infection with cytomegalo-virus or aspergillus, which follow a more subacute course. Infections with mycobacteria and mycoses, however, exhibit a more chronic course. Opportunistic pulmonary infections are the preferred choice for the differential diagnosis in patients who develop a temperature during a state of granulocytopenia (Figs. 4, 5). This is due to either the disease itself or to the drug-induced immune suppression. The chest X-ray may be normal in these patients, but treatment can only commence based on the symptoms or a higher degree of suspected infection. Patients most likely affected are those with malignant lymphoma, plasmocytoma, HIV-associated tumors, bone marrow recipients and those receiving multiple courses of aggressive chemotherapy. The most frequent microbiotic agents are *Enterobacter*, *Pseudomonas*, *Streptococcus*, and fungi. Recent literature states the incidence of pneumocystis carinii infections as 25% in patients with leukemia; the incidence of *Legionella* infection

Table 6. Most probable diagnosis as guaged by duration of onset and course of pulmonary disease

Onset	*Course*
Acute (hours-days)	Bacterial pneumonia Pneumocystis pneumonia
Subacute (1–2 weeks)	CMV pneumonia Aspergillosis
Chronic (weeks-months)	Mycotic pneumonia Tuberculosis Drug reaction Radiation pneumonitis Tumor manifestation

CMV, cytomegalovirus.

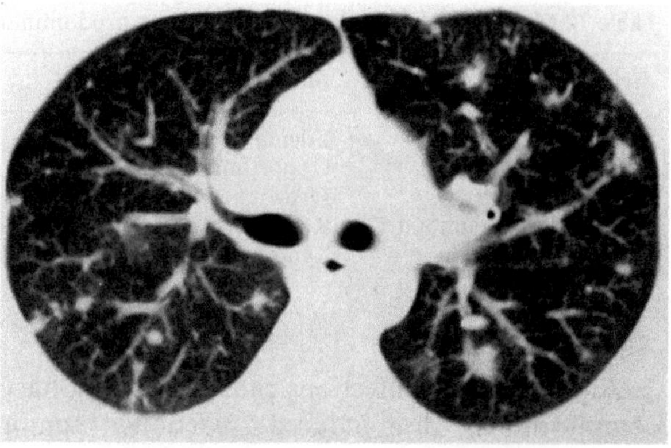

Fig. 4. Pulmonary candidiasis in an immunocompromised patient undergoing cancer chemotherapy

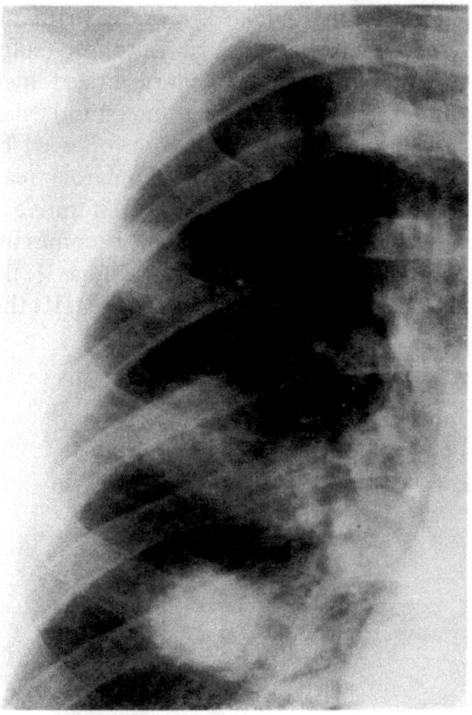

Fig. 5. Multiple coin lesions in a patient with fungal pneumonia simulating metastatic disease

is 22% in patients with myeloproliferative disease (LINK et al. 1986). However, based on previous experience the causative microbiotic agent can only be defined in one third of the cases. Irrespective of both definite proof of the microbiotic agent and of the radiographic findings this endangered group of patients must be treated immediately according to a graduated treatment plan consisting of antibiotic, antimycotic, antiviral and tuberculostatic drugs (PETERS et al. 1986).

Table 7. Most probable diagnosis as guaged by predominant X-ray pattern

Alveolar/acinar	*Interstitial*	*Nodular/miliary*
Edema	Edema	Metastases
Pneumonia	Opportunistic infection	Granulomas
Drug reaction	Drug reaction	Opportunistic infection
Radiation pneumonitis	Radiation pneumonitis	Tumor manifestation
	Lymphatic carcinomatosis	

Among the noninfectious causes of pulmonary complications, drug-induced reactions, tumor manifestations and radiation-induced reactions appear to have a longer latent period and a more chronic course (Table 6).

Once a radiation therapy has begun, a radiation-induced pulmonary reaction to the therapy would, at the earliest, take 2 months to manifest itself. Pneumonitis appears at its onset (stage I: early pneumonitis) and is characterized histologically and radiographically as interstitial edema (acute exudative phase). Stage I is followed by a florid interstitial or alveolar inflammatory reaction with serofibrinous exudation (proliferative stage). If allowed to progress the tissue becomes increasingly fibrous and begins to shrink (stage II: florid pneumonitis). After a transition stage (III) the endstage of pulmonary fibrosis is reached within the course of 9 months maximally after commencement of radiation therapy (Slanina et al. 1982; Rubin and Casarett 1968).

During the florid stage there are interstitial opacities intermixed with patchy opacities of lower density. Clinical symptoms such as a nonproductive cough (50%), fever (40%), dyspnea (30%) and chest pain (12%) may or may not occur during this stage.

Frequency and severity of a radiogenic pneumonitis and the fibrosis which follows may show considerable individual variability. This depends mainly on the dose, dose rate, fractionation, size and location of the radiated field, and the irradiation volume. An average one-sided fractionation usually consists of 30 Gy. This level is normally well

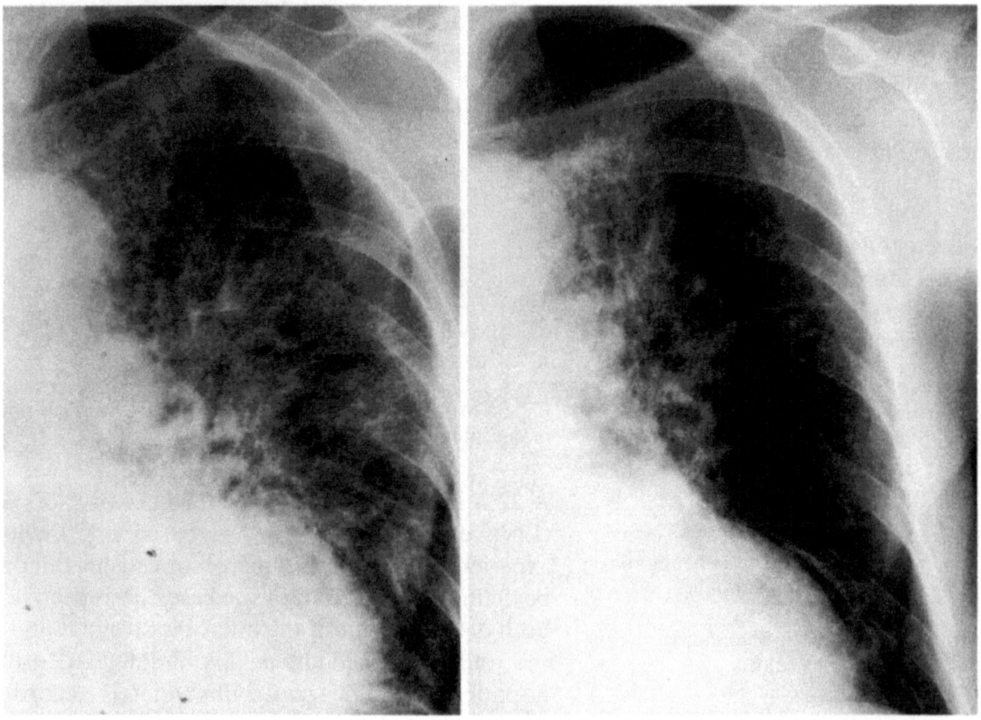

Fig. 6. Typical appearances in a patient with radiation pneumonitis in the acute phase and in the regressive phase. In this particular patient, who received radiation for an esophageal carcinoma, the changes resolved without resultant fibrosis

tolerated. With a dose above 40 Gy a radiogenic pneumonitis is likely to occur (DAVIS et al. 1992; ZERHOUNI 1989). For a fractionated irradiation of the total lung, the tolerable dose threshold lies at 20 Gy. For a total body irradiation the threshold level lies at 10 Gy (COX 1972; MOLLS et al. 1986). Irradiation with 10 Gy in one fraction leads to pneumonitis in a rather high percentage (80%) of patients (VAN DYK et al. 1981). The threshold dose for myocardial damage lies at 40 Gy (JOHN et al. 1988). Predisposing factors for a radiogenic pneumonitis are preexisting cardiopulmonary diseases such as emphysema or cardiac failure, in addition to advancing age. The importance of these factors, however, is not a measurable entity. Preceding or accompanying treatment with cytostatic agents (especially bleomycin and adriamycin) present considerable risks. A so-called recall phenomena exhibited by pneumonitis can occur when radiation therapy has taken place years ago and with the onset of a new chemotherapy (bleomycin, doxorubicin).

Important diagnostic hints for a radiogenic pneumonitis are the temporary context during which the radiation therapy is given, the exact topographic location of the radiated field and the characteristic stages through which the radiogenic pneumonitis may course (Fig. 6). Initially, there are edematous-like interstitial opacities, which become confluent alveolar opacities of relatively low density. With increasing fibrosis more course, more dense and better defined linear to reticular opacities are seen. Signs of shrinking and accompanying pleural scarring may also be noted. Pulmonary diseases due to other etiological causes are easily differentiated. In doubtful cases computed tomography can support the diagnosis by exactly defining the location of the infiltrates and by illustrating an existing or absent association of the borders of the pulmonary infiltrate with those of the radiated field (straight edge sign). Rarely do the pulmonary infiltrates (due to radiogenic pneumonia) exceed the radiation field and fall on to the contralateral side. The reason for such a generalized reaction is unknown. A hypersensitivity reaction or a generalization by hematogenic mediators has been suggested.

5 Clinical Symptoms

In some cases the clinical symptoms are important for the correct interpretation of radiographic findings. In patients with interstitial lung disease without any clinical symptoms, the first choice for differential diagnosis should be a simple interstitial edema, excluding causes such as a radiogenic pneumonia. Interstitial edema is a frequent finding in those multimorbid patients and is due to a fluid, electrolyte or albumin imbalance as a result of a renal or cardiac failure or of an infusion therapy accompanying chemotherapy. The same is true for asymptomatic alveolar opacities. They should preferably be interpreted as nonhomogeneous edema or as pulmonary hemorrhage. The latter is especially true in patients with thrombocytopenia (REED 1984).

6 Analysis and Interpretation of Radiographic Findings

The interpretation of a chest X-ray is only useful if the findings are based on systematic image analysis and are correlated with clinical data and practical experience. The following questions should always be addressed: What is the predominant radiographic morphology? Is or was the patient treated with a lung toxic drug? Is the course of the disease acute or chronic? Does the patient have fever? Can pulmonary edema be excluded (REED 1984)?

With respect to the radiographic morphology it was found to be useful to differentiate three types of opacities: an alveolar type, an interstitial type, and a nodular type. Hence, a rough classification of the pathology is possible (Table 8).

6.1 Interstitial Opacities

The most frequent cause of asymptomatic interstitial opacities is edema. In a patient with fever, the most diagnosis is an opportunistic infection (see Fig. 2). In a patient with no or slowly appearing symptoms, a drug-induced pneumonia, radiogenic pneumonia or lymphatic spread of tumor are all possible causes. The diagnosis of lymphatic spread of tumor can be reliably made with HRCT. In patients with malignant lymphoma, lymphatic spread of tumor is frequently associated with tumors of enlarged lymph nodes.

6.2 Alveolar Opacities

The radiographic morphology mostly consists of a mixed alveolar/interstitial pattern. In an acutely ill

Table 8. Most probable diagnosis as guaged by predominant X-ray pattern, onset of manifestation and course

	Predominantly interstitial	Predominantly alveolar	Predominantly nodular
Relatively asymptomatic	Edema	Drug reaction Pulmonary hemorrhage	
Acute/febrile	Opportunistic infection	Edema Viral pneumonia	Opportunistic infection Septic emboli
Subacute-chronic	Drug reaction Radiation pneumonitis	Opportunistic infection Bacterial, viral, or fungal pneumonia	
Chronic	Lymphatic carcinomatosis		Metastases Granulomas Fungal pneumonia Tuberculosis

patient the mot likely diagnosis is edema or fulminant viral pneumonia (see Fig. 4). Drug- induced pulmonary disease and pulmonary hemorrhage have fewer symptoms and a less flamboyant course. For subacute or chronic disease, an opportunistic infection would be the most obvious choice, the cause of which is due to bacterial, viral, or mycotic agents depending on the immune status of the patient.

6.3 Nodular Opacities

Nodular opacities may be due to a granulmatous inflammatory process such as a mycotic infection, miliary tuberculosis, or hematogenic metastases (if the opacities develop slowly and the disease follows a chronic course) (see Fig. 5). In more acutely ill patients, such as those with an elevated temperature, septic emboli or an opportunistic viral or mycotic infection are the more likely causative agents. For a predominantly miliary pattern the differential diagnosis should include septic emboli, a metastatic hematogenic spread of tumor and leukemic tumor.

7 Summary

There is a growing number of drugs that exhibit lung toxicity, and radiologists are increasingly confronted with nonspecific patterns of possibly therapy-induced lung disease. This chapter has reviewed clinical symptoms, radiographic features and differential diagnosis associated with lung disease occurring during tumor therapy. Clinical, pathological and radiological findings are nonspecific in the majority of cases, and clinicians and radiologists can only hope to assess the probability of drug-induced lung disease by correlating radiographic and clinical data. Drug-induced lung disease frequently simulates disseminated opportunistic infections (particularly pneumocystis carinii) and must be differentiated from these because the treatment is completely different. Useful clinical data include respiratory symptoms, results of respiratory function tests, dose and schedule of drug administration, and information concerning tumor activity and concomitant or previous administration of drugs or radiation therapy. Roentgen morphological categorization is based on the predominant pattern and distinguishes three types of pulmonary opacities: interstitial disease, air space consolidation and nodular opacities. Altogether, the radiological features, clinical data and patient's history enable the clinician to find the most likely diagnosis in most cases.

References

Cooper JAD, White DA, Matthay RA (1986) Drug- induced pulmonary disease: cytotoxic drugs. Am Rev Respir Dis 133: 321–340

Cox JD (1972) Total pulmonary irradiation for metastases from testicular carcinoma. Radiology 105: 163–167

Davis SD, Yankelevitz DF, Henschke CI (1992) Radiation effects on the lung: clinical features, pathology, and imaging findings. Am J Roentgenol 159: 1157–1164

Drings P (1988) Kardiorespiratorische Spätfolgen nach Chemo- und Radiotherapie. Med Klin 83: 408–416

Janzen DL, Padley SPG, Adler BD, Müller NL (1993) Acute pulmonary complications in immunocompromised non-AIDS patients: comparison of diagnostic accuracy of CT and chest radiography. Clin Radiol 47: 159–165

John V, Müller RD, Reiners C, Löhr E (1988) Radiologisch-diagnostische Aspekte zu Späteffekten an den Thoraxorganen nach Chemo- und/oder Strahlentherapie sowie nach Behandlung mit Radionukliden. Strahlenther Onkol 164: 619–628

Kreisman H, Wolkove N (1992) Pulmonary toxicity of antineoplastic therapy. In: Perry MC (ed) The chemotherapy source book. Williams and Wilkins, Baltimore 598–619

Link H, Reinhard U, Walter E, Wernet P, Schneider EM, Fischbach H, Blaurock M, Wilms K, Niethammer D, Ostendorf P (1986) Lung diseases after bone marrow transplantation. Klin Wochenschr 64: 595–614

McLeod TC, Müller NL (1990) Chronic diffuse lung disease. In: Putman CE (ed) Diagnostic imaging of the lung. Dekker, New York 443–490

Molls M, Budach V, Bamberg M (1986) Total body irradiation: the lung as critical organ. Strahlenther Onkol 162: 226–232

Müller NL, Miller RR (1990) Acute diffuse lung disease. In: Putman CE (ed) Diagnostic imaging of the lung. Dekker, New York, pp 337–441

Munk PL, Müller NL, Miller RR, Ostrow DN (1988) Pulmonary lymphatic carcinomatosis: CT and pathologic findings. Radiology 166: 705–709

Naidich DP, Zerhouni EA, Siegelman SS (1991) Computed tomography and magnetic resonance of the thorax. Raven, New York

Oken MM, Creech RH, Tormey DC (1982) Toxicity and response criteria of the Eastern Cooperative Oncology Group. Am J Clin Oncol 5: 649–655

Padley SPG, Adler B, Hansell DM, Müller NL (1992) High resolution computed tomography of drug induced lung disease. Clin Radiol 46: 232–236

Pennington JE (1983) Respiratory infections – Diagnosis and management. Raven, New York

Peters HD, Fink U, Schmoll HJ (1986) Toxizitäten. In: Schmoll HJ, Peters HD, Fink U (eds) Kompendium Internistische Onkologie. Springer, Berlin Heidelberg New York

Reed JC (1984) Chest radiology. Patterns and differential diagnoses. Year Book Medical Publishers, Chicago

Rosenow EC (1972) Spectrum of drug-induced pulmonary disease. Ann Intern Med 77: 977–991

Rosenow EC, Wilson WR, Cockerill FR (1985) Pulmonary disease in the immunocompromised host. Mayo Clin Proc 60: 473, 610–631

Rubin P, Casarett GW (1968) Clinical radiation pathology. Saunders, Philadelphia

Schaefer C, Prokop M, Galanski M (1990) Medikamenteninduzierte Lungenveränderungen. Radiologe 30: 564–573

Slanina J, Wannenmacher M, Bruggmoser G, Krüger HU (1982) Die pulmonale Strahlenreaktion im Röntgenbild. Radiologe 22: 74–82

van Dyk J, Keane TJ, Kan S, Rider WD, Fryer CJH (1981) Radiation pneumonitis following large single dose irradiation: a re-evaluation based on absolute dose to lung. Int J Radiat Oncol Biol Phys 7: 461–467

Zerhouni EA (1989) Computed tomography of the pulmonary parenchyma. An overview. Chest 95: 901–907

5 Cardiotoxicity

5.1 Evaluation of Late Cardiotoxicity by Pulsed Doppler Echocardiography in Patients Treated for Hodgkin's Disease

ERNST-D. KREUSER, HEINZ VÖLLER, ALEXANDER UHRIG, ANGELA BESSERER, and ECKHARD THIEL

CONTENTS

1 Advances 163
2 Patients and Methods 163
2.1 Patients and Treatment 163
2.2 Irradiation 165
2.3 Diagnostic Procedures 165
2.4 Echocardiography 165
2.5 Doppler Echocardiography 165
2.6 Statistical Analysis 166
2.7 Control Subjects 166
3 Results 166
3.1 Clinical Findings 166
3.2 Physical Examination 166
3.3 ECG Findings 167
3.4 Chest X-rays 167
3.5 M-mode and Two-Dimensional Echocardiography 167
3.6 Pulsed Doppler Echocardiography 167
4 Discussion 167
5 Summary and Conclusions 171
References 172

1 Advances

In the treatment of all stages of Hodgkin's disease, intensified chemotherapy, irradiation and bone marrow transplantation have led to the expectation of long-term survival in more than 70% of patients. The 5-year survival rate is approximately 90% in stages I and II and about 60% in stages III and IV (SANTORO et al. 1987; HENKELMAN et al. 1988; LOEFFLER et al. 1988; LONGO 1990). This therapeutic success has focused attention on chronic or irreversible side effects such as secondary cancer (QALDOR et al. 1990; SANTORO et al. 1987), gonadal toxicity (SANTORO et al. 1987), (DA CUNHA et al. 1984; KREUSER et al. 1988, 1992), thyroid diseases (HANCOCK et al. 1991), and psychosocial sequelae (FOBAIR et al. 1986). Although considerable data have been published on late cardiotoxicity associated with treatment for Hodgkin's disease, including mediastinal irradiation and various chemotherapeutic regimens (Table 1; RUCKDESCHEL et al. 1975; MARTIN et al. 1975; BROSIUS et al. 1981; APPLEFELD et al. 1981, 1982; GOTTDIENER et al. 1983; KRAMER et al. 1984; LA MONTE et al. 1986; WATCHIE et al. 1987; GREEN et al. 1987; POHJOLA-SINTONEN et al. 1987; GUSTAVSON et al. 1990), there is currently only limited information available about the impact of myocardial, valvular, and pericardial abnormalities on cardiac hemodynamic parameters. However, the influence of therapy-induced cardiac abnormalities on altered hemodynamics would probably reflect their clinical significance.

We therefore evaluated the influence of myocardial, valvular and pericardial abnormalities on early and late transvalvular and hepatic flow velocities using pulsed Doppler echocardiography in patients 1–8 years after their successful treatment for Hodgkin's disease.

2 Patients and Methods

2.1 Patients and Treatment

A total of 49 patients and Hodgkin's disease were evaluated 1–8 years after chemotherapy. All eligible patients were asked to participate in this study on the late effects of therapy. Patient fulfilling the following selection criteria were included: histologically confirmed Hodgkin's disease, age at diagnosis 14–60 years in men and 14–50 in women, complete remission > 1 year. Exclusion criteria consisted of radiation therapy only, Karnofsky index status < 50%, and relapse < 1 year. Further patient characteristics are summarized in Table 2.

ERNST-D. KREUSER, Prof. Dr., ECKHARD THIEL, Prof. Dr., Klinik für Innere Medizin, Universitätsklinikum Steglitz, Abteilung Hämatologie/Onkologie, Hindenburgdamm 30, 12203 Berlin, FRG
HEINZ VÖLLER, Dr., ALEXANDER UHRIG, Dr., Klinik für Innere Medizin, Universitätsklinikum Steglitz Abteilung Kardiologie, Hindenburgdamm 30, 12203 Berlin, FRG
ANGELA BESSERER, Dr., Universitätsklinikum Steglitz, Abteilung Radiologie, Hindenburgdamm 30, 12203 Berlin, FRG

Table 1. Acute and late cardiotoxicity in patients treated for Hodgkin's disease: a review of the literature

Therapy	*Patients (n)*	*Interval (months)*	*Methods*	*Results (%)*	*Reference*
Radiation[a] ± CT	81		ECG, CC	PT (30.9)	Ruckdeschel et al. 1975
Radiation	81	5	ECG, CC	PE (29.6) PTP (6)	Martin et al. 1975
Radiation ± CT	16	55	Autopsy	PT (94) MF (50) FME (75) VT (81)	Brosius et al. 1981
Radiation ± CT	9	88	ECG, echo (M-mode)	CP (50)	Applefield et al. 1981
Radiation ± CT	25	96	ECG, RV, CC, echo (M-mode)	CHD (12) PT (64) CMP (4)	Applefield et al. 1982
Radiation	25	130	ECG, echo (2-D)	LVED↓(50) FS↓(19)	Gottdiener et al. 1983
Radiation ± CT	37	48	ECG, echo (2-D, M-mode)	PT (24) PE (9)	Kramer et al. 1984
Radiation ± CT	19	39	ECG, echo (M-mode)	LVEF↓(16) LVEF↑(11)	LaMonte et al. 1986
Radiation ± CT	57	60	ECG	ECG pathology (13)	Watchie et al. 1987
Radiation	28	90	ECG, echo (2-D, M-mode)	LVED↑(19) LA↑(15) LVEF↓(15) PT (43)	Green et al. 1987
Radiation	28	103	ECG, stress test, CC, echo (2-D, M-mode)	Total pathology (43; serious 11) ECG pathology (46) CHD (7) PE (38) LVED↓(7) PT (34) LVED↑(7)	Pohjola-Sintonen et al. 1987
Radiation	25	180	MS, ECG, stress test, echo (Doppler, 2-D, M-mode)	CHD (15) LVED↓(28) LVED↓(8) LA↓(24) E/A < 1(50) VT (40) MR (36)	Gustavsson et al. 1990
Radiation ± CT	49	48	History, ECG, stress test Pulsed Doppler, 2-D, M-mode, echo	PE (0) PT (39) FS (18) VT (42)	Present study

Abbreviations: CT, chemotherapy; RV, radionuclide ventriculography; CC, cardiac catheterization; CHD, coronary heart-disease; PT, pericardial thickening; PTP, pericardial tamponade; MF, myocardial fibrosis; FME, fibrous thickening of mural endocardium; CMP, cardiomyopathy; MS, myocardial scintography; LA, left atrial dimension; FS, fractional shortening; E/A, ratio of early to late flow velocity; PE, pericardial effusion; LVED, left ventricular end-diastolic diameter; VT; valvular thickening; LVEF, left ventricular ejection fraction; CP, constrictive pericarditis; MR, mitral regurgitation.
[a]Mantle field irradiation.

The study population was derived from a group of patients consecutively enrolled in the German Hodgkin Study Group protocols. From July 1983 to March 1988, 20 patients with Hodgkin's disease classified as stage IIIB or stage IVA/B, according to the Ann Arbor criteria, received the COPP/ABVD (cyclophosphamide, vincristine, procarbazine, prednisone, adriamycin, bleomycin, vinblastine, dacar-

Table 2. Demographic and clinical features of the patients with Hodgkin's disease evaluated for late cardiotoxicity

Evaluable patients	49
Age at the time of study	
Median	39
Range	21–65
Age at the time of diagnosis	
Median	35
Range	15–58
Sex	
Male	27
Female	22
Chemotherapy	
COPP/ABVD[a]	26
COPP	23
Mantle field irradiation	31
Number of courses	
Median	6
Range	3–9
Time of evaluation (months)	
Median	4.37
Range	2–12

[a]COPP/ABVD regimen: cyclophosphamide, vincristine, procarbazine, prednisone, adriamycin, bleomycin, vinblastine dacarbazine.

bazine) regimen ± irradiation at our institution. The complete HD3 treatment program of the prospective randomized trial was published previously (Loeffler et al. 1988). Administration of three double cycles of alternating COPP/ABVD was followed by complete restaging. Patients in complete remission were randomized for consolidation radiotherapy (20 Gy to involved field) or chemotherapy (one double cycle COPP/ABVD). COPP was given as a modification of the MOPP regimen, mustargen being replaced by cyclophosphamide. Six patients were treated according to the ongoing HD6 protocol of the German Hodgkin Study Group. Patients with Hodgkin's disease classified as stage IIIB, IVA/B were randomized to receive COPP/ABVD × 4 or COPP/ABV/IMEP × 4 + 30 Gy to bulk or slow-responding areas. A total of 23 patients treated according to the COPP regimen were also examined in order to compare the toxicity of the anthracycline-based regimen with that of COPP chemotherapy.

The COPP/ABVD regimen consisted of: cyclophosphamide, 650 mg/m^2 i.v. days 1 + 8; vincristine, 1.4 mg/m^2 i.v. days 1 + 8; procarbazine, 100 mg/m^2 p.o. days 1–14; prednisone, 40 mg/m^2 p.o. days 1–14; doxorubicin, 25 mg/m^2 i.v. days 29 + 43; bleomycin, 10 mg/m^2 i.v. days 29 + 43; vinblastine, 6 mg/m^2 i.v. days 29 + 43; and DTIC, 375 mg/m^2 i.v. days 29 + 43. The recycle was started at day 57.

2.2 *Irradiation*

In ten patients, mediastinal irradiation was applied with a 33 MeV betatron from an anterior rectangular field, and the anterior cardiac dose was 1.25 times the tumor dose. In 21 patients, the mediastinal irradiation was applied by an 8 MeV linear accelerator from two opposing irregular fields, where cut blocks were used to shield the heart. The radiation volume comprised 60%–70% of the total heart volume, as calculated from the chest X-ray by planimetry. Radiotherapy was delivered through cobalt-60 teletherapy or a 6 MeV linear accelerator. Supradiaphragmatic nodal sites weree irradiated through A-P, P-A mantle fields tailored to each patient, after planning set up at a simulator, and the daily dose was 0.85 + 0.85 Gy.

2.3 *Diagnostic Procedures*

The cardiac evaluation included a history, physical examination and chest radiograph. The noninvasive cardiac examination comprised an ECG at rest and a symptom-limited exercise bicycle stress test. Additionally, M-mode, 2-D, and Doppler echocardiography was performed. The examiner was blinded to the details of prior therapy for Hodgkin's disease. The patients did not receive any drugs in the last 4 weeks before investigation.

2.4 *Echocardiography*

Two-dimensional and M-mode echocardiograms were obtained from the parasternal and apical view by placing the patients in the left lateral decubitus position and utilizing a Toshiba SSH-160 A ultrasound system with a 2.5 MHz transducer. Recordings were assessed for chamber sizes, left ventricular wall thickness, and percent fractional shortening. The patterns of pericardial thickening described by Schnittger et al. (1978) were used as a guide in evaluating the posterior pericardium. Additionally, the morphology of valvular and subvalvular structures was analyzed.

2.5 *Doppler Echocardiography*

Doppler ultrasound recordings were made with a 2.5 MHz transducer from the apical four-chamber view during quiet respiration. Mitral and tricuspid

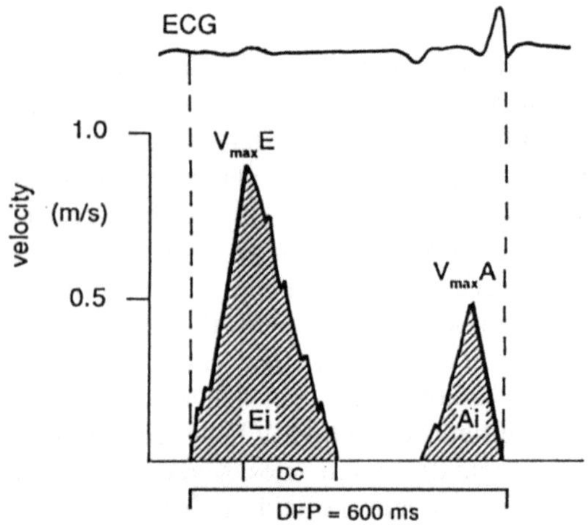

Fig. 1. Mitral flow velocity recorded by pulsed-wave Doppler echocardiography and simultaneous electrocardiography (*ECG*). Variables measured include peak ($V_{max}E$) and integrated (*Ei*) velocity of early mitral filling, peak ($V_{max}A$) and integrated (*Ai*) velocity at a trial contraction, deceleration time (*DC*) measured by extending a line from peak flow along the deceleration slope to the baseline and the diastolic filling period (*DFP*)

flow velocities were recorded using the pulsed wave Doppler technique with the sample volume placed between the leaflet tips to record maximal velocity of anterograde flow. The following Doppler parameters (average of at least five cardiac cycles) were analyzed: peak early (E) and late (A) diastolic flow velocities across mitral and tricuspid valves were measured, and the E/A ratio was calculated. Additionally, flow velocity integrals for early (Ei) and late (Ai) diastolic filling and their ratio (Ei/Ai) for transmitral flow were calculated. The deceleration time (Dc) of the E wave and the diastolic filling period (DFP) were measured (Fig. 1). Since heart rate is one of the most common variables affecting mitral and tricuspid flow, filling indices were corrected by dividing the parameters by the diastolic filling period. Hepatic vein recordings were obtained from the subcostal view with a 2 mm wide sample volume in the hepatic vein 2 cm proximal to its junction with the inferior vena cava. The deceleration times of forward flow were measured during systole (Dc sys) and diastole (Dc dias) (ms) in apnea and inspiration. The pulsed Doppler ECG was displayed with spectral analysis and a simultaneous ECG at a paper speed of 50 mm/s.

Valvular regurgitation was identified by recording systolic or diastolic reversal of flow across the valve with the pulsed wave sample volume placed just proximal to the valvular orifice. Continuous wave Doppler ultrasound was used to detect valvular stenosis and record the maximal velocity of regurgitation by adjusting the orientation of the interrogating beam guided by the auditory and visual Doppler outputs (Hatle and Angelsen 1985).

2.6 Statistical Analysis

The study design was retrospective with age- and sex-matched controls. A two-tailed unpaired *t* test was used for intergroup comparisons. Values are expressed as mean ± SD. When $p < 0.05$, the difference was considered to be statistically significant.

2.7 Control Subjects

The control group consisted of 25 sex- and age-matched volunteers (mean age ± SD 43.4 ± 10.8 years, range 21–59 years) who showed no evidence of cardiac disease. They were screened by physical examination, questionnaire of their personal and family histories, serum electrolyte determinations, blood pressure measurements at rest and during exercise, 12-lead ECG, symptom-limited exercise ECG in a supine position, 24 h Holter monitoring with ST-segment analysis, 2-D echocardiography and continuous wave, color flow, and pulsed Doppler echocardiography.

3 Results

3.1 Clinical Findings

An analysis of the history of the 49 patients treated for Hodgkin's disease revealed coronary heart disease in only one patient, who had undergone triple coronary artery bypass grafting 3 years previously. However, pathological ECG findings were already present before the initiation of chemotherapy. No patient reported symptoms related to heart failure indicating cardiomyopathy.

3.2 Physical Examination

The physical examination of the heart and lungs was not remarkable except in one patient. This 55-year-old female patient had a 2/6 holodiastolic murmur first detected 2 years after completion of chemotherapy. All patients had a regular cardiac rhythm. No patient had tachycardia (heart rate > 100/min on physical examination). Five of the 49 patients had mild or moderate hypertension according to the third Joint National Committee classification of blood pressure (Joint National Committee on Detection, Evaluation and Treatment of High Blood Pressure 1984).

3.3 *ECG Findings*

Altogether 44 of the 49 patients had normal ECGs. Five patients with hypertension had ECG patterns related to left ventricular hypertrophy. The bicycle stress test carried out in all 49 patients disclosed no pathological findings with respect to significant horizontal or descending ST-segment depression, arrhythmias, or chest pain.

3.4 *Chest X-rays*

No patient had an enlarged right or left ventricle. There were 5/49 patients with mild to moderate pulmonary fibrosis.

3.5 *M-mode and Two-Dimensional Echocardiography*

No pericardial effusion was found in any of the patients (Table 3). Pericardial thickening, defined as a pericardial thickness of ≥ 4 mm, was identified in 19 of 49 patients (38.8%). It occurred in only five of 49 (9%) patients given chemotherapy alone but in fourteen of 49 (28%) of those treated with chemotherapy and mantle field irradiation ($p < 0.05$). The left atrial diameter was slightly increased in six of 49 (12%) patients. Either LVED or LVES was increased in only wo cases whereas fractional shortening was reduced in nine of 49 (18%) (Table 3). Left ventricular hypertrophy was found in six patients (12%).

Table 3. Frequency of echocardiographic findings of the patients treated for Hodgkin's disease in the present study

Pathological parameters	*n*	(%)
Pericardial thickening	19/49	(38.8)
Pericardial effusion	0/49	(0.0)
Enlarged diameter of LA	6/49	(12.0)
Reduced fractional shortening	9/49	(18.4)
Left venticular hypertrophy	6/49	(12.0)
Valvular thickening	21/49	(42.0)

LA, left atrium.

Valvular thickening was seen in 21 patients (43%). Small areas exhibited increased echo intensity in the basal parts of the aortic cusps and/or the anterior mitral leaflet in 16 patients. A more extensive thickening affecting the aortic and mitral ring as well was seen in the remaining five patients. Three patients additionally showed thickening of a chorda to the mitral valve.

3.6 *Pulsed Doppler Echocardiography*

Since diastolic filling abnormalities have been reported in various types of heart disease, eight patients had to be excluded from Doppler evaluation of right and left ventricular filling: six with left ventricular hypertrophy, one with proven coronary heart disease and one with moderate aortic insufficiency. Slight tricuspid insufficiency was demonstrated in three of the remaining 41 patients by color flow and continuous wave Doppler. There was no evidence of valvular stenosis in any of the patients.

Regarding left ventricular filling, neither the peak early and late diastolic filling velocities nor their ratio differed among the groups (Table 4). The same results were seen with regard to the integrated filling velocities and the deceleration time. As for of heart rate-dependent alteration of transmitral filling (significantly longer DFP in group I, 417 ± 98 m/s, group II, 346 ± 42 m/s, and group, III 308 ± 60 m/s; $p \leq 0.05$), the normalization for heart rate changes did not reveal any new significantly different transmitral filling patterns among the groups (Table 5).

Regarding right ventricular filling, the early and late peak flow velocities, the E/A ratio and the deceleration time of the early diastolic filling did not significantly differ among the three groups (Table 4). Also the amount of change made in correcting by the diastolic filling period provided no striking differences (Table 5). Figure 2 shows the mean values for the hepatic vein flow velocity variables with no significant differences among the control group and patients treated for Hodgkin's disease during either apnea or inspiration.

4 Discussion

Although a considerable number of studies have previously been published regarding the impact of

Table 4. Doppler echocardiography-derived parameters for transmitral flow, transtricuspid flow and hepatic vein flow

			Transmitral flow				Transtricuspid flow				
	HR (1/min)	DFP (m/s)	E (m/s)	A (m/s)	E/A	Ei/Ai	Dc (m/s)	E (m/s)	A (m/s)	E/A	Dc (m/s)
Normal	70	417	0.77	0.55	1.47	2.27	176	0.59	0.30	1.73	158
($n=25$)	±10	±98	±0.09	±0.11	±0.42	±0.67	±23	±0.19	±0.02	±0.30	±37
Chemo-	72	346*	0.75	0.56	1.35	2.37	164	0.50	0.32	1.60	147
therapy	±5	±42	±0.14	±009	±0.23	±0.40	±27	±0.06	±0.03	±0.24	±27
($n=15$)											
Mantle field	79*	308*	0.81	0.63	1.36	2.42	158	0.51	0.37	1.47	165
irradiation	±11	±60	±0.19	±0.20	±0.43	±0.51	±32	±0.12	±0.09	±0.40	±44
($n=27$)											

HR, heart rate; DFP, diastolic filling period; E, A, peak early and late diastolic flow velocities, respectively; Ei, Ai, flow velocity integrals for early and late diastolic filling, respectively; Dc, deceleration time.
$*p < 0.05$ compared to controls.

Table 5. Doppler echocardiography-derived diastolic filling parameters, normalization for heart rate changes

			Transmitral		Transtricuspid	
	HR (1/min)	DFP (ms)	(E/A)/DFP (1/ms)	Dc/DFP	(E/A)/DFP (1/m)	Dc/DFP
Controls	70±10	417±98	0.0036	0.44	0.0046	0.43
($n=25$)			±0.0011	±0.9	±0.0013	±0.8
Chemotherapy	72±5	346±42*	0.0042	0.47	0.0045	0.46
($n=15$)			±0.0011	±0.05	±0.001	±0.3
Mantle field	79±11*	308±60*	0.0047	0.51	0.0045	0.47
irradiation ($n=27$)		±0.0021	±0.11	±0.02	±0.9	

HR, heart rate; DFP, diastolic filling period; E, A, peak early and late diastolic flow velocities, respectively; Dc, deceleration time.
$*p < 0.05$ compared to controls.

mantle field irradiation and chemotherapy on cardiac functions in patients treated for Hodgkin's disease, there is conflicting evidence concerning both the frequency and clinical significance of late cardiac toxicity (Table 1; RUCK DESHCHEL et al. 1975; MARTIN et al. 1975; BROSIUS et al. 1981; APPLEFELD et al. 1981, 1982; GOTTDIENER et al. 1983; KRAMER et al. 1984; LAMONTE et al. 1986; WATCHIE et al. 1987; GREEN et al. 1987; POHJOLA-SINTONEN et al. 1987; GUSTAVSSON et al. 1990). This survey of available literature on acute and late cardiac effects after mediastinal irradiation and/or chemotherapy in patients successfully treated for Hodgkin's disease showed that various cardiac abnormalities have been reported. Pericardial thickening occurred in 24%–47%, valvular thickening in 40%–81%, reduced fractional shortening in 20%–44%, cardiomyopathy in 0%–4% and coronary heart disease in 0%–%15% (Table 1). At variance with the high incidence of these abnormalities is the recently documented finding that, though patients treated for Hodgkin's disease still showed a higher risk of dying of leukemia and solid tumors, their risk of dying of cardiovascular complications and myocardial infarction was not increased (VAN RIJSWIJK et al. 1987; HANCOCK et al. 1988). The most striking features in our study were valvular thickening in 42%, pericardial thickening in 39%, and reduced fractional shortening in 18% (Table 3). However, no patient suffered from cardiomyopathy and only one of 49 from coronary heart disease. Since the hemodynamic impact of cardiac abnormalities detected by pulsed Doppler echocardiography had not previously been examined, we conducted this study in order to evaluate their clinical significance.

Pulsed Doppler echocardiography was used to determine the impact of pericardial and valvular thickening and reduced fractional shortening on early and late peak flow velocities across the mitral and tricuspid valves. It was also used to measure hepatic venous flow patterns (APPLETON et al. 1988a; VON BIBRA et al. 1989). Doppler echocardiography is a new approach which enables us to study

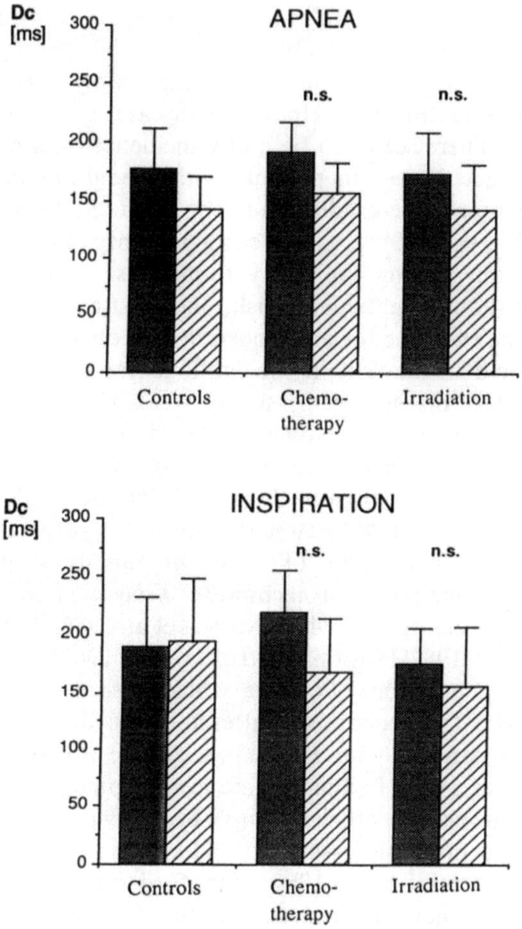

Fig. 2. Systolic and diastolic deceleration time of the hepatic vein in patients treated for Hodgkin's disease with chemotherapy ± irradiation. *Black bars* indicate systolic and *dotted bars* diastolic deceleration time (ms); *bars* are means ± SEM

noninvasively and directly the functional effect of structural changes by measuring blood flow velocities. Moreover, it has recently been shown that pulsed Doppler echocardiography is a sensitive and noninvasive method for assessing right and left ventricular filling (ROKEY et al. 1985; APPLETON et al. 1988b; STODDARD et al. 1989).

Historically, the noninvasive pattern considered typical of diastolic dysfunction was delayed and reduced early ventricular filling, manifested as a shift in the Doppler profile to a lower E wave and a higher atrial contribution to filling. The reduced E/A ratio thus became the principal Doppler index of hemodynamic impairment in coronary artery disease (WIND et al. 1987; FUJII et al. 1985; LABOVITZ et al. 1987), hypertension (PHILLIPS et al. 1989), valvular heart disease (OH et al. 1989) and cardiomyopathies of the dilated type (TANENAKA et al. 1986; AGUIRRE et al. 1989) and hypertrophic varieties (TAKENAKA et al. 1986a; BRYG et al. 1987). However, recent reports have described a Doppler pattern of diastolic dysfunction quite different from the classic E/A reversal. This pattern is characterized by a narrow E wave with a high peak velocity and steep deceleration, and a small A wave. This pattern has been observed in connection with low ventricular compliance, as in constrictive pericarditis (HATLE et al. 1989) and restrictive cardiomyopathy (APPLETON et al. 1988a). Since pericardial restraint influences diastolic performance, determination of both the right and left ventricular filling pattern and central venous flow parameters might be a sensitive noninvasive screening method detecting occult constrictive pericarditis.

Our patients treated for Hodgkin's disease with chemotherapy alone or in combination with mantle field irradiation did not differ significantly from control subjects with respect to the peak early and late diastolic right and left ventricular filling velocities (Tables 4, 5). Thus, there was no evidence of subclinical or clinical constrictive pericarditis in the present study despite the demonstration of pericardial thickening in 39% of these patients (Table 3). Previous studies have reported pericardial thickening in 24%–47% (Table 1), while clinically apparent pericarditis was only demonstrated in a minority of patients (0%–7%) with Hodgkin's disease using an equally weighted, anterior-posterior mantle technique in both adults and children (APPLEFIELD et al. 1981; GOMEZ et al. 1983; DONALDSON and KAPLAN 1982). Recently GREEN et al. (1987) reported that none of 28 patients treated during childhood and adolescence for Hodgkin's disease had symptoms of constrictive pericarditis 19–182 months after mediastinal irradiation. Compared to the low frequency of constrictive pericarditis reflecting late cardiac toxicity after mantle field irradiation in patients successfully treated for Hodgkin's disease, the incidence of pericarditis and pericardial fluid related to acute or delayed cardiac toxicity seems to be relatively high.

During the first 6 months after mediastinal irradiation, pericardial fluid has been reported in 40% (IKÄHEIMO et al. 1985). Delayed pericardial disease is the most important and most common category of RIHD (radiation-induced heart disease) (STEWART and FAJARDO 1984). The interval between mediastinal radiation and the onset of pericarditis ranges from about 4 months to several years with the majority of cases occurring within the first 12 months (STEWART and FAJARDO 1984).

Delayed pericarditis clears spontaneously with only mild supportive care in most instances, but there is occasional progression to symptomatic constriction requiring pericardiectomy. The high frequency(24%–47%) of pericardial thickening in this study and others (Table 1) can be explained as an echocardiographic residuum from acute or delayed pericarditis and pericardial fluid occurring often asymptomatic in patients who have undergone mediastinal irradiation with or without chemotherapy.

A decreased fractional shortening was measured in 18% of our study group (Table 3). Except in one patient, this was accompanied by normal or small left ventricular end-diastolic dimensions. Thus these findings are compatible with restrictive cardiomyopathy (APPLETON et al. 1988; HATLE et al. 1989). Although patients with proven coronary artery disease (one patient) and left ventricular hypertrophy (five patients) were excluded from this analysis, which reduced the E/A ratio, the study groups did not show a significantly higher E/A ratio or significantly shorter deceleration times of early peak flow velocities than controls. With increasing heart rate, the transvalvular flow velocity at the start and as a result of atrial contraction progressively increased and subsequently diminished the E/A ratio (APPLETON et al. 1991). Our patients revealed significantly higher heart rates probably due to fear of pathologic results. But the amount of change made in correcting by the diastolic filling period provided no striking differences. Only one of the previous studies listed in Table 1 used pulsed Doppler to assess late cardiac effects in patients treated for Hodgkin's disease. GUSTAVSSON et al. (1990) applied the conventional cutoff value of 1.0 for the E/A to identify an abnormal ventricular filling due to restrictive cardiomyopathy. They reported a diastolic dysfunction in 50% of their patients. However, the recently described "restrictive pattern" of diastolic dysfunction was quite different from the classic E/A reversal.

To rule out the hemodynamic effects of valvular lesions, we used color flow and continuous wave Doppler to determine both valvular stenosis and insufficiency (HATLE and ANGELSEN 1985). None of the patients showed an acceleration of peak flow across the valves due to valvular stenosis. Only one patient disclosed a moderate diastolic reversal of flow across the aortic valve which might be related to the treatment for Hodgkin's disease. A slight regurgitant flow was recorded at the tricuspid valve in three patients. This coincides with regurgitant flow patterns of normal valves described by KOSTUCKI et al. (1986). Thus, the regurgitant lesions found in our study are probably not due to the treatment for Hodgkin's disease.

There seems to be a low incidence of coronary heart disease in patients with Hodgkin's disease who received radiation to the heart (STEWART and FAJARDO 1984). Considering the rarity of such cases from among the many thousands of previously irradiated patients at risk, one must conclude that the evidence for an important role of prior mantle field irradiation in the pathogenesis of coronary heart disease seems to be weak (STEWART and FAJARDO 1984). However, the frequency of coronary heart disease reported in patients treated for Hodgkin's disease during childhood and adolescence ranges between 0% and 12% after mediastinal irradiation following the equally weighted, anterior-posterior technique (GREEN et al. 1987; KRAMER et al. 1984; LAMONTE et al. 1986; WATCHIE et al. 1987; POHJOLA-SINTONEN et al. 1987). A rather high incidence of coronary heart disease (12%) has recently been reported after mantle field irradiation in patients with Hodgkin's disease (GUSTAVSSON et al. 1990). Irradiation induced coronary heart disease has recently been published in two definite and one probable case among 28 patients (POHJODA-SINTONAN et al. 1987). Stanford reported a low frequency of irradiation-induced coronary heart disease, 2/160 in children and 1/377 adults (CARMEL and KAPLAN 1976). In a report from Harvard, the relative death rate estimate was 1.5 among 957 patients with Hodgkin's disease and did not differ significantly from the general population (BOIVIN and HUTCHISON 1982). A study revealed five confirmed and one probable case of irradiation-induced coronary heart disease among 48 patients examined by the exercise test and angiography (APPLEFELD et al. 1981). Coronary artery stenoses may be due to intimal proliferation or atherosclerotic lesions (MC ENIEY et al. 1987). It has been shown that coronary arteries receiving larger radiation doses were more likely to develop stenosis (ANNEST et al. 1983). In the previously reported cases, the radiation dose ranged from 15 to 51 Gy, suggesting no clear dose dependency.

A review of available literature regarding myocardial infarctions after mediastinal irradiation reveals 25 case reports on patients under the age of 40 (GUSTAVSSON et al. 1990). Nevertheless, despite these reports in contrast to the thousands of cases without clinical symptoms related to coronary heart disease, there is convincing evidence that irradiation and chemotherapy do not significantly increase the risk of myocardial infarction. Moreover, it has been shown that, although patients treated for Hodgkin's disease still showed an increased risk of dying, their risk of dying of cardiovascular complications was not increased (VAN RIJSWIJK et al. 1987).

In the present study, none of the 49 patients treated for Hodgkin's disease exhibited signs of cardiomyopathy. The incidence of cardiomyopathy reported in the literature is low (Table 1). Anthracycline-based chemotherapy is known to produce cardiomyopathy. Successful development of the ABVD plus doxorubicin regimen (BONADONNA and SANTORO 1982) for treatment of patients with Hodgkin's disease has raised concern about the occurrence of drug-induced cardiomyopathy. Comparisons of large groups of patients treated for Hodgkin's disease with radiotherapy and either the MOPP or ABVD regimen have not demonstrated an increased risk of cardiac death in patients receiving ABVD chemotherapy (SANTORO et al. 1987; LA MONTE et al. 1986). It thus seems unlikely that the incidence would differ from that in the general population. This low frequency of anthracycline-induced cardiomyopathy is clearly related to the low cumulative doxorubicin dose of only 300 mg per m^2 in patients receiving six cycles of the ABVD regimen. These findings are in keeping with those recently published at the Memorial Hospital (New York) evaluating 19 of 41 patients treated with the MOPP/ABV regimen and mediastinal irradiation (LA MONTE et al. 1986). Furthermore, SANTORO et al. (1987) reported cardiomyopathy in only 1/232 patients submitted to the MOPP or ABVD regimen with or without mediastinal irradiation cardiomyopathy. Taken together, these results suggest that clinically apparent cardiomyopathy is very rare in patients treated for Hodgkin's disease.

In conclusion, our results indicate that, though valvular and pericardial abnormalities are frequent in patients treated for Hodgkin's disease with mantle field irradiation and chemotherapy, they have no significant impact on early and late transvalvular and hepatic flow velocities. The normal hemodynamic parameters may reflect the minor clinical relevance of valvular and pericardial lesions. The risk of cardiomyopathy does not appear to be increased after successful treatment with mediastinal irradiation and chemotherapy. The incidence of coronary artery disease and subsequent myocardial infarction does not seem to be significantly increased, although therapy-related coronary heart disease may occur in patients with further risk factors. Successful treatment for Hodgkin's disease still involves an increased risk of dying, but not of late cardiac toxicity. Therefore routinely assessed Doppler echocardiography does not seems to be indicated in such cases.

5 Summary and Conclusions

In view of the favorable prognosis for patients with Hodgkin's disease, treatment toxicity has become an important issue. Chemotherapy with and without mediastinal radiation can induce both acute and late myocardial, valvular, and pericardial abnormalities in patients treated for Hodgkin's disease. Only limited data are currently available about therapy-related cardiac toxicity on hemo-dynamic parameters probably reflecting their clinical significance.

The impact of valvular, myocardial and pericardial abnormalities on cardiac hemodynamics in patients treated for Hodgkin's disease with COPP/ABVD ± radiation was determined by submitting 49 patients to cardiac evaluation 2–10 years (median 5.37 years) after they had completed induction therapy. Diagnostic procedures to evaluate cardiac functions consisted of history, physical examination, bicycle exercise stress test, M-mode and 2-D echocardiography, and pulsed Doppler echocardiography, including the peak and integrated early (E, Ei) and late (A, Ai) diastolic flow velocities across the mitral and tricuspid valve and their ratios (E/A) and Ei/Ai). The assessment also covered the diastolic filling period and the deceleration times of early diastolic transmitral, transtricuspid, and hepatic vein flows. Doppler indices were compared to those of 25 age- and sex-matched control subjects.

No patient reported symptoms related to cardiomyopathy or coronary heart disease. Pericardial thickening was demonstrated on echocardiograms in 19/49 (38.8%), valvular thickening in 21/49 (42.9%) and reduced fractional shortening in 9/49 (18.4%) patients. The Doppler-derived mean E and A (± SD) of transmitral flow were 0.75 ± 0.14 m/s and 0.56 ± 0.09 m/s, respectively in patients receiving chemotherapy and 0.81 ± 0.19 m/s and 0.63 ± 0.20 m/s, respectively, in those with additional mantle field irradiation. There was no statistically significant difference between mean E and A of transmitral flow of patients treated for Hodgkin's disease and control subjects. Furthermore, the transtricuspid and hepatic vein flow velocities did not differ significantly.

Although the present study demonstrates a high frequency of pericardial and valvular thickening in patients treated for Hodgkin's disease with the COPP/ABVD regimen ± mediastinal irradiation, these findings had no impact on cardiac flow velocities and may be thus of minor clinical relevance in cured patients.

Acknowledgments. We would like to thank Susanne Carl for excellent editorial assistance. This work was supported by a grant from Deutsche Krebshilfe, Bonn, Contract No. M 34/88 Kr 1.

References

Aguirre FV, Pearson AC, Lewen MK et al. (1989) Usefulness of Doppler echocardiography in the diagnosis of congestive heart failure. Am J Cardiol 63: 1098–1102

Annest LS, Anderson RP, Li W, Hafermann MD (1983) Coronary artery disease following mediastinal radiation therapy. J Thorac Cardiovasc Surg 85: 257–263

Applefield MM, Cole JF, Pollock SH et al. (1981) The late appearance of chronic pericardial disease in patients treated by radiotherapy for Hodgkin's disease. Ann Intern Med 94: 338–341

Applefield MM, Slawson RG, Sicer KM et al. (1982) Long-term cardiovascular evaluation of patients with Hodgkin's disease treated by thoracic mantle radiation therapy. Cancer Treat Rep 66: 1003–1013

Appleton CP, Hatle LK, Popp RL (1988a) Demonstration of restrictive ventricular physiology by Doppler echocardiography. JACC 11: 757–768

Appleton CP, Hatle LK, Popp RL et al. (1988b) Relation of transmitral flow velocity patterns to left ventricular diastolic function: new insights from a combined hemodynamic and Doppler echocardiographic study. J Am Coll Cardiol 12: 426–440

Appleton CP, Carucci MJ, Henry CP et al. (1991) Influence of incremental changes in heart rate on mitral flow velocity: assessment in lightly sedated, conscious dogs. J Am Coll Cardiol 17: 227–236

Boivin J-F, Hutchison GB (1982) Coronary heart disease mortality after irradiation for Hodgkin's disease. Cancer 49: 2470–2475

Bonadonna G, Santoro A (1982) ABVD chemotherapy in the treatment of Hodgkin's disease. Cancer Treat Rev 9: 21–35

Brosius FC, Waller BF, Robert WC (1981) Radiation heart disease. Am J Med 70: 519–530

Bryg RJ, Pearson AC, Williams, GA et al. (1987) Left ventricular systolic and diastolic flow abnormalities determined by Doppler echocardiography in obstructive hypertrophic cardiomyopathy. Am J Cardiol 59: 925–931

Carmel RJ, Kaplan HS (1976) Mantle irradiation in Hodgkin's disease. Cancer 37: 2813–2815

da Cunha MF, Meistrich ML, Fuller LM et al. (1984) Recovery of spermatogenesis after treatment for Hodgkin's disease: limiting dose of MOPP chemotherapy. J Clin Oncol 2: 571–577

Donaldson SS, Kaplan HS (1982) Complications of treatment of Hodgkin's disease in children. Cancer Treat Rep 66: 977–989

Fobair P, Hoppe RT, Bloom J et al. (1986) Psychosocial problems among survivors of Hodgkin's disease. J Clin Oncol 4: 805–814

Fujii J, Yazaki Y, Sawada H et al. (1985) Noninvasive assessment of left and right ventricular filling in myocardial infarction with a two-dimensional Doppler echocardiographic method. J Am Coll Cardiol 5: 1155–1160

Gomez GA, Park JJ, Panahon AM et al. (1983) Heart size and function after radiation therapy to the mediastinum in patients with Hodgkin's disease. Cancer Treat Rep 67: 1099–1103

Gottdiener JS, Katin MJ, Borer JS et al. (1983) Late cardiac effects of therapeutic mediastinal irradiation. N Engl J Med 308: 569–572

Green DM, Gingell RL, Pearce J et al. (1987) The effect of mediastinal irradiation on cardiac function of patients treated during childhood and adolescence for Hodgkin's disease. J Clin Oncol 5: 239–245

Gustavsson A, Eskilsson J, Landberg T et al. (1990) Late cardiac effects after mantle radiotherapy in patients with Hodgkin's disease. Ann Oncol 1: 355–363

Hancock SL, Hoppe RT, Horning SJ et al. (1988) Intercurrent death after Hodgkin's disease therapy in radiotherapy and adjuvant MOPP trials. Ann Intern Med 109: 183–189

Hancock SL, Cox RS, McDougall IR (1991) Thyroid diseases after treatment of Hodgkin's disease. N Engl J Med 325: 599–605

Hatle L, Angelsen B (1985) Doppler ultrasoun in cardiology, physical principles and clinical applications, 2nd edn Lea and Febiger, Philadelphia, pp 110–188

Hatle LK, Appleton CP, Popp RL (1989) Differentiation of constrictive pericarditis and restrictive cardiomyopathy by Doppler echocardiography. Circulation 79: 357–370

Henkelmann GC, Hagemeister FB, Fuller LM (1988) Two cycles of MOPP and radiotherapy for stage III_1A and stage III_1B Hodgkin's disease. J Clin Oncol 6: 1293–1302

Ikäheimo M, Niemelä K, Linnaluota M et al. (1985) Early cardiac changes related to radiation therapy. Am J Cardiol 56: 943–946

Joint National Committee on Detection, Evaluation and Treatment of High Blood Pressure (1984) The 1984 report of the Joint National Committee on Detection, Evaluation and Treatment of High Blood Pressure. Arch Intern Med 144: 1045

Kaldor JM, Day NE, Clarke EA et al. (1990) Leukemia following Hodgkin's disease. N Engl J Med 322: 7–13

Kostucki W, Vandenbossche JL, Friart A et al. (1986) Pulsed Doppler regurgitant flow patterns of normal values. Am J Cardiol 58: 309–313

Kramer W, Cibis W, Krieger H et al. (1984) Herzerkrankungen als Spätkomplikation nach kombinierter Polychemo- und Radiotherapie bei Morbus Hodgkin. Med Welt 35: 1098–1102

Kreuser ED, Hetzel WD, Heit W et al. (1988) Reproductive and endocrine gonadal functions in adults following multidrug chemotherapy for acute lymphblastic or undifferentiated leukemia. J Clin Oncol 6: 588–595

Kreuser ED, Felsenberg D, Behles C et al. (1992) Long-term gonadal dysfunction and its impact on bone mineralization in patients following COPP/ABVD chemotherapy for Hodgkin's disease. Ann Oncol (in press)

Labovitz AJ, Lewen MK, Kern M et al. (1987) Evaluation of left ventricular systolic and diastolic dysfunction during transient myocardial ischemia produced by angioplasty. J Am Coll Cardiol 10: 748–755

LaMonte CS, Yeh SDJ, Straus DJ (1986) Long-term follow-up of cardiac function in patients with Hodgkin's disease treated with mediastinal irradiation and combination chemotherapy including doxorubicin. Cancer Treat Rep 70: 439–444

Loeffler M, Pfreundschuh M, Hasenclever D et al. (1988) Prognostic risk factor in advanced Hodgkin's lymphoma. Blut 56: 273–281

Longo DL (1990) The use of chemotherapy in the treatment of Hodgkin's disease. Semin Oncol 17: 716–735

Martin RG, Ruckdeschel JC, Chang P et al. (1975) Radiation-related pericarditis. Am J Cardiol 35: 216–220

Mc Eniery PT, Dorosti K, Schiarone WA et al. (1987) Clinical and angiographic features of coronary artery disease after chest irradiation. Am J Cardiol 60: 1020–1024

Oh JK, Hatle LK, Sinak LJ et al. (1989) Characteristic Doppler echocardiographic pattern of mitral inflow velocity in severe aortic regurgitation. J Am Coll Cardiol 14: 1712–1717

Phillips RA, Goldman ME, Ardeljan M et al. (1989) Determinants of abnormal left ventricular filling in early hypertension. J Am Coll Cardiol 14: 979–985

Pohjola-Sintonen S, Tötterman KJ, Salmo M et al. (1987) Late cardiac effects of mediastinal radiotherapy in patients with Hodgkin's disease. Cancer 60: 31–37

Ruckdeschel JC, Chang P, Martin RG et al. (1975) Radiation-related pericardial effusions in patients with Hodgkin's disease. Medicine 54: 245–259

Rokey R, Kuo LC, Zoghbi WA et al. (1985) Determination of parameters of left ventricular diastolic filling with pulsed Doppler echocardiography: comparison with cineangiography. Circulation 71: 543–550

Santoro A, Bonadonna G, Valagussa P et al. (1987) Long-term results of combined chemotherapy-radiotherapy approach in Hodgkin's disease: superiority of ABVD plus radiotherapy versus MOPP plus radiotherapy. J Clin Oncol 5: 27–37

Schnittger I, Bowden RE, Abrams J et al. (1978) Echocardiography: pericardial thickening and constrictive pericarditis. Am J Cardiol 42: 388–395

Stewart JR, Fajardo LF (1984) Radiation-induced heart disease: an update. Prog Cardiovasc Dis 27: 173–194

Stoddard MF, Pearson AC, Kern MJ et al. (1989) Left ventricular diastolic function: comparison of pulsed Doppler echocardiographic and hemodynamic indexes in subjects with and without coronary artery disease. JACC 13: 327–336

Takenaka K, Dabestani A, Gardin JM et al. (1986a) Left ventricular filling in hypertrophic cardiomyopathy: a pulsed Doppler echocardiographic study. J Am Coll Cardiol 7: 1263–1271

Takenaka K, Dabestani A, Gardin JM (1986b) Pulsed Doppler echocardiographic study of left ventricular filling in dilated cardiomyopathy. Am J Cardiol 58: 143–147

van Rijswijk REN, Verbeek J, Haanen C et al. (1987) Major complications and causes of death in patients treated for Hodgkin's disease. J Clin Oncol 5: 1624–1633

von Bibra H, Schober K, Jenni R et al. (1989) Diagnosis of constrictive pericarditis by pulsed Doppler echocardiography of the hepatic vein. Am J Cardiol 63: 483–488

Watchie J, Coleman CN, Raffin TA et al. (1987) Minimal long-term cardiopulmonary dysfunction following treatment for Hodgkin's disease. Int J Radiat Oncol Biol Phys 13: 517–524

Wind BE, Snider AR, Buda AJ et al. (1987) Pulsed Doppler assessment of left ventricular diastolic filling in coronary artery disease before and immediately after coronary angioplasty. Am J Cardiol 59: 1041–1046

Ward RL, Sabbar AH, ... (198[illegible]) ... Doppler assessment of left ventricular diastolic filling in coronary artery disease before and immediately after coronary angioplasty. Am J Cardiol 58: [illegible]

... parameters of left ventricular diastolic filling ... Doppler echocardiography: comparison with ... angiography. Circulation 71: 543–550

Santoro A, Bonadonna G, Valagussa P et al. (1987) Long-term results of combined chemotherapy-radiotherapy ...

5.2 Anthracycline-Induced Cardiotoxicity in Children: Pathophysiology and Prevention

STEFAN BIELACK and RUDOLF ERTTMANN

CONTENTS

1 Introduction 175
2 Mechanisms of Cardiac Damage 175
3 Myocardial Pathology 175
4 Incidence of Anthracycline Cardiotoxicity 175
4.1 Clinical Evidence 175
4.2 Subclinical Evidence 176
5 Documented and Potential Risk Factors 176
5.1 Cumulative Dose 176
5.2 Peak Drug Levels 176
5.3 Mediastinal Irradiation 176
5.4 Time After Anthracycline Treatment 176
5.5 Young Age 177
5.6 Additional Stress to the Heart 177
6 Prevention 177
6.1 Schedule Alterations 177
6.2 Modified Anthracyclines 178
6.3 Other Modifications of Anthracycline Pharmacology 178
6.4 Cardioprotective Agents 178
6.5 Monitoring for Early Signs of Cardiotoxicity . . 178
7 Treatment 179
8 Summary and Therapeutic Recommendations . . 179
References 179

1 Introduction

The anthracyclines are among the most effective and most widely used cytostatic agents in pediatric oncology. Apart from drug resistance, cardiotoxicity is the most important factor limiting their therapeutic success. Clinically, cardiotoxicity is characterized by the progressive development of a chronic cardiomyopathy leading to congestive heart failure and death. With an increasing number of pediatric cancer patients surviving many years after successful anthracycline therapy, this potentially deleterious side effect is now of major concern. In this chapter, we will try to review the characteristics of anthracycline cardiotoxicity and approaches to avoid this disabling and possibly lethal complication.

STEFAN BIELACK, Dr., RUDOLF ERTTMANN Prof. Dr., Universitätskinderklinik Hamburg, Abteilung für pädiatrische Hämatologie und Onkologie, Martinistraße 52, 20251 Hamburg, FRG

2 Mechanisms of Cardiac Damage

The exact mechanism by which anthracyclines damage the heart is still a matter of debate. Most authors favor the hypothesis that free radicals are responsible for the cardiac side effects seen (OLSON and MUSHLIN 1990). The heart is especially vulnerable to oxidative damage, since it has a low potential to detoxify radicals (OLSON et al. 1981). Anthracyclines are capable of producing free radicals due to one electron reduction of their quinone ring by flavin reductases. Alternatively, free radicals can be produced nonenzymatically by an anthracycline-iron complex (BASSER and GREEN 1993; OLSON and MUSHLIN 1990). The alterations in calcium handling and the diminished capacity for ATP generation frequently observed in heart muscle cells after exposure to anthracyclines might then be due to oxidative damage of lipid membranes, especially those of the sarcoplasmatic reticulum (MYERS and CHABNER 1990).

3 Myocardial Pathology

Morphological changes induced by anthracyclines can be graded by electron microscopy in tissue obtained by endomyocardial biopsy. Loss of myofibrils, swelling of the sarcoplasmatic reticulum and mitochondria give way to cell necrosis. Finally, diffuse myocardial fibrosis develops (BILLINGHAM et al. 1978).

4 Incidence of Anthracycline Cardiotoxicity

4.1 *Clinical Evidence*

How common are these cardiotoxic effects? Early reports, mainly dealing with adult patients during or immediately after anthracycline treatment, reported the incidence of congestive heart failure to be only a few percent. For example, two very large retrospective studies by VON HOFF et al., each evaluating thousands of patients, found a 2.2% incidence of congestive heart failure after doxorubicin chemotherapy and 1.16% after daunorubicin chemotherapy (VON HOFF et al. 1979; VON HOFF and LAYARD 1981). Heart failure has also been observed in children and adolescents treated with anthracyclines: we saw a 2.2% incidence of congestive heart failure in 785 young patients after doxorubicin treatment for osteosarcoma (GEIDEL et al. 1991). GOORIN et al. (1981) found a 4% incidence of congestive heart failure in 389 doxorubicin-treated children. At first glance, these percentages of clinical cardiac events may seem acceptable when taking into account the important contribution of anthracyclines against many cancers; however, caution is necessary, as discussed below.

4.2 Subclinical Evidence

Subclinical cardiotoxicity is much more common than clinical signs of congestive heart failure (GEIDEL et al. 1991; LIPSHULTZ et al. 1991; STEINHERZ et al. 1991). Various invasive and noninvasive methods have been used to measure the extent of cardiac damage. Depending on the sensitivity of the method employed, the proportion of hearts found to be damaged has varied widely. In some studies, almost all hearts showed measurable treatment-related changes (DRUCK et al. 1984; MAIONE et al. 1988; MARCHANDISE et al. 1989; STEIN et al. 1989). Echocardiography is probably the most widely used tool in the evaluation of anthracycline-induced cardiac damage. Usually, systolic function is estimated by measuring the fractional shortening rate of the left ventricle. Using this parameter, we found a 21% incidence of abnormal values in 29 young patients after doxorubicin therapy (mean: 342 mg) for osteosarcoma (GEIDEL 1991). STEINHERZ et al. (1991) investigated 201 patients 4–20 years after anthracycline therapy for pediatric malignancies and found a 23% incidence of abnormal cardiac function on noninvasive testing, while only nine of these 201 had late clinical symptoms. LIPSHULTZ et al. (1991) found decreased contractility in 23% of 115 children treated with doxorubicin for acute lymphoblastic leukemia. Left ventricular afterload, however, was increased in 57% of patients. As HAUSDORF et al. (1988), from our institution, and others (LEE et al. 1987; MAIONE et al. 1988; MARCHANDISE et al. 1989) have reported, changes in diastolic function seem to be common even before contractility is measurably impaired. Accordingly, decreases in the peak filling rate have been shown to precede congestive heart failure which develops despite serial monitoring of systolic cardiac function (GANZ et al. 1993).

What do these subclinical but measurable alterations of cardiac function after anthracycline therapy mean for any given patient? How many and which of the patients with such changes will develop heart failure? Unfortunately, nobody knows. It seems that there is no method, be it invasive or noninvasive, that can unequivocally predict or exclude anthracycline cardiomyopathy. As congestive heart failure can develop after just a single dose, all anthracycline-treated patients should be considered to be at risk. Measurable impairments of contractility might then have to be considered as a sign of more imminent danger.

5 Documented and Potential Risk Factors

5.1 Cumulative Dose

A very close correlation between cumulative anthracycline dose and risk of heart failure has been well documented in series including thousands of patients (VON HOFF et al. 1979; VON HOFF and LAYARD 1981).

5.2 Peak Drug Levels

Administration schedules leading to reduced peak drug levels will cause less cardiac damage at any given cumulative anthracycline dose (reviewed in BIELACK et al. 1989).

5.3 Mediastinal Irradiation

While many other risk factors for clinical anthracycline cardiomyopathy are still being debated, mediastinal irradiation unquestionably enhances cardiac damage (BILLINGHAM et al. 1978).

5.4 Time After Anthracycline Treatment

It is very important to keep in mind that there is no reason to believe that anthracycline-induced cardiac damage is reversible. On the contrary, evidence has accumulated that heart function will continue to deteriorate even long after anthracyclines have been discontinued. Various authors have reported cases of cardiac decompensation years or even decades after anthracycline treatment in childhood or adolescence (GOORIN et al. 1990; GOTTLIEB et al. 1980; STEINHERZ et al. 1991). We saw initial manifestations of congestive heart failure as late as 436 weeks after the final doxorubicin dose (GEIDEL et al. 1991). An early study in rabbits showed progression of morphological damage long after doxorubicin was withdrawn (JAENKE 1974). Several reports have stressed that subclinical indices of heart function continue to worsen with time after treatment. For example, we saw deteriorations of systolic function parameters in eight of nine osteosarcoma patients studied after recovering from their last anthracycline dose and then again after a treatment-free interval of several years. Also, echocardiography and radionuclide ventriculography showed subnormal function more commonly in patients followed for more than 80 months than in patients studied earlier after cessation of anthracycline therapy (GEIDEL et al. 1991). The same negative influence of time after treatment was found by STEINHERZ et al. In their study on survivors of childhood malignancy, they saw 56 patients at least 10 years after a median anthracycline dose of 495 mg/m^2 and found an incidence of 38% abnormal findings, compared with 18% of 145 patients evaluated after less than 10 years (STEINHERZ et al. 1991). Afterload increased progressively in 24 of 34 patients evaluated serially by LIPSHULTZ et al. (1991).

5.5 Young Age

Patients treated early in life may be at an increased risk to eventually suffer from cardiotoxic effects of anthracyclines. For example, VON HOFF and LAYARD saw an incidence of 6% congestive heart failure at 500 mg/m^2 daunorubicin in children younger than 15 years compared to only 1.3% for patients age 15–40 years (VON HOFF and LAYARD 1981). In another study, an age of less than 4 years at treatment predicted increased afterload in children evaluated 6.4 years after treatment for childhood acute lymphoblastic leukemia (LIPSHULTZ et al. 1991). STEINHERZ et al., by contrast, saw no influence of age at anthracycline treatment on cardiac function in 201 survivors after 4–20 years (STEINHERZ et al. 1991). Why might children have an increased risk for anthracycline cardiomyopathy? Failure of growth of cardiac mass to match the patient's somatic growth has been proposed to predispose children for late anthracycline-induced congestive heart failure (GOORIN et al. 1990). Accordingly, LIPSHULTZ et al. (1991) saw an inappropriately small increase of left ventricular wall thickness in relation to somatic growth. A second reason why persons treated during childhood could have a higher likelihood of manifesting late cardiac changes is their greater life expectancy, giving heart function more time to deteriorate.

5.6 Additional Stress to the Heart

Cardiac decompensation can be triggered by unusual stress to the heart, such as pregnancy and delivery (DAVIS and BOROW 1988), or isometric exercise, such as active weight lifting (STEINHERZ and STEINHERZ 1988). Patient management might influence which patients will experience congestive heart failure. SCHWARTZ et al. (1987) reported that fewer patients with subclinical cardiotoxicity developed cardiomyopathy when given "appropriate" medical therapy.

6 Prevention

How can anthracycline cardiotoxicity be avoided when replacing anthracyclines by other agents is usually not feasible? The problem can be approached in several ways, as discussed below.

6.1 Schedule Alterations

Several authors have been able to show convincingly that both the risk of developing heart failure and the incidence and severity of subclinical cardiac alterations decrease markedly when anthracyclines are given in split doses (VON HOFF et al. 1979; WEISS et al. 1976; review: BIELACK et al. 1989) or by prolonged infusion (LEGHA et al. 1982), thereby reducing peak durg levels without compromising the area under the plasma concentration curve. While reduced cardiotoxicity compared to bolus administration has been demonstrated for infusions as short as 6 h (SHAPIRA et al. 1990), the fact is that the longer the time allowed for infusion, the smaller the risk of cardiac damage (reviewed in BIELACK et al. 1989). While most other toxicities remain unaltered, mucositis becomes dose limiting with these prolonged infusions (GREEN et al. 1984). Whether antitumor efficacy is reduced by these schedule alterations is still unclear. Judging from the available evidence, however, a major negative impact on therapeutic efficacy is unlikely (BIELACK et al. 1989; CASPER et al. 1991; ZALUPSKI et al. 1991). Schedule alterations are therefore a realistic way of minimizing the harmful effects of anthracyclines.

6.2 Modified Anthracyclines

The search for anthracyclines with reduced cardiotoxic potential but unimpaired (or even better) antitumor activity has been going on ever since the discovery of the classical anthracyclines daunorubicin and doxorubicin over 30 years ago. While several other anthracyclines are currently commercially available (e.g., epirubicin, aclacinomycin A, idarubicin) or under clinical investigation (e.g., several morpholinyl-anthracyclines), none of these analogues has been shown to be more than moderately less cardiotoxic at equieffective dosages (WEISS 1992).

6.3 Other Modifications of Anthracycline Pharmacology

Several other methods to modify the pharmacokinetics of anthracyclines, such as liposome encapsulation (HERMAN et al. 1983) and coupling of the molecule to microspheres (NAPOLI et al. 1992), have been developed in order to increase their therapeutic efficacy. While promising in some respects, none of these has yet become standard clinical practice.

6.4 Cardioprotective Agents

Based on the free radical hypothesis of cardiac damage, several compounds have been evaluated as protective agents. Classical anti-oxidants such as vitamin E or *n*-acetylcysteine have not shown cardioprotection in humans (BASSER and GREEN 1993). This lack of activity is probably because hydroxyl radicals generated by membrane- or DNA-bound anthracycline-iron complexes are formed right at their target sites, making it impossible for free radical scavengers to intervene (MYERS and CHABNER 1990). A very important contribution to the prevention of anthracycline cardiotoxicity, however, has been made by the bispiperazinedione ICRF-187 (ADR 529, dexrazoxane). Its mechanism of action seems to be intracellular iron chelation, possibly by forming a ternary anthracycline-iron-ICRF-187 complex, thereby disabling oxidative damage by anthracycline-iron complexes (SOBOL et al. 1992). A randomized clinical trial in women with advanced breast cancer receiving doxorubicin in combination with fluorouracil and cyclophosphamide or the same regimen preceded by ICRF-187 showed that ICRF-187 permitted significantly greater doses of doxorubicin to be administered to patients with greater safety. While cardiotoxicity was markedly reduced, response rates were not (SPEYER et al. 1992). The same was true in a randomized trial of pediatric soft tissue sarcoma (WECHSLER et al. 1993). ICRF-187 is not without side effects itself; myelosuppression can be dose limiting (HOCHSTER et al. 1992). As with continuous infusion, coadministration of ICRF-187 with anthracyclines is a realistic way to prevent damage to the heart. The drug is already available in several European countries.

6.5 Monitoring for Early Signs of Cardiotoxicity

The development of anthracycline-induced congestive heart failure might be avoided by premature termination of anthracycline therapy upon the development of subclinical changes in heart function. In patients undergoing chemotherapy, sequential monitoring of cardiac function, for example by echocardiography or radionuclide ventriculography, has been advocated to identify such subclinical cardiotoxicity. It is thought that monitoring could guide modifications of chemotherapy in order to minimize cumulative cardiotoxicity. The Cardiology Committee of the Childrens Cancer Study Group proposed recommendations for standardized noninvasive monitoring of children during and after chemotherapy and has published guidelines for modifications of chemotherapy (STEINHERZ et al. 1992). However, these recommendations are somewhat arbitrary, since there is as yet no method which will unequivocally predict which patient will develop clinical cardiotoxicity with continued anthracycline treatment and for whom the next dose is safe (see Sect. 4.2). During chemotherapy, many confounding variables other than drug toxicity, such as anemia or sepsis, can influence cardiac function parameters, making interpretation of these tests even more difficult.

7 Treatment

The questions when and how anthracycline-induced cardiomyopathy should be treated are still unanswered. Should measurable alterations of systolic function without clinical symptoms be treated? Are changes in loading conditions, which precede depression of systolic function (HAUSDORF et al. 1988; LIPSHULTZ et al. 1991), an indication for therapy? In view of the trend towards continued deterioration of heart function even late after anthracyclines, the decision whether to treat should not be made too late.

Which drug or drugs could prevent or at least slow down the disease process? This question, which has not at all been answered for anthracycline cardiomyopathy, is still fervently debated for heart failure in general. So far, only angiotensin converting enzyme inhibitors have had well-documented positive effects on survival in patients with heart failure (COHN 1992). Skepticism prevails regarding the value of positive inotropic agents (PACKER 1993). In extreme cases, heart transplantation may be a therapeutic option (LUTHY et al. 1992).

8 Summary and Therapeutic Recommendations

Late anthracycline cardiotoxicity is a disturbing side effect of otherwise successful treatment for childhood cancer. Heart function has been shown to deteriorate further with longer time after treatment. Anthracycline-induced damage of the myocardium seems to be mediated by free radicals. Its extent is related to both peak drug levels and cumulative dose. Monitoring for subclinical signs of cardiac dysfunction during therapy may help to define those patients at risk for severe toxicity. Schedule alterations which lead to decreased peak drug levels and the iron chelator ICRF-187 can both be used to significantly decrease anthracycline cardiotoxicity.

References

Basser RL, Green MD (1993) Strategies for prevention of anthracycline cardiotoxicity. Cancer Treat Rev 19: 57–77

Bielack S, Erttmann R, Winkler K, Landbeck G (1989) Doxorubicin: effect of different schedules on toxicity and anti-tumor efficacy. Eur J Cancer Clin Oncol 25: 873–882

Billingham ME, Mason JW, Bristow MR, Daniels JR (1978) Anthracycline cardiomyopathy monitored by morphological changes. Cancer Treat Rep 62: 865–872

Casper ES, Gaynor JJ, Hajdu SI, Magill GB, Tan C, Friedrich C, Brennan MF (1991) A prospective randomized trial of adjuvant chemotherapy with bolus versus continuous infusion of doxorubicin in patients with high-grade extremity soft tissue sarcoma and an analysis of prognostic factors. Cancer 68: 1221–1229

Cohn JN (1992) The prevention of heart failure – A new agenda. N Engl J Med 327: 725–727

Davis LE, Borow CEL (1988) Peripartum heart failure in a patient treated previously with doxorubicin. Obstet Gynecol 71: 506–508

Druck MN, Gulenchyn KY, Evans WK, Gottlieb A, Srigley JR, Bar-Shlomo BZ, Feiglin DH, McEwan P, Silver MD, Millband L, Winter K, Hilton JD, Jablonsky G, Morch JE, McLaughlin P (1984) Radionuclide angiography and endomyocardial biopsy in the assessment of doxorubicin cardiotoxicity. Cancer 53: 1667–1674

Ganz WI, Sridhar KS, Forness TJ (1993) Detection of early anthracycline cardiotoxicity by monitoring the peak filling rate. Am J Clin Oncol 16: 109–112

Geidel S, Garn M, Grävinghoff L, Hausdorf G, Morf G, Bielack S, Knop J, Winkler K (1991) Cardiomyopathy after treatment for osteosarcoma: a contribution to cardiotoxicity of adriamycin. Klin Pädiatr 203: 257–261

Goorin AM, Borow KM, Goldman A, Williams RG, Henderson C, Sallan S, Cohen H, Jaffe N (1981) Congestive heart failure due to adriamycin cardiotoxicity: it's natural course in children. Cancer 47: 2810–2816

Goorin AM, Chauvenet AR, Perez-Atayde AR, Cruz J, McKone R, Lipshultz SE (1990) Initial congestive heart failure, six to ten years after doxorubicin chemotherapy for childhood cancer. J Pediatr 116: 144–147

Gottlieb SL, Edminston WA, Haywood LJ (1980) Late, late doxorubicin cardiotoxicity. Chest 78: 880–882

Green MD, Speyer JS, Bottino JC, Blum RH, Wernz JC, Muggia FM (1984) Phase I–II study of the continuous infusion of doxorubicin in the treatment of non-small cell lung cancer. Cancer Treat Rep 60: 681–682

Hausdorf G, Morf G, Beron G, Erttmann R, Winkler K, Landbeck G, Keck EW (1988) Long-term doxorubicin cardiotoxicity in childhood: Non-invasive evaluation of the contractile state and diastolic filling. Br Heart J 60: 309–315

Herman EH, Rahman H, Fermans VJ, Vick JA, Schein PS (1983) Prevention of chronic doxorubicin cardiotoxicity in beagles by liposomal encapsulation, Cancer Res 43: 5427–5432

Hochster H, Liebes L, Wadler S, Oratz R, Wernz JC, Meyers M, Green M, Blum RH, Speyer JL (1992) Pharmacokinetics of the cardioprotector ADR-529 (ICRF-187) in escalating doses combined with fixed-dose doxorubicin. J Natl Cancer Inst 84: 1725–1730

Jaenke RS (1974) An anthracycline antibiotic-induced cardiomyopathy in rabbits. Lab Invest 30: 302–304

Lee BH, Goodenday LS, Muswick GJ, Yasnoff WA, Leighton RF, Skeel RT (1987) Alterations in left ventricular diastolic function with doxorubicin therapy. J Am Coll Cardiol 9: 184–188

Legha SS, Benjamin RS, Mackay B, Ewer M, Wallace S, Valdivieso M, Rasmussen SL, Blumenschein GR, Freireich EJ (1982) Reduction of doxorubicin cardiotoxicity by prolonged continuous intravenous infusion. Ann Intern Med 96: 133–139

Lipshultz SE, Colan SD, Gelber RD, Perez-Atayde AR, Sallan SE, Sanders SP (1991) Late cardiac effects of doxorubicin therapy for acute lymphoblastic leukemia in childhood. N Engl J Med 324: 808–815

Luthy A, Furrer M, Waser M, Maggiorini M, Pluess HJ, Real F, Weiss B, Gallino A, Turina M (1992) Orthotopic heart transplantation: an efficient treatment in a young boy with doxorubicin-induced cardiomyopathy. J Heart Lung Transplant 11: 815–816

Maione S, Giunta A, Tuccillo B, Biagini R, del Rosso P, Pezza A, de Blasio F (1988) Doppler echocardiographic assessment of left ventricular function in patients with primary lung cancer treated with doxorubicin. Tumori 74: 725–729

Marchandise B, Schroeder E, Bosly A, Doyen C, Weynants P, Kremer R, Pouleur H (1989) Early detection of doxorubicin cardiotoxicity: interest of Doppler echocardiographic analysis of left ventricular filling dynamics. Am Heart J 118: 92–98

Myers CE, Chabner BA (1990) Anthracyclines. In: Chabner BA, Collins JM (eds) Cancer chemotherapy. Principles and practice. Lippincott, Philadelphia, pp 356–381

Napoli S, Burton MA, Martins IJ, Chen Y, Codde JP, Gray BN (1992) Dose response and toxocity of doxorubicin microspheres in a rat tumor. Anticancer Drugs 3: 47–53

Olson RD, Mushlin PS (1990) Doxorubicin cardiotoxocity: analysis of prevailing hypothesis. FASEB J 4: 3076–3086

Olson RD, Boerth RC, Gerber JG, Nies AS (1981) Mechanism of adriamycin cardiotoxocity: evidence for oxidative stress. Life Sci 29: 1393–1401

Packer M (1993) The search for the ideal positive inotropic agent. N Engl J Med 329: 201–202

Schwartz RG, McKenzie WB, Alexander J, Sager P, D'Souza A, Manatunga A, Schwartz PE, Berger HJ, Setaro J, Surkin L Wackers FJT, Zarret BL (1987) Congestive heart failure and left ventricular dysfunction complicating doxorubicin therapy. Seven year experience using serial radionuclide angiocardiography. Am J Med 82: 1109–1118

Shapira J, Gotfried M, Lishner M, Ravid M (1990) Reduced cardiotoxicity of doxorubicin by a 6-hour infusion regime. A prospective randomized evaluation. Cancer 65: 870–873

Sobol MM, Amiet RG, Green MD (1992) In vitro evidence for direct complexation of ADR-529/ICRF-187 [(+)-1, 2-bis-(3,5-dioxopiperazin1-yl)propane] onto an existing ferric-anthracycline complex. Mol Pharmacol 41: 8–17

Speyer JL, Green MD, Zeleniuch-Jacquotte A, Wernz JC, Rey M, Sanger J, Kramer E, Ferrans V, Hochster H, Meyers M, Blum RH, Feit F, Attubato M, Burrows W, Muggia F (1992) ICRF-187 permits longer treatment with doxorubicin in women with breast cancer. J Clin Oncol 10: 117–127

Stein JI, Langevin A, Benson LN, Souza MD, Wilson G, Chan H (1989) Serial determination of anthracycline poisoning in children. Wiener Klin Wochenschr 101: 45–48

Steinherz LJ, Steinherz P (1988) Cardiac failure more than six years post anthracyclines. Am J Cardiol 62: 505

Steinherz LJ, Steinherz PG, Tan CTC, Heller G, Murphy ML (1991) Cardiotoxicity 4–20 years after completing anthracycline therapy. JAMA 266: 1672–1677

Steinherz LJ, Graham T, Hurwitz R, Sondheimer HM, Schwartz RG, Shaffer EM, Sandor G, Benson L, Williams R (1992) Guidelines for cardiac monitoring of children during and after anthracycline therapy: report of the Cardiology Committee of the Children's Cancer Study Group. Pediatrics 89: 942–949

von Hoff DD, Layard M (1981) Risk factors for development of daunorubicin cardiotoxocity. Cancer Treat Rep 65 [Suppl 4]: 19–23

von Hoff DD, Layard MW, Basa P, Davis HL, von Hoff AL, Rosencweig M, Muggia FM (1979) Risk factors for doxorubicin-induced congestive heart failure. Ann Intern Med 91: 710–717

Wechsler LH, Berg S, Andrich M, Chen C, Dilsizian V, McClure L, Venzon D, Jarosinski P, DeLaney T, Balis F, Poplack D, Horowitz ME (1993) ICRF-187 reduces doxorubicin-induced cardiotoxicity with no impact on response to chemotherapy. Proc Am Soc Clin Oncol 29: A1434

Weiss AJ, Metter GE, Fletcher WS, Wilson WL, Grage TB, Ramirez G (1976) Studies on adriamycin using a weekly regimen demonstrating its clinical effectiveness and lack of cardiac toxicity. Cancer Treat Rep 60: 813–822

Weiss RB (1992) The anthracyclines: will we ever find a better doxorubicin? Semin Oncol 19: 670–686

Zalupski M, Metch B, Balcerzak S, Fletcher WS, Chapman R, Bonnet JD, Weiss GR, Ryan J, Benjamin RS, Baker LH (1991) Phase III comparison of doxorubicin and decarbazine given by bolus versus infusion in patients with soft tissue sarcomas: a southwest oncology group study. J Natl Cancer Inst 83: 926–932

5.3 Radiation-Induced Cardiotoxicity: Experimental Data

SUSANNE SCHULTZ-HECTOR

CONTENTS

1 Introduction 181
2 Time Course of Events and Dose Response 181
3 Hemodynamics and Pathophysiology 183
4 Morphology 184
5 Pathogenesis 185
References 188

1 Introduction

The myocardium is included in the treatment field of radiation therapy of mediastinal tumors, breast and lung cancer. While early clinical and experimental observations focused on radiation-induced pericarditis, more recent reports show that with modern radiotherapy techniques the incidence of pericardial disease has dropped below 5% (CARMEL and KAPLAN 1976; WATCHIE et al. 1987; MORGAN et al. 1985). However, increasing survival rates and follow-up times of relatively young patients reveal that heart irradiation can cause chronic impairment of cardiac pump function. Systematic cardiological evaluation of patients 5–20 years after mediastinal radiotherapy for Hodgkin's disease revealed an abnormally low left ventricular ejection fraction in 4%–29% of the patients (MORGAN et al. 1985; GOMEZ et al. 1983; BURNS et al. 1983; GOTTDIENER et al. 1983; APPLEFELD and WIERNIK 1983; SAVAGE et al. 1990; GUSTAVSSON et al. 1990). Although nearly all of these patients were free of clinical symptoms of heart disease, it is conceivable that latent cardiomyopathy will predispose them to cardiotoxic effects during further tumor therapy and to overt heart disease from other causes. Several experimental models have been developed with the aim of studying the radiobiology, pathophysiology and pathogenesis of radiation-induced cardiomyopathy.

SUSANNE SCHULTZ-HECTOR, Privatdozent, Dr., GSF-Foschungszenrum für Umwelt und Gesundheit GmbH, Institut für Strahlenbiologie, 85764 Oberschleißheim, FRG

2 Time Course of Events and Dose Response

Experimental heart irradiations have been carried out in rats, rabbits and dogs. Since the heart is surrounded by relatively radiosensitive tissues, the radiation field has to be carefully limited to the heart. The radiation doses administered experimentally are usually just above the clinical dose range, in order to produce a measurable degree of heart disease in all treated animals. Similar to patients, higher doses of radiation can produce a transient pericarditis in experimental animals (SCHULTZ-HECTOR 1992). However, since the clinical problem of radiation-induced pericarditis has been successfully overcome by modifying treatment techniques, it will not be considered in the following.

Figure 1 gives a schematic representation of the time course of events after heart irradiation in Wistar rats with a single dose of 20 Gy. After a delay of about 3–4 weeks, functional and ultrastructural alterations of the capillary network set in. Morphological damage in cardiomyocytes follows, rapidly increasing in extent and severity. However, myocardial degeneration appears to reach its maximum long before clinical symptoms of heart disease are detecable. This phase of functional compensation of structural damage is attributed to up-regulation of adrenergic receptors. Finally, cardiac function decompensates and dilated heart failure requires that the animals be killed. Each of these phases will be adressed in detail in the following. The sequence of events was similar for different dose groups or fractionation schedules and for different strains of rat (LAUK et al. 1985; SCHULTZ-HECTOR et al. 1992a). Of course, the detailed observations and interpretations differ between experimental groups and models, but in principle this sequence of events is compatible with other experimental reports (YEUNG and HOPEWELL 1985; GAVIN and GILLETTE 1982; GILLETTE et al. 1985; MCCHESNEY et al. 1988a; WONDERGEM et al. 1991; FRANKEN et al. 1993).

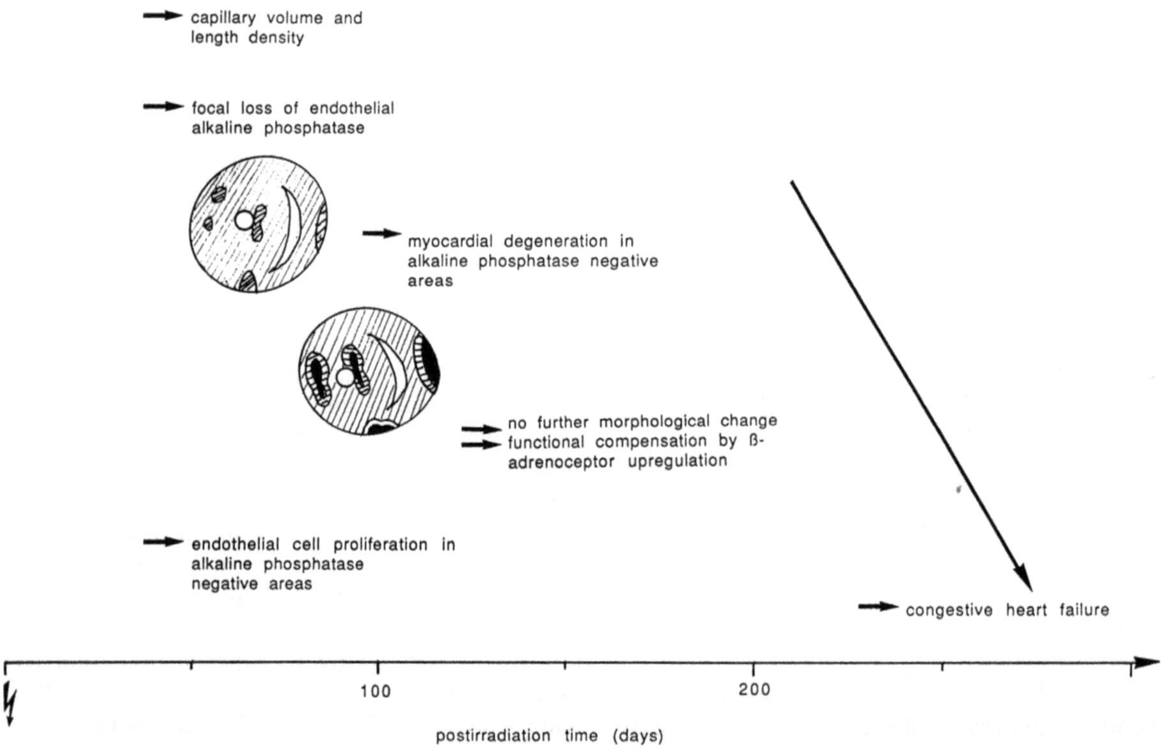

Fig. 1. Sequence of events observed after local heart irradiation in the rat. Simultaneous to a reduction in capillary density, there is a focal loss of endothelial alkaline phosphatase, represented as *hatched areas* in the drawing of a cross-section through both ventricles of a rat heart. Then, myocardial degeneration develops within enzyme negative foci (*black areas*). By 100 days after 20 Gy, morphological changes have reached their maximum extent. Hemodynamic function in vivo is moderately reduced at this time and is compensated by up-regulation of adrenergic receptors. Finally, after dose-dependent latent times, congestive heart failure sets in. After lower doses of radiation, which do not cause clinical heart failure, myocardial degeneration and alkaline phosphatase loss appear to persist

The incidence of heart failure shows a very steep dose-response after single dose irradiation. While 15 Gy did not cause symptomatic heart disease in a single animal even after observation times of nearly 2 years, 17.5 Gy led to fatal heart failure in all animals (LAUK et al. 1985). Again, a very similar dose response was found in dogs (GAVIN and GILLETTE 1982). For quantitative comparison of the effectiveness of different fractionation schedules, we therefore chose the latent time of heart failure, i.e., the average survival time as endpoint. After single dose or fractionated irradiation, the survival time decreases with increasing radiation dose. A quantitative comparison of morphometric and enzyme-histochemical parameters indicates that the histopathological changes underlying clinical heart failure are very constant, i.e., that latent time is the main dose-dependent variable. The effect of dose fractionation can be quantified in terms of the linear quadratic model (THAMES et al. 1986) by performing a nonparametric regression of dose-survival time curves according to the Cox proportional hazard model. A relatively low α/β ratio of 3.4 Gy with a 95% confidence level of 1.3–6 Gy can be derived (SCHULTZ-HECTOR et al. 1992a) (Fig. 2).

In a dog model, the effect of dose fractionation was assessed by comparison of various histological and physiological parameters at fixed observation times of 3 and 6 months (GILLETTE et al. 1985). The derived α/β ratios ranged from 2.8 to 5 Gy and are in good agreement with our own observations, in spite of the fundamental difference in experimental design.

The applicability of the linear quadratic model for analysis of complex, chronic radiation effects which can be only partly understood in terms of cell survival is questionable. However, the results indicate a significant increase in radiation tolerance of the myocardium with increasing dose fractionation and suggest that the rate of clinical complications can be minimized by keeping the dose per fraction low.

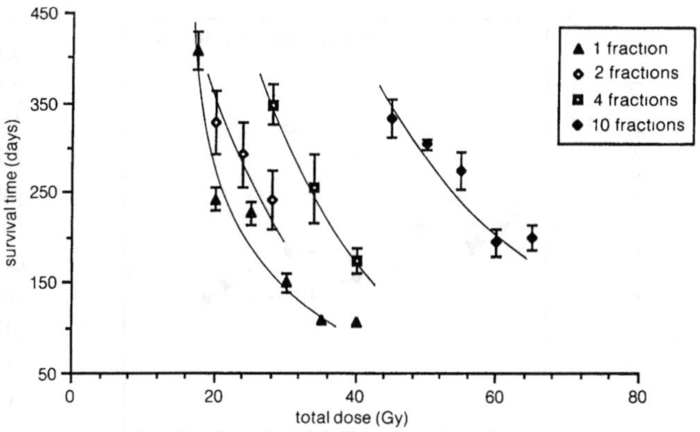

Fig. 2. Average latent time of heart failure in rats after local heart irradiation as a function of total radiation dose, given in one, two, four or ten fractions within an overall treatment time of 4 weeks. Error bars represent standard errors of the mean (sem). With increasing dose fractionation, there is a considerable increase in survival time, i.e., tolerance of the myocardium. The curves can be fitted by the Cox proportional hazard model, yielding an α/β ratio of 3.4 Gy with 95% confidence limits of 1.3–6 Gy (SCHULTZ-HECTOR et al. 1992a)

3 Hemodynamics and Pathophysiology

In vivo hemodynamic studies in rats revealed a continuous, dose-dependent decrease in cardiac output (YEUNG and HOPEWELL 1985). In dog studies, it was demonstrated that a reduction in left ventricular stroke volume is due to heart irradiation and is not secondary to lung irradiation (MCCHESNEY et al. 1991). In our own experiments, radionuclide ventriculography in rats showed a parallel reduction in left ventricular ejection fraction (SCHULTZ-HECTOR et al. 1992b). In biochemical studies of the energy metabolism in irradiated rat hearts, the overall myocardial oxidative energy production (state 3 respiration) was found to be reduced (FRANKEN et al. 1993). However, hemodynamic function is maintained at this reduced level for months. When heart failure finally develops in individual animals, clinical symptoms such as dyspnea at rest, apathy and subcutaneous edema rapidly develop, simultaneous to a significant increase in end-diastolic ventricular volume (SCHULTZ-HECTOR et al. 1992b). When cardiac output and ventricular fractional shortening are assessed in isolated working heart preparations in vitro, a much earlier, more rapid deterioration of hemodynamic function is observed (WONDERGEM et al. 1991). Figure 3 illustrates the diverging time course of cardiac output in vivo and in vitro. In vivo measurement of cardiac output was carried out in two different laboratories using different equipment and methods of analysis (YEUNG and HOPEWELL 1985; SCHULTZ-HECTOR et al. 1992b). Nevertheless, the time course of relative cardiac output in both investigations is in very good agreement, supporting the suggestion that differences between in vivo and in vitro measurements are, in fact, of biological significance and do not merely reflect variability between experimental setups. One possible explanation for a discrepancy between hemodynamic parameters measured in vivo and in vitro would be the existence of compensatory mechanisms which are effective in vivo but not in vitro. In biochemical receptor binding studies, a radiation-induced increase in the density of both α- and β-adrenoceptors can be observed (LAUK et al. 1989; FRANKEN et al. 1992; SCHULTZ-HECTOR et al. 1992b). The time course of adrenoceptor up-regulation is similar in the different experimental models (Fig. 3). The radiation-induced incrase in α- and β-adrenergic receptors that has been consistently observed in different laboratories and using different radioligands would be expected to result in an increased positive inotropic response to intermittent adrenergic stimulation. Both α- and β-adrenoceptors mediate positive inotropy (BÖHM et al. 1988a, b). An increased receptor concentration on the surface of functional cardiomyocytes therefore mediates a stronger positive inotropic response to intermittent adrenergic stimulation. Adrenergic stimulation will occur in vivo in response to stress conditions, but not in the isolated heart preparation. Quantitative autoradiographic studies confirm that the biochemically measured increase in adrenoceptors does take place in areas of morphologically intact and presumably functional myocardium, while ligand binding was very much reduced in areas of degeneration and necrosis (SCHULTZ-HECTOR et al. 1994). Thus adrenoceptor up-regulation in intact cardiomyocytes appears to be effective in maintaining hemodynamic function for a significant time period after full development of structural myocardial damage.

The cause of adrenoceptor up-regulation appears to be a radiation-induced alteration of myocardial catecholamine metabolism. Biochemical studies show that myocardial norepinephrine concentrations are reduced due to a reduction in the rate-limiting enzyme of catecholamine synthesis, tyrosine dehydroxylase (SCHULTZ-HECTOR et al.

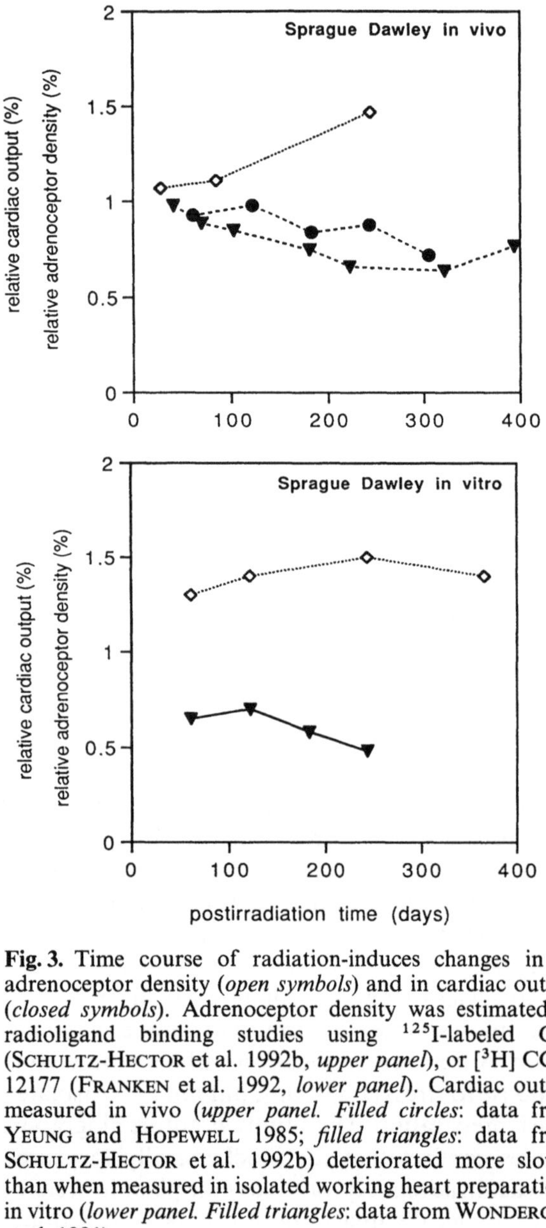

Fig. 3. Time course of radiation-induces changes in β-adrenoceptor density (*open symbols*) and in cardiac output (*closed symbols*). Adrenoceptor density was estimated in radioligand binding studies using ^{125}I-labeled Cyp (SCHULTZ-HECTOR et al. 1992b, *upper panel*), or [^{3}H] CGP-12177 (FRANKEN et al. 1992, *lower panel*). Cardiac output measured in vivo (*upper panel. Filled circles*: data from YEUNG and HOPEWELL 1985; *filled triangles*: data from SCHULTZ-HECTOR et al. 1992b) deteriorated more slowly than when measured in isolated working heart preparations in vitro (*lower panel. Filled triangles*: data from WONDERGEM et al. 1991)

1992b; FRANKEN et al. 1992). Preliminary results from morphometric studies indicate that, parallel to the increase in adrenoceptors, there is structural damage to myocardial sympathetic nervous endings, which are the physiological site of myocardial catecholamine synthesis (SCHULTZ-HECTOR et al. 1994a).

Although the pathophysiology of radiation-induced cardiomyopathy is still not understood, these results show that it is quite different from ischemic or idiopathic dilated cardiomyopathy. It is well documented that in these types of heart disease there is increased norepinephrine production associated with adrenoceptor down-regulation and a reduced positive inotropic responsiveness (CHIDSEY et al. 1962; HEILBRUNN et al. 1989; WAAGSTEIN et al. 1989). Unfortunately, there are no clinical data on pathophysiology of radiation-induced cardiomyopathy such as receptor binding studies which could reveal whether the mechanisms consistently observed in irradiated rat myocardium are also effective in patients. Since the sympathetic nervous system is not only essential in physiological regulation of cardiac performance, but is also an important target of therapeutic intervention, such information would be of clinical interest.

4 Morphology

Light microscopic studies in animal models and human autopsy material show that radiation-induced heart failure is associated with myocardial degeneration and necrosis, and interstitial fibrosis. The severity of fibrosis is quite variable in different species. It is described as very pronounced in rabbit and human hearts (FAJARDO and STEWART 1970), as moderate in dogs (GAVIN and GILLETTE 1982; MCCHESNEY et al. 1988b) and nearly absent in rat hearts (LAUK et al. 1985). Biochemical studies indicated a radiation-induced disturbance of both collagen synthesis and degradation, suggesting that measurement of the overall resulting collagen content may be a relatively insensitive parameter (MURRAY and PARKINS 1988). Electron microscopic studies show that myocardial vacuoles are formed by mitochondrial degeneration, i.e., loss of cristae and swelling of empty mitochondrial membranes (HARPER et al. 1991; SCHULTZ-HECTOR and BALZ 1994b). In rats, quantitative measurements of the relative extent of foci of degeneration in the ventricular myocardium showed that foci started to appear at 70 days after 20 Gy, then rapidly increased in size and number and reached a maximum extent of 23% ± 4% at around 100 days after 20 Gy. Following a lower dose of 15 Gy, the onset of degeneration was delayed and reached its maximum of 7.5% ± 3% at about 200 days postirradiation.

The degree of morphological changes appears to be significantly more severe in the atria than in the ventricles (GAVIN and GILLETTE 1982; MCCHESNEY et al. 1988b; CILLIERS et al. 1989; HARPER et al. 1991). However, the atrium cannot be shielded during radiotherapy of mediastinal tumors and, in contrast to the tip of the heart and lower ventricles, receives a radiation dose very close to the tumor dose.

5 Pathogenesis

Early electron microscopic studies already revealed that radiation damage to cardiomyocytes is preceded by capillary endothelial cell swelling and protrusion of cytoplasmic projections into the lumen (MORGENROTH et al. 1968). While these alterations in endothelial cell morphology are at least partly reversible (FAJARDO and STEWART 1973; SCHULTZ-HECTOR and BALZ 1994b), the number of capillaries, i.e., the volume and length density of capillaries, is found to be persistently reduced in irradiated hearts. Following single doses of 15 or 20 Gy, there is a rapid loss in both volume and length density of capillaries starting at 25 days postirradiation. After 15 Gy, both parameters are reduced to about 64% of normal values throughout an observation time of more than 600 days, i.e., throughout the remaining lifespan of the animals (SCHULTZ-HECTOR 1993). Besides capillary density, the staining pattern of endothelial marker enzymes such as alkaline phosphatase and 5′-nucleotidase are altered following heart irradiation. While in untreated myocardium all capillaries show a strong alkaline phosphatase reaction (Fig. 4), there was a focal loss of endothelial enzyme activity in irradiated hearts (LAUK 1987). Enzyme negative pathes are evident weeks before myocardial degeneration can be detected light microscopically (Fig. 5) and when foci of myocardial degeneration appear, they are exclusively found within enzyme negative areas. The maximum extent of enzyme loss was dose-dependent (LAUK 1987). In cell kinetic studies, alkaline phosphatase negative endothelial cells show a radiation-induced increase in proliferation (Fig. 6), while in enzyme positive areas, endothelial cell [^{3}H]thymidine labeling indices remain unchanged (LAUK and TROTT 1990). These observations indicate that the loss of endothelial alkaline phosphatase represents a significant step in the pathogenesis of radiation-induced cardiomyopathy.

This hypothesis is indirectly supported by comparison of different strains of rat. The average survival time in Sprague Dawley rats is always about twice as long as in Wistar rats, for a range of different single doses (LAUK 1986). Again, very similar results were obtained when Sprague Dawley rats were studied in different laboratories (YEUNG et al. 1989) (Fig. 7). A corresponding difference is found for all significant pathogenetic steps such as onset of alkaline phosphatase loss, endothelial cell proliferation or myocardial degeneration (LAUK 1987; LAUK and TROTT 1990). We concluded that these two strains of rat therefore must differ in some

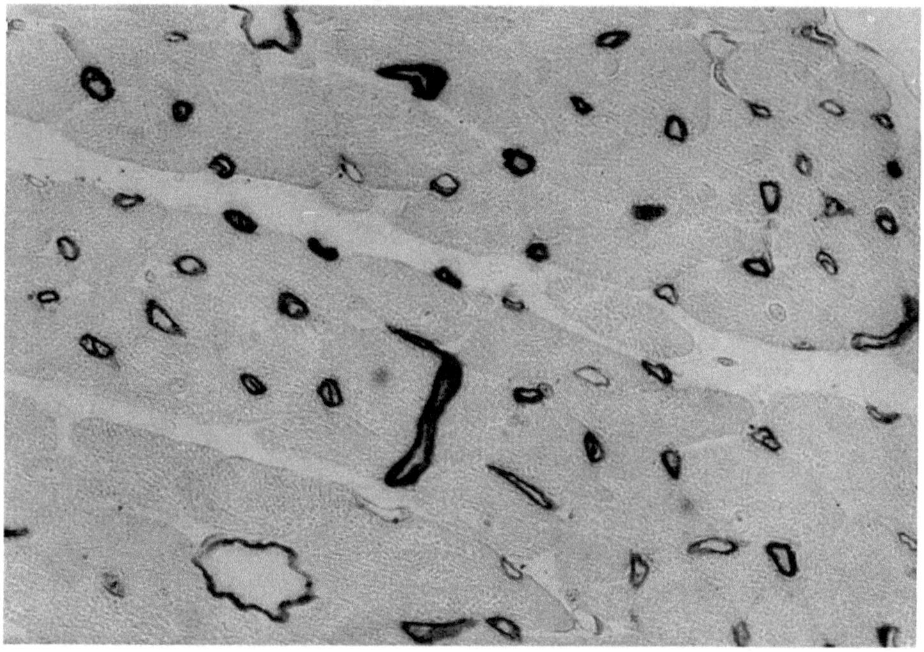

Fig. 4. Micrograph of an untreated rat heart. All capillaries show a strong, dark alkaline phosphatase reaction. × 375

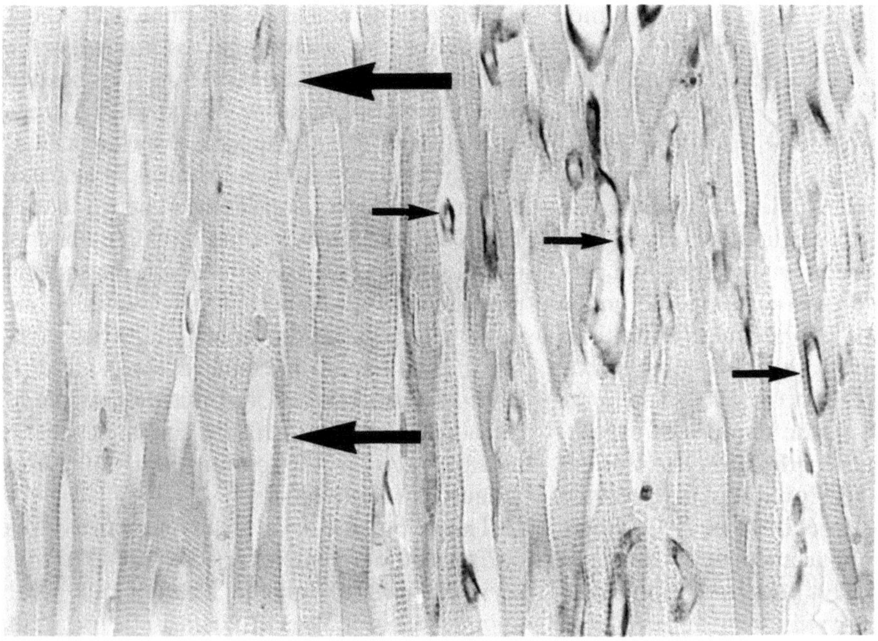

Fig. 5. Micrograph of an irradiated rat heart, 50 days after 20 Gy. There are areas in the myocardium, where capillaries have lost their alkaline phosphatase activity (*large arrows*), while in other areas (*small arrows*), enzyme reaction appears unchanged. × 375

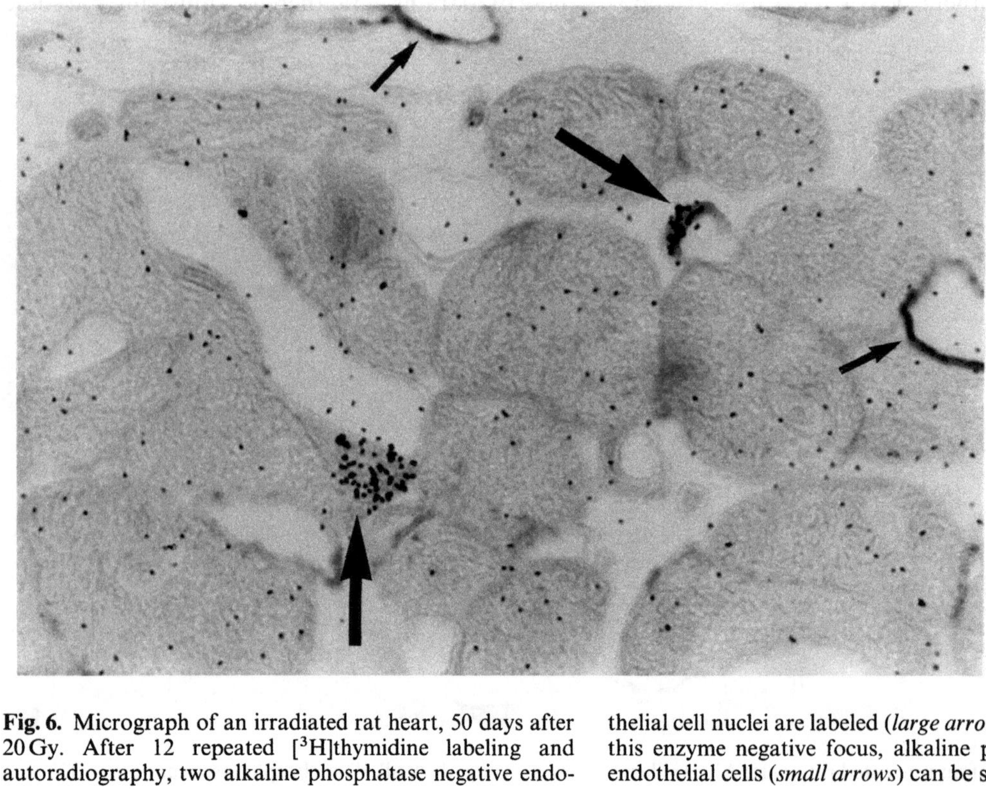

Fig. 6. Micrograph of an irradiated rat heart, 50 days after 20 Gy. After 12 repeated [^{3}H]thymidine labeling and autoradiography, two alkaline phosphatase negative endothelial cell nuclei are labeled (*large arrows*). At the border of this enzyme negative focus, alkaline phosphatase positive endothelial cells (*small arrows*) can be seen. × 1500

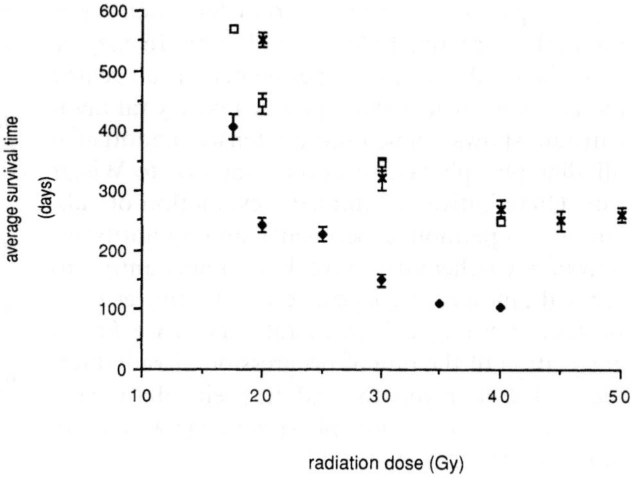

Fig. 7. Average latent time of heart failure (±sem) as a function of radiation dose, given in single doses. In two different institutions, experiments were carried out in Sprague Dawley rats (*x*, data from YEUNG and HOPWELL 1985; *open squares*, data from LAUK 1986), yielding very similar survival times. In Wistar rats (*filled diamonds*, data from SCHULTZ-HECTOR et al. 1992a) heart failure developed much more quickly at all dose levels

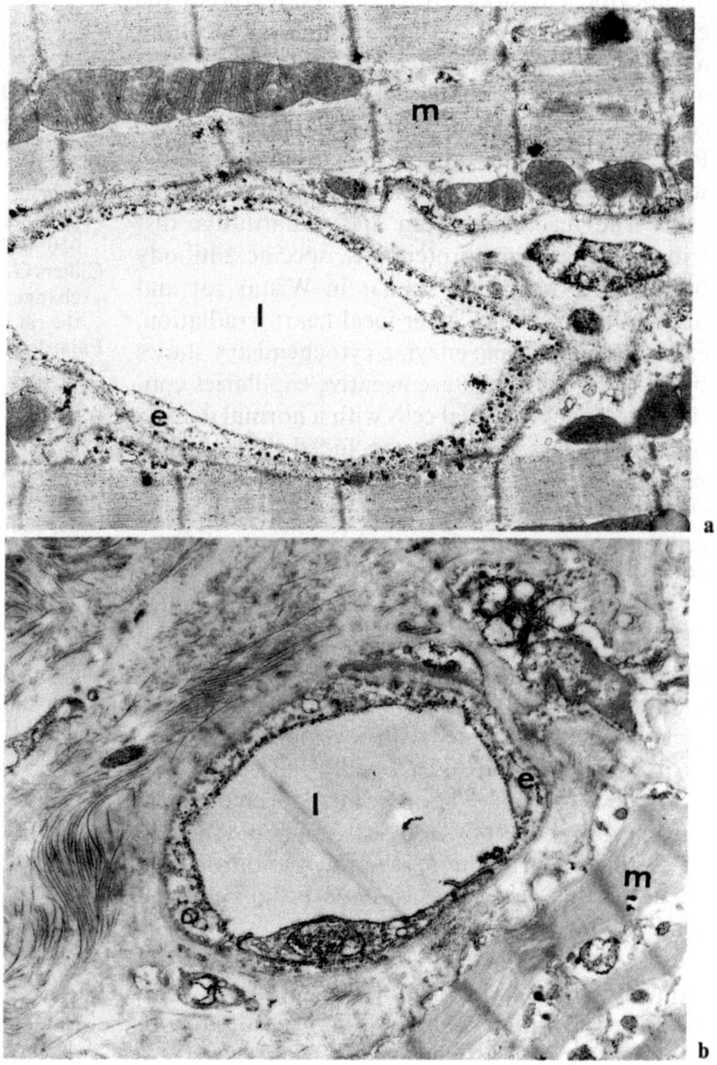

Fig. 8a, b. Electron micrographs showing a capillary endothelial cell. Alkaline phosphatase reaction product is labeled with lead precipitates. **a** untreated Wistar rat heart and **b** human myocardium, from a patient receiving cardiac transplantation for dilated heart failure (data from SCHULTZ-HECTOR et al. 1994). In both rat and human heart, enzyme reactivity is located along the abluminal and luminal endothelial cell membrane and in cytotic vesicles. *l*, lumen; *e*, endothelial cell; *m*, myocyte. ×1400

physiological or anatomical parameter which determines their reaction to heart irradiation. In enzyme histochemical staining experiments in untreated animals it is obvious that Sprague Dawley rat myocardium shows a much more intensive endothelial alkaline phosphatase reaction compared to Wistar rats. Quantitative densitometric evaluation of substrate competition experiments and quantitative immunocytochemistry reveal a significantly increased amount of enzyme reactivity and enzyme protein in Sprague Dawley rats. Thus we find a correlation of the rate of progression of radiation-induced cardiomyopathy and the preirradiation expression level of alkaline phosphatase (LAUK 1986; SCHULTZ-HECTOR et al. 1993).

Although the endothelial alkaline phosphatase is well characterized on a biochemical and molecular genetic level, very little is known about its physiological function in vivo. In enzyme and immunocytochemical electron microscopy studies, the enzyme reaction product and protein are localized along the abluminal and luminal cell membrane and in cytoplasmic vesicles of capillary endothelial cells of both rat and human myocardium (Fig. 8). Pericytes also show above background labeling, which is, however, much weaker than in endothelial cells. The reaction pattern and quantitative distribution of enzyme protein, i.e., specific antibody binding sites, are very similar in Wistar rat and human myocardium. After local heart irradiation, electron microscopic enzyme cytochemistry shows that alkaline phosphatase negative capillaries consist of intact endothelial cells with a normal density of cytosolic vesicles. It is concluded that alkaline phosphatase loss is unrelated to cell death or to structural damage of normal enzyme bearing cellular components (SCHULTZ-HECTOR and BALZ 1994).

Local heart irradiation causes both a quantitative loss of capillary endothelial cells and an alteration of specific cell function unrelated to cell death. This radiation-induced loss of alkaline phosphatase activity is closely associated with development of myocardial degeneration and probably plays a key role in its development. The molecular mechanism of enzyme loss and its physiological function remain to be clarified. Furthermore, the interaction or connection between changes in endothelial cells and sympathetic nerve endings needs to be established. However, the pathogenetic principle of radiation-induced changes in cell metabolism, ultimately leading to deterioration of organ function, could be of considerable clinical relevance, since disturbances or dysregulation of cell function should be much more amenable to therapeutic intervention than cell loss.

Acknowledgment. This work was supported by the Deutsche Forschungsgemeinschaft, grant La 576/4-1.

References

Applefield MM, Wiernik PH (1983) Cardiac disease after radiation therapy for Hodgkin's disease: analysis of 48 patients. Am J Cardiol 51: 1679–1681

Böhm M, Beuckelmann D, Brown L, Feiler G, Lorenz B, Näbauer M, Kemkes B, Erdmann E (1988a) Reduction of β-adrenoceptor density and evaluation of positive inotropic responses in isolated, diseased human myocardium. Eur Heart J 9: 844–852

Böhm M, Diet F, Feiler G, Kemkes B, Erdmann E (1988b) α-adrenoceptors and α-adrenoceptor-mediated positive inotropic effects in failing human myocardium. J Cardiovasc Pharmacol 12: 357–364

Burns RJ, Bar-Shlomo B-Z, Druck MN, Herman JG, Gilbert BW, Perrault DJ, McLaughlin PR (1983) Detection of radiation cardiomyopathy by gated radionuclide angiography. Am J Med 74: 297–302

Carmel RJ, Kaplan HS (1976) Mantle irradiation of Hodgkin's disease: an analysis of technique, tumor eradication and complications. Cancer 37: 2813–2825

Chidsey CA, Harrison DC, Braunwald E (1962) Augmentation of plasma norepinephrine response to exercise in patients with congestive heart failure. N Engl J Med 267: 650–654

Cilliers GD, Harper IS, Lochner A (1989) Radiation-induced changes in the ultrastructure and mechanical function of the rat heart. Radiother Oncol 16: 311–326

Fajardo LF, Stewart JR (1970) Experimental radiation-induced heart disease. I. Light microscopic studies. Am J Pathol 59: 299–315

Fajardo LF, Stewart JR (1973) Pathogenesis of radiation-induced myocardial fibrosis. Lab Invest 29: 244–257

Franken NAP, van der Laarse A, Bosker FJ, Reynart IWC, van Ravels FJM, Strootman E, Wondergem J (1992) Time dependent changes in myocardial norepinephrine concentration and adrenergic receptor density following X-irradiation of the rat heart. Int J Radiat Oncol Biol Phys 24: 721–727

Franken NAP, Hollaar L, Bosker FJ, van Ravels FJM, van der Laarse A, Wondergem J (1993) Effects of in vivo heart irradiation on myocardial energy metabolism in rats. Radiat Res 134: 79–85

Gavin PR, Gillette EL (1982) Radiation response of the canine cardiovascular system. Radiat Res 90: 489–500

Gillette EL, McChesney SL, Hoopes PJ (1985) Isoeffect curves for radiation-induced cardiomyopathy in the dog. Int J Radiat Oncol Biol Phys 11: 2091–2097

Gomez GA, Park JJ, Panahon AM, Parthasarathy KL, Pearce J, Reese P, Bakshi S, Henderson ES (1983) Heart size and function after radiation therapy to the mediastinum in patients with Hodgkin's disease. Cancer Treat Rep 67: 1099–1103

Gottdiener JS, Katin MJ, Borer JS, Bacharach SL, Green MV (1983) Late cardiac effects of therapeutic mediastinal irradiation. Assessment by echocardiography and radionuclide angiography. N Engl J Med 308: 569–588

Gustavsson A, Eskilsson J, Landberg T, Svahn-Tapper G, White T, Wollmer P, Akerman M (1990) Late cardiac effects after mantle radiotherapy in patients with Hodgkin's disease. Ann Oncol 1: 355–363
Harper IS, Williams K, Cilliers GD, Lochner A (1991) Ultrastructural injury in the atrium after radiation of the rat heart. J Appl Physiol 6: 41–49
Heilbrunn SM, Shah, P, Bristow MR, Valantine HA, Ginsburg, Flower MB (1989) Increased β-receptor density and improved hemodynamic response to catecholamine stimulation during long-term Metoprolol therapy in heart failure from dilated cardiomyopathy. Circulation 79: 483–490
Lauk S (1986) Strain differences in the radiation response of the rat heart. Radiother Oncol 5: 333–335
Lauk S (1987) Endothelial alkaline phosphatase activity loss as an early stage in the development of radiation-induced heart disease in rats. Radiat Res 110: 118–128
Lauk S, Trott K-R (1990) Endothelial proliferation in the rat heart following local heart irradiation. Int J Radiat Biol 57: 1017–1030
Lauk S, Kiszel Z, Buschmann J, Trott K-R (1985) Radiation induced heart disease in rats. Int J Radiat Oncol Biol Phys 11: 801–808
Lauk S, Böhm M, Feiler G, Geist BJ, Erdmann E (1989) Increased number of cardiac adrenergic receptors following local heart irradiation. Radiat Res 119: 157–165
McChesney SL, Gillette EL, Orton EC (1988a) Canine cardiomyopathy after whole heart and partial lung irradiation. Int J Radiat Oncol Biol Phys 14: 1169–1174
McChesney SL, Gillette EL, Powers BE (1988b) Radiation-induced cardiomyopathy in the dog. Radiat Res 113: 120–132
McChesney SL, Gillette S, Powers BE, Orton EC, Gillette EL (1991) Early radiation response in the canine heart and lung. Radiat Res 125: 34–40
Morgan GW, Freeman AP, McLean RG, Jarvie BH, Giles RW (1985) Late cardiac, thyroid and pulmonary sequelae of mantle radiotherapy for Hodgkin's disease. Int J Radiat Oncol Biol Phys 11: 1925–1931
Morgenroth K, Junge-Hülsing G, Hauss WH (1967) Über Veränderungen am Rattenherzen nach gezielter Röntgenbestrahlung. Strahlentherapie 133: 610–620
Murray JC, Parkins CS (1988) Collagen synthesis in CBA mouse heart after total thoracic irradiation. Radiother Oncol 13: 137–143
Savage DE, Constine LS, Schwartz RG, Rubin P (1990) Radiation effects on left ventricular function and myocardial perfusion in long term survivors of Hodgkin's disease. Int J Radiat Oncol Biol Phys 19: 721–727
Schultz-Hector S (1992) Radiation-induced heart disease: review of experimental data on dose response and pathogenesis. Int J Radiat Biol 61: 149–160
Schultz-Hector S, Sund M, Thames HD (1992a) Fractionation response and repair kinetics of radiation-induced heart failure in the rat. Radiother Oncol 23: 33–40
Schultz-Hector S, Böhm M, Blöchel A, Dominiak P, Erdmann E, Müller-Schauenburg W, Weber A (1992b) Radiation-induced heart disease in rats: morphology, changes in catecholamines, β-adrenoceptor binding sites and hemodynamic function. Radiat Res 129: 281–289
Schultz-Hector S (1993) Experimental studies on radiation damage in the heart. In: Hinkelbein W, Braggmoser G, Frommhold H, Wannenmacher M (eds) Acute and long-term side-effects of radiotherapy. Springer, Berlin Heidelberg New York, pp 145–157 (Recent results in cancer research, vol 130)
Schultz-Hector S, Balz K, Böhm M, Ikehara Y, Rieke L (1993) Cellular localization of endothelial alkaline phosphatase reaction product and enzyme protein in the myocardium. J Histochem Cytochem 41: 1813–1821
Schultz-Hector S, Beilharz C, Rothermel F, Gais P (1994a) Topographic analysis of radiation-induced changes in β-adrenoceptor density and sympathetic nerve fibers in rat myocardium. Int J Radiat Biol Oncol Phys (submitted)
Schultz-Hector S, Balz K (1994b) Radiation-induces loss of endothelial alkaline phosphatase activity and development of myocardial degeneration: an ultrastructural study. Lab Invest (submitted)
Thames HD, Rozell ME, Tucker SL, Ang KK, Fisher DR, Travis EL (1986) Direct analysis of quantal radiation response data. Int J Radiat Biol 49: 999–1009
Waagstein F, Caidahl K, Wallentin I, Bergh C-H, Hjalmarson A (1989) Long-term β-blockade in dilated cardiomyopathy. Circulation 80: 551–563
Watchie J, Coleman N, Raffin T, Cox R, Rauibitschek A, Fahey T, Hoppe R, Venkessel A (1987) Minimal long-term cardiopulmonary dysfunction following treatment for Hodgkin's disease. Int J Radiat Oncol Biol Phys 13: 517–524
Wondergem J, van der Laarse A, van Ravels FJM, Wermeskerken AM, Verhoeve HR, de Graaf BW, Leer JWH (1991) In vitro assessment of cardiac performance after irradiation using an isolated working heart preparation. Int J Radiat Biol 59: 1053–1068
Yeung TK, Hopewell JW (1985) Effects of single doses of irradiation on cardiac function in the rat. Radiother Oncol 3: 339–345
Yeung TK, Lauk S, Simmonds RH, Hopewell JW, Trott K-R (1989) Morphological and functional changes in the rat heart after X-irradiation: strain differences. Radiat Res 119: 489–499

5.4 Cardiotoxicity After Megavoltage Irradiation and Chemotherapy for Hodgkin's Disease with Special Emphasis on Coronary Heart Disease Mortality – The Freiburg Experience 1940–1992

JOACHIM SLANINA, KARL HENNE, NORBERT HODAPP, GISELA MOOG, and HERMANN FROMMHOLD

CONTENTS

1 Introduction and Study Population 191
2 Results 191
3 Discussion 193
3.1 Risk of Fatal Myocardial Infarction 193
4 Conclusions 194
References 194

1 Introduction and Study Population

From 1940 to 1992, 1735 patients with Hodgkin's disease were treated in the Department of Radiotherapy of the University of Freiburg. A retrospective evaluation was carried out in 1537 of these patients. The object of the study was cardiotoxicity occurring after mediastinal (cardiac) irradiation which was of clinical-symptomatic relevance. The analysis showed that heart disease was observed only after megavoltage irradiation of the mediastinum. As a result of these findings, cardiotoxicity was associated solely with megavoltage irradiation, which in Freiburg has been applied exclusively in wide-field technique for 29 years and is prescribed as mandatory in all modern treatment studies. Since the issue addressed was long-term cardiotoxicity, only those patients who reached complete or partial remission (CR, PR) after mediastinal megavoltage irradiation were included in the analysis. The control group consisted of those patients who had not received mediastinal irradiation and who were in remission (CR, PR) after treatment.

Mediastinal irradiation had been performed in 1255 of the 1587 patients. Of these, 949 (76%) had received megavoltage (telecobalt or linear accelerator photons with 4–6 MeV), 282 (22%) orthovolt irradiation, and 24 (2%) both types. Patient selection and characteristics in terms of mean age, sex, and primary stage distribution according to the Ann Arbor classification (CARBONE et al. 1971) are presented in Table 1.

Table 1. Selection of patient groups and initial characteristics

Patients	*N*	Mean age (years)	M:F	Stages (%) I	II	III	IV
Evaluable (total)	1587	34	1.17:1	21	45	28	6
With mediastinal irradiation	1256	33	1.04:1	18	47	30	5
With mediastinal megavoltage irradiation	971	33	1.07:1	18	43	34	5
With mediastinal megavoltage irradiation in CR or PR	859	32	1.02:1	19	43	34	4
With mediastinal megavoltage irradiation in CR or PR with heart disease	40	34	1:1	18	47	35	0
Without mediastinal irradiation	331	40	1.88:1	33	34	22	11

CR, complete remission, PR, partial remission.

The cumulative (actuarial) probability of heart disease occurring in a patient was calculated by the method of KAPLAN and MEIER (1958).

2 Results

Of the 859 patients who had received mediastinal megavoltage irradiation and who had attained CR or PR, 40 patients (4.7%) were found to have various diseases of the heart (Table 2). The mediastinal midline dose in equally weighted dorsoventral opposing fields was 26 and 35 Gy in two of the 40 patients, respectively, 40–44 Gy in 28 patients, 45–50 Gy in eight patients, and 60 and 66 Gy in two patients, respectively. Two of the 40 patients had received chemotherapy alone with procarbazine

JOACHIM SLANINA, Prof. Dr., KARL HENNE, Dr., NORBERT HODAPP, Dr. rer. nat., GISELA MOOG., HERMANN FROMMHOLD, Prof. Dr., Radiologische Universitätsklinik, Abteilung Strahlentherapie, Hugstetter Straße 55, 79106 Freiburg, FRG

Table 2. Different kinds of heart disease ($N = 40$ patients)

Disease	*N*
Coronary heart disease	18
Infarction	15
Mycardinal heart disease	18
Myocarditis	4
Cardiomyopathy/insufficiency	14
Pericarditis	13
Cor pulmonale	7
Valvular heart disease	7
Arrhythmias	5

and vinblastine, respectively, 15 received combined therapy: nine of 15 MOPP, one of 15 ABVD+C-MOPP, one of 15 adriamycin+C- MOPP, and four of 15 C-MOPP.

With the exception of one case each of acute pericarditis (after 3 days) and myocardinal infarction (after 2 months), the various types of cardiac disorders consisted of delayed and late delayed reactions of the heart (Fig. 1). Table 2 shows the frequency of heart disease and Table 3 shows the different possible combinations per patient.

The cumulative risk of heart disease was 3%, 4%, 12%, 16%, and 16% after 5, 10, 15, 20, and 25 years, respectively. The cumulative risk of death from coronary heart disease (CHD) with myocardial infarction was 0%, 1%, 2%, 4%, and 4% after 5, 10, 15, 20, and 25 years, respectively.

In the smaller control group of 331 patients without mediastinal irradiation, in which there was a higher percentage of women than in the study population (Table 1), no heart disease following therapy was observed.

Of the 40 patients developing heart disease, 21 were still alive at the time of the study. They had survived a mean period of 16.1 years after the diagnosis of Hodgkin's disease and 8.2 years after the development of the first cardiac symptoms (Table 4). Of the 19 deceased patients, two deaths were obviously caused by advanced Hodgkin's disease, in one case the cause of death was uncertain. The remaining 16 patients died of heart disorders. The mean survival time of these patients was 12.8 years after the diagnosis of Hodgkin's disease and 4.5 years after the development of the first cardiac symptoms. The most frequent heart-related cause of death was myocardial infarction (67%), the primary infarction being fatal in seven out of ten patients. Of the ten patients who died of myocardial infarction, one additionally suffered from myocardiopathy and one from arrhythmia. The absolute incidence of fatal infarctions was ten out of 859

Table 3. Different kinds of heart disease and their combinations per patient ($N=40$ patients)

N	CHD ($N=18$)	IF ($N=15$)	CMP/IS ($N=14$)	M ($N=4$)	P ($N=13$)	CP ($N=7$)	VD ($N=7$)	RD ($N=5$)
5			×					
1	×							
1				×				
1							×	
1								×
12	×	×						
3			×		×			
1			×					×
1				×	×			
1				×		×		
1					×			×
1					×		×	
1					×	×		
1	×					×		
2			×		×	×		
1	×	×					×	
1	×	×						×
1			×		×		×	
1				×	×		×	
1					×	×	×	
1	×	×	×			×		
1	×		×		×		×	×
40	18	15	14	4	13	7	7	5

N, number of patients; CHD, Coronary heart disease; IF, infarction; CMP/IS, cardiomyopathy/insufficiency; M, myocarditis; P, pericarditis; CP, cor pulmonale; VD, Valvular heart disease; RD, arrhythmias.

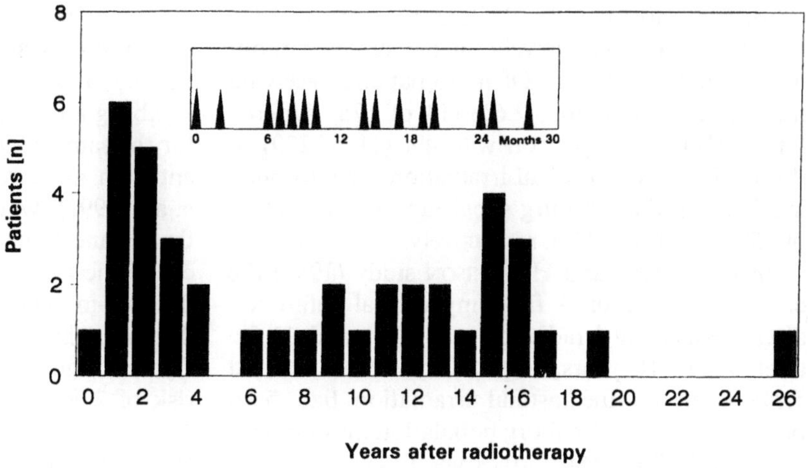

Fig. 1. Latency of heart diseases

Table 4. Survival, causes of death ($N=40$ patients)

		Mean survival (years)	
	N	After diagnosis	After occurrence of heart disease
Alive	21	15.6	7.9
Deceased	19		
Cause of death			
Hodgkin's disease	2		
Unknown	1		
Cardiac	16	12.8	4.5
Myocardial infarction	10[a]	13.2	1.7
Cardiomyopathy	6	12.1	6.8

[a] Seven died of myocardial infarction.

(1.1%). Six patients (6/859, 0.7%) died of manifest cardiac insufficiency due to cardiomyopathy (Table 4).

3 Discussion

The three most frequent types of heart diseases found in the study population were coronary heart disease (with and without myocardial infarction), cardiomyopathy (with cardiac insufficiency), and pericarditis. In the Freiburg study 18 patients had coronary heart disease, 15 of whom had one or more myocardial infarctions; 18 patients had myocardial heart disease, four of whom had transient myocarditis and 14 who had manifest cardiac insufficiency due to cardiomyopathy. Pericarditis, which is described in the literature as being the most frequent adverse effect of irradiation on the heart (Applefield et al. 1980, 1981; Byhardt et al. 1975; Carmel and Kaplan 1976; Ruckdeschel et al. 1975; Steward and Fajardo 1971), ranked third in frequency of heart disorders. It was observed in 13 patients and was associated with fatal cardiomyopathy in three patients.

3.1 Risk of Fatal Myocardial Infarction

A number of case studies indicate that mediastinal irradiation in the treatment for Hodgkin's disease is associated with increased coronary heart disease (CHD) mortality (Applefield et al. 1983; Carmel and Kaplan 1976; Hagemeister et al. 1982; Hellman et al. 1978; McReynolds et al. 1976; Nissen et al. 1980; Prosnitz et al. 1982; Yahalom et al. 1983). Furthermore, Boivin and Hutchison (1982) conducted a retrospective study designed to evaluate this hypothesis. Their report describes 957 patients diagnosed with Hodgkin's disease between 1942 and 1975 and analyzes follow-up findings through December 1977. Of these patients, 678 had received mediastinal (cardiac) irradiation, 279 patients had not. Though no information is given on the type of irradiation, from the dates 1942–1975 we would assume that orthovoltage irradiation was used. The ratio of men to women was 1.25 : 1 in both subsets. The percentage of patients under 44 years of age was 81% among those with mediastinal irradiation and 38% among those without mediastinal irradiation. The stage distribution is not necessarily comparable with that of the Freiburg population, since it was carried out according to the Rye classification (Rosenberg 1966). This distribution was 40%, 27%, 24%, and 9% for stages I, II, III, and IV, respectively, in the subset receiving mediastinal irradiation and 20%, 13%, 31%, and 36% for stages I, II, III, and IV, respectively, in the subset without mediastinal irradiation. Of those patients receiving mediastinal irradiation, 2.6% (14 of 678) suffered fatal CHD in comparison with 4% (11 of 279) of those without mediastinal irradiation. The absolute incidence in the Freiburg subgroups was 1.1% (ten of 859) and 0% (0/331), respectively.

In the BOIVIN and HUTCHISON study (1982) the cumulative risk of a fatal myocardial infarction after mediastinal irradiation was 8.8% and 11.5% after 5 and 10 years, respectively, and 5.7% and 5.7% when no mediastinal irradiation had been performed. In the Freiburg population the cumulative risk of a fatal heart attack was 0% and 1% after 5 and 10 years, respectively, in the group of patients treated with mediastinal megavoltage irradiation and 0% and 0%, respectively, in those not receiving mediastinal irradiation, which means that the cumulative risk was considerably lower.

The absolute incidence and cumulative risk of a fatal myocardial infarction were considerably higher in the BOIVIN and HUTCHISON study. One explanation for this could be the larger percentage of male and older patients and the considerably higher percentage of patients with stages III–IV, hence an increased morbidity in the group of patients not treated with mediastinal irradiation. A more important reason, however, is the fact that according to the National Institute of Health (EPSTEIN and PISA 1979) the rate of fatal myocardial infarction is twice as high in the United States as in Germany. In the USA between 1968 and 1976, the mortality associated with myocardial infarction was about 0.1% in men aged 40–44 years and 0.04% in women of the same age, as compared with 0.06% and 0.01%, respectively, in former West Germany. These figures show that women are at a far lower risk for fatal myocardial infarction and this might be the reason why there were no deaths in the Freiburg control group, not irradiated to the heart, in which there were twice as many women as men.

Of special interest is the relative risk of fatal myocardial infarction in patients with mediastinal irradiation in comparison with the normal population. The epidemiological data from the National Institute of Health (CARMEL and KAPLAN 1976) for the observation period between 1968 and 1976 allow the risk of fatal myocardial infarction to be estimated for an age- and sex-adjusted normal population in Germany, according to which their cumulative risk of fatal heart attack would be 0.1%, 0.3%, 0.6%, 1.2%, and 2.3% after 5, 10, 15, 20, and 25 years, respectively. This yields a relative (RR observed/expected) risk of fatal infarction of 0, 3.3, 3.3, 3.3, and 1.7, respectively, for the patients in the Freiburg group treated with mediastinal irradiation for the same period of time. This relation is consistent with more recent findings obtained by BOIVIN et al. (1992), who conducted a follow-up study of the connection between mediastinal irradiation, chemotherapy, and mortality from coronary artery disease in 4,665 patients treated for Hodgkin's disease. The average duration of follow-up was 7 years. Significantly increased age-adjusted relative risk of 2.56 was observed after mediastinal irradiation. These results are similar to those of the Freiburg study.

4 Conclusions

The results of the Freiburg retrospective study show that patients treated with megavoltage mediastinal irradiation are at a greater risk for fatal myocardial infarction than patients not treated with mediastinal irradiation and in comparison with a sex- and age-adjusted normal population. This is consistent with the literature. The results illustrate that based on a 1% risk of suffering fatal myocardial infarction in the normal population, patients undergoing mediastinal irradiation are at a threefold-higher risk after 6–15 years and a two- to threefold higher risk after 20–25 years (1%–2% in the normal population). Considering the low risk of spontaneous fatal myocardial infarction, the relative risk of fatal infarction in the study population must be assessed as low. Taking into account other nonfatal heart disorders does not alter this assessment in a way that would question the use of mediastinal irradiation for Hodgkin's disease. However, the results show that all measures available today must be taken to reduce treatment-induced cardiotoxicity, for example, by reducing the total dose in the scope of combined radiotherapy/chemotherapy, by reducing the dose of single fractions, and by reducing the volume load on the heart and controlling this by means of computer-assisted irradiation planning.

References

Applefield MM, Cole FJ, Pollock H, Sutton JF, Slawson RG, Singleton RT, Wiernik PH (1981) The late appearance of chronic pericardial disease in patients treated by radiotherapy for Hodgkin's disease. Ann Intern Med 94: 338–341

Applefield MM, Pollock SH (1980) Cardiac disease in patients who have malignancies. Curr Probl Cardiol 4: 1–37

Applefield MM, Wiernik PH (1983) Cardiac disease after radiation therapy for Hodgkin's disease. Analysis of 48 patients. Am J Cardiol 51: 1679–1681

Boivin J-F, Hutchinson GB (1982) Coronary heart disease mortality after irradiation for Hodgkin's Disease. Cancer 49: 2470–2475

Boivin J-F, Hutchison GB, Lubin JH, Mauch P (1992) Coronary artery disease mortality in patients treated for Hodgkin's disease. Cancer 69: 1241–1247

Byhardt R, Brace K, Ruckdeschel J, Chang P, Martin R, Wiernik P (1975) Dose and treatment factors in radiation-related pericardial effusion association with the mantle technique for Hodgkin's disease. Cancer 35: 795

Carbone PP, Kaplan HS, Musshoff K, Smithers DW, Tubiana M (1971) Report of the committee on Hodgkin's disease staging classification. Conference on staging in Hodgkin's disease. Ann Arbor, 26–28 April. Cancer Res 31: 1860–1861

Carmel RJ, Kaplan HS (1976) Mantle irradiation in Hodgkin's disease. An analysis of technique, tumor eradication and complications. Cancer 37: 2813–2825

Epstein FH, Pisa Z (1979) International comparisons in ischemic heart disease mortality. In: Havlik RJ Feinleib M (eds) Proceedings of the conference on the decline in coronary heart disease mortality. NIH no 79–1610, May 1979: 61 (Fig. 1) and 70 (Fig. 16)

Hagemeister FB, Fuller LM, Sullivan JA, Johnston D, North L, Butler JJ, Velasquez WS, Shullenberger CC (1982) Treatment of patients with stages I and II nonmediastinal Hodgkin's disease. Cancer 50: 2307–2313

Hellman S, Mauch P, Goodman RI, Rosenthal DS, Moloney WC (1978) The place of radiation therapy in the treatment of Hodgkin's disease. Cancer 42: 971–978

Kaplan EL, Meier P (1958) Nonparametric estimation from incomplete observations. J Am Stat Assoc 58: 457–481

Mc Reynolds RA, Gold GL, Roberts WC (1976) Coronary heart disease after mediastinal irradiation for Hodgkin's disease. Am J Med 60: 39

Nissen NI, Nordentoft AM, Brincker H, Andersen E, Krogh Jensen M, Nielsen JB, Pedersen-Bjergaard J, Jensen TS, Jensen KB, Videbaek AA, Pedersen M, Walbom- Jörgensen S (1980) Radiotherapy versus radiotherapy plus chemotherapy in stages I and II Hodgkin's disease. Scand J Haematol 25: 35–44

Prosnitz LR, Farber LR, Kapp DS, Bertino JR, Nordlund M, Lawrence R (1982) Combined modality therapy for advanced Hodgkin's disease. Long-term follow up data. Cancer Treat Rep 66: 871–879

Rosenberg SA (1966) Report of the Staging Committee of Hodgkin's disease. Cancer Res 26: 1310

Ruckdeschel JC, Chang P, Martin RG, Byhardt RW, O'Connel MJ, Sutherland JC, Wiernick PH (1975) Radiation related pericardial effusion in patients with Hodgkin's disease. Medicine 54: 245–259

Stewart JR, Fajardo LF (1971) Dose response in human and experimental radiation-induced heart disease. Radiology 99: 403

Yahalom J, Hasin Y, Fuks Z (1983) Acute myocardial infarction with normal coronary arteriogram after mantle field radiation therapy for Hodgkin's disease. Cancer 52: 637–641

5.5 Cardiac Morbidity and Mortality Following Radiotherapy

SEYMOUR H. LEVITT

CONTENTS

1 Introduction 197
2 Experimental Data 197
3 Clinical Data 198
4 Studies of Hodgkin's Disease Patients 199
5 Studies of Breast Cancer Patients 200
6 Importance of Radiation Technique 201
7 Conclusion 202
References 202

1 Introduction

With increasing evidence in recent years of radiation-induced cardiac morbidity and mortality, it is ironic that fewer than 50 years ago the heart was considered resistant to radiation. One of the first reports on radiation-induced myocardial infarction was by PEARSON in 1957. Since then, several other studies have examined the effect of radiation on the heart (COHN et al. 1967; JONES and WEDGWOOD 1960; LEACH 1943; LINDAHL et al. 1983, RUBIN and CASARETT 1968; WHITFIELD et al. 1963). The rapid increase in knowledge is partially due to advances in and beneficial outcomes of cancer treatments, especially of Hodgkin's disease. Careful follow-up of patients successfully treated for Hodgkin's disease, from Stanford (HANCOCK et al. 1993b; STEWART and FAJARDO 1984), the Joint Center for Radiation Therapy (MAUCH et al. 1988; TARBELL et al. 1990), the University of Minnesota (LEE et al. 1990) and other institutions (JOENSUU 1993), along with overviews of individual studies (HENRY-AMAR and SOMERS 1990a), have added to our knowledge of the potential harmful effects of radiation on the heart.

New more recent evidence of cardiac complications secondary to radiation has come from studies on breast cancer. An early study by Host demonstrated an increased risk of cardiac damage in stage I patients treated with radiation (HOST and BRENNHOVD 1977). More recent follow-up studies by Rutqvist (RUTQVIST et al. 1992; RUTQVIST and JOHANSSON 1990) and also by Fuller (FULLER et al. 1992) have confirmed the potential of cardiac disease induced by radiation following breast cancer treatment.

This chapter examines the experimental and clinical data of radiation-induced cardiac disease and discusses the incidence found in patients treated for Hodgkin's disease and breast cancer.

2 Experimental Data

STEWART and FAJARDO (1971) documented the development of radiation-induced heart disease observed in experiments done on rabbits. During the first 2 days following a single dose of 2000 rad, a transient acute exudate of granulocytes was noted in all tissues of the heart including the valves. No morphologic alterations or clinical manifestations of disease were evident 3–70 days following this acute inflammatory exudate; however, ultrastructural damage of the microcirculation was found to occur in the myocardium during this time. Progressive irreversible fibrosis of the pericardium and myocardium occurred at 70 days. Treatment of groups of rabbits with single doses ranging from 1200 rads to 8250 rads indicated that the incidence of pericarditis and myocardial fibrosis was dose-dependent.

A more recent study by SHULTZ-HECTOR (1992) noted that a single dose of radiation greater than 15 Gy leads to reversible exudative pericarditis in rabbits, dogs, and rats 100 days after exposure. Chronic congestive myocardial failure may develop, dependent on dose, after a longer period. Histological examination of the myocardium revealed degeneration and necrosis, which may be accompanied by interstitial fibrosis in some species. Decrease in capillary density and ultrastructural endothelial cell degeneration also have been noted. In hemo-

SEYMOUR H. LEVITT, Dr., Department of Therapeutic Radiology, Box 494, UMHC, University of Minnesota, Minneapolis, Minnesota 55455, USA

dynamic studies in rats, cardiac output has been shown to decrease of 64% and then maintain a steady state after 20 Gy.

Schultz-Hector noted that radiation-induced heart disease conforms in many respects to radiobiological concepts of the late responding tissues with a chronic progressive time course and a pronounced fractionation effect (Schultz-Hector 1992). She found that experimental evidence indicated the importance of alterations of regulatory mechanisms and that pathogenesis cannot be understood in terms of target cell depletion alone. She notes that "in spite of different experimental end points used, α/β ratios derived according to the linear quadratic model were very similar and were lower in the heart than most other organs investigated. In view of the fact that the target cell population for radiation cannot be defined in the myocardium, the pathogenesis of radiation-induced cardiomyopathy cannot sufficiently be described in terms of cell survival. The applicability of the linear-quadratic model could be questioned." (Schultz-Hector 1992).

In another study on the fractionation response and repair kinetics of radiation-induced heart failure in rats, Schultz-Hector noted that from experiments giving 1, 2, 4, or 10 dose fractions, a low α/β ratio of 3.7 Gy could be calculated and that when the time interval between dose fractions is varied, time intervals up to 3 h did not significantly increase survival time (Schultz-Hector et al. 1992). She concluded that repair of sublethal damage was very slow, but that pathogenic mechanisms independent of cell death could contribute to this effect, making it difficult to interpret the α/β ratio in terms of cell survival parameters of a target cell population.

Another recent study by Gillette on canine mediastinal radiation reported on the treatment of 70 adult beagle dogs irradiated with doses ranging from 24 to 68 Gy giving 2 Gy, 3 Gy, and 4 Gy fractions (Gillette et al. 1992). Evaluation included echocardiography, electrocardiography, and hemodynamic cardiac output of the right heart. In addition, histomorphometric analysis of all tissues were done 2 years after the experiments. Some of the dogs died due to pericardial infusion or constrictive pericarditis. Heart failure was reported at doses of 62 Gy given in 2 Gy fractions, 60 Gy given in 3 Gy fractions, and 52 Gy given in 4 Gy fractions. The ED_{50} values for pericardial fibrosis for 2 Gy, 3 Gy, and 4 Gy fractions were 46.1 Gy, 43.9 Gy, and 26.6 Gy, respectively. An α/β ratio of 2.5 Gy was calculated by a direct quantal response analysis. There were small foci of myocytolytic lesions noted in 11 dogs. The calculated ED_{50} values for myocytolytic lesions were 70.4 Gy given in 2 Gy fractions and 50.8 Gy given in 4 Gy fractions. The estimated α/β ratio was 3.2 Gy. Heart rates determined from physical examination and frequency of S-T segment changes increased with increasing dose. However, no other dose related changes were found in any of the other functional parameters. Functional changes were detected in 14 dogs with clinical signs of heart failure.

From this data, the authors concluded that the lung was the most sensitive area in the mediastinum radiated and that damage to the lung contributed to the cardiac problems. Although myocardial lesions were noted with higher ED_{50} values, they were not found to be functionally significant at 2 years after radiation. The authors concluded that longer observation periods were needed for development of these lesions in humans. Finally, the authors found that all α/β ratios calculated in this study fell within the range expected for late responding tissues, further emphasizing the sparing function of late normal tissue injury by reducing dose per fraction. However, they also noted that is it not clear whether additional sparing can be achieved by decreasing the dose per fraction below that conventionally used.

3 Clinical Data

Each of the layers of the heart can be affected by irradiation and can produce symptoms that are typical of radiation changes (Schultz-Hector 1992), including acute pericarditis during radiotherapy, delayed pericarditis, pancarditis, valvular and conduction defects, and coronary artery disease (Stewart and Fajardo 1984). Studies show that pericarditis is the most frequently reported radiation effect (Schultz-Hector 1992; Stewart and Fajardo 1984) and pancarditis the most severe complication (Stewart and Fajardo 1984). Exudative pericarditis, which was reported in 25%–60% of Hodgkin's disease patients in the 1960s and 1970s, has been noted to occur generally in acute form only and usually resolves; however, some cases of progressive disease leading to severe and sometimes fatal constrictive pericarditis have been reported (Schultz-Hector 1992).

Follow-up studies of cardiac function in Hodgkin's disease patients show an abnormally low resting left ventricular ejection fraction in about

20% of the patients, which appears to be related to the increasing radiation dose to the heart (SCHULTZ-HECTOR 1992). A decrease in the left ventricular ejection fraction associated with the myocardial volume included in the treatment beam has also been noted in some studies, with the majority of patients not reporting clinical symptoms of heart disease. A moderate reduction of left ventricular fraction, along with ECG abnormalities, after completion of radiotherapy are usually reversible within 2–6 months and have not shown predictive or pathogenic importance for radiation-induced cardiomyopathy. Schultz-Hector noted that the early phase of reversible effusive pericarditis and late phase of reduced left ventricle ejection fraction characterizing the time course of experimental radiation-induced heart disease is similar to that observed in patients who underwent mediastinal radiotherapy (SCHULTZ-HECTOR 1993).

A study by CARLSON et al. (1991) of valvular injury following mediastinal irradiation reported a continual valvular disease following radiation that begins with mild asymptomatic valvular thickening and progresses to severe valvular fibrosis with hemodynamic compromise requiring surgery. This study documented one patient who underwent a successful aortic and mitral valve replacement associated with valvular disease. In an analysis of 15- to 20-year survivors after adjuvant breast cancer irradiation, Gyenes found a significant difference between cineangiographic findings of patients treated to the heart and those not treated. Patients were evaluated by echocardiography, bicycle ergometry stress tests, technetium 99m, Sesta MIBI, myocardial perfusion, and myocardial scintigraphy. A significant difference of ischemic heart disease was noted in the treated patients, while echocardiography did not show any deterioration in left ventricular systolic or diastolic function (GYENES et al. submitted).

Myocardial and coronary artery disease following radiation treatment of Hodgkin's disease or of breast cancer has also been reported. In a overview of cardiac morbidity following radiotherapy, JOENSUU (1993) focused on the less reported and more controversial incidence of radiation-induced myocardial infarction and coronary artery disease. He reported at least 17 published cases of coronary artery disease in patients younger than 30 years old treated for Hodgkin's disease, and at least 22 patients between 30 and 39, who prior to treatment did not have symptoms of heart disease. The study noted that a high incidence of left main coronary artery and right ostial coronary disease appears to characterize radiation-induced coronary artery disease and that cobalt-60 was used to treat many of the patients who developed coronary artery disease. The incidence of myocardial infarction also was noted in patients treated for Hodgkin's disease and breast cancer, as described in the following studies.

4 Studies of Hodgkin's Disease Patients

Data from studies on Hodgkin's disease provide most of the information on specific cardiac complications due to irradiation showing that pericarditis and myocardial infarction are major risk factors, along with accelerated coronary artery disease and valvular injury (COSSET et al. 1991, HANCOCK et al. 1993b). In the most recent study of 2232 Hodgkin's disease patients treated at Stanford University Medical Center from 1960 to 1991, 88 patients died of heart disease: 55 from acute myocardial infarction and 33 from other cardiac diseases. The relative risk of cardiac death was 3.1. The relative risk of cardiac death was found to increase significantly with duration after treatment for both acute myocardial infarction ($p = 0.02$) and other cardiac diseases ($p = 0.04$) (HANCOCK 1993b). A study by the Institute Gustave-Roussy of 499 patients treated by mediastinal radiation for Hodgkin's disease reported a statistically significant 10-year cumulative incidence rate of 3.9% of acute myocardial infarction and 9.5% of pericarditis compared to no incidence of myocardial infarction ($p < 0.05$) or pericarditis ($p < 0.005$) in 138 patients treated without radiation (COSSET et al. 1991). The risk of pericarditis was significantly increased with total dose of greater than or equal to 41 Gy and with dose per fraction greater than or equal to 3.0 Gy, while the risk of myocardial infarction was not found to be related to dose or fractionation. However, the lack of significant statistical finding could be the result of the small number of patients treated and evaluated.

Myocardial infarction was reported as the most frequent cardiovascular complication following both standard and radical radiotherapy in a series of patients treated between 1970 and 1983 at the University of Minnesota (LEE et al. 1990). Thirteen patients had myocardial infarction: ten of 119 patients without large mediastinal mass who received standard radiotherapy and three of 60 patients with large mediastinal mass, hilar disease, or splenic involvement who received radical radiation therapy. Similarly, unpublished data of 253 patients treated for Hodgkin's disease at the Radiumhemmet Karolinska Hospital between 1973 and 1985 suggest a significant increased incidence of myocardial infarction in patients treated with radiation doses of 40 Gy (2.9 Gy daily) and without subcarinal blocking (LEVITT, unpublished data).

Long-term cardiac effects following treatment of Hodgkin's disease are a major concern because many patients treated for the disease are young and can expect to live longer because of improvements in treatment. Studies from the European Organization for Research on Treatment of Cancer (EORTC) showed that the proportion of death resulting from progression of Hodgkin's disease, treatment side effects, and intercurrent diseases decreased with time, whereas second cancer and cardiac failure peaked during the 10–12 years posttreatment (HENRY-AMAR et al. 1990, HENRY-AMAR and SOMERS 1990b). This delayed occurrence of myocardial infarction is consistent with other studies reporting a time-lag for onset of radiation-induced heart disease and the need for careful follow-up of irradiated patients because of such delayed complications (O'DONNELL et al. 1986).

Several studies have shown an increased incidence of myocardial infarction in young patients following irradiation. POHJOLA-SINTONEN et al. (1987) evaluated cardiac function in a series of 28 patients younger than 40 years of age treated with mediastinal irradiation and found that 19 of the 28 patients had some abnormal cardiac findings. A pericardial event after irradiation occurred in 43% of the patients. ECG abnormalities occurred in 13 of 28 patients, and two patients had myocardial infarction, one of whom died. A study from Stanford University of 635 patients younger than 21 years old treated with high dose irradiation for Hodgkin's disease showed a relative risk of death from acute myocardial infarction of 41.5 and 29.6 for any cardiac disease (HANCOCK et al. 1993a). An earlier 14-year median follow-up study from Stanford of 326 patients showed that, although only nine patients died from acute myocardial infarctions 2–19 years after therapy, five of the nine patients were under 45 years of age and had no known cardiac risk factors (HANCOCK et al. 1988). The fact that myocardial infarction may remain undiagnosed and unreported because of its rare occurrence in young patients must also be considered. This was noted by JOENSUU (1989) in a study of 47 patients younger than 40 years old treated with irradiation to the mediastinum for Hodgkin's disease in which a myocardial infarction occurred in two male patients, 24 and 28 years old.

5 Studies of Breast Cancer Patients

Follow-up studies of breast cancer patients who received irradiation as part of treatment have also reported cardiac complications due to irradiation, although the results of these studies are quite recent and more information is needed to make analyses comparable to those made with Hodgkin's disease.

Several studies indicate changes to the heart due to irradiation but note that the changes are reversible and have not been proven a major risk factor. One study by STRENDER et al. (1985) of a 10-year follow-up of 197 patients treated with irradiation for breast cancer found a low incidence of serious cardiac complications in both autopsies of deceased patients and in patients examined still living. A high incidence of ECG T-wave change was noted in 62 of the 102 patients living who were examined, but the authors concluded that the changes were reversible and that no functionally significant damage was noted to the perimyocardium. Another study, by FARAGO and GYENES (1991), showed that more than one third of 54 breast cancer patients treated by postoperative telecobalt or electron therapy showed signs of pericardial irritation, which usually disappeared in 6–12 months. The authors concluded that ionizing radiation, mainly telecobalt therapy, may be a risk factor for cardiovascular disease and needs to be considered in treatment planning.

Other studies do show an increased risk of major cardiac complications, especially myocardial infarction in early breast cancer patients, particularly those with left lesions, treated with irradiation. A study by RUTQVIST and JOHANSSON (1990) of 54,617 breast cancer patients reported to the Swedish Cancer Registry between 1970 and 1985 found that patients with left-sided tumors treated with irradiation had a higher mortality due to myocardial infarction than did patients with right-sided tumors ($p < 0.01$). No difference was found in total intercurrent mortality. These results were confirmed in a more recent study by Rutqvist of a long-term follow-up (mean time of 16 years) of 960 breast cancer patients randomized between pre- or post-operative radiotherapy versus surgery alone (RUTQVIST et al. 1992). This study showed that, again, although there was no increase in intercurrent mortality in any of the patients, the patients who received the highest radiation dose to the myocardium (i.e., patients treated with tangential ^{60}Co fields for left-sided tumors) had a significant increase in the risk of death from ischemic heart disease compared to the patients treated by surgery alone or the patients who received less radiation to the myocardium (i.e., patients treated with electrons to chest wall and internal mammary nodes or those with right-sided tumors). The authors concluded that radiation-induced cardiovascular mortality for early breast cancer is associated with a biological dose of radiation to the heart and the irradiated volume. This study highlights the importance of the laterality of the tumor, portal arrangements, radiation energy, fractionation, and total dose in treatment planning to avoid excess treatment.

A recent study of GYENES et al. evaluated the hypothesis set forth by Rutqvist, that breast cancer patients treated with irradiation for left-sided lesions were at higher risk of developing cardiac problems (GYENES et al. submitted publication). The authors noted several drawbacks to their study (e.g., retrospective study of a relatively small number of 37 patients), but did find that 25% of the patients who received radiotherapy to left-sided early breast cancer exhibited scintigraphic defects that were significant when compared to none found in the control group ($p < 0.05$). The authors concur with previous studies, that left-sided adjuvant radiotherapy for early breast cancer may contribute to the risk of ischemic heart disease.

A study by FULLER et al. (1992) verifies the importance of radiation technique to reduce the risk of cardiac morbidity and mortality. This study compared patients treated by mastectomy followed mainly by orthovoltage radiation an patients treated with conservative surgery followed by a modern two- or four-field megavoltage technique. The authors found that for patients with left-sided tumors, the heart volume irradiated to a minimum extrapolated target dose of 5 Gy was significantly decreased for patients treated with a modern technique when compared with those patients treated with the earlier technique using orthovoltage. Haybittle also found an increased risk of cardiac complications in patients treated to the left breast with orthovoltage technique (HAYBITTLE et al. 1989). Megavoltage techniques have been shown to reduce the total heart dose and to spare the left circumflex and right coronary arteries; new radiation techniques are needed to reduce the dose to the left anterior descending artery (FULLER et al. 1992).

6 Importance of Radiation Technique

The above studies of Hodgkin's disease and breast cancer show that the risk of radiation-induced heart disease increases with inappropriate radiation technique. STEWART and FAJARDO (1984) reported that the use of cobalt and anterior weighted beams, or treating one field daily, led to complications because of daily inhomogeneity and large dose to the heart per fraction on days that the anterior port was treated. This has been substantiated in more recent studies (JOENSUU 1993). STEWART and FAJARDO (1984) also showed that the effects of radiation on cardiac disease are dose-related. In one study the authors found that low doses of up to 4000 rads in 20F/4W to a large heart volume were well-tolerated, but higher doses resulted in a sharp rise in cardiac complications. A small heart volume was able to tolerate a dose of 6000 rad in 30F/6W, with a rapid increase in problems at higher doses. The authors speculated that less than a 5% incidence of pericarditis was expected in patients with large heart volumes treated (60% of the heart treated) with doses of 40 Gy or less in 20F/4W. For small volumes (20%–30% of the heart treated) the corresponding tolerance was about 60 Gy in 30F/6W.

More recent studies confirm the importance of reducing dose to the heart and modifying irradiation techniques (i.e., shielding the heart, treating equally weighted anterior and posterior fields), to reduce radiation-induces heart disease (AUQUIER et al. 1992; BOIVIN et al. 1992; HANCOCK et al. 1993b, JOENSUU 1993; LEVITT and FLETCHER 1991; MAUCH et al. 1988, STRAUS and GLATSTEIN 1992; TARBELL et al. 1990). An updated study by BOIVIN et al. (1992) of 4665 Hodgkin's disease patients showed that the relative risk of acute myocardial infarction was reduced from 6.33 (reported in an earlier study with older irradiation techniques) to 1.97 in patients treated with equally weighted anterior and posterior fields, with daily doses of 200 cGy or less, and with the use of subcarinal blocking after 3000 cGy. The recent Stanford study found that lower doses to the mediastinum (30 Gy or less) did not increase relative risk of cardiac death, whereas higher doses (above 30 Gy) increased the relative risk to 3.5. The study found that limiting cardiac exposure through blocking reduced the relative risk for other cardiac disease (5.3 vs 1.4) but not for myocardial infarction (3.7 vs 3.4) (HANCOCK et al. 1993b). An updated report from the Joint Center for Radiation Therapy of 590 Hodgkin's patients showed that cardiac complications following mantle irradiation were uncommon, with pericarditis as the most common complication occurring in 2.2% of patients (TARBELL et al. 1990). However, an overall 6.7 standardized mortality ratio for myocardial infarction was found in this study, although in a previous study from the same institution only three cases of fatal myocardial infarction were reported in 315 patients treated with mantle irradiation (9-year median follow-up) (MAUCH et al. 1988).

The varied reports on the effect of modern radiation technique on reducing myocardial disease indicates the need to further study ways to decrease radiation-induced myocardial disease. In a combined study of the Oslo and Stockholm breast cancer trials, the authors showed that although long-term effects, such as myocardial disease, among patients with node-negative breast cancers have been associated with megavoltage treatment, such negative effects are assumed to be dependent on the given dose and dose distribution to the heart. These negative effects may be prevented by minimizing irradiation to the lungs and heart by treating the chest wall with electron beams versus tangential ports, by decreasing the extent of irradiation to the internal mammary nodes, (LEVITT and FLETCHER 1991), and by avoiding large fraction sizes (AUQUIER et al. 1992). The above studies show that modifying irradiation technique, such as careful shielding of the heart with subcarinal blocks, reduces the frequency of cardiac sequelae, and several of the studies indicate that reducing total dose to the heart decreases myocardial sequelae (BOIVIN et al. 1992; LEVITT and FLETCHER 1991). These findings suggest that a combination of technique modification and dose reduction could decrease all cardiac sequelae.

7 Conclusion

Experimental and clinical data show that radiation produces a variety of changes to the heart, including acute pericarditis, delayed pericarditis, pancarditis, valvular and conduction defects, coronary artery disease, and myocardial infarction. Studies of patients treated for Hodgkin's disease have provided the most substantial information regarding the association between irradiation and cardiac complications; more recently studies of patients treated for breast cancer also indicate a correlation. As evidence for radiation-induced cardiac complications increases, the need to adjust radiotherapeutic techniques to balance this risk with the increased potential for cure also increases. Using modern radiotherapeutic techniques is important to minimize the risks of radiation-induced cardiac disease.

Acknowledgments. I wish to thank Mary Beth Nierengarten for her major contributions to editing this paper.

References

Auquier A, Rutqvist LE, Host H, Rotstein S, Arriagada R (1992) Post-mastectomy megavoltage radiotherapy: The Oslo and Stockholm Trials. Eur J Cancer 28: 433–437

Boivin JF, Hutchison GB, Lubin JH, Mauch P (1992) Coronary artery disease mortality in patients treated for Hodgkin's disease. Cancer 69: 1241–1247

Boivin JF, Hutchinson GB (1982) Coronary heart disease mortality after irradiation for Hodgkin's disease. Cancer 49: 2470–2475

Carlson RG, Mayfield WR, Norman S, Alexander JA (1991) Radiation-associated valvular disease. Chest 99: 538–545

Cohn KE, Stewart JR, Fajardo LF, Hancock EW (1967) Heart disease following radiation. Medicine 46: 281–298

Cosset JM, Henry-Amar M, Pellae-Cosset B, Carde P, Girinski T, Tubiana M, Hayat M (1991) Pericarditis and myocardial infarctions after Hodgkin's disease therapy at the Institute Gustave-Roussy. Int J Radiat Oncol Biol Phys 21: 447–449

Farago K, Gyenes G (1991) Pericardial irritation in breast cancer patients treated by curative postoperative radiotherapy – early results. Strahlenther Onkol 167: 207–210

Fuller SA, Haybittle JL, Smith REA, Dobbs HJ (1992) Cardiac dose in postoperative breast irradiation. Radiotherapy and Oncology 25: 19–24

Gillette SM, Gillette EL, Shida T, Boon J, Miller CW, Powers BE (1992) Late radiation response of canine mediastinal tissues. Radiotherapy and Oncology 23: 41–52

Gyenes G, Fornander T, Carlens P, Rutqvist LE (submitted) Morbidity of ischemic heart disease in early breast cancer 15–20 years after adjuvant radiotherapy

Hancock SL, Hoppe RT, Horning SJ, Rosenberg SA (1988) Intercurrent death after Hodgkin's therapy in radiotherapy and adjuvant MOPP trials. Ann Intern Med 109: 183–189. Corrections in: Hancock SL, Cox RS, Rosenberg SA (1991) Death After Treatment of Hodgkin's Disease. Ann Intern Med 114: 810

Hancock SL, Donaldson SS, Hoppe RT (1993a) Cardiac disease following treatment of Hodgkin's disease in children and adolescents. J Clin Oncol 11: 1208–1215

Hancock SL, Tucker MA, Hoppe RT (1993b) Factors affecting late mortality from heat disease after treatment of Hodgkin's disease. JAMA 270: 1949–1955

Haybittle JL, Brinkley D, Houghton J, A'Hern RP, Baum M (1989) Postoperative radiotherapy and late mortality: evidence from the Cancer Research Campaign trial for early breast cancer. Br Medical Journal 289: 1611–1614

Henry-Amar M, Hayat M, Meerwaldt JH, Burgers M, Carde P, Somers R, et al. (1990) Causes of death after therapy for early stage Hodgkin's disease entered on EORTC protocols. Int J Radiat Oncol Biol Phys 19: 1155–1157

Henry-Amer M, Somers R (1990a) Survival outcome after Hodgkin's disease: A report from the international data base on Hodgkin's disease. Semin Oncol 17: 758–768

Henry-Amar M, Somers R (1990b) Long-term survival in early stages Hodgkin's disease: The EORTC experience. In: Somers R, Henry-Amar M, Meerwaldt JH, Carde P, (eds) Treatment Strategy in Hodgkin's Disease. London, Paris: Colloque/INSERM/John Libbey Eurotext, 146: 151–166

Host H, Brennhovd IO (1977) The effect of postoperative radiation therapy in breast cancer. Int J Radiat Oncol Biol Phys 2: 1061–1067

Joensuu H (1989) Acute myocardial infarction after heart irradiation in young patients with Hodgkin's disease. Chest 95: 338–390

Joensuu H (1993) Myocardial infarction after irradiation in Hodgkin's disease: A review. In: Hinkelbein W, Bruggmoster G, Frommhold H, Wannenmacher M (eds.) Recent Results in Cancer Research. Acute and Long Term Side-Effects of Radiotherapy. Springer-Verlag, Heidelberg, pp 157–173

Jones A, Wedgwood J (1960) Effects of radiations on the heart. Br J Radiol 33: 138–158

Leach JE (1943) Effect of roentgen therapy on the heart. Arch Intern Med 72: 715–745

Lee CKK, Aeppli DM, Bloomfield CD, Levitt SH (1990) Curative radiotherapy for laparotomy-staged IA, IIA, IIIA Hodgkin's disease: An evaluation of the gains achieved with radical radiotherapy. Int J Radiat Oncol Biol Phys 19: 547–559

Levitt SH, Fletcher GH (1991) Trials and tribulations: Do clinical trials prove that irradiation increases cardiac and secondary cancer mortality in the breast cancer patient? Int J Radiat Oncol Biol Phys 20: 523–527

Lindahl J, Strender LE, Larsson LE, Unsgaard B (1983) Electrocardiographic changes after radiation therapy for carcinoma of the breast. Acta Radiol Oncol 22: 433–440

Mauch P, Tarbell N, Weinstein H, Silver B, Goffman T, Osteen R, et al. (1988) Stage IA and IIA supradiaphragmatic Hodgkin's disease: Prognostic factors in surgically staged patients treated with mantel and paraaortic irradiation. J Clin Oncol 6: 1576–1583

O'Donnell L, O'Neill T, Toner M, O'Brien S, Graham I (1986) Myocardial hypertrophy, fibrosis, and infarction following exposure of the heart to radiation for Hodgkin's disease. Postgraduate Medical Journal 62: 1055–1058

Pearson HES (1957) Coronary occlusion following thoracic radiotherapy. Proc R Soc Med 50: 516

Pohjola-Sintonen S, Totterman KJ, Salmon M, Siltanen P (1987) Late cardiac effects of mediastinal radiotherapy in patients with Hodgkin's disease. Cancer 60: 31–37

Rubin P, Casarett GW (1968) Clinical radiation pathology. Philadelphia, WB Saunders Company, 471–517

Rutqvist LE, Johansson H (1990) Mortality by laterality of the primary tumour among 55,000 breast cancer patients from the Swedish Cancer Registry. Br J Cancer 61: 866–868

Rutqvist LE, Lax I, Fornander T, Johansson H (1992) Cardiovascular mortality in a randomized trial of adjuvant radiation therapy versus surgery alone in primary breast cancer. Int J Radiat Oncol Biol Phys 22: 887–96

Schultz-Hector S, Sund M, Thames HD (1992) Fractionation response and repair kinetics of radiation-induced heart failure in the rat. Radiother Oncol 23: 33–40

Schultz-Hector S (1992) Radiation-induced heart disease: review of experimental data on dose response and pathogenesis. Int J Radiat Biol 61: 149–160

Schultz-Hector S (1993) Experimental studies on the pathogenesis of damage in the heart. Recent Results in Cancer Research, Vol. 130, Springer Verlag, Berlin-Heidelberg, pp 145–156

Stewart JR, Fajardo LF (1971) Dose response in human and experimental radiation-induced heart disease. Application of the nominal standard dose (NSD) concept. Radiology 99: 403–408

Stewart JR, Fajardo LF (1984) Radiation-induced heart disease: An update. Progress in Cardiovascular Diseases Vol XXVII(3): 173–194

Straus KL, Glatstein E (1992) Hodgkin's disease and non-Hodgkin's lymphoma. In: Levitt SH, Khan FM, Potish RA (eds) Levitt and Tapley's Technological Basis of Radiation Therapy: Practical Clinical Applications, second edition. Pennsylvania, Lea and Febiger, p 370

Strender LE, Lindahl J, Larsson LE (1985) Incidence of heart disease and functional significance of changes in the electrocardiogram 10 years after radiotherapy for breast cancer. Cancer 57: 929–934

Tarbell NJ, Thompson L, Mauch P (1990) Thoracic irradiation in Hodgkin's disease: disease control and long-term complications. Int J Radiat Oncol Biol Phys 18: 275–281

Whitfield AGW, Bond WH, Kunkler PB (1963) Radiation damage to thoracic tissues. Thorax 18: 371–380

6 Nephrotoxicity

6.1 Nephrotoxicity of Ifosfamide in Children

RAINER ROSSI and JOACHIM BOOS

CONTENTS

1 Ifosfamide 207
1.1 Indication 207
1.2 Side Effects 207
2 Renal Fanconi's Syndrome 207
3 Renal Side Effects of Ifosfamide 208
3.1 Fanconi's Syndrome After Ifosfamide 208
3.2 Subclinical Impairment of Renal Function . . . 208
3.3 Histological Findings 209
3.4 Risk Factors of Ifosfamide-Induced Nephrotoxicity 209
3.4.1 Cumulative Ifosfamide Dose 209
3.4.2 Reduction in Nephron Number 209
3.4.3 Platinum Compounds 210
3.4.4 Age of Primary Diagnosis 210
3.4.5 Concomitant Medication/Mode of Administration 210
3.5 Pathomechanism 211
3.6 Prognosis 211
4 Summary and Therapeutic Recommendations . 211
References 211

1 Ifosfamide

1.1 Indication

Ifosfamide, a structural isomer of cyclophosphamide, was introduced into clinical studies in 1972. Ifosfamide is an alkylating substance and has to be activated by hepatic metabolism similar to cyclophosphamide (LOEHRER 1992). The antitumoral properties of ifosfamide take effect in a number of sarcomas, lymphomas and other tumors, and it is also effective in patients pretreated with cyclophosphamide due to only partial cross-resistance (BRADE et al. 1986). Following these findings ifosfamide has been incorporated into treatment schedules not only for relapsed but also for newly diagnosed patients. It has also been widely used in treating a variety of childhood malignancies including Ewing's sarcoma, rhabdomyosarcoma, osteosarcoma, neuroblastoma and B cell neoplasia or recurrent leukemias, Wilms and germ cell tumors, hepato- and retinoblastomas (JÜRGENS et al. 1989). This widespread use of ifosfamide has, however, been challenged (SHAW and EDEN 1990) due to doubts about its superior activity in comparison to that of cyclophosphamide.

1.2 Side Effects

Acute side effects of ifosfamide include nausea, vomiting and alopecia in virtually every patient treated. It has a myelotoxic potential and combination chemotherapy employing ifosfamide is generally followed by distinct leuco- and thrombocytopenia and anemia requiring substitution therapy. A rather specific effect seems to be CNS toxicity, which leads to disturbances of mental state, motor system, cranial nerves and cerebellar function or seizures (PRATT et al. 1986).

Hemorrhagic cystitis, as seen after both cyclophosphamide and ifosfamide, was attributed to the metabolite acrolein (COX 1979), but this side effect can be controlled with mesna (MUNSHI et al. 1992). After the introduction of mesna into chemotherapeutic regimens employing ifosfamide, dose escalation has become possible.

2 Renal Fanconi's Syndrome

Renal Fanconi's syndrome can occur together with inborn errors of metabolism like cystinosis or be an acquired disease secondary to a variety of nephrotoxic agents. It may be reversible, as in galactosemia, or persist, as in cystinosis. Its pathobiochemical mechanism is not uniform and has been clarified only in part (BRODEHL 1992). Findings in the maleate model indicate mitochondrial damage and a defective energy supply of proximal tubular cells. The resulting cell damage leads to a complex impairment of tubular transport capacity mainly

RAINER ROSSI, Dr., JOACHIM BOOS, Dr., Universitätskinderklinik, Pädiatrische Hämatologie/Onkologie, Albert-Schweitzer-Straße 33, 48129 Münster, FRG

located at the proximal tubular site. Reabsorption of solutes filtrated by the glomerulus will be impaired leading to urinary loss of glucose, amino acids, phosphate, bicarbonate, sodium, and potassium. In addition, there will be tubular low molecular weight proteinuria or loss of concentrating capacity. While increased urinary glucose, amino acid, and protein excretion will not precipitate metabolic disturbances, phosphate and bicarbonate loss will result in metabolic bone disease – rickets in children, osteomalacia in adults – and renal tubular acidosis. The renal sodium loss, together with diminished concentrating capacity, may render a patient at risk for dehydration episodes. Glomerular function, initially normal, will be impaired secondary to the tubulopathy. Causal therapy beside avoidance of the causative agent is not possible. Hallmarks of therapy are phosphate and bicarbonate supplementation, sometimes in combination with vitamin D. In addition, balanced fluid and salt intake is mandatory.

3 Renal Side Effects of Ifosfamide

3.1 Fanconi's Syndrome After Ifosfamide

Since the first case report in 1974 (DE FRONZO et al. 1974) approximately 40 reports have been published on pediatric cancer patients who developed renal Fanconi's syndrome secondary to ifosfamide containing chemotherapy regimens. Among these patients there is only one additional adult (ROSSI et al. 1992a), but the majority of patients were comparatively young, i.e., <5 years of age, and had received a rather high cumulative dose of ifosfamide. Approximately half of the patients with clinically apparent renal Fanconi's syndrome secondary to ifosfamide had been treated with platinum compounds as well, some had undergone unilateral nephrectomy or had received abdominal radiotherapy including the kidneys. In the two patients reported on by ROUSSEL et al. (1990) tumor-related bilateral hydronephrosis was thought to aggravate ifosfamide nephrotoxicity. Overall, acquired renal Fanconi's syndrome after ifosfamide was reported to affect between 1.7% (three of 218) (PRATT et al. 1991) and 5% (four of 74) (SUAREZ et al. 1991) of treated patients. In our own series examining 120 patients from a single institution who had received ifosfamide as part of their chemotherapeutic regimens (range of cumulative dose 2–95 g/m^2), eight patients were identified who had renal Fanconi's syndrome (6.7%).

From these case reports it was concluded that

- Nephrotoxicity after ifosfamide is mainly related to high cumulative doses.
- There is an additive effect of other potentially nephrotoxic therapeutic modalities, namely, therapies with platinum compounds, reduction of kidney mass by nephrectomy, or preexisting renal damage on ifosfamide nephrotoxicity.
- Young children are more susceptible to ifosfamide-induced tubular toxicity.

3.2 Subclinical Impairment of Renal Function

Subclinical impairment of proximal tubular reabsorption was first noted by PATTERSON and KHOJASTEH (1989), who observed hyperaminoaciduria, glucosuria, renal proteinuria and bicarbonate loss after ifosfamide. In a series by SKINNER et al. (1990a) 11 patients after high-dose ifosfamide chemotherapy were all found to have proximal tubular damage, and six patients showed distal tubular impairment as indicated by decreased morning urine osmolarity. In addition, the glomerular filtration rate was reduced in six of these patients. A prospective study by CARON et al. (1992) showed 12 of 15 patients had developed tubular toxicity during ongoing therapy. In seven patients the tubulopathy resulted in renal Fanconi's syndrome requiring supplementation therapy. Improvement from this condition was recorded in three of these patients after extended follow-up. Hyperaminoaciduria was identified to predict severe tubular damage. In our own series we clearly demonstrated the predominance of proximal tubular damage over both distal impairment and reduction in glomerular filtration rate. Again, hyperaminoaciduria, as indicated by a low percent reabsorption of amino acids, was the parameter impaired most frequently. Renal phosphate loss was expressed as fractional reabsorption of phosphate (BRODEHL et al. 1982), as this parameter is the renal determinant of the serum phosphorus level; low fractional reabsorption will render a patient at risk of developing hypophosphatemic bone disease. In fact, a decreased value was seen in 38% of our patients and, accordingly, 37% presented with hypophosphatemia. Consequently, fractional phosphate reabsorption is the single most important parameter to examine. Renal tubular acidosis which may result from both proximal and distal tubular losses of bicarbonate was diagnosed in only seven patients all of whom had severe renal damage.

Reductions in the glomerular filtration rate were rarely seen (ten patients), and again all these patients had severe proximal tubular damage indicating that the reduction in glomerular filtration rate was a secondary event. Other studies and these data as well suggest that ifosfamide has no direct toxic effect on the glomerulus, and any reduction in glomerular filtration rate observed after ifosfamide seems to be secondary to a proximal tubulopathy.

Apart from the impairment of solute reabsorption, measurements of tubular enzyme excretion (GOREN et al. 1989) or combined enzyme and globulin excretion (BRANDIS et al. 1992) also showed the predominance of proximal tubular impairment after ifosfamide. This finding was confirmed (ROSSI and EHRICH 1993) in a subset of patients from our study in whom glomerular and tubular proteinuria were distinguished using transferrin and immunoglobulin G excretion as indicators of glomerular impairment and α_1-microgolobulin and *N*-acetyl-β-D-glucosaminidase as indicators of proximal tubular dysfunction.

3.3 Histological Findings

The majority of histological examinations after ifosfamide treatment was done post mortem. Tubular cell necrosis (DE FRONZO et al. 1974) or degenerative changes of the tubular system (PRATT et al. 1991) were reported. A biopsy from an adult patient with renal insufficiency secondary to ifosfamide (WILLEMSE et al. 1989) showed focal atrophy and interstitial fibrosis but no interstitial nephritis. Similar findings were shown in another patient (ROSSI et al. 1992a) with loss of cortical tubular cells in the S1 and S2 segments of the proximal tubule. Glomerulus, juxtaglomerular apparatus and distal tubular cells were normal. Electron microscopy revealed irregularly distributed remnant microvili, loss of mitochondria, and interdigitating membrane infoldings in the basilar cytoplasm. Neither by conventional nor immunostaining could any hint of interstitial nephritis be identified. Thus, histological findings indicate primary epithelial damage to the proximal tubular system without any sign of interstitial nephritis.

3.4 Risk Factors of Ifosfamide-Induced Nephrotoxicity

3.4.1 Cumulative Ifosfamide Dose

The majority of case reports described renal Fanconi's syndrome or severe tubular damage only after a high cumulative dose of ifosfamide, an observation confirmed for both the occurrence of renal Fanconi's syndrome (SUAREZ et al. 1991) and the occurrence of subclinical tubular dysfunction (SKINNER et al. 1990a). The findings in our patients are in good agreement with these studies, as only four out of the 22 patients with severe tubular dysfunction (overt renal Fanconi's syndrome and generalized tubulopathy) received ifosfamide chemotherapy without concomitant cisplatin or operative reduction in kidney mass. Cumulative ifosfamide doses had been high in those patients, ranging from 51 to 95 g/m^2. However, a number of patients have been reported to develop ifosfamide-induced renal Fanconi's syndrome after only short-lasting chemotherapy with rather low cumulative doses (HENEY et al. 1989). These patients presented with a very abrupt onset of the renal disease, severe tubular acidosis and dehydration episodes due to diminished concentrating capacity. They probably represent a distinct entity, and an idiosyncratic reaction to the drug might be speculated upon; this fact though has never been examined.

The cumulative ifosfamide dose, especially if very high (>80 g/m^2), was shown to be of great importance (SKINNER et al. 1993b). The correlation of fractional phosphate reabsorption and cumulative ifosfamide dose seen in our patients after exclusion of all patients with nephrectomy and cisplatin therapy ($n=63$) was linear, although only weak ($r=-0.37$), indicating that other risk factors beside the cumulative dose might be of importance.

3.4.2 Reduction in Nephron Number

The highest frequency of renal Fanconi's syndrome after ifosfamide in one series of patients was reported to be 11.4% (BURK et al. 1990). All those patients had relapsed Wilms tumors and ifosfamide had been administered following unilateral nephrectomy. A high rate of renal Fanconi's syndrome after unilateral nephrectomy was recently confirmed (ROSSI et al. 1993). Operative reduction of kidney mass seems to be the single most important risk factor of ifosfamide-induced nephrotoxicity. The resulting higher single nephron load of any toxin applied after unilateral nephrectomy might explain this phenomenon, as shown for cisplatin-mediated nephrotoxicity in a rat model (JONGEJAN et al. 1986). Similarly, radiation-induced interstitial fibrosis leading to reduced glomerular filtration rates (WILLETT et al. 1986) may also lead to higher single nephron concentrations of toxic metabolites and thus further aggravate nephrotoxicity.

3.4.3 Platinum Compounds

Numerous case reports and retrospective (PRATT et al. 1991; ROSSI 1994) and prospective (CARON et al. 1992) studies have proposed the aggravation of ifosfamide-mediated nephrotoxicity by concomitant therapy with platinum compounds. Platinum has itself a nephrotoxic potential which is distinctly different from the "Fanconi-like" tubulopathy induced by ifosfamide (DAUGAARD and ABILDGAARD 1989) and mainly results in long-lasting reductions of glomerular filtration rate and renal magnesium loss (BIANCHETTI et al. 1990). The reduction of glomerular filtration rate after cisplatin can be avoided or diminished by salt load prior to cisplatin infusion (OZOLS et al. 1988) and this procedure has been incorporated into most of the chemotherapeutic regimens used. The glomerular filtration rate in our patients was not lower after ifosfamide/cisplatin combination chemotherapy compared to ifosfamide chemotherapy alone. Thus, reduced clearance of toxic ifosfamide metabolites cannot explain the aggravated ifosfamide-mediated toxicity in the presence of cisplatin. To date, the pathophysiological explanation for the influence of cisplatin in the aggravation of ifosfamide-mediated nephrotoxicity remains unclear. It may be noteworthy that carboplatin, although less nephrotoxic than cisplatin (HANNEMANN and BAUMANN 1990), was found to aggravate ifosfamide-mediated nephrotoxicity in a similar way as cisplatin (CARON et al. 1992).

3.4.4 Age of Primary Diagnosis

In the majority of case reports patients with overt renal Fanconi's syndrome after ifosfamide were less than 5 years of age, and even less than 2.5 years for the 4 patients reported by SUAREZ et al. (1991). Two studies (SHORE et al. 1992; SKINNER et al. 1992) supported this impression. In contrast, we were unable to find an influence of age of ifosfamide-induced nephrotoxicity of any grade, i.e., clinically apparent renal Fanconi's syndrome or tubulopathy, by multivariate analysis on 120 patients. In the series reported by SHORE et al. (1992) mean age for the "nephrotoxic" and "nonnephrotoxic" group was 87.1 ± 64.1 vs 103.8 ± 66.6 months. Applying the same statistical methods on our population of nephrotoxic ($n = 22$, renal Fanconi's syndrome and generalized tubulopathy) and nonnephrotoxic group mean ages for the nephrotoxic patients turned out to be even slightly higher (135 vs 118 months), but differences were not statistically significant. SKINNER et al. (1992) compared patients above ($n = 12$) and below ($n = 6$) 5 years of age after ifosfamide therapy only and found statistically significant lower values for the serum phosphorus level and percent glucose reabsorption, but not for five additional parameters of proximal tubular transport including fractional phosphate reabsorption. Applying the same statistical methods on our group (<5 years: $n = 12$; >5 years: $n = 51$) for patients after ifosfamide only there were no significant differences of tubular function but a higher serum phosphorus level in younger children and a corresponding trend for higher fractional phosphate reabsorption; these are physiological differences as younger children have higher values for both the serum phosphorus level and the fractional phosphate reabsorption (BRODEHL et al. 1982). To clarify the influence of age on ifosfamide-mediated nephrotoxicity greater studies including children of various ages after identical chemotherapy are necessary.

3.4.5 Concomitant Medication/Mode of Administration

Beside ifosfamide and cisplatin, potentially nephrotoxic medication in pediatric cancer patients may include methotrexate or supportive antibiotic therapy with gentamicin. These drugs both have a distinct nephrotoxic potential (methotrexate: FILLASTRE et al. 1988; gentamicin: KALOYANIDES and PASTORIZA-MUNOZ 1980) different from proximal tubulopathies induced by ifosfamide. In our series we did not find any influence of concomitant methotrexate medication on ifosfamide-induced nephrotoxicity of any grade (57 of 120 patients). Gentamicin may induce tubular enzyme excretion (STEINKAMP et al. 1986) in a similar way as ifosfamide (GOREN et al. 1989), but gentamicin therapy in 68 of 120 patients did not contribute to ifosfamide nephrotoxicity. A possible influence of other potentially nephrotoxic medication such as acyclovir or amphotericin B on renal function after ifosfamide has not been described to date, as these patients represent a very small subset of the populations in all studies published.

The administration mode of ifosfamide (i.v. push vs continuous infusion) has been thought to influence the nephrotoxicity of ifosfamide, but to date there are no convincing data that any particular administration mode may be less toxic. The rate of renal Fanconi's syndrome after high-dose ifosfamide was four of 47 patients (median cumulative dose 60 g/m^2) (SUAREZ et al. 1991), but two of 33 patients in our series (median cumulative dose 66 g/m^2). This rate is similar to that of SUAREZ et al. (1991), who gave ifosfamide as a bolus 1 h infusion (2 × 3 g/m^2 days 1 and 2), as opposed to the 6 g/m^2, given as a 48 h continuous infusion, reported here.

3.5 *Pathomechanism*

Ifosfamide is the only alkylating agent with this type of nephrotoxicity which suggests differences in metabolism to be a possible explanation: Side chain oxidation, virtually nonexistent for cyclophosphamide metabolism, accounts for approximately 20% of administered doses (BOOS et al. 1991) and may generate the nephrotoxic metabolite acrolein. The latter has not only been shown to be the cause of hemorrhagic cystitis (COX 1979) but was also found to be directly nephrotoxic to tubular cells (MOHRMANN et al. 1992). The urothelial toxicity of acrolein can virtually be abolished by mesna (MUNSHI et al. 1992) but molar concentrations of acrolein in both tubular lumen and cells have not been established. Acrolein is generated in cyclophosphamide metabolism as well and if it were the causative agent the described type of proximal tubular toxicity should, in principle, also be expected after cyclophosphamide. To date no single such report has been published. Chloroacetaldehyde is another metabolite thought to be responsible for ifosfamide-mediated nephrotoxicity (SKINNER et al. 1993a). It is generated during side chain oxidation, but so far proof confirming the relevance of this metabolite in ifosfamide-mediated nephrotoxicity is lacking.

3.6 *Prognosis*

The majority of patients who developed a clinically apparent renal Fanconi's syndrome after ifosfamide did not show normalization of their renal function. A few patients, though, have been reported to show complete recovery of renal dysfunction leading to healing of rickets (CARON et al. 1992, VAN GOOL et al. 1992). On repeated examination of subclinical impairment of renal function (SKINNER et al. 1990b) a trend towards deterioration was observed. Reexamination of the fractional phosphate reabsorption again indicated deterioration of this function over time in once established tubular damage (ROSSI et al. 1992b). Thus, the majority of reports seem to indicate a rather poor prognosis of once established renal tubular dysfunction after ifosfamide.

4 Summary and Therapeutic Recommendations

Ifosfamide should be regarded to be potentially nephrotoxic to every patient. Beside the cumulative ifosfamide dose, unilateral nephrectomy seems to be the single most important risk factor to precipitate ifosfamide-induced nephrotoxicity, and this drug should possibly be withheld in patients after operative reduction of kidney mass or tumorous infiltration of one kidney leading to a reduced nephron number. Platinum compounds have been shown to significantly enhance ifosfamide–mediated renal damage; consequently, the advisability of combination chemotherapy employing both ifosfamide and cisplatin should be discussed with reference to the prognosis of the malignant disease, definite proof of efficacy of both drugs for the given malignancy, and possible renal side effects.

Follow-up examinations of patients treated with ifosfamide are necessary over a prolonged period of time in order to identify patients at risk for the development of metabolic bone disease and to prevent growth failure by early supplementation therapy. Beside other tests, fractional phosphate reabsorption and serum biocarbonate level are most important to assess, as renal phosphate and bicarbonate loss are both directly related to the development of metabolic bone disease.

Future studies on ifosfamide nephrotoxicity should further define risk groups of patients, find a simple to use test to predict severe renal damage and, finally, clarify the pathomechanism of ifosfamide-induced renal damage.

References

Bianchetti MG, Kanaka C, Ridolfi-Lüthy A, Wagner HP, Hirt A, Paunier L, Peheim E, Oetliker OH (1990) Chronic renal magnesium loss, hypocalciuria and mild hy-

pokalaemic metabolic alkalosis after cisplatin. Pediatr Nephrol 4: 219–222
Boos J, Welslau U, Ritter J, Blaschke G, Schellong G (1991) Urinary excretion of the enantiomers of ifosfamide and its inactive metabolites in children. Cancer Chemother Pharmacol 28: 455–460
Brade W, Seeber S, Herdrich K (1986) Comparative activity of ifosfamide and cyclophosphamide. Cancer Chemother Pharmacol 18: [Suppl 2]: 1–9
Brandis M, Mohrmann M, van den Hardt K, Zimmerhackl LB (1992) Ifosfamide nephrotoxicity (abstract). Pediatr Nephrol 6: C90
Brodehl J, Gellissen K, Weber HP (1982) Postanatal development of tubular phosphate reabsorption. Clin Nephrol 17: 163–171
Brodehl J (1992) The Fanconi syndrome. In: Edelmann CM (ed) Pediatric kidney disease 2nd edn. Little and Brown, Boston, pp 1841–1871
Burk CD, Restaino I, Kaplan BS, Meadows AT (1990) Ifosfamide-induced renal tubular dysfunction and rickets in children with Wilms tumor. J Pediatr 117: 331–335
Caron HN, Abeling N, van Gennip A, de Kraker J, Voute PA (1992) Hyperaminoaciduria identifies patients at risk of developing renal tubular toxicity associated with ifosfamide and platinate containing regimes. Med Pediatr Oncol 20: 42–47
Cox PJ (1979) Cyclophosphamide cystitis – identification of acrolein as the causative agent. Biochem Pharmacol 28: 2045
Daugaard G, Abildgaard U (1989) Cisplatin nephrotoxicity – a review. Cancer Chemother Pharmacol 25: 1–9
de Fronzo RA, Abeloff M, Braine H, Humphrey RL, Davis PJ (1974) Renal dysfunction after treatment with isophosphamide (NSC 109724) Cancer Chemother Rep 58: 375–382
Fillastre JP, Viotte G, Morin JP, Moulin B (1988) Nephrotoxicity of antitumoral agents. Adv Nephrol 17: 175–218
Goren MP, Pratt CB, Viar MJ (1989) Tubular nephrotoxicity during longterm ifosfamide and Mesna therapy. Cancer Chemother Pharmacol 25: 70–72
Hannemann J, Baumann K (1990) Nephrotoxicity of cisplatin, carboplatin and transplatin. Arch Toxicol 64: 393–400
Heney D, Lewis IJ, Bailey CC (1989) Acute ifosfamide-induced tubular toxicity (letter to the editor). Lancet II: 103–104
Jongejan HTM, Provoost AP, Wolff ED, Molenaar JC (1986) Nephrotoxicity of cisplatin comparing young and adult rats. Pediatr Res 20: 9–14
Jürgens H, Treuner J, Winkler K, Göbel U (1989) Ifosfamide in pediatric malignancies. Semin Oncol 16: [Suppl 3] 46–50
Kaloyanides GJ, Pastoriza-Munoz E (1980) Aminoglycoside nephrotoxicity. Kidney Int 18: 571–582
Loehrer PJ Sr (1992) The history of ifosfamide. Semin Oncol 19: 2–6
Mohrmann M, Pauli A, Ritzer M, Schonfeld B, Seifert B, Brandis M (1992) Inhibition of sodium-dependent transport systems in LLC-PK1 cells by metabolites of ifosfamide. Renal Physiol Biochem 15(6): 289–301
Munshi NC, Loehrer PJ Sr, Williams SD, Langefeld C, Sledge C, Nichols CR, Roth BJ, Neumann A, Walsh WB, Einhorn LH (1992) Comparison of N-acetylcysteine and mesna as uroprotectors with ifosfamide combination chemotherapy in refractory germ cell tumors. Invest New Drugs 10(3): 159–163
Ozols RF, Cordon BJ, Jacobs J, Wesley M, Ostchega Y, Young RC (1988) High-dose cisplatin in hypertonic saline. Ann Intern Med 100: 19–24
Patterson WP, Khojasteh A (1989) Ifosfamide-induced renal tubular defects. Cancer 63: 649–651
Pratt CB, Green AA, Horowitz ME, Meyer WH, Etcubanas E, Douglass E, Hayes FA, Thompson E, Williams J, Igarashi M, Kovnar E (1986) Central nervous system toxicity following the treatment of pediatric patients with ifosfamide/mesna. J Clin Oncol 4: 1253
Pratt CB, Meyer WH, Jenkins JJ, Avery L, McKay CP, Wyatt RJ, Hancock ML (1991) Ifosfamide, Fanconi's syndrome and Rickets. J Clin Oncol 9: 1495–1499
Rossi R, Ehrich JHH (1993) Partial and complete de Toni-Debré-Fanconi syndrome after ifosfamide chemotherapy of childhood malignancy. Eur J Clin Pharmacol 44 (Suppl 1): S43–S45
Rossi R, Helmchen U, Schellong G (1992a) Tubular function and histological findings in ifosfamide-induced renal Fanconi syndrome – a report of two cases. Eur J Pediatr 151: 384–387
Rossi R, Ehrich JHH, Ullrich K, Riepenhausen M, Jürgens H (1992b) Ifosfamide and cisplatinum-induced tubular dysfunction – irreversible (abstract)? Proc Am Soc Clin Oncol 11: 130
Rossi R, Kleinebrand A, Gödde A, Rath B, Jürgens H (1993) Increased risk of ifosfamide-induced renal Fanconi's syndrome after unilateral nephrectomy. Lancet (letter to the editor) 341: 755
Rossi R, Danzebrink S, Hillebrand D, Linnenbürger K, Ullrich K, Jürgens H (1994) Ifosfamide-induced subclinical nephrotoxicity and its potentiation by cisplatinum. Med Pediatr Oncol 22: 27–32
Roussel B, Munzer M, Daoud S, Pennaforte F (1990) The de Toni-Debre-Fancone Syndrome in two children treated with ifosfamide (abstract). Pediatr Nephrol 4: C3
Shaw PJ, Eden T (1990) Ifosfamide in pediatric oncology: tried but not tested? Lancet 335: 1022–1023
Shore R, Greenberg M, Geary D, Koren G (1992): Iphosphamide-induced nephrotoxicity in children. Pediatr Nephrol 6: 162–165
Skinner R, Pearson ADJ, Price L, Coulthard MG, Craft AW (1990a) Nephrotoxicity after ifosfamide. Arch Dis Child 65: 732–738
Skinner R, Pearson ADJ, Price L, Coulthard MG, Craft AW (1990b) A follow-up study of Ifosfamide nephrotoxicity in children and adolescens (abstract). Med Pediatr Oncol 18: 5: 422
Skinner R, Pearson ADJ, Price L, Coulthard MG, Craft AW (1992) The influence of age on nephrotoxicity following chemotherapy in children. Br J Cancer 66: S30–S35
Skinner R, Sharkey IM, Pearson ADJ, Craft AW (1993a) Ifosfamide, mesna, and nephrotoxicity in children. J Clin Onocl 11: 173–190
Skinner R, Pearson ADJ, Price L, Wyllie RA, Coulthard MG, Craft AW (1993b) Cumulative dose is a major risk factor for the development of ifosfamide nephrotoxicity in children. International conference on the late effects of treatment for childhood malignancy, Manchester, 5–7 May (abstract O20)
Steinkamp G, Lütge M, Wurster U, Schulz-Baldes JG, Gröne HJ, Ehrich JHH (1986) Renal function in cystic fibrosis: proteinuria and enzymuria before and after tobramycin therapy. Eur J Pediatr 145: 526–531
Suarez A, McDowell H, Niaudet P, Comoy E, Flamant F (1991) Long-term follow-up of ifosfamide renal toxicity

in children treated for malignant mesenchymal tumors: an International Society of Pediatric Oncology report. J Clin Oncol 9: 2177–2182

van Gool S, Brock P, Wijndaele G, van de Casseye W, Kruger M, Proesmans W, Casteels-van Daele M (1992) Reversible hypophosphatemic rickets following ifosfamide treatment. Med Pediatr Oncol 20: 254–257

Willemse PHB, Jong PE de, Elema JD, Mulder NH (1989) Severe renal failure following high-dose ifosfamide and mesna. Cancer Chemother Pharmacol 23: 329–330

Willett CG, Tepper JE, Orlow EL, Shipley WU (1986) Renal complications secondary to radiation treatment of upper abdominal malignancies. Int J Radiat Oncol Biol Phys 12: 1601–1604

6.2 Radiation Nephritis

Michael Flentje

CONTENTS

1 Historical Background 215
2 Pathohistological Changes Related to Pathogenesis 215
3 Radiobiological Models 216
4 Clinical Manifestation 218
5 Clinical Implications 222
References 223

1 Historical Background

As early as the first decade of this century subacute nephritis and renal failure were observed after radiotherapy and attributed to radiation exposure of the kidneys (Baermann and Linser 1904). Whartin described three cases of eventually fatal renal impairment after abdominal irradiation for leukemia in 1907. However, two of his patients died within weeks, possibly due to uric acid nephropathy. Experimental studies looking at early effects after large single doses of radiation showed only minor histologic changes and mild proteinuria. More or less concealed was the fact that radiation-induced nephrotoxicity is rather of a delayed type and that the kidneys are probably the most radiosensitive structure in the abdomen.

In the 1920s it was acknowledged that radiation damage to the kidney histologically resembles chronic interstitial nephritis, and the typical clinical presentation of nephritis and hypertension, occurring 4–12 months after irradiation, was described (Domagk 1927; Doub et al. 1927; Hartman et al. 1927). In 1994 late-occurring hypertension, developing years after radiotherapy, was correlated with radiation injury (Dean and Abels 1944). Experimental studies in dogs showed that this condition was a distinct entity (Zollinger 1957). However, up to the early 1950s reports of radiation injury were anecdotal and not without controversy (Stephan 1920; Zuelzer et al. 1950). No exact dosimetry was available and, especially, no dose-volume response relationship was provided before the classical publications from the Christie Hospital in Manchester. In 1952 Paterson and also Kunkler et al. (1952) reported on how the long-term results of seminoma treatment actually deteriorated in the process of "optimizing" radiation treatment technique. This was related to the development of fatal renal complications as a consequence of increasing the radiation dose to the kidney. Luxton and Kunkler (1964) and Luxton (1961) retrospectively reconstructed the putative isodose distributions for the kidneys, described distinct clinical entities related to bilateral renal irradiation and deduced by and large still accepted tolerance doses for whole organ irradiation. The original approximated dose distributions, combined with incidences of nephrotoxicity, are given in Fig. 1.

2 Pathohistological Changes Related to Pathogenesis

Considerable controversy has arisen on the pathophysiological changes and the dominant target cell population in radiation-induced nephrotoxicity. In the first reported experimental study, atrophy of both glomeruli and renal tubules, associated with interstitial fibrosis, was described in the late stage of damage evolution. Looking at the time course of events, Bolliger and Laidley (1930) demonstrated that in the first 6 months after irradiation progressive degeneration of the tubulus epithelium with an interstitial proliferative reaction is prevalent. Sclerosis and atrophy of the glomeruli, seen in later stages, were thought to be secondary to the tubular damage. This conclusion is supported by recent work, particularly by Jordan et al. (1978), Phillips and Ross (1973) and Michalowski et al. (1986), who observed loss of tubulus epithelium starting at the most proximal parts in the renal

Michael Flentje, Prof. Dr., Strahlentherapeutische Klinik, Josef-Schneider-Straße 11, 97080 Würzburg, FRG

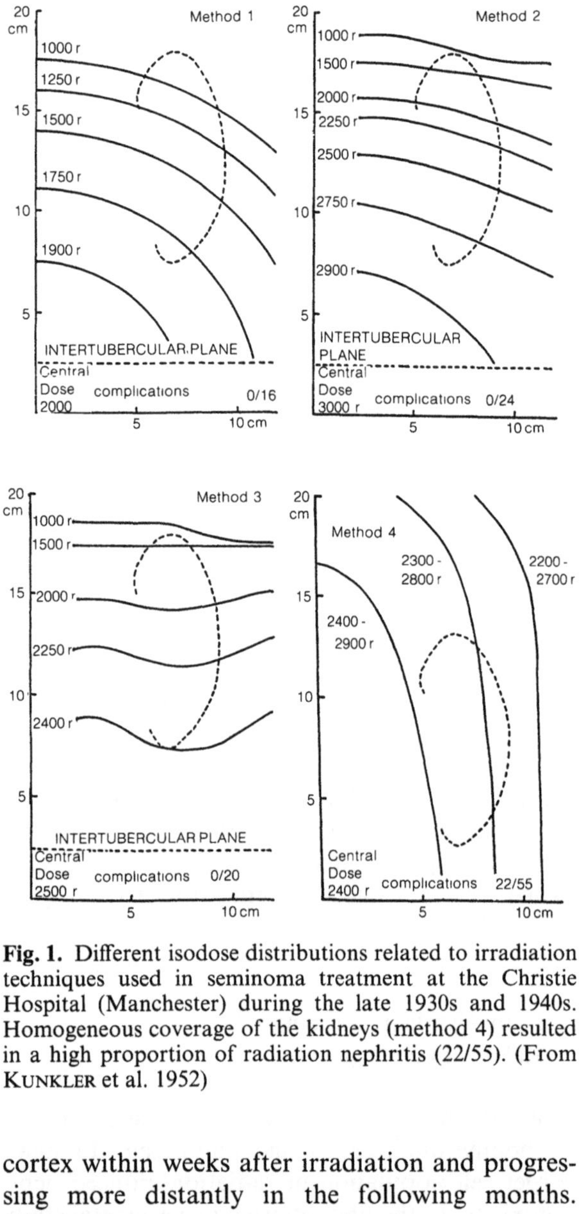

Fig. 1. Different isodose distributions related to irradiation techniques used in seminoma treatment at the Christie Hospital (Manchester) during the late 1930s and 1940s. Homogeneous coverage of the kidneys (method 4) resulted in a high proportion of radiation nephritis (22/55). (From KUNKLER et al. 1952)

cortex within weeks after irradiation and progressing more distantly in the following months. Glomerular changes were minor or nonexistent (JORDAN et al. 1978). Consistently the tubulus portion of the renal medulla seemed to be less affected. Whether this related to a physiologically lower oxygen tension in this part of the kidney or to the functional organization of the proliferative compartment is unknown.

Histopathologic changes suggesting that cellular damage in the glomerular apparatus is the most important cause of renal impairment were described by several authors (FAJARDO et al. 1976; GLATSTEIN et al. 1977), and MADRAZO and CHURG (1976) reported a simultaneous evolution of degeneration and sclerosis in the tubuli and glomeruli. There is no doubt that at a certain stage of injury vascular changes at the arteriolar and capillary level are an important facet of organ injury. Mesangial thickening due to fibrinoid deposits, cell degeneration and necrosis and areas of endothelial proliferation lead to vessel occlusion and rarefication paralleled by interstitial fibrosis. These findings form one of the fundamentals in the theories of RUBIN and CASARETT (1968), that damage to the interstitial connective tissue and especially the fine vasculature is the general mechanism in late radiation toxicity.

Notwithstanding the fact that radiation-induced damage and histopathologic changes seem to be progressive and functionally irreversible, proliferation of tubulus epithelium and even regeneration tubules have been commonly observed in irradiated kidneys (BOLLIGER and LAIDLEY 1930; SORANSON and DENEKAMP 1986; WITHERS et al. 1986). Typically these events take place in the time period in which clinical signs of radiation nephritis develop. It may well be that a damage related compensatory proliferation of "doomed" cells leads to an accelerated damage progression. This phenomenon, termed the "avalanche effect" by Michalowski et al., ties damage manifestation to the turnover time of a relevant cell type and readily explains the clinically observed, time-dependent "waves" of radiation injury (MICHALOWSKI 1986). A comprehensive review on experimental approaches and results in radiation-induced kidney damage has recently been given by STEWART and WILLIAMS (1991).

3 Radiobiological Models

The kidney has been used as a model system for studying tissues presenting a parallel architecture of independent substructures which maintain organ function. In radiation nephritis, this situation seems to be characterized by a behavior typical to radiation injury (WITHERS et al. 1988). WITHERS et al., using the concept of functional subunits (FSUs), postulated that the nephrons behave as biologically self-contained entities and that survival of a critical number of clonoges (cells with sufficient proliferative potential) within this subunit determines whether functional regeneration will occur after radiation exposure. If the FSUs act independently, one expects a threshold volume below which clinically detectable radiation damage is not present or only occurs at extremely high doses (leading to tissue necrosis). Above the threshold, the clinical complication probability should increase as a low-order function of the irradiated volume, corresponding to the increasing number of irradiated nephrons, whose independent individual complication probabilities contribute additively to the normal tissue complication probability (NTCP). If a certain number of FSUs are inactivated, the reserve capacity of the organ is exhausted and clinically relevant impairment is seen. This kind of volume dependence can be described by a power law relation as used in the currently employed algorithms by LYMAN and WOLBARST (1989), KUTCHER et al. (1991) and NIEMIERKO and GOITEIN (1991). Thus, a good representation of clinical tolerance data for whole kidney irradiation is obtained (BURMAN et al. 1991; EMAMI et al. 1991). For partial volume irradiation a better fit seems to be reached with models explicitly incorporating parallel architecture and functionally derived values for reserve capacity and heterogeneity within a patient population (YORKE et al. 1993). Interestingly, modeling of tissue tolerance using Poisson statistics leads to extremely steep dose-response relationships. YORKE et al. (1993) estimated that NTCP for lung should theoretically rise from 5% to 95% between 24.25 and 24.76 Gy. The considerably shallower relationship seen in clinical practice stresses the importance of individual variations in sensitivity (both regarding radiosensitivity and organ reserves) and confounding variables (dose reporting fractionation, volume and radiotherapy technique).

Three-dimensional spatial information on dose distributions was used in a historical series of 142 patients irradiated to the paraaortic region using predominantly rotational techniques, which led to variable, but partly substantial, exposure of the kidneys. Three-dimensional dose distributions were reconstructed retrospectively (FLENTJE et al. 1993). NTCPs for the kidneys were generated from the individual dose volume histograms for each patient using published algorithms.

Figure 2 shows that the rate of observed complications vs median dose and the best fit for NTCPs vs "ideal" median dose were in close correlation and well within the area between two logit curves representing modified dose distributions to allow for uncertainties in the retrospective analysis. The observed complication rate seemed to be placed slightly to the left from the predicted NTCP curve using the original power law relationship, possibly indicating a modest underestimation by this model and supporting predictions based on a parallel architecture model (YORKE et al. 1993) when inhomogeneous dose distributions are present. Alternatively, there may have been a slight but systematic underestimation of kidney exposure by the retrospective approach.

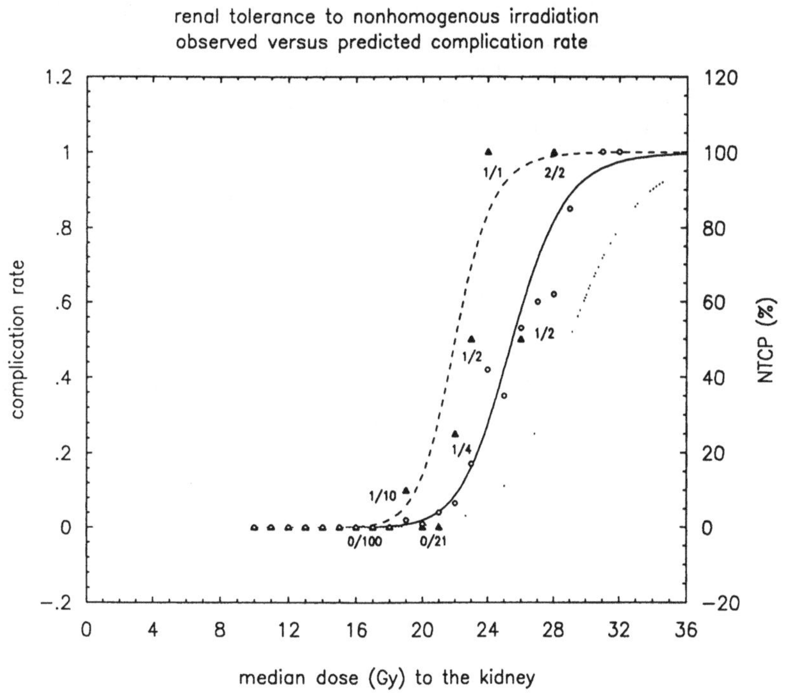

Fig. 2. Predicted (*open circles*) and observed (*filled triangles*) complication rate vs median dose to the kidneys. The estimates according to the Lyman algorithm are given. The number of complications vs persons at risk for each data point is also shown: Normal tissue complication probability (*NTCP*) points without related patient data have been calculated theoretically by using the dose volume histograms and changing the reference dose. (From FLENTJE et al. 1993)

This retrospective study showed the possibility to relate assumptions inherent in biophysical models to clinical data sets with regard to radiation nephritis. It has to be stressed that total organ irradiation with only a limited degree of inhomogeneity was present in the relevant patient group showing complications ($n = 7$). This may be the reason for the better immediate conformity between complication rate and NTCP estimate, for instance, in contrast to the data of LAWRENCE et al. (1992) on liver tolerance, in which considerable dose inhomogeneity was present.

However, due to the radiation techniques used, the dose per fraction to the kidney was considerably lower than the prescribed dose and in the range of 1 Gy and below. In theory, a considerable increase in tolerance should have resulted. The kidney has a marked capacity for repair of radiation damage during fractionated radiotherapy and numerous experimental studies have demonstrated that the isoeffect relationship is described by a linear quadratic function using an α/β of about 2.5 Gy for doses per fraction between 2 and 10 Gy (for review: STEWART and WILLIAMS 1991). Applying this relation to the data cited above in order to derive an isoeffective dose would require a $TD_{50/5}$ of about 22 Gy for conventional fractionation to yield an equivalent fit. This seems unreasonably low. A linear quadratic response relationship for single doses lower than 2 Gy is less feasible for the kidneys. Experiments using small doses per fraction suggested that there are major deviations from the linear quadratic model in this dose range and that X-ray effectiveness might be considerably larger than predicted (JOINER and JOHNS 1988; STEWART et al. 1987).

Furthermore, data on $TD_{50/5}$ rely mainly on the reports from KUNKLER, FARR and LUXTON (1952) and KIM et al. (1984). In both series dose per fraction to the kidneys for homogeneous irradiation was in the range of 1 Gy and below. These data, and our series with NTCPs for nonhomogeneous irradiation, suggest that the dose response for kidney tolerance to bilateral irradiation is very steep and that a $TD_{50/5}$ of 28 Gy for conventional fractionation irradiation may even slightly underestimate complication probabilities. Conversely, it is obvious that there is not enough clinical evidence to support the view that reducing the dose per fraction well below 2 Gy will allow an increase of total dose beyond the accepted tolerance doses.

4 Clinical Manifestation

Different syndromes, both in terms of latency and clinical presentation, are encountered. LUXTON and KUNKLER (1964) have separated four clinical entities after bilateral renal irradiation:

1. Acute radiation nephritis: latency period 6–12 months, with hypertension, edema, anemia and retention of urea and creatinine
2. Chronic radiation nephritis: latency 2–4 years, with proteinuria and loss of concentrating ability
3. Benign hypertension: latency 2–5 years, in combination with proteinuria
4. Late malignant hypertension: latency 1.5–11 years.

These syndromes were seen in a group of seminoma patients treated with 2500–3250 rads to the paraaortics using a technique that resulted in a homogeneous exposure of both kidney to approximately the same doses. Of the 55 patients, 22 developed severe renal complications. By comparing these data to previous treatments resulting in very inhomogeneous irradiation of the kidneys (Fig. 1) and preserved function they deducted the considerable influence of the irradiation volume factor. They concluded that doses between 27 and 25 Gy to a third of the kidneys were tolerated without nephritis if the dose to the upper third was below 17 Gy (KUNKLER et al. 1952). However, in a subsequent publication they noted that late hypertension might be caused also by partial kidney irradiation (LUXTON and KUNKLER 1964).

Overt radiation nephritis is diagnosed by relating a nephritic syndrome to previous radiotherapy at doses >20 Gy and the typical time interval. Anemia is hypochromic and throught to be both caused by erythroprotein deficiency and a hemolytic component. Clinical elevation of BUN and creatinine points to considerable impairment of renal function.

Hypertension after unilateral nephropathy is usually due to kidney atrophy and hypersecretion of renin (SHAPIRO et al. 1977). However the rare case of radiation-induced renal artery stenosis should be excluded, since management might be different.

Isotope techniques are particularly able to detect more subtle changes with high sensitivity. Creatinine clearance, loss of concentration ability, microalbuminuria as a sign of glomerular damage and excretion of small proteins (like retinol binding protein) suggesting tubular dysfunction can also be used to look for subclinical damage.

Reports in the literature of clinically observed dose-incidence relationships do not aid in establishing a correlation between higher doses and earlier presentation of damage or a more severe course of injury. This may reflect the fact that the threshold for radiation-induced nephrotoxicity is low and the dose-response is very steep. However, it should be kept in mind that the rather low number of reported cases and the range of doses received may preclude clinical recognition of subtle differences. Both in experimental kidney radiotoxicity and in terms of the general progression of late effects in normal tissues has a dependence of progression rate on dose been described (STEWART and WILLIAMS 1991; TURESSON 1989).

Delayed renal toxicity after total body irradiation (TBI) in the conditioning for allogeneic bone marrow transplantation (BMT), originally described by KAMIL et al. (1978), has been reported from several institutions. Doses used in TBI are considerably lower than the commonly accepted tolerance doses for renal injury (DEAN and ABELS 1944) and have been in the range of 12–14 Gy in six to nine fractions with dose rates between 0.05 and 0.2 Gy/min in the series commenting on nephrotoxicity. Clearly, a combination effect between kidney irradiation and: (1) high dose chemotherapy, (2) subclinical graft vs host disease, (3) renal toxicity of anti-fungal agents used in case of infection, and, (4) especially, cyclosporine, used for immunosuppression, has to be considered. Children seem to be at an increased risk. TARBELL et al. (1988) reported that six of 17 children transplanted for leukemia (conditioning regime Ara-C, cyclophosphamide and teniposide) and five of seven children with neuroblastoma (receiving cisplatin as part of their conditioning regime) developed renal dysfunction 4–7 months after TBI. Renal biopsies performed in two patients were compatible with radiation nephropathy.

In an experimental BMT model MOULDER and FISH (1991) found a shortened latency and a lowered threshold for radiation-induced nephritis when drugs such as BCNU or cisplatin were administered. Typically, cisplatin nephrotoxicity is enhanced when given 3–12 months after irradiation. This could be explained by additional drug-related damage superimposed on the progressive course of radiation injury (STEWART and WILLIAMS 1991). However, altered cisplatin excretion in an irradiated kidney has to be considered, and use of this drug after relevant kidney irradiation should be contemplated with caution. Nonetheless, the typical time course (onset 6–12 months after irradiation) and the histopathologic picture of TBI-related nephropathy point to a dominant role of radiotherapy, with total dose of particular importance. LAWTON et al. (1992) reported that the incidence of late renal dysfunction decreased from 26% to 6% in a series of 143 BMT patients when radiation to the kidneys was reduced from 14 to 12 Gy (in nine fractions) by partial shielding.

Renal tolerance to irradiation seems to be lowered in young children, especially after unilateral nephrectomy for Wilms' tumor. Delayed radiation nephritis has been reported at doses of 14 Gy to the remaining kidney (O'MALLEY et al. 1963). Hypertension, partly as a consequence of postirradiation renal artery stenosis (LANDMAN-PARKER et al. 1991), decreased glomerular filtration rate and proteinuria have also been reported.

LEVITT et al. (1992) studied 53 survivors after nephroblastoma treatment with a mean follow-up of 13 years. Children receiving >12 Gy to the remaining kidney did not show compensatory renal hypertrophy and had a statistically significant reduction in glomerular filtration rate. Four of 17 were treated for arterial hypertension. Interestingly, a group of children treated at an age <2 years and not irradiated also had compromised renal function. It was speculated that genetic abnormalities linked to nephroblastoma might cause predisposition to glomerular pathology. In a prospective study renal function was studied in 34 children 12–15 months after treatment for nephroblastoma. Glomerular filtration rate was, on average, 71% of normal in ten irradiated children (10–15 Gy to the kidney) vs 89% of normal in nonirradiated children with unilateral nephrectomy ($p = 0.03$). However, there were no clinical signs of kidney damage (DEGRAAF et al. 1990). Both in the ongoing NWTS and SIOP studies in Wilms' tumor, radiation dose to the remaining kidney is explicitly restricted to 12 Gy, requiring proper shielding if whole abdominal irradiation is necessary.

Long-term consequences of unilateral or partial renal irradiation are less well defined. Inclusion of the left kidney in treatment fields used for irradiation of the spleen, retroperitoneal malignancy and especially gastric lymphoma is commonly employed.

WILLET et al. (1986) reported on a series of 86 patients irradiated for different malignancies with a median follow-up of 3 years (1–9 years). The patients had received doses between 25 and >60 Gy to at least 50% of the left kidney. In four of 13 patients preexisting hypertension deteriorated and two patients developed arterial hypertension after radiotherapy. Using an indirect determination of creatinine clearance, the authors found that the mean clearance decreased about 10% in patients who had 50% of the kidney irradiated vs about 25% in patients in whom the entire left kidney was in the treatment field. There were no cases of overt renal failure. PÖTTER et al. (1993) studied 20 children with Hodgkin's disease (mean age 10 years at diagnosis, 7 year follow-up) and noted that local clearance was reduced after a dose of 30–40 Gy to the upper third of the left kidney and abolished at doses >40 Gy. Overall clearance was normal irrespective of the dose to the left upper pole in patients in whom the dose to both kidneys (rotational technique) was <15 Gy. However, total clearance was diminished about one standard deviation when the dose to both kidneys was >15 Gy. There were no cases of overt renal dysfunction or hypertension.

In summary, giving 40 Gy to the left kidney results in profound morphological damage and atrophy. Renal function assessed by isotope techniques and functional assays show a decrease of tubular function (Tc-DMSA uptake) and glomerular filtration rate in the irradiated kidney starting about 4–6 months after irradiation. However, no global renal impairment developed although the function of the left kidney was reduced to 20%–30%. In the series of 74 patients reported on by LEBOURGEOIS et al. (1979) the major part of the left kidney (30%–80%) received 40–45 Gy in 5.5 weeks. No cases of arterial hypertension were seen and plasma renin was normal in the five patients investigated. This finding is paralleled by the results of DEWIT et al. (1990), who did not see impairment of renal function in 27 patients studied prospectively and only a trend for increased blood pressure in patients irradiated with 40 Gy to the upper part ($n = 7$) or the whole left kidney ($n = 5$). Follow-up in both series was limited to 3–5 years and DEWIT et al. noted a progressive decline of scintigraphically determined parameters of tubular function during the observation period. This may explain the difference with the findings of THOMPSON et al. (1971) with a patient follow-up of up to 19 years after irradiation of the left kidney in the course of treatment of gastric ulcer with doses between 1500 and 3500 rads (most patients received 2000 rads). Hypertension and other signs of renal damage were seen in 31 of 84 patients with a median latency of 11 years. In only four patients did disease present within 5 years

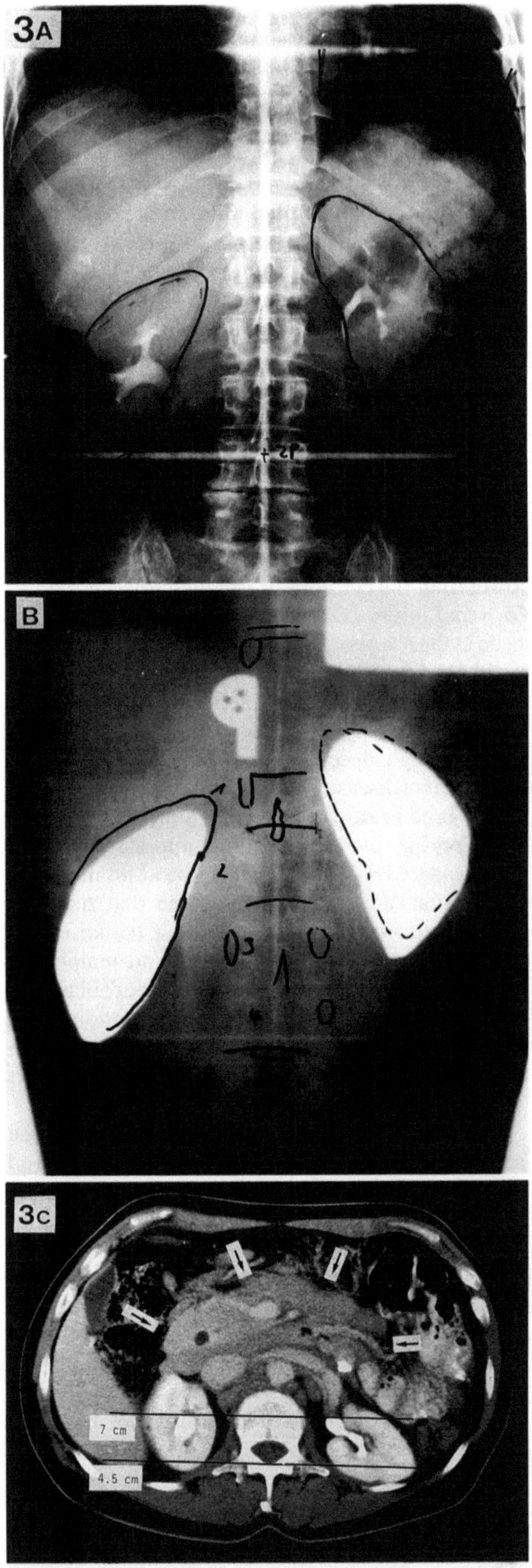

Fig. 3A–C.

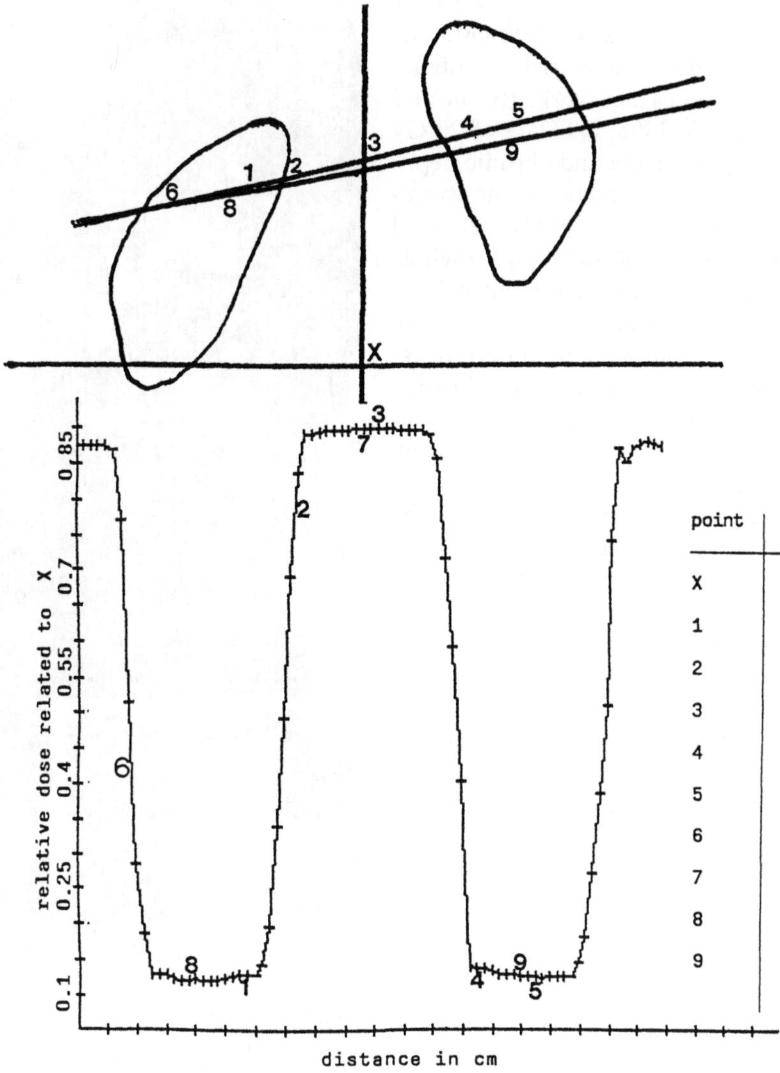

point	relative dose
X	1.00
1	0.12
2	0.79
3	0.96
4	0.13
5	0.11
6	0.42
7	0.93
8	0.15
9	0.14

D

Fig. 3A–D. Kidney shielding in radiotherapy of the whole abdomen in a patient with lymphocytic lymphoma (*arrows*). The kidneys are shielded from posterior and 20 Gy are given with opposing AP/PA fields. Then 10 Gy are given using a 3-field box. **A** The kidneys are localized using urography during simulation. **B** Correct positioning of the satellites is verified using subtrascopic comparison with the simulator radiograph. **C** Dose distribution in a central plane through the kidneys with shielding blocks. **D** Reconstructed dose profile by treatment planning program and relative doses measured in a phantom using a ionization chamber (1–6 depths 4.5 cm from posterior surface; 7–9 depths 7 cm from posterior surface). Transmitted and scattered radiation result in exposure of the tissue under the satellites of about 12%–15%

of irradiation. The very high incidence of hypertension and renal disturbances may in part be explained by reported additional noxes like gout nephritis ($n = 2$), analgesics abuse ($n = 5$) and diabetes ($n = 2$). No cases of arterial hypertension were observed in a retrospective analysis of 3000 patients irradiated for peptic ulcer over a period of 30 years (dose to the major part of the left kidney in the range of 16 Gy; Clayton et al. 1968). This result, however, seems at variance with the prevalence of idopathic hypertension in the adult population.

From these data it may be concluded that global excretory function is not compromised by unilateral or partial kidney irradiation as clearance is preserved by the unirradiated organ parts which may show functional and even anatomical hypertrophy. This supports current radiotherapy practice if partial kidney exposure cannot be reasonably avoided. However, hypertension may be a long-term sequela and only studies with considerable follow-up can adequately adress this question. The true risk is still a matter of some uncertainty.

The reported data have been employed to define tolerance doses. A summary of the available literature in 1983 was used by Cohen and Creditor to test their cell kinetic model for radiation-induced tissue damage. They derived a TD5/5 between 21 and 31 Gy in 4–6 weeks for daily treatment. The authors stressed the considerable risk of higher fraction doses. Based on earlier work, RUBIN and WASSERMAN described, in 1988, a TD5/5 of 20 Gy and TD50/5 of 25 Gy for acute and chronic nephrosclerosis using conventional fractionation. By updating these reports EMAMI et al. (1991) reported a TD 5/5 of 23 Gy and a TD 50/5 of 28 Gy for whole kidney irradiation and extrapolated tolerance doses for partial volume irradiation. These doses are not truly measured data but have been derived by analyzing reports from the literature (partly historical and representing remarkable diversity in techniques, doses and fractionation) and by using personal experience and opinion. Uncertainties regarding dosimetry and follow-up have to be considered and are discussed by EMAMI et al. (1991).

5 Clinical Implications

The kidneys are obviously the most sensitive tissue to be considered in radiotherapy of the abdomen (excluding the gonads). In radiotherapy practice, 20 Gy to the kidneys, including irradiation contributed from scattering, seem to be the maximum dose justifiable, requiring appropriate shielding in radiotherapy of the whole abdomen as performed in treatment of lymphoma or ovarian cancer. Even lower doses are close to tolerance in small children and in TBI conditioning for bone marrow transplantation. The interaction with nephrotoxic anticancer chemotherapy, cyclosporine and antibiotics should be carefully considered.

Different shielding techniques have been described. Total doses of 25–30 to the whole abdomen are tolerated using parallel opposing AP/PA fields and fraction doses of about 1.5 Gy if the kidneys are shielded from posterior (6 HVL) during the whole course of treatment. In our institution open fields are used until a dose of 13.5 Gy is reached. After this, both AP and PA shielding is employed. Treatment planning using urography during simulation, verification of correct position of blocks during treatment and dosimetry is shown in Fig. 3. No cases of renal impairment have been encountered in our institution using this setup.

Treatment of paraaortic lymph nodes typically involves the most medially located parts of the kidneys. Clinical practice proves that this form of partial volume irradiation is tolerated without sequelae. Inclusion of the spleen and the splenic

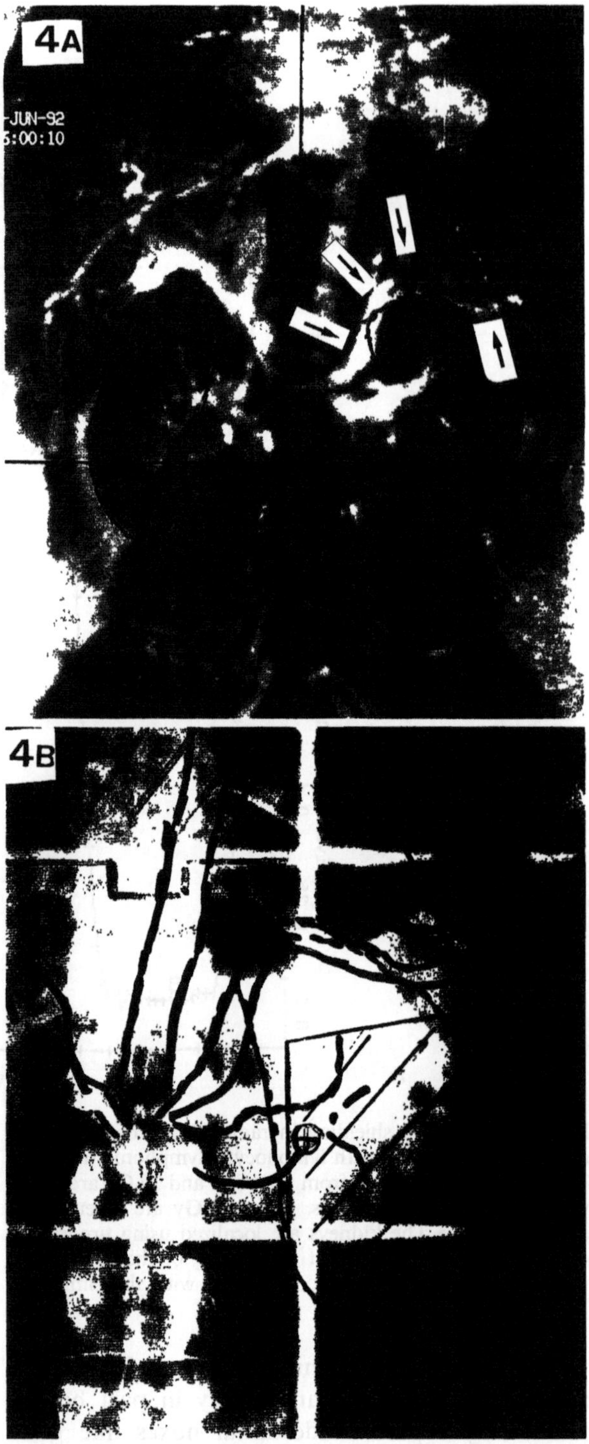

Fig. 4A, B. Magnetic resonance (MR)-based localization of the spleen and the splenic vessels. Structures from an electronically generated coronary MR of the abdomen (composed of a T1-weighted sequence and MR angiography) (**A**) are superimposed onto the simulator radiograph using a subtrascope (**B**). The position of the splenic pedicle with regard to the left kidney is clearly visualized (*arrows*)

pedicle, as often employed in radiotherapy of Hodgkin's disease, generally demands inclusion of the upper parts of the left kidney in the treatment field. As the long-term consequences in terms of hypertension are still debatable, meticulous treatment planning to spare as much kidney as possible seems warranted. Localization of the splenic vessels can be done either by use of conventional angiography (PÖTTER et al. 1989) or magnetic resonance (MR) based techniques (KÖSTER et al. 1992; Fig. 4). The value of these procedures is supported by the finding that location of the splenic vessels with regard to the left kidney shows considerable anatomical variability. KÖSTER et al. described that the splenic pedicle projected onto the upper third of the left kidney only in 24 of 38 studied cases (in eight patients position below, in six above) and on average 32% of the left kidney volume could be spared by use of individual localization.

Functional mobility during breathing excursions and topographic changes in supine and prone position have been determined by VOSS et al. (1975). They found maximum variations between 2 and 7 cm in the longitudinal axis. As most patients tend to keep a midline respiratory state during radiation treatment, this seems of less practical concern. However, change between prone and supine position for opposing field treatment requires very exact localization of the respective kidney position and should be avoided, if possible.

Current knowledge of kidney tolerance levels and attention to appropriate treatment techniques will prevent overt radiation nephritis. Avoidance of more insidious long-term sequelae of dimished organ reserve and the development of late hypertension after cure of malignancy demands even greater effort to spare as much renal tissue as possible from high dose irradiation.

References

Baermann G, Linser P (1904) Über die lokale und allgemeine Wirkung der Röntgenstrahlen. Münch Med Wochenschr 51: 996–999

Bolliger A, Laidley JWS (1930) Experimental renal disease produced by X-rays. Histological changes in the kidney exposed to a measured amount of unfiltered rays of medium wavelength. Med J Aust 1: 136–147

Burman C, Kutcher GJ, Emami B, Goitein M (1991) Fitting of normal tissue tolerance to an analytic function. Int J Radiat Oncol Biol Phys 21: 123–135

Clayman CB, Palmer WL, Kirsner JB (1968) Gastric irradiation in the treatment of peptic ulcer. Gastroenterology 55: 403–407

Cohen L, Creditor M (1983) Iso-effect tables for tolerance of irradiated normal human tissues. Int J Radiat Oncol Biol Phys 9: 223–241

Deal AL, Abels JC (1944) Study by the newer renal function tests of an unusual case of hypertension following irradiation of the kidney and the relief of the patient by nephrectomy. J Urol 52: 497–501

deGraaf SSN, van Luyk WHJ, Tamminga RYJ, Mehta DM (1990) Prospective study of renal function in Wilams' tumor patients. Proc AACR 31: 202

Dewit L, Anninga JK, Hoefnagel CA, Nooijen WJ (1990) Radiation injury in the human kidney: a prospective analysis using specific scientigraphic and biochemical endpoints. Int J Radiat Oncol Biol Phys 19: 977–983

Domagk G (1927) Röntgenstrahlenschädigung der Niere beim Menschen. Med Klin 23: 345–347

Doub HP, Bolliger A, Hartman EW (1927) The relative sensitivity of the kidney to irradiation. Radiology 8: 142–148

Emami B, Lyman J, Brown A, Coia L, Goitein M, Munzenrider JE, Shank B, Solin LJ, Wesson M (1991) Tolerance of normal tissue to therapeutic irradiation. Int J Radiat Oncol Biol Phys 21: 109–122

Fajardo LF, Brown JM, Glatstein E (1976) Glomerular and juxtaglomerular lesions in radiation nephropathy. Radiat Res 68: 177–183

Flentje M, Hensley F, Gademann G, Menke M, Wannenmacher M (1993) Renal tolerance to nonhomogenous irradiation. Comparison of observed effects to predictions of normal tissue complication probability from different biophysical models. Int J Radiat Oncol Biol Phys 27: 25–30

Glatstein E, Brown RC, Fajardo LF, Brown JM (1977) Radiation injury in the mouse kidney. Int J Radiat Oncol Biol Phys 2: 933–943

Hartman EW, Bolliger A, Doub P (1927) Functional studies throughout the course of roentgen-ray nephritis. JAMA 88: 139–145

Joiner MC, Johns H (1988) Renal damage in the mouse: the response to very small doses per fraction. Radiat Res 114: 385–398

Jordan SW, Key CR, Gomez LS, Agnew J, Barton SL (1978) Late effects of radiation on the mouse kidney. Exp Mol Pathol 29: 115–129

Kamil ES, Latta H, Johnston WH, Feig SA, Bergstein JM (1978) Radiation nephritis following bone marrow transplantation. Kidney Int 14: 713

Kim TH, Somerville PJ, Freeman CR (1984) Unilateral nephropathy – the longterm significance. Int J Radiat Biol Oncol Phys 10: 2053–2059

Köster A, Kimmig B, Müller-Schimpfle M, Brix G, Semmler W, Wannenmacher M (1992) MR-Tomographie und MR-Angiographie- eine neue Methode zur Bestrahlungsplanung abdomineller Großfelder. Strahlenther Onkol 168: 230–236

Kunkler PB, Farr RF, Luxton RW (1952) The limit of renal tolerance to X-rays. Br J Radiol 25: 190–201

Kutcher GJ, Burman C, Brewster MS, Goitein M, Mohan R (1991) Histogram reduction method for calculating complication probabilities for 3-D treatment planning evaluations. Int J Radiat Oncol Biol Phys 21: 137–146

Lawrence TS, TenHaken RK, Kessler ML, Robertson JM, Lyman JT, Lavigne ML, Brown MB, DuRoss DJ, Andrews JC, Ensminger WD, Lichter AS (1992) The Use of 3-D dose volume analysis to predict radiation hepatitis. Int J Radiat Oncol Biol Phys 23: 781–788

Lawton CA, Barber-Derus SW, Murray KJ, Cohen EP, Ash RC, Moulder JE (1992) Influence of renal shielding on the incidence of late renal dysfunction associated with T-lymphocyte deplete bone marrow transplantation in adult patients. Int J Radiat Oncol Biol Phys 23: 681–686

LeBourgeois JP, Meignan M, Parmentier C, Tubiana M (1979) Renal consequences of irradiation of the spleen in lymphoma patients. Br J Radiol 52: 52–60

Landman-Parker J, Tournade MF, Habrand JL, Raquin M, Lemerle J (1991) Late renal sequelae after unilateral nephrectomy for Wilms'tumor treatment; 20 year follow-up. Proc ASCO 10: A1084

Levitt GA, Yeomans E, Dicks Mireaux C, Breatnach F, Kingston J, Pritchard J (1992) Renal size and function after cure of Wilms' tumor. Br J Cancer 66: 877–882

Luxton RW, Kunkler PB (1964) Radiation nephritis. Acta Radiol Ther Phys Biol 2: 169–176

Luxton RW (1961) Radiation nephritis: a longterm study of 54 patients. Lancet II: 1221–1224

Lyman J, Wolbarst B (1989) Optimization of radiation therapy, IV: a dose-volume histogram reduction algorithm. Int J Radiat Oncol Biol Phys 17: 433–436

Moulder JE, Fish BL (1991) Influence of nephrotoxic drugs on the late renal toxicity associated with bone marrow transplant conditioning regimens. Int J Radiat Oncol Biol Phys 20: 333–337

Madrazo A, Churg J (1976) Radiation nephritis: chronic changes following moderate doses of radiation. Lab Invest 34: 283–290

Michalowski A (1986) The pathogenesis of the late side effects of radiotherapy. Clin Radiol 37: 203–207

Michalowski A, Cullen BM, Burgin J, Rogers MA (1986) Development of structural renal damage and its quantitation. Br J Cancer 53 (S7): 295–298

Niemierko A, Goitein M (1991) Calculation of normal tissue complication probability and dose-volume reduction schemes for tissues with a critical element architecture. Radiother Oncol 20: 166–176

O'Malley B, D'Angio GJ, Vawter GJ (1963) Late effects of roentgen therapy given in infancy. AJR 89: 1067–1074

Paterson R (1952) Renal damage from radiation during treatment of seminoma testis. J Fac Radiol 3: 370–374

Phillips TL, Ross G (1973) A quantitative technique for measuring renal damage after irradiation. Radiology 109: 457–462

Pötter R, Sank J, Haverkamp U (1989) Digital subtraction angiography (iv DSA) in treatment planning of subdiaphragmatic Hodgkin's disease. Int J Radiat Oncol Biol Phys 17: 389–396

Pötter R, Roes F, Schellong G, Bartenstein P, Brämswig JH, von Lengerke HJ, Rath B, Mohring R, Rossi R (1993) Subclinical impairment of renal function after radiotherapy for Hodgkin's disease in children. In: Hinkelbein W et al. (eds) Acute and long-term side effects of radiotherapy. Springer, Berlin Heidelberg New York, pp 259–277 (Recent results in cancer research, vol 130)

Rubin P, Casarett GW (1968) The kidney. In: Rubin P, Casarett GW (eds) Clinical radiation pathology. Saunders, Philadelphia, pp. 293–333

Rubin P, Wasserman TH (1988) The late effects of toxicity scoring. Int J Radiat Oncol Biol Phys 14(S): 29–38

Shapiro AP, Cavallo T, Cooper W, Lapenas D, Bron K, Berg G (1977) Hypertension in radiation nephritis. Arch Intern Med 137: 848–851

Soranson J, Denekamp J (1988) Recipitation of latent renal radiation injury by unilateral nephrectomy. Br J Cancer 53: 268–272

Stephan O (1920) Über die Steigerung der Zellfunktion durch Röntgenenergie. Strahlentherapie 11: 517–562

Stewart FA, Oussoren Y, Luts A, Begg AC, Dewit L, Lebesque J, Bartelink H (1987) Repair of sublethal damage radiation injury after multiple small doses in mouse kidney: an estimate of flexure dose. Int J Radiat Biol Oncol Phys 13: 765–772

Stewart FA, Williams MV (1991) The urinary tract. In: Scherer E, Streffer CH, Trott KR (eds) Radiopathology of organs and tissues. Springer, Berlin Heidelberg New York, pp 405–432

Tarbell NJ, Guinan EC, Niemeyer C, Mauch P, Sallan SE, Weinstein HJ (1988) Late onset of renal dysfunction in survirors of bone marrow transplantation. Int J Radiat Oncol Biol Phys 15: 99–104

Thompson PL, Mackay IR, Robson GSM, Wall AJ (1971) Late radiation nephritis after gastric x-irradiation for peptic ulcer. Q J Med 40: 145–157

Turesson I (1989) The progression rate of late radiation effects in normal tissue and its impact on dose response relationships. Radiother Oncol 15: 217–226

Voss AC, Wöllgens P, Rey G (1975) Untersuchungen über die Lageveränderung der Nieren und Folgerungen für die Strahlentherapie der Nierentumoren zur Optimierung der Bestrahlungsplanung. Strahlentherapie 150: 551–556

Warthin AS (1907) The changes produced in the kidneys by roentgen irradiation. Am J Med Sci 133: 736–746

Willett CG, Tepper JE, Orlow EL, Shipley WU (1986) Renal complications secondary to radiation treatment of upper abdominal malignancies. Int J Radiat Oncol Biol Phys 12: 1601–1604

Withers HR, Mason KA, Thames HD (1986) Late radiation response of kidney assayed by tubule cell survival. Br J Radiol 59: 587–597

Withers HR, Taylor JMG, Maciejewsky B (1988) Treatment volume and tolerance. Int J Radiat Biol Oncol Phys 14: 751–759

Yorke ED, Kutcher GJ, Jackson A, Ling CC (1993) Probability of radiation induced complications in normal tissues with parallel architecture under conditions of uniform whole or partial organ irradiation. Radiother Oncol 26: 226–237

Zollinger HU (1951) Hypertonie nach experimenteller Röntgenbestrahlung der Nieren. Schweiz Z Pathol Bakteriol 14: 366

Zuelzer NW, Palmer HD, Newton WA (1950) Unusual glomerulonephritis in young children, probably radiation nephritis; reorts of three cases. Am J Pathol 26: 1019–1039

7 Gonadal Toxicity

7.1 Long-Term Gonadal Dysfunction and Its Impact on Bone Mineralization in Patients Following COPP/ABVD Chemotherapy for Hodgkin's Disease

ERNST-D. KREUSER, DIETER FELSENBERG, CHRISTIAN BEHLES, and ECKHARD THIEL

CONTENTS

1 Introduction 227
2 Material and Methods 227
2.1 Patients and Treatment 227
2.2 Diagnostic Procedures for Assessing Gonadal Toxicity 228
2.3 Diagnostic Procedures for Assessing Bone Mineralization 228
2.4 Statistical Methods 228
3 Results 229
3.1 Hormonal Evaluation 229
3.2 Semen Analysis 229
3.3 Questionnaire 229
3.4 Bone Mineral Density Measurements 229
4 Discussion 230
5 Summary 231
References 233

1 Introduction

Advances in the treatment of all stages of Hodgkin's disease with chemotherapy and irradiation have led to the expectation of long-term survival of more than 70% of patients (LONGO 1990). This recent success of multimodal treatment has focused attention on long-term adverse effects, including second malignancies (KALDOR et al. 1990; CIMINO et al. 1991) and gonadal toxicity (KREUSER et al. 1987; BONADONNA et al. 1984). More than three cycles of MOPP (mechlorethamine, vincristine, procarbazine, prednisone), COPP, (cyclophamide, vincristine, procarbazine, prednisone), or similar regimens are known to produce significant and mostly irreversible testicular failure (DA CUNHA et al. 1984), whereas ovarian and testicular dysfunction is considerably less severe after the ABVD (adriamycin, bleomycin, vinblastine, dacarbazine) regimen (BONADONNA et al. 1984). The impact on gonadal functions, however, of chemotherapy combining the COPP and ABVD regimen has not yet been carefully examined.

The implications of cytotoxically induced gonadal injury in patients cured of Hodgkin's disease go beyond potential infertility and involve impaired gonadal steroid synthesis, which may lead to metabolic or cardiovascular dysfunctions. Among the metabolic disorders, bone loss after prematurely induced ovarian failure merits pronounced consideration in order to estimate the risk of osteoporosis and fractures in long-term survivors (REDMANN et al. 1988). A large body of information supports the causal role of estrogen deficiency in the pathogenesis of bone demineralization (JOHNSTON et al. 1991).

Bone mass can be measured safely, accurately, and precisely by a number of techniques calculating bone density on the basis of tissue absorption of photons derived from either a radionuclide or an X-ray tube (JOHNSTON et al. 1991). However, the various methods for predicting fracture risk in patients treated for Hodgkin's disease have not been applied so far. The present study was therefore conducted to evaluate the impact of the COPP/ABVD regimen on gonadal functions and bone density in patients treated for Hodgkin's disease.

2 Material and Methods

2.1 *Patients and Treatment*

A total of 49 patients with Hodgkin's disease were evaluated 1–8 years after chemotherapy. All eligible patients were asked to participate in this study on the late effects of therapy. Patients fulfilling the following selection criteria were included: histologically confirmed Hodgkin's disease, age at diagnosis 14–60 years in men and 14–50 in women, complete remission >1 year. Exclusion criteria consisted of radiation therapy only, Karnofsky

ERNST-D. KREUSER, Prof. Dr., CHRISTIAN BEHLES, Dr., ECKHARD THIEL, Prof. Dr., Klinik für Innere Medizin, Universitätsklinikum Steglitz, Abteilung Hämatologie und Onkologie, Hindenburgdamm 30, 12203 Berlin, FRG
DIETER FELSENBERG, Dr., Universitätsklinkum Steglitz, Abteilung Radiologie, Hindenburgdamm 30, 12203 Berlin, FRG

Table 1. Demographic and clinical features

Characteristics	*n*
Evaluable patients	49
Age at the time of study	
Median	39
Range	21–60
Age at the time of diagnosis	
Median	35
Range	15–58
Sex	
Male	27
Female	22
Chemotherapy	
COPP/ABVD	26
COPP	23
Mantle field irradiation	31
Number of courses	
Median	6
Range	3–9
Time of evaluation (years)	
Median	4.3
Range	1–10

COPP, cyclophosphamide, vincristine, procarbazine, prednisone; ABVD, adriamycin, bleomycin, vinblastine, dacarbazine.

performance status < 50%, and relapse < 1 year. Further patient characteristics are summarized in Table 1.

The study population was derived from a group of patients consecutively enrolled in the German Hodgkin Study Group protocols. From July 1983 to March 1988, 20 patients with Hodgkin's disease classified as stage IIIB or stage IVA/B according to the Ann Arbor criteria received the COPP/ABVD regimen ± irradiation at our institution. The complete HD3 treatment program of the prospective randomized trial was published previously (Loeffler et al. 1991). Patients received three double cycles of alternating COPP + ABVD followed by complete restaging. Patients in complete remission were randomized to receive consolidation treatment by radiotherapy (involved field) with 20 Gy or chemotherapy (one double cycle COPP/ABVD). COPP was given as a modification of the MOPP regimen, mechlorethamine being replaced by cyclophosphamide.

Six patients were treated according to the ongoing HD6 protocol of the German Hodgkin Study Group. Patients classified as stage IIIB, IVA/B were randomized to receive COPP/ABVD × 4 or COPP/ABV/IMEP (ifosfamide, methotreate etoposide, prednisone) × 4 + 30 Gy to bulk or slow-responding areas. In addition, 23 patients treated according to the COPP regimen were examined in order to compare the toxicity of the anthracycline-based regimen with that of COPP chemotherapy.

The COPP/ABVD regimen consisted of: cyclophosphamide (650 mg/m^2 i.v. days 1 + 8), vincristine (1.4 mg/m^2 i.v. days 1 + 8), procarbazine (100 mg/m^2 po days 1–14), prednisone (40 mg/m^2 po days 1–14), doxorubicin (25 mg/m^2 i.v. days 29 + 43), bleomycin (10 mg/m^2 i.v. days 29 + 43), (vinblastine (6 mg/m^2 i.v. days 29 + 43), and decarbazine (375 mg/m^2 i.v. day 295 + 43); recycle day 57.

2.2 Diagnostic Procedures for Assessing Gonadal Toxicity

In order to evaluate gonadal toxicity in men, blood samples were tested for follicle-stimulating hormone (FSH), luteinizing hormone (LH), inhibin-α subunits, and testosterone. In women, FSH, LH, 17β-estradiol, and progesterone were measured. Semen analysis was performed in 15 men treated with the COPP/ABVD regimen. Furthermore, all patients were asked to answer questions regarding fertility, sexuality, and symptoms related to hormone deficiency.

2.3 Diagnostic Procedures for Assessing Bone Mineralization

To evaluate the impact of multidrug chemotherapy on bone mineralization, we measured bone density using dual-energy quantitative computed tomography (DEQCT) on a SOMATOM DR scanner (Siemens, Erlangen, Germany) at lumbar vertebrae L_1-L_3 and single-energy quantitative computed tomography (SEQCT) on an SCT 900 (Stratec, Munich, Germany) at the radius. At the calcaneus, we used single-photon absorptiometry (SPA) with ^{125}I as the source of photons and a nuclear detector DATA ND 555 (Fa. Nuclear Data, Frankfurt, Germany).

2.4 Statistical Methods

The design of the present study was a retrospective one with age- and sex-matched controls. The Wilcoxon test (two-sided) for unpaired samples was carried out in order to compare hormone levels and bone densities in different subgroups. Raw data (means ± SEM) are presented. In multiple comparisons, the Bonferroni correction was applied to the levels of significance. When $p < 0.05$, the difference was considered to be statistically significant. Uni- and multivariate analyses were done using logistic regression models.

3 Results

3.1 Hormonal Evaluation

Serum FSH levels were increased in 21 of 27 (80%) men, ranging from 6–44 U/l (median 17 U/l) 1–8 years after therapy. Median FSH levels did not differ significantly between men with COPP and those with COPP/ABVD chemotherapy (Fig. 1). In contrast, the median FSH level was significantly higher than in 20 healthy males (Fig. 1; $p = 0.003$). Testosterone values were within normal limits in all men with no statistically significant difference compared to age-matched controls (data not shown). Therapy-induced ovarian failure occured in 17 of 22 (77%) women 1–8 years after therapy. There was a statistically significant difference in FSH levels between women with normal ovarian function and those suffering from therapy-induced ovarian failure with or without estrogen replacement (Fig. 1). All women with primary ovarian failure had increased FSH and LH levels and decreased 17β- estradiol and progesterone values. Five of 22 (23%) women retained normal ovarian function after chemotherapy with the COPP/ABVD regimen. All these women were under the age of 30 at the time of therapy.

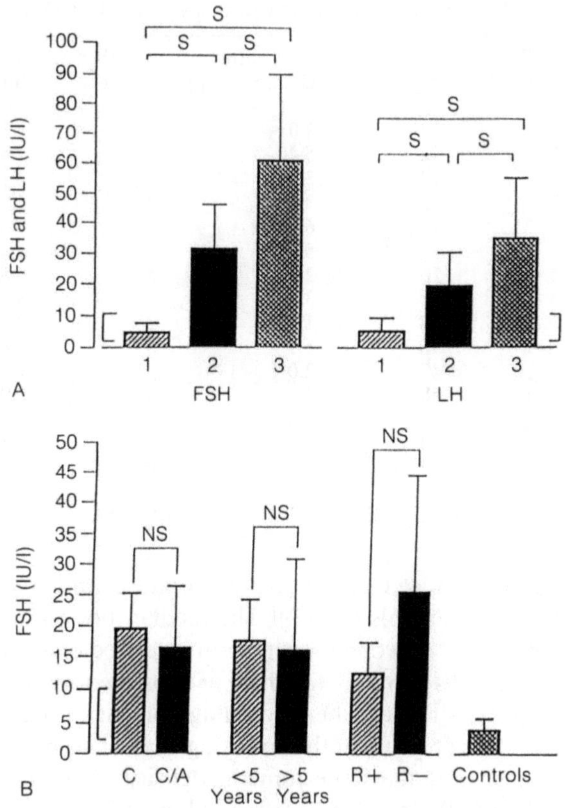

Fig. 1A, B. **A** Serum FSH and LH levels in female patients who received chemotherapy for Hodgkin's disease. FSH and LH levels are within normal limits in female patients with normal ovarian function (1) and significantly increased in women with ovarian failure (*2*, + estrogen; *3*, − estrogen). **B** Serum FSH levels in male patients treated for Hodgkin's disease. FSH levels are significantly increased in all subgroups compared to controls. *C*, COPP chemotherapy; *C/A*, COPP/ABVD chemotherapy; *< 5 years*, interval between chemotherapy and this study less than 5 years; *> 5 years* more than 5 years; *R +*, infradiaphragmatic radiation: *R-*, no infradiaphragmatic radiation

3.2 Semen Analysis

Semen analysis was performed in 15 patients treated according to the COPP/ABVD regimen. As presented in Table 2, 13 of 15 (86%) showed azoospermia and two of 15 (13%) severe oligozoospermia. In six of 15 patients, the interval between therapy and the time point of this study exceeded 5 years, thus suggesting stem cell depletion during COPP/ABVD chemotherapy without evidence of a recovery of spermatogenesis.

3.3 Questionnaire

All men and women completed the questionnaire. None of the women became pregnant after chemotherapy. Two men fathered two healthy children each after chemotherapy for Hodgkin's disease. Normal sexual functions were reported in 80% of men. Analysis of menstrual history revealed that only five of 22 (23%) women retained normal ovarian function after therapy. All of them were under the age of 30 at the time of therapy, indicating an age-related risk of treatment-induced ovarian failure. Although 11 of 17 (64%) women with therapy-induced ovarian failure suffered from premature menopausal symptoms, only six received estrogen replacement therapy.

3.4 Bone Mineral Density Measurements

We found a statistically significant difference ($p = 0.001$) in bone densities between women with

Table 2. Semen analyses of patients treated with the COPP/ABVD regimen for Hodgkin's disease

Patient	Age	Years after chemotherapy	Number of cycles	Volume (ml)	Density (10^6/ml)	Motility (%)	FSH (IU/ml)	LH (IU/ml)
1	29	4.0	4	1.7	5.2	58	12.2	5.3
2	42	5.4	6	0.8	0	–	16.9	5.2
3	47	3.9	8	2.1	0	–	9.9	3.7
4	32	3.6	4	4.7	0	–	14.7	7.9
5	43	6.0	6	0.3	0	–	17.3	6.3
6	32	5.8	6	0.8	0	–	10.8	4.2
7	20	2.0	8	6.8	0	–	19.4	5.7
8	28	3.0	6	3.2	1	67	9.2	8.0
9	38	1.1	2	0.7	0	–	18.9	8.1
10	36	5.5	8	1.8	0	–	25.7	7.8
11	47	2.0	8	1.3	0	–	3.7	2.1
12	58	5.9	6	0.9	0	–	18.3	9.7
13	28	4.4	2	2.8	0	–	12.9	4.8
14	53	1.5	4	1.1	0	–	14.8	4.6
15	32	6.8	6	3.0	0	–	12.9	5.1

Reference values: FSH 2–10 IU/ml, LH 2–10 IU/ml.

therapy-induced premature menopause and age-matched controls (Fig. 2). The median bone mineral density of women with therapy-related ovarian failure was similar to that of postmenopausal controls, although the median age of our patients was 35 vs 66 years in the control group. It seems of interest that the bone mineral density of women suffering from treatment-related ovarian failure shows no statistically significant difference with or without estrogen replacement (Fig. 2). This contradictory result may be due to the fact that most patients did not receive adequate hormone replacement. Estrogen substitution was not adequate because of its late initiation (median 2.6 years) after ovarian failure was diagnosed.

Furthermore, ten of 17 women with ovarian impairment suffered from postmenopausal symptoms resulting from too low a dosage of estrogen replacement. Men showed no statistically significant difference in bone mineral density compared to age-matched controls, indicating that chemotherapy has no impact on bone density. The serum levels of parathormone, calcitonin and 1,25 dihydroxy-vitamin D were normal in all patients. However, women with ovarian failure after treatment for Hodgkin's disease had increased levels of osteocalcin indicating increased bone turnover. Osteocalcin serum levels in men were within normal limits (data not shown).

4 Discussion

The most important findings of the present study in patients successfully treated for Hodgkin's disease with the COPP/ABVD regimen were the high incidence of gonadal impairment in both men and women and the significant impact on bone mineralization in women with drug-induced premature ovarian failure.

Gonadal toxicity has been intensively studied in male Hodgkin's disease patients receiving MOPP or COPP chemotherapy (Table 3). Testicular failure following MOPP or COPP treatment has been reported as 86%–100% (Table 3). It has been shown that more than three cycles of the MOPP regimen produce significant and irreversible germ cell aplasia (Da Cunha et al. 1984). After the ABVD regimen, however, testicular dysfunction occurred in only 33% with a high recovery rate (Bonadonna et al. 1984). The present study clearly demonstrates that a combined COPP and ABVD regimen leads to germ cell aplasia with subsequent sterility in 86% and no evidence of recovery after a median follow-up of 4.3 years. It seems of interest, however, that none of these men had decreased testosterone levels, indicating normal Leydig cell function, which suggests dissociated gonadopathy.

Some 17 of 22 (77%) of our female patients treated with the COPP/ABVD regimen developed ovarian failure. None of these women recovered normal ovarian function up to 8 years after chemotherapy. The reported incidence of therapy-induced ovarian dysfunction after MOPP or COPP chemotherapy ranged from 46% to 80% (Table 4). This wide range is clearly explained by an age-related ovarian sensitivity to cytotoxic agents based on the physiological decrease of follicles in the course of life (for review: see Kreuser et al. 1987). There is convincing evidence of a minimal sterility risk in

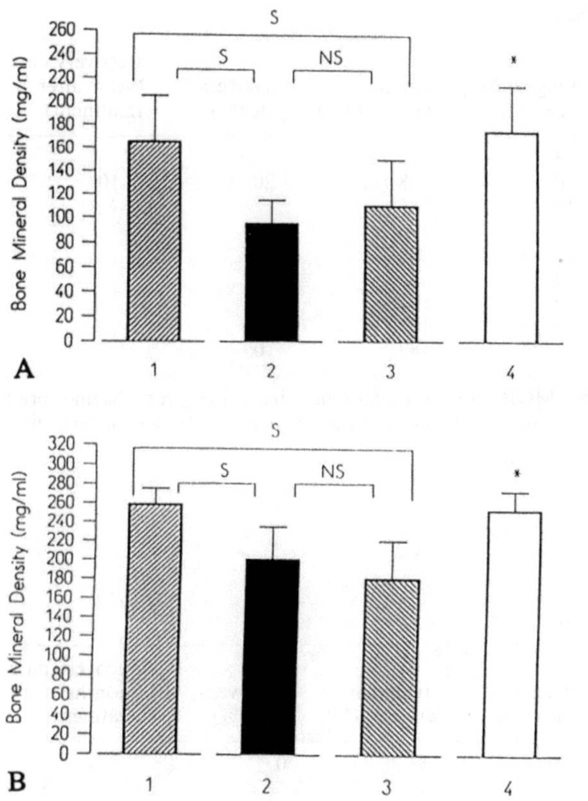

Fig. 2. A Lumbar bone density in female patients with Hodgkin's disease, as determined by dual-energy computed tomography. There was a significant (*S*) bone loss in female patients with ovarian failure (*2*, + estrogen; *3*, − estrogen) compared to women with normal ovarian function (*1*) and premenopausal control subjects (*4*) **B** Radial bone mineral density in female patients with Hodgkin's disease. There was also a significant decrease of bone mass compared to control subjects (*asterisk*)

female patients receiving the ABVD regimen alone (Bonadonna et al. 1984). The present study, however, has shown that a combined COPP and ABVD regimen produces significant and irreversible ovarian failure in 77% of the women, the quality of life thus being significantly influenced by premature menopausal symptoms in most patients.

Since only limited data are currently available on the impact of chemotherapy on bone mineralization, bone mass was measured at different sites using different methods in patients treated for Hodgkin's disease. This investigation has demonstrated a significant decrease in bone density in women with drug-induced ovarian failure (Fig. 2). The severity of the bone loss demonstrated in these patients, with a median age of 39 years, is comparable to that in the postmenopausal control group, with a median age of 66 years. Furthermore, there was a statistically significant correlation between trabecular and cortical bone loss ($v = 0.831$, $p = 0.0001$) in women with ovarian failure, indicating a similar trabecular and cortical bone loss due to drug-induced ovarian failure. Bone density measurements at the lumbar spine, the radius, and the calcaneus showed a highly significant correlation in female patients treated for Hodgkin's disease. This means that bone density screening can be carried out safely and accurately at any of these sites. However, since abdominal computed tomography has to be done routinely during staging and restaging procedures, we propose the measurement of bone density at the lumbar spine during staging procedures for high-risk patients. Furthermore, this study has demonstrated for the first time that COPP or COPP/ABVD chemotherapy including prednisone has no adverse effect on bone mineralization in men (Fig. 3).

In conclusion, our data suggest that germ cell aplasia with subsequent sterility occurs in 86% of the men treated with the COPP/ABVD regimen, suggesting identical toxicity with the COPP or MOPP schedule alone. In contrast, there was no evidence of androgen deficiency in men treated with the COPP/ABVD regimen. Chemotherapy-induced ovarian failure occurred in 77% of the women and had a significant impact on bone mineralization. Early hormone replacement is therefore strongly indicated in women with drug-induced ovarian failure in order to stop or slow down bone loss. Bone density screening by quantitative computed tomography is a feasible technique for predicting the risk of fractures in patients successfully treated for Hodgkin's disease.

5 Summary

Only limited data are currently available on long-term gonadal toxicity and its impact on bone mineralization in men and women treated for Hodgkin's disease. The present study was therefore conducted to evaluate gonadal toxicity and bone loss in 49 patients with Hodgkin's disease 1–8 (median 4.3) years after chemotherapy. A total of 26 patients were treated with the COPP/ABVD regimen ± irradiation according to the protocols (HD3, HD6) of the German Hodgkin Study Group. There were 23 patients who were treated with the

Table 3. Testicular failure following treatment for Hodgkin's disease

Reference[c]	Number of patients	Regimen	Oligozoo-spermia (%)	Azoo-spermia (%)	Recovery rate (%)	Recovery date (years after treatment)
CHAPMAN et al. 1981	64	MOPP	23	77		
WAXMAN et al. 1982	46	MOPP	0	88	20	2–10
WHITEHEAD et al. 1982	49	MOPP	10	86		
BONADONNA et al. 1984	27	MOPP	0	96	8	3
	18	ABVD	17	33	100	1
DACUNHA et al. 1984	14	MOPP[a]	22	35		
KREUSER et al. 1987	11	MOPP[b]	9	91	9	3
	19	COPP	0	100	0	3
Present study	15	COPP/ABVD	13	87	0	

COPP, cyclophosphamide, vincristine, procarbazine, prednisone; MOPP, mechlorethamine, vincristine, procarbazine, prednisone; MVPP, as MOPP but with vinblastine instead of vincristine; ABVD, adriamycin, bleomycin, vinblastine, dacarbazine.
[a]One to three cycles of MOPP.
[b]Six cycles of MOPP.
[c]See KREUSER et al. 1987.

Table 4. Ovarian failure following treatment for Hodgkin's disease

Reference[a]	Number of patients	Regimen	Amenor-rhea (%)	Irregular menses (%)	Recovery rate (%)	Recovery date (months after treatment)
CHAPMAN et al. 1981	36	MVPP	49	34	0	
	19	TNI	6	47		
HORNING et al. 1981	34	MOPP	15	29		
	50	MOPP + TNI	52	28		
SCHILSKY et al. 1981	24	MOPP	46			
WAXMAN et al. 1982	28	MOPP	79	0	0	
WHITEHEAD et al. 1983	44	MOPP	39	23	0	
BONADONNA et al. 1984	36	MOPP	17	0	3	6
	24	ABVD	0	0	—	
KREUSER et al. 1987	14	COPP	57	15	0	
Present study	22	COPP/ABVD	77	0	0	

TNI, total nodal irradiation; MVPP, mechlorethamine, vinblastine, procarbazine, prednisone; MOPP, mechlorethamine, vincristine, procarbazine, prednisone; COPP, cyclophosphamide, vincristine, procarbazine, prednisone; ABVD, adriamycin, bleomycin, vinblastine, dacarbazine.
[a]KREUSER et al. 1987.

COPP regimen to compare toxicity with the anthracycline-based COPP/ABVD protocol. Blood samples were tested for gonadotropins (FSH, LH), gonadal steroids, inhibin-α, parthyroid hormone, osteocalcin, and calcitonin. Bone mineral density was measured using single- and dual-energy quantitative computed tomography and single-photon absorptiometry. FSH serum levels were significantly increased in 21 of 27 (80%) men, demonstrating germ cell aplasia. Some 13 of 15 (86%) men showed azoospermia after the COPP/ ABVD regimen. In contrast, testosterone levels were within normal limits in all men tested, suggesting normal Ledyig cell function. Some 17 of 22 (77%) women exhibited increased FSH and LH levels, indicating premature ovarian failure. Women with therapy-induced ovarian failure had a significantly lower trabecular (98 ± 34 mal/cm^3) and cortical (292 ± 48 mg/cm^3) spinal bone density than those with normal ovarian function. Men showed no evidence of bone loss after therapy. These data suggest severe gonadal toxicity in both men and women treated with the COPP/ABVD regimen. In female patients, drug-induced ovarian failure has a significant impact on bone mineralization.

Acknowledgment. This work was supported by a grant from the Deutsche Krebshilfe, contract no. M34/88 Ke1.

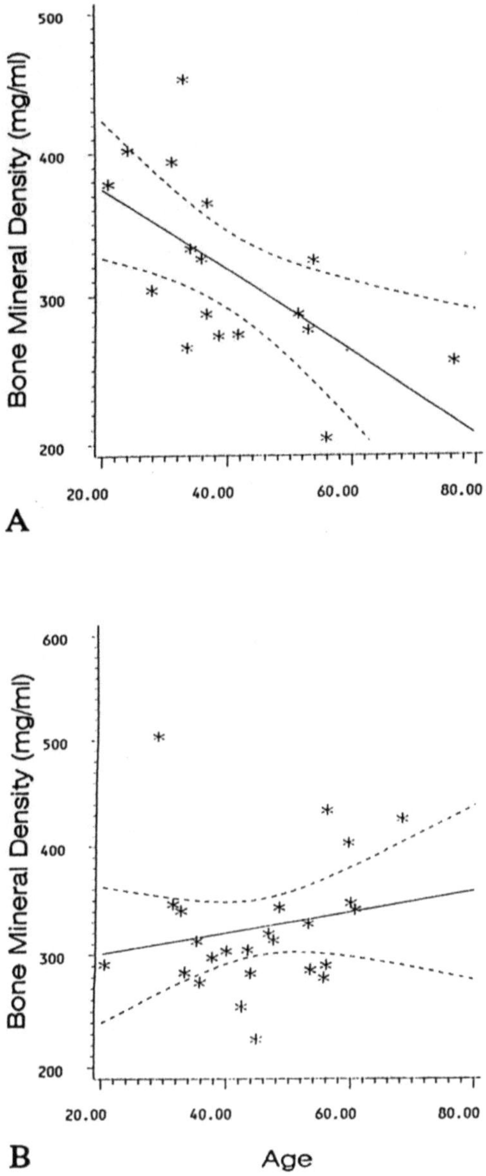

Fig. 3. A Lumbar bone mineral density and age in female patients. There was a marked bone loss in women. **B** Lumbar bone mineral density and age in male patients. There was no evidence of decreased bone mineralization in men treated for Hodgkin's disease

References

Bonadonna G, Santoro A, Viviani S, Lombardi C, Ragni G (1984) Gonadal damage in Hodgkin's disease from cancer chemotherapeutic regimens. Arch Toxicol 7: 140–145

Chapman RM, Sutcliffe SB, Malpas JS (1981) Male gonadal dysfunction in Hodgkin's disease: a prospective study. JAMA 245: 1323–1328

Cimino G, Biti GP, Anselmo AP (1991) Second primary cancer following Hodgkin's disease: updated results of an Italian multicentric study. J Clin Oncol 9: 432–437

Da Cunha MF, Meistrich ML, Fuller LM, Cundiff JH, Hagemeister FB, Velasquez WS, McLaughlin P, Riggs SA, Cabanillas FF, Salvador PG (1984) Recovery of spermatogenesis after treatment for Hodgkin's disease: limiting dose of MOPP chemotherapy. J Clin Oncol 2: 571–577

Horning SJ, Toppe RT, Kaplan HS, Rosenberg SA (1981) Female reproductive potential after treatment for Hodgkin's disease. N Engl J Med 304: 1377–1382

Johnston F, Slememda CW, Melton LJ (1991) Clinical use of bone densitometry. N Engl J Med 324: 1105–1109

Kaldor JM, Day NE, Clarke EA, van Leeuwen FE, Henry-Amar M, Fiorentino MV, Bell J, Pedersen D, Band P, Assouline D, Koch M, Choi W, Prior P, Blair V, Langmark F, Kirn VP, Neal F, Peters D, Pfeiffer R, Karjalalainen S, Cuzick J, Sutcliffe SB, Somers R, Pellae-Cosset B, Pappagallo GL, Fraser P, Storm H, Stovall M (1990) Leukemia following Hodgkin's disease. N Engl J Med 322: 7–13

Kreuser E-D, Xiros N, Hetzel WD, Heimpel H (1987) Reproductive and endocrine gonadal capacity in patients treated for Hodgkin's disease. J Cancer Res Clin Oncol 113: 260–266

Loeffler M, Pfreundschuh M, Hasenclever D, Hiller E, Gerhartz H, Wilmanns W, Rohloff R, Rühl U, Kühn G, Fuchs R, Kirchner H, Teichmann J, Schoppe W, Petsch S, ilhelmy W, Worst P, Pflüger KH, Hecht T, Bartels H, Gassmann W, Krüger G, Schmitz G, Oertel W, Diehl V (1991) Prognostiĉ risk factor in advanced Hodgkin's lymphoma. Blut 56: 273–281

Longo DL (1990) The use of chemotherapy in the treatment of Hodgkin's disease. Semin Oncol 17: 716–735

Redman JR, Bajorunas DR, Wong G, McDermott K, Gnecco C, Schneider R, Lacher MJ, Lange JM (1988) Bone mineralization in women following successful treatment of Hodgkin's disease. Am J Med 85: 65–72

Schillsky RL, Sherins RJ, Hubbard SM, Wesley MN, Young RC, DeVita VT (1981) Long-term follow-up of ovarian function in women treated with MOPP chemotherapy for Hodgkin's disease. Am J Med 71: 552–556

Waxman JH, Terry YA, Wrigley PF, Malpas JS, Ress LH, Besser GM, Lister TA (1982) Gonadal function in Hodgkin's disease: long-term follow-up of chemotherapy. Br J Med 285: 1612–1613

Whitehead E, Shalet SM, Blackledge G, Crowther D, Beardwell CG (1982) The effect of Hodgkin's disease and combination chemotherapy and gonadal function in the adult male. Cancer 49: 418–422

Whitehead E, Shalet SM, Blackledge G, Crowther D, Beardwell CG (1983) The effect of combination chemotherapy on ovarian function in women treated for Hodgkin's disease. Cancer 52: 988–993

7.2 Gonadal Dysfunction After Radiotherapy

MICHAELA RIEPL and SILVIA REITZ

CONTENTS

1	Introduction	235
2	Influences of Radiation Therapy on Gonadal Function	235
2.1	Radiation of the Hypothalamic and Pituitary Region	235
2.2	Direct Exposure During Total Body Irradiation	236
2.3	Radiation of the Infradiaphragmal Region	236
3	Influence of Radiation on Male Gonadal Function	236
3.1	Irradiation Effects on Spermatogenesis	237
3.1.1	Single Dose Irradiation	237
3.1.2	Fractionated Irradiation	237
3.2	Fertility Outcome After Radiotherapy	237
3.3	Effects of Irradiation on Leydig Cell Function	237
4	Influence of Radiation on Female Gonadal Function	238
4.1	Irradiation Effects on Ovarian Function	238
4.2	Pregnancy Outcome After Radiation Therapy	238
5	Possibilities for the Protection of Gonadal Function	239
5.1	Protection of Testicular Function	239
5.1.1	Testicular Shielding During Radiotherapy	239
5.2	Protection of Ovarian Function	240
5.2.1	Medial Ovaropexy	240
5.2.2	Lateral (High) Abdominal Overopexy	240
6	Summary and Therapeutic Recommendations	241
	References	241

1 Introduction

Up to now there has been little attention paid to the long-term side effects of cancer treatment on gonadal function. However, there are now more long-time survivors, particularly younger patients, who worry about their sexual function and fertility. Gonadal dysfunction following cancer therapy is influenced not only by radiotherapy to the tumor itself, but also by anatomic, physiological and endocrine processes as well as by the patient's psychology and behavior. The tumor may involve the gonads or the hormone producing glands. Surgical therapy may include ovarectomy, (semi) castration, or resection of pituitary tissue, impairing sexual function or hormonal status. Radical retroperitoneal lymph node dissection may cause retrograde ejaculation or impotence in men (GERL et al. 1993). Most therapy regimens also include chemotherapy and many cytotoxic drugs, particularly alkylating agents (VIVIANI et al. 1985; CHAPMAN et al. 1979), cause severe and permanent disturbances in both testicular and ovarian function (WAXMAN et al. 1982). Moreover, psychological aspects, such as family, relationships, and social responses to the tumor also play an important role.

MICHAELA RIEPL, Dr., Strahlentherapeutische Klinik und Poliklinik, Universität Erlangen-Nürnberg, Universitätsstraße 27, 91054 Erlangen, FRG
SILVIA REITZ Dr., Institut und Poliklinik für Strahlentherapie, Technische Universität, Ismaninger Straße 15, 81675 München, FRG

2 Influences of Radiation Therapy on Gonadal Function

Radiotherapy impairs gonadal function by a variety of mechanisms: (1) radiation of the hypothalamic and pituitary region; (2) direct exposure during total body irradiation preceding bone marrow transplantation; (3) direct or indirect exposure of the gonads during radiation of the infradiaphragmal region, for example, irradiation of the paraaortal and iliac lymphnodes or the pelvis.

2.1 Radiation of the Hypothalamic and Pituitary Region

Apart from radiotherapy of pituitary gland tumors, there are other tumor entities, particularly brain tumors and nasopharyngeal carcinomas, in which the hypothalamus or the pituitary gland may be situated in or at the margin of the radiation field. Thus, side effects such as hormone deficiencies leading to gonadal dysfunction have to be taken into account.

Table 1. Differences in radiosensibility

	Testis	Ovary
Repopulation ability	+	–
Effect of fractionation	Increased radiation effects	Protection
Hormonal function	Resistant; independent of germ cell damage	Sensitive; dependent on germ cell damage
Sensitive cells	Type A/B spermatogonia, Stem cells during mitosis, (early stage of differentiation)	Primary oocytes, (mature cells)
Relation to age	No relation	Corresponds with age

From Fritz-Niggli (1991) and Oakberg (1956).

Lam et al. (1991) found that 30% patients with nasopharyngeal carcinoma treated with radiotherapy had deficiencies in gonadotropin secretion, suggesting a defect in the release of gonadotropin releasing hormone within 2 years. The estimated average dose to the hypothalamus was 39.8 Gy. Constine et al. (1993) studied endocrine function in 32 patients with brain tumors. The irradiation dose to the pituitary and hypothalamic region ranged from 39.6 to 70.2 Gy. Overall, 61% of the post-pubertal patients showed evidence of hypogonadism, combined with a varying pattern of other hormonal deficits, particularly hypothyroidism. Blatt et al. (1981) reported no evidence of impaired gonadal function after cranial irradiation with a dose of 24 Gy in children with lymphoblastic leukemia. However, an exact correlation between dose and type or extent of hypothalamic or pituitary hormone deficiencies has not yet been described.

2.2 Direct Exposure During Total Body Irradiation

Total body irradiation (TBI) combined with chemotherapy prior to bone marrow transplantation is known to have relevant toxic side effects. After TBI in 21 adults with doses between 10 Gy and 13.2 Gy in five or six fractions, all females suffered amenorrhea within 3 months with low estradiol levels requiring estrogen replacement. Some women show recovery of gonadal function; in a few cases even pregnancies after chemotherapy and TBI with 12 Gy – fractionated in single doses of 2 Gy – have been reported (Giri et al. 1992). In males severe oligo- or azoospermia was noted, the testosterone levels in the serum were normal. There was no evidence of direct damage to the hypothalamic-pituitary axis (Littley et al. 1991). After TBI in 31 children most showed evidence of gonadal dysfunction. All pubertal girls had ovarian failure, with one recovery. The boys showed evidence of damage to the germinal epithelium and two of three in early puberty had raised FSH concentrations. Children undergoing such procedures are considered to require long-term endocrine management (Ogilvy-Stuart et al. 1992).

2.3 Radiation of the Infradiaphragmal Region

The consequences of direct or indirect irradiation of the gonads during radiation of the infradiaphragmal region will be discussed more extensively. Generally, gonadal dysfunction after radiation is determined by dose and fractionation and is inversely related to the distance from the gonads to the irradiated field (Byne et al. 1987; Hamre et al. 1987). The effects of radiation on male and female gonads differ because of the different germ cell evolution (Table 1).

3 Influence of Radiation on Male Gonadal Function

Depending on their degree of differentiation and maturation the germinal cells are highly sensitive. In spermatogenesis the most sensitive cell stages are the type A spermatogonia, particularly the more differentiated stages A_{2-4}, stem cells in the mitotic phase (Oakberg 1956), and the type B spermatogonia (Fritz-Niggli 1991; Ash 1980). These susceptible cells are killed by an acute irradiation of 0.15 Gy (Ash 1980; Greiner 1982, 1985). Following irradiation, the surviving stem cells (early type A spermatogonia) develop into these more radiosensitive stages. Thus fractionated irradiation may be more harmful, emptying the stem cell pool, even the total dose applied is less (Ash 1980;

GREINER 1982). Only the type A spermatogonia are able to repopulate in the tubuli seminiferi. If a sufficient number of these cells stay alive there will be recovery of spermatogenesis even if it requires up to several years (HAHN et al. 1982). Later cell stages, i.e., spermocytes, spermatids and spermatozoa, are less sensitive.

3.1 Irradiation Effects on Spermatogenesis

3.1.1 Single Dose Irradiation

Concerning acute radiation delivered in a single dose, experimental irradiation of human testes of prisoners with doses ranging from 0.08 to 6 Gy showed that doses of 0.5–0.78 Gy produced marked oligospermia and decreased sperm concentration in the semen to about two millions per ml 11 weeks post irradiation. Complete recovery took place within 9–19 months after less than 0.1 Gy as a single dose, 30 months after 2 Gy and 5 or more years after 4–6 Gy as an acute dose (HELLER et al. 1966; ROWLEY et al. 1974). Moreover, damage of spermatocytes after 2.0–3.0 Gy of acute irradiation was shown by their inability to complete maturation division. Spermatids seemed to be damaged after 4.0–6.0 Gy, since the number of agile spermatozoa was significantly decreased afterwards.

3.1.2 Fractionated Irradiation

GREINER (1982) investigated the recovery of spermatogenesis in 58 patients with seminoma treated postoperatively with irradiation. After a total dose to the testis of less than 1 Gy, with daily fractions of 3–5 cGy, spermatogenesis is completely recovered; for a total dose between 1 Gy and 1.5 Gy partial recovery – with an azoospermic interval of 5 or 6 months; for a total dose higher than 1.5 Gy (GREINER 1982) or 2.0 Gy (SANDEMANN 1966), permanent azoospermia has to be presumed. In individual cases, recovery following an overall dose of 3 Gy has been reported (SANDEMANN 1966). The change from temporary oligospermia to temporary aspermia took place at about 0.35 Gy total dose (SANDEMANN 1966).

For fractionated postoperative radiotherapy in patients with seminoma and a total dose to the testis of between 1.4 and 1.6 Gy, the threshold from partial recovery to permanent azoospermia concerning the single dose delivered appeared to be 8.6 cGy (GREINER 1982). Generally, the length of the sterile period varies with the overall exposure dose, the single dose, and the time intervals between fractions. It has been reported that the sperm count starts to decrease approximately after 4 weeks (UNSCEAR 1988). The beginning of the oligo- or azoospermic interval, in contrast to duration, seems to be dose-dependent and is to be expected 2–5 months after radition therapy (GREINER 1982).

3.2 Fertility Outcome After Radiotherapy

The recovery of sperm usually takes place during the first 24 months after radiotherapy. GREINER (1982) showed in 50 patients that with sustained azoospermia after this period no relevant further repopulation took place within the next 5 years. In contrast, SANDEMANN (1966) noted two patients with recovery after azoospermia lasting 12 and 14 years. Afterwards, even with oligospermia, normal children may be conceived (GREINER 1982; HAHN et al. 1982). Due to the delayed decrease in sperm count and the risk of genetic damage to the stem cells, the patients should be advised regarding contraception throughout the first year after radiotherapy (KIMMIG et al. 1980; KUBO and SHIPLEY 1982).

A very important factor in assessing the fertility of males after radiotherapy is the gonadal function before radiotherapy. For example, in patients with seminoma, after semicastration alone, 60% of the patients may have a transient oligo- or azoospermia; 25% remaia infertile no matter what treatment follows (FOSSA et al. 1980; JEWETT et al. 1983; WEISSBACH et al. 1974). Furthermore, the patients' age is probably also an important factor. Older men more often show a persistent disturbance of their fertility (GERL et al. 1993). The age at diagnosis seems to be inversely correlated with fertility, although some authors deny this (FRITZ-NIGGLI 1991).

A study of 2283 cancer survivors showed that radiation below the diaphragm depressed fertility in males by about 25%; chemotherapy with alkylating agents, however, resulted in a fertility deficit of 60% no matter whether combined with radiotherapy or not (BYRNE et al. 1987).

3.3 Effects of Irradiation on Leydig Cell Function

The function of the Leydig cells seems to remain unchanged in adult males within the scope of radiation doses resulting from indirect exposure. Greiner (1982) and Barth and Hums (1990) reported normal testosterone production in seminoma patients after postoperative radiotherapy. Brauner et al. (1983), however, evaluated boys with acute lymphoblastic leukemia and testicular irradiation (24 Gy in 12 fractions) and found in ten out of 17 patients inadequate Leydig cell function, in three cases even without chemotherapy containing cyclophosphamide or cytarabine, known to have toxic side effects on Leydig cell function (Shalet et al. 1981). The severity of the disturbances appeared to be variable, probably slowly occurring over a matter of years (Brauner et al. 1983; Shalet et al. 1989). After fractionated testicular irradiation with doses between 27.5 and 30 Gy prepubertal boys showed much more severe Leydig cell dysfunction than adult males, suggesting an age-dependent vulnerability (Shalet et al. 1989).

4 Influence of Radiation on Female Gonadal Function

In contrast to males, there is no stem cell comparable to the spermatogonium initiating repopulation. The preliminary stages of oogenesis are completely shortly after birth, the major part of the cell population consists of oocytes in their resting stage of prophase (Lintern-Moore et al. 1974). The repair capacity of each oocyte determines the preservation of ovarian function, thus fractionation with lower single doses has a positive effect (Greiner 1985). Depending on the age at treatment, younger patients are supposed to have more oocytes and are therefore more likely to keep ovarian function (Horning et al. 1981; Lushbaugh and Casarett 1976; Unscear 1988).

In most cases the irradiation exposure to the ovaries is higher than to the male testis because the ovaries are situated in the pelvis, within or near the target volume. Not only the direct beam has to be taken into account but also scatter radiation, particularly in the case of ovarian transposition.

4.1 Irradiation Effects on Ovarian Function

An important source of information is the former use of low fractionated irradiation to induce early menopause. The results have been summarized by Ash (1980): radiation of the ovaries with a total dose of 4–7 Gy in four fractions to achieve sterilization was recommended for women older than 40 years and with 12.5–15 Gy if younger.

In women with Hodgkin's disease undergoing fractionated irradiation after medial ovaropexy, transient menstrual irregularities occurred after an ovarian dose of 1.5 Gy. Temporary sterility is induced by doses up to 4 Gy, prolonged sterility by 4–10 Gy. In the age range of 18 to 36 years, after 5–6 Gy total dose to the ovary, most patients remain amenorrheic (Thomas et al. 1976). Ash (1980) estimated that 60% of the women who receive a minimal ovarian dose of 2.5–5.0 Gy will develop ovarian failure. Chambers et al. (1991) noted that in patients with pelvic irradiation for cervical cancer after ovarian transposition almost 90% of the women are likely to keep their ovarian function if the total dose to the ovary is 3 Gy or less, in contrast to only 40% preservation with higher doses delivered. Horning et al. (1981) reported that women younger than 20 years have an about 70% chance of persisting gonadal function after medial ovaropexy and total nodal irradiation, in contrast to the 20% of the women beyond an age of 30.

In an analysis of multiple values including age, ovarian dose, dose per fraction and total treatment time, Ray et al. (1970) found neither a threshold dose for ovarian failure nor a single predictive factor for radiation sterilization. It is generally believed, however, that ovarian failure after radiotherapy is both dose- and age-dependent, with no reliable prediction of outcome for the dose range of 3–10 Gy (Chapman and Sutcliffe 1986). Haie-Meder et al. (1993) recently presented new results with three progonstic factors of ovarian castration: age over 25, MOPP chemotherapy and a total dose to the ovaries higher than 5 Gy after lateral ovaropexy. Based on their results, Grabenbauer et al. (1991) presume, for infradiaphragmal irradiation after lateral high abdominal ovaropexy (see Sect. 5.2.2), that ovarian failure occurs only in women older than 30 years or treated with polychemotherapy.

4.2 Pregnancy Outcome After Radiation Therapy

Byrne et al. (1987) found that female long-term cancer survivors, after radiation below the diaphragm, had a fertility rate about 25% lower than normal. Horning et al. (1981), examining 103 women after treatment for Hodgkin's disease, found that with ovaropexy the probability of becoming pregnant, if attempted, was about 77% (20 out of 26). The least reported pregnancies occurred in the group with both total nodal irradiation and chemotherapy (MOPP or PAVe). The 21 pregnancies resulted in normal babies with two premature and one low birth weight infants. No birth defects or developmental abnormalities occurred. In 134 women who underwent radiation after lateral ovaropexy – in 72 cases combined with chemotherapy – HAIE-MEDER et al. (1993) noted a significantly lower birth rate than normal, again without abnormalities among the offspring. Concerning the total dose, a successful pregnancy after radiotherapy even after a fractionated ovarian dose of 6.5 Gy has been reported (THOMAS et al. 1976).

In contrast, NICHOLSON and BYRNE (1993) suggested that females who had radiation to the abdomen should be followed as high-risk obstetrical patients, because they have a slightly increased risk of adverse pregnancy outcomes such as miscarriages or preterm deliveries. The corresponding studies presume that there may be radiotherapy-induced changes in the uterus (BYRNE et al. 1988; HAWKINS and SMITH 1989).

5 Possibilities for the Protection of Gonadal Function

5.1 Protection of Testicular Function

One method discussed is the suppression of gonadotropin with administration of testosterone, but there is no clinical relevance up to now (REDMAN et al. 1986). Concerning fertility, for men cryopreservation of sperm can be performed prior to radiotherapy. It is not feasible for every patient because cancer patients quite often show a reduced sperm count or sperm quality prior to radiotherapy (JEWETT et al. 1983). Nevertheless cryopreservation should be offered. If there is oligospermia after the treatment there are two supporting techniques: direct intrauterine placement of the sperm, or, in case of a severely reduced sperm count, in vitro fertilization (SHERINS 1993).

5.1.1 Testicular Shielding During Radiotherapy

The testicular dose delivered results from a number of sources: accelerator head leakage, scattering from the collimator and the field-shaping blocs, air scattering, scattering from the abdomen within the patient and from the thighs (KUBO and SHIPLEY 1982). Field size, irradiated volume and distance from the field edge are also important (KIMMIG et al. 1980). The aim of gonadal protection is to keep the testicular dose below 1% of the prescribed dose. It should be used whenever the dose to the testis is larger than 0.5 Gy (FRAAS et al. 1985). For the reasons mentioned above, our technique includes not only a gonadal shield, but also two additional blocs, in each case on the caudal field edge, one about 10 cm above the patient and the other 20 cm beyond the accelerator head (Fig. 1), to minimize scatter radiation (GRABENBAUER and SAUER 1991).

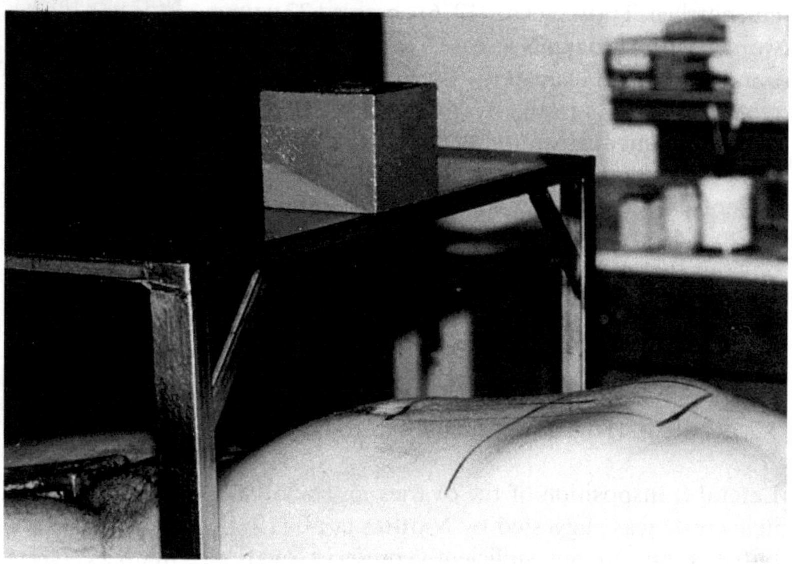

Fig. 1. Threefold testicular shielding (GRABENBAUER and SAUER 1991), including a gonadal shield and two additional blocks on the caudal field edge. One is positioned about 10 cm above the patient, as shown here, the other beyond the accelerator head

5.2 Protection of Ovarian Function

In premenopausal women the ovarian function should be preserved if possible to avoid menopausal symptoms and to maintain the chance of pregnancy. One of the methods that has been discussed is suppression of gonadotropin with oral contraceptives in order to inhibit germ cell proliferation, thus reducing gonadal toxicity. Comparable to the results in men, this has, however, not yet been shown to be effective (CHAPMAN and SUTCLIFFE 1981).

A hardly feasible technique has been described in a case report by LEPORRIER et al. (1987): Subcutaneous heterotopic transplantation of the ovary to the inner upper arm before radiotherapy. After treatment, puncture of the ovary showed mature oocytes and normal follicle growth was seen.

A method proven to be effective is ovaropexy – the ovaries are transposed to a region, where they either can be shielded during radiotherapy or lie outside the radiation field – with two different techniques. These are described below.

5.2.1 Medial Ovaropexy

In the case of medial ovaropexy the ovaries are moved to the midline of the pelvis and are fixed on the posterior wall of the uterus. The position is marked with clips and the ovaries are shielded during radiotherapy. With 40.6–45 Gy delivered to the pelvis, RAY et al. (1970) described minimal ovarian doses ranging from 2.63 Gy to 6.6 Gy, with nine of 22 patients suffering from permanent amenorrhea. THOMAS et al. (1976) observed 22 young women with Hodgkin's disease treated with irradiation after medial ovaropexy. Twelve of the patients received 6–35 Gy to the ovaries, nine of them had persisting amenorrhea (75%). GRABENBAUER et al. (1991) also reported ovarian failure in three of four patients, with doses to the ovaries ranging from 3.9 to 5 Gy (median dose 4.9 Gy). Therefore it is obvious that medial ovaropexy may yield sufficient preservation of endocrine function only in about 25%–60% of all patients.

5.2.2 Lateral (High) Abdominal Ovaropexy

Lateral transposition of the ovaries just below the iliac crests was suggested by NAHHAS et al. (1971), but it seems to not sufficiently preserve ovarian function, particularly in the case of pelvic irradiation (CHAMBERS et al. 1991). As a modification to this technique, laterial high abdominal ovaropexy is performed. The ovaries are transposed beyond the iliaci crests, anterior to the superior renal pole and lateral to the right or left colic flexures, and marked with clips (BELINSON et al. 1984; GAETINI et al. 1988). Despite extensive mobilization of the ovary, the operative complication rate seems to be low (GAETINI et al. 1988: 0/27; BELINSON et al. 1984: 0/13); CHAMBERS et al. (1991), however, noted a threefold increased risk to develop symptomatic ovarian cysts.

BELINSON et al. (1984) showed that three patients, out of three with an ovary positioned above the iliac crest had no evidence of ovarian failure after infradiaphragmal radiotherapy. GAETINI et al. (1988)

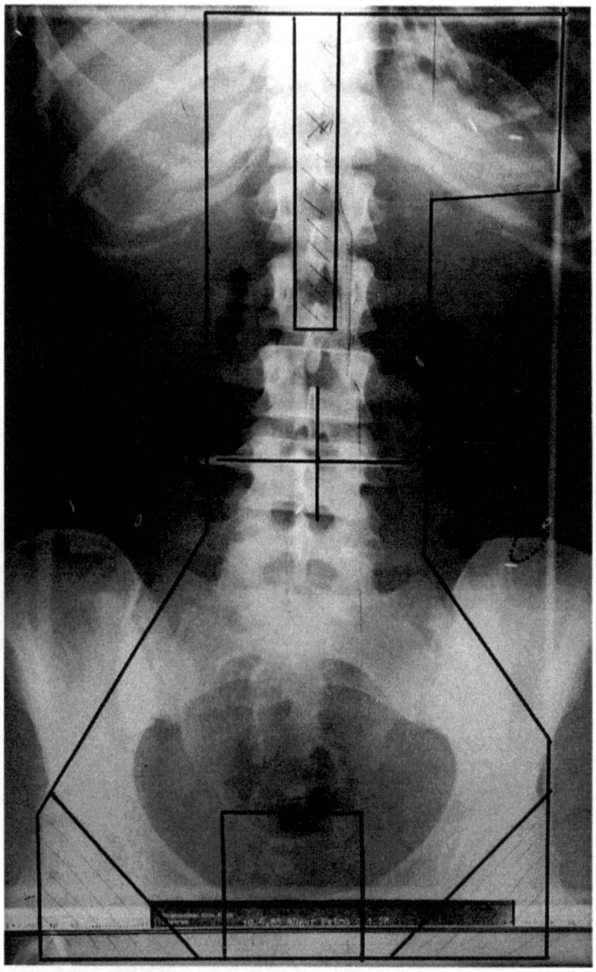

Fig. 2. The site of the transposed ovary (marked with *clips*) in relation to the irradiation field after lateral high abdominal ovaropexy (GRABENBAUER et al. 1991)

reported on five out of six women (83%) with pelvic irradiation during treatment for Hodgkin's disease who showed no ovarian failure with doses to the ovary ranging between 1.28 and 4.40 Gy. The one amenorrheic patient was one of those who received six cycles of chemotherapy (MOPP). GRABENBAUER et al. (1991) also showed that seven out of nine women (78%) treated with total nodal irradiation including pelvic and inguinal lymph nodes had normal ovarian function after lateral high abdominal ovaropexy (Fig. 2). The doses to the ovary ranged between 2.6 and 5 Gy (median dose 3.25 Gy), the two women with ovarian failure in this group had polychemotherapy with COPP/ABVD before. Therefore, lateral high abdominal ovaropexy is the method of choice if protection of gonadal function is desired. Successful pregnancies after lateral high abdominal ovaropexy and radiation have also been reported (GAETINI et al. 1988; GRABENBAUER et al. 1991).

6 Summary and Therapeutic Recommendations

In premenopausal females, a lateral high abdominal ovaropexy should be performed during primary operation if the planned therapy regimen is likely to include radiotherapy of the pelvis or the infradiaphragmal lymph nodes (GRABENBAUER et al. 1991). Symptoms of ovarian failure after cancer treatment require an accurate determination of the menstrual and hormonal status and adequate hormonal replacement if necessary.

In young male patients and those concerned about their fertility a cumulative dose of 0.5 Gy to the testis can be accepted, but requires effective gonadal shielding (FRAAS et al. 1985; KUBO and SHIPLEY 1982), as mentioned above (GRABENBAUER and SAUER 1991). The patient should be counseled regarding additional possibilities to preserve fertility, such as sperm conservation prior to treatment or in vitro fertilization afterwards.

References

Ash P (1980) The influence of radiation on fertility in man. Br J Radiol 53: 271–278

Barth V, Hums R (1990) Serumhormone und Spermiogrammveränderungen bei Patienten mit malignen Hodentumoren nach Strahlen- und Zytostatikatherapie. Z Urol Nephrol 83: 291–295

Belinson JL, Doherty M, McDay JB (1984) A new technique for ovarian transposition. Surg Gynecol Obstet 139: 157–160

Blatt J, Poplack DG, Sherins RJ (1981) Testicular function in boys after chemotherapy for acute lymphoblastic leukemia. N Engl J Med 304: 1121–1124

Brauner R, Czernichow P, Cramer P, Schaison G, Rappaport R (1983) Leydig-cell function in children after direct testicular irradiation for acute lymphoblastic leukemia. N Engl J Med 309: 25–28

Byrne J, Mulvihill JJ, Myers MH et al (1987) Effects of treatment on fertility. N Engl J Med 317: 1315–1321

Byrne J, Mulvihill JJ, Conelly RR et al (1988) Reproductive problems and birth defects in survivors of Wilm's tumor and their relatives. Med Pediatr Oncol 16: 233–240

Chambers SK, Chambers JT, Kier R, Peschel RE (1991) Sequelae of lateral ovarian transposition in irradiated cervical cancer patients. Int J Radiat Oncol Biol Phys 20: 1305–1308

Chapman RM, Sutcliffe SB (1981) Protection of ovarian function by oral contraceptives in women receiving chemotherapy for Hodgkin's disease. Blood 58: 849–851

Chapman RM, Sutcliffe SB (1986) The effects of chemotherapy and radiotherapy on fertility and their prevention. Rec Adv Clin Oncol 2: 239–251

Chapman RM, Sutcliffe SB, Malpas JS (1979) Cytotoxic-induced ovarian failure in women with Hodgkin's disease. I. Hormone function. JAMA 242: 1877–1881

Constine LS, Woolf PD, Cann D, Mick G, McCormick K, Raubertas RF, Rubin P (1993) Hypothalamic-pituitary dysfunction after radiation for brain tumors. N Engl J Med 328: 87–94

Fossa SD, Klepp O, Aakvaag A, Molne K (1980) Testicular function after combined chemotherapy for metastatic testicular cancer. Int J Androl 3: 59–65

Fraas BA, Kinsella TJ, Harrington FS, Glatstein E (1985) Peripherical dose to the testes: the design and clinical use of a practical and effective gonadal shield. Int J Radiat Oncol Biol Phys 11: 609–615

Fritz-Niggli H (1991) Strahlengefährdung/Strahlenschutz. Ein Leitfaden für die Praxis, 3rd edn. Huber, Bern

Gaetini A, DeSimone M, Urgesi A, Levis A, Resegotti A, Ragona R, Anglesio S (1988) Lateal high ovaropexy: An original surgical technique for protection of the ovaries during curative radiotherapy for Hodgkin's disease. J Surg Oncol 39: 22–28

Gerl A, Clemm C, Wilmanns W (1993) Gonadale Funktionsstörungen nach Therapie von Hodentumoren. Dtsch Med Wochenschr 118: 683

Giri N, Vowels MR, Barr AL, Mameghan H (1992) Successful pregnancy after total body irradiation and bone marrow transplantation for acute leukaemia. Bone Marrow Transplant 10: 93–95

Grabenbauer GG, Sauer R (1991) Hodenseminome – Zielvolumen, Dosierung und Technik der externen Radiotherapie. Bildgebung 58 [Suppl 1]: 53–55

Grabenbauer GG, Girke P, Wildt L, Müller RG, Herbst M, Sauer R (1991) Ovaropexie und die Behandlung des Morbus Hodgkin. Strahlenther Oncol 167: 273–276

Greiner R (1982) Die Erholung der Spermatogenese nach fraktionierter, niedrig dosierter Bestrahlung der männlichen Gonaden. Strahlentherapie 158 (6): 342–355

Greiner R (1985) Wirkung der Strahlen- und Chemotherapie auf die Gonadenfunktion. Münch Med Wochenschr 127: 870–874

Hahn EW, Feingold SM, Simpson L, Batata M (1982) Recovery from aspermia induced by low-dose radiation in seminoma patients. Cancer 50: 337–340

Haie-Meder C, Mlika-Cabanne N, Michel G et al (1993) Radiotherapy after ovarian transposition: ovarian function and fertility preservation. Int J Radiat Oncol Biol Phys 25: 419–424

Hamre MR, Robinson LL, Nesbit ME, Sather HN, Meadows AT, Ortega JA (1987) Effects of radiation on ovarian function in long-term survivors of childhood acute lymphoblastic leukemia: a report from the Childrens Cancer Study Group. J Clin Oncol 5: 1759–1765

Hawkins MM, Smith RA (1989) Pregnancy outcomes in childhood cancer survivors: probable effects of abdominal irradiation. Int J Cancer 43: 399–402

Heller CG, Wootton P, Rowley MJ, Lalli M, Brusca DR (1966) Action of radiation on human spermatogenesis. Exc Med Found Int Congr Ser 112: 408–410

Horning SJ, Hoppe RT, Kaplan HS, Rosenberg SA (1981) Female reproductive potential after treatment for Hodgkin's disease. N Engl J Med 304: 1377–1382

Jewett MA, Thachil JV, Harris JF (1983) Exocrine function of testis with germinal testicular tumor. Br Med J 286: 1849–1850

Kimmig B, Kober B, Fehrentz D (1980) Gonadenbelastung bei der Strahlentherapie des retroperitonealen Lymphsystems. Therapiewoche 30: 3445–3448

Kubo H, Shipley WU (1982) Reduction of the scatter dose to the testicle outside the radiation treatment fields. Int J Radiat Oncol Biol Phys 8: 1741–1745

Lam KS, Tse VK, Wang C, Veung RT, Ho JH (1991) Effects of cranial irradiation on hypothalamic-pituitary function – a 5-year longitudinal study in patients with nasopharyngeal carcinoma. Q J Med 78 (287): 165–176

Leporrier M, von Theobald P, Roffe JL, Muller G (1987) A new technique to protect ovarian function before pelvic irradiation. Cancer 60: 2201–2204

Lintern-Moore S, Peters H, Moore GPM, Faber M (1974) Follicular development in the infant human ovary. J Reprod Fertil 39: 53–64

Littley MD, Shaley SM, Morgenstern GR, Deakin DP (1991) Endocrine and reproductive dysfunction following fractionated total body irradiation in adults. Q J Med 78 (287): 265–274

Lushbaugh CC, Casarett GW (1976) The effects of gonadal irradiation in clinical radiation therapy: a review. Cancer 37: 1111–1120

Nahhas WA, Nisce LZ, D'Angio GJ, Lewis JL (1971) Lateral ovarian transposition. Obstet Gynecol 38: 785–788

Nicholson HS, Byrne J (1983) Fertility and pregnancy after treatment for cancer during childhood or adolescence. Cancer 71: 3392–3399

Oakberg EF (1956) A description of spermatogenesis in the mouse and the use in analysis of the cycle of the seminiferous epithelium. Am J Anat 99: 507–516

Ogilvy-Stuart AL, Clark DJ, Wallace WH, Gibson BE, Stevens RF, Shalet SM, Donaldson MD (1992) Endocrine deficit after fractionated total body irradiation. Arch Dis Child 67: 1107–1110

Ray GR, Trueblood HW, Enright LP, Kaplan HS, Nelsen TS (1970) Oophoropexy: a means of preserving ovarian function following pelvic megavoltage radiotherapy for Hodgkin's disease. Radiology 96: 175–180

Redman J, Davis R, Evenson D et al (1986) Prospective randomized trial of testosterone cypionate to prevent sterility in men treated with chemotherapy for Hodgkin's disease: Preliminary results. In: Proceedings of the 14th international cancer congress, Budapest. Karger, Basel, p 440

Rowley MJ, Leach DR, Warner GA, Heller CG (1974) Effects of graded doses of ionizing radiation on the human testis. Radiat Res 59: 665–678

Sandemann TF (1966) The effects of X-irradiation on male human fertility. Br J Radiol 39: 901–907

Shalet SM, Hann IM, Lendon M, Morris Jones PH, Beardwell CG (1981) Testicular function after combination chemotherapy in childhood for acute lymphoblastic leukemia. Arch Dis Child 56: 275–278

Shalet SM, Tsatsoulis A, Whitehead E, Read G (1989) Vulnerability of the human Leydig cell to radiation damage is dependent upon age. J Endocrinol 120: 161–165

Sherins RJ (1993) Gonadal dysfunction. In: DeVita, Hellman, Rosenberg (eds) Cancer, principles and practice in oncology, 4th edn. Lippincott, Philadelphia, pp 2395–2406

Thomas PRM, Winstantly D, Peckham MJ, Austin DE, Murray MAF, Jacobs HS (1976) Reproductive and endocrine function in patients with Hodgkin's disease: effects of oophoropexy and irradiation. Br J Cancer 33: 226–231

UNSCEAR – United Nations Scientific Committee on the Effects of Atomic Radiation (1988) Sources, effects and risks of ionizing radiation. Report to the General Assembly, with annexes. United Nations Publications, New York, p 35

Viviani S, Santoro A, Ragni G, Bonfante V, Bestetti O, Bonadonna G (1985) Gonadal toxicity after combination chemotherapy for Hodgkin's disease: comparative results of MOPP and ABVD. Eur J Clin Oncol 21: 601–605

Waxman JH, Terry YA, Wrigley PFM, Malpas JS, Rees LH, Besser GM, Lister TA (1982) Gonadal function in Hodgkin's disease: long-term follow-up of chemotherapy. Br Med J 285: 1612–1613

Weissbach L, Lange CE, Rodermund CE, Zwicker A, Gropp A, Pothmann W (1974) Fertilitätsstörungen bei behandelten Hodentumorpatienten. Urologe [A] 13: 80–85

8 Disturbances of Sceletal Growth

8.1 Dose-Time Considerations for Skeletal Growth Disturbances After Radiotherapy

HORST ALHEIT

CONTENTS

1 Background 245
2 Parameters Influencing Damage to Growing Bones 245
2.1 Total Dose 245
2.2 Age at Irradiation 246
2.3 Fractionation 246
2.4 Radiation Quality 247
3 Clinical Findings in Radiation-Induced Growth Damage 247
4 Radiobiology of Growth Damage 247
5 Summary and Therapeutic Recommendations . . 249
References 249

1 Background

The radiation-induced growth arrest of bones after radiotherapy in childhood is a side effect well known to pediatric oncologists. In 1903, PERTHES described growth retardation which occurred after irradiation of the wings of 1 day old chicks and noted an influence of dose and fractionation. Later on, many case reports appeared regarding radiation-induced damage of growing bones after radiation therapy for tumors and for benign childhood diseases. A very detailed study was published by DAHL (1936), who irradiated 12–14 day old rats with doses of 0.8–40 Gy. The degree of growth arrest was found to be dependent on the dose and indirectly correlated with the age at the time of irradiation. Furthermore fractionation was found to produce a lesser degree of damage than signle dose irradiation.

GALL et al. (1940) studied the effect of increasing radiation doses on the long bones of rats and observed the relationship of histologic changes in the epiphyseal plate to the total dose, time elapsed since irradiation, and energy of the external beam. Using doses ranging from 6 to 30 Gy, the severity of the damage was noted to be directly related to the dose, up to 18 Gy. At higher doses the degree of severity was no longer proportional to dose, but the histologic changes were relatively uniform throughout the range to 30 Gy.

Studies by HINKEL (1943), BARR et al. (1943), and REIDY et al. (1947) also demonstrated the shortening of long bones of experimental animals. In addition, when the epiphysis was exposed to single doses of 6 Gy or more some growth retardation occurred, while complete inhibition of growth was produced by doses greater than 12 Gy.

GAUWERKY (1960) and RAUSCH et al. (1964) showed, in a catamnestic study of children who were irradiated for benign processes such as hemangioma with Chaoultherapy or brachytherapy, that single doses of 6 Gy and cumulative doses of 12 Gy on the surface should not be administered, to avoid severe damage of growing bone. PROBERT et al. (1973) discussed a greater radiation sensitivity of growing bone in children younger than 6 years and during the pubertal growth spurt in patients with acute leukemia, medulloblastoma and Hodgkin's disease.

More recently, PROBERT and PARKER (1975), HARTSELL et al. (1989), EIFFEL (1988), EIFFEL et al. (1990) and MASUDA et al. (1990) reported avoidance of growth retardation by unconventional fractionated radiotherapy with lower doses per fraction.

2 Parameters Influencing Damage to Growing Bones

2.1 Total Dose

One of the most important parameters is the total dose delivered to the epiphyseal plate. For single fractionated experiments in animals a dose of about 6 Gy or more was found to produce growth retardation and 12 Gy to cause complete growth

HORST ALHEIT, Dr., Universitätsklinikum Carl Gustav Carus, Technische Universität Dresden, Klinik und Poliklinik für Strahlentherapie, Fetscherstraße 74, 01307 Dresden, FRG

inhibition (HINKEL 1943; BARR et al. 1943; REIDY et al. 1947). GALL et al. (1940) found that a dose of 18 Gy was necessary to produce complete growth inhibition. In the dose range from 6 to 18 Gy GALL et al. (1940) found a proportional dose-effect relationship, whereas with doses greater than 18 Gy the growth inhibition was no longer proportional to the dose increment.

The existence of a "stunting dose," below which no damage to the cartilage will occur, remains controversial. Some authors (HINKEL et al. 1942; BARR et al. 1943; REIDY et al. 1947; WELLS 1969) found such a dose in the range of about 5 Gy, whereas RAUSCH (1964) maintained that a stunting dose was between 4 and 7 Gy. WELLS (1969) and GONZALEZ and VAN DIJK (1983) reported a dose of about 2.5 Gy; other authors reported a deficit in growth after an exposure to 1 Gy or less (PHILLIPS and KIMELDORF 1964, 1966).

In interpreting these findings, it must be noted that the authors used different animals and that the effect of irradiation below doses of 5 Gy was very small; differences between irradiated and nonirradiated control animals were not significant.

In 1952, NEUHAUSER et al. noted that, for fractionated therapy, more than 20 Gy delivered to the spine caused the most severe damage, independent of the age at irradiation, and that at doses below 10 Gy no damage occurred. These data show that there is indeed a dose above which no further damage occurs in response to further dose increments. This dose limit was found by GALL et al. (1940) to be about 18 Gy and by HINKEL (1943), BARR et al. (1943) and REIDY et al. (1947) to be 12 Gy for single dose irradiation. WELLS (1969) and GONZALEZ and VAN DIJK (1983) found that at about 20 Gy no further shortening of the bones occurred. This could be explained as a saturation effect and seemed to be correlated with sterilization of the epiphyseal proliferative cells.

RISEBOROUGH et al. (1976) concluded that there is a definite dose relationship in the development of scoliosis after fractionated radiation therapy. None of the 81 patients who received less than 26 Gy developed scoliosis, whereas the others with a dosage over 30.7 Gy had scoliosis with a scoliotic angle of more than 25°.

2.2 Age at Irradiation

Today most investigators agree that there is an inversely proportional relation between growth retardation after irradiation and age at the time of radiotherapy (HINKEL 1942; NEUHAUSER 1952; PHILLIPS and KIMELDORF 1964, 1966; VAETH et al. 1962; STASEK et al. 1965; SHALET et al. 1987).

PROBERT et al. (1973) reported that irradiation of children at the time of their most active growth caused especially marked retardation of spinal growth. NEUHAUSER et al. (1952) concluded that in conventionally fractionated radiotherapy with 200 kV X-rays in a dose range lower than 10 Gy no or less changes in the spine occur, whereas doses of more than 20 Gy regularily produce severe deformities of the vertebral bodies. In the dose range between 10 and 20 Gy, the severity of damage was dependent on the age of the child at the time of irradiation. More severe changes occurred in patients younger than 2 years of age.

GONZALEZ and VAN DIJK (1983) found a relationship between the absolute shortening of the growing tibia after irradiation and the age of the animal at the time of treatment, but they also showed that, if the growth remaining at the moment of irradiation is taken into account, no significant differences in effect occur with age. They reanalyzed data from the literature of various authors, who used different species and only found a dependence of the relative growth arrest on total dose but not on age. Thus, the dose and the time which the individual has left to grow until adolescence, i.e., the growth potential at the time of irradiation, are the most important factors in determining the end points of radiation damage to growing bone. Similar findings were reported by STASEK et al. (1965) and SCHAEFER et al. (1965). RISEBOROUGH et al. (1976) pointed out that definitive conclusions about the progression and severity of spinal deformity can only be made after skeletal maturity.

2.3 Fractionation

PERTHES (1903) had concluded that dose fractionation caused less severe damage to normal tissues than a single dose. This is now a well known fact in radiation biology. In 1936 DAHL found less damage in irradiated 12–14 days old rats if the dose was given in five equal fractions. He tried to find equivalent single doses in a dose range from 2 to 40 Gy. In a reanalysis of this data, GAUWERKY (1960) found fractionation factors between 1.6 and 3.77 without any correlation to the severity of damage or to the dose range.

HARTSELL et al. (1989) investigated the influence of the dose per fraction on the degree of growth retardation in spine (short sitting stature) by irradiating Sprague-Dawley rats with a total dose of 25 Gy. The fraction dose ranged from 1.0 to 1.8 Gy, and the authors found significantly more growth of the vertebral bodies in the treated fields using smaller doses per fraction (1.0 to 1.25 Gy) rather than larger fraction sizes (1.5 or 1.8 Gy). They concluded that there is a protective effect on bone growth by using a hyperfractionated irradiation regimen.

2.4 *Radiation Quality*

Many of the early investigations on skeletal alterations by ionizing radiation were done with conventional roentgen rays of about 200 kV. The first clinical observations were made following therapy of benign processes, most hemangiomas, with Chaoul or low energy X-ray therapy.

SHAEFER et al. (1965) reported greater effectiveness in shortening of the long bones in rabbits using 35 MV electron beams instead of 200 kV X-rays. However, in low energy irradiation the amount of absorbed energy in the bony tissue may be higher than occurs using higher beam energies.

3 Clinical Findings in Radiation-Induced Growth Damage

RUBIN and CASARETT (1968) gave a summary of clinical findings in radiation induced damage of growing bones. They distinguished an acute and subacute phase from a chronic phase in the clinical course.

In the acute and subacute phases there are no clinical symptoms detectable, but many of structural changes in the epiphyseal plate can be found by histologic methods. In the chronic phase roentgenologic symptoms such as shortening of the extremities and of the vertebral bodies, with delays in sitting and standing up, gibbosity and scoliosis, deformities of the bony surface, asymmetries of pelvis, ribs or face and epiphyseolysis, mostly of the femoral head, can be found. The severity of changes depends on dose, age at irradiation and the time between radiation and observation. The microscopic findings in the epiphyseal plates of irradiated long bones were carefully described by SISSONS (1955), MELANOTTE and FOLLIS (1961), KEMBER (1967), and KEMBER and SADEK (1970) The earliest histopathologic effects on the growing cartilage are substantially evident within a few days to one or more weeks, depending upon the dose regimen. The most prominent changes are to be found in the zone of proliferating chondroblasts, in the so called columns. These include reduction of mitotic activity among the chondroblasts, degeneration and necrosis, reduction in the number of chondroblasts, enlargement of lacunae, and a relatively increase of the intercolumnar matrix with destruction of the columnar structure. Due to these changes, islands of isolated cells surrounded by an edge of chondroitin matrix develop. There is excessive mineralization and osteoid or osseous material replaces the primary cartilaginous trabeculae and is deposited in the metaphyseal trabeculae. Dependent on the dosage, the bone marrow and the fine vasculature are also effected, whereas the osteoblastic and osteclastic processes seem to be less involved.

In the subacute phase the histologic picture depends upon the delivered dose and the degree of initial damage. With a smaller dosage, recovery of the cartilage is possible. The reserve chondroblasts in the epiphyseal part of the growth plate begin to proliferate and replace the destroyed chondroblasts in the proliferation zone. If the dose was low enough and the initial damage was mild or moderate a nearly complete restitution is possible. At most a slight reduction in the width of the cartilage plate, a slight reduction in cellularity and a disorientation of the columns are to be seen.

At the other extreme, higher doses cause permanent residual damage which may be observed histologically. This damage shows marked narrowing of the cartilage plate, marked reduction in cellularity, irregular metaphyseal chondroclastic and osteoclastic processes and deposition of osteoid or pseudobone material on the metaphyseal spongiosa.

4 Radiobiology of Growth Damage

From the radiobiological point of view the influence of dose per fraction and time between two fractions is of the most interest. WHITEHOUSE and LAMPE (1953) observed that smaller daily doses led to less bone damage in children treated for renal tumors.

Figure 1 shows our own data of fractionation experiments in young rats from 1991 to 1993. With increasing total dose, the ratio of potential growth decreases; that is, with increasing dose the damage to the growing cartilage increases. This effect is seen

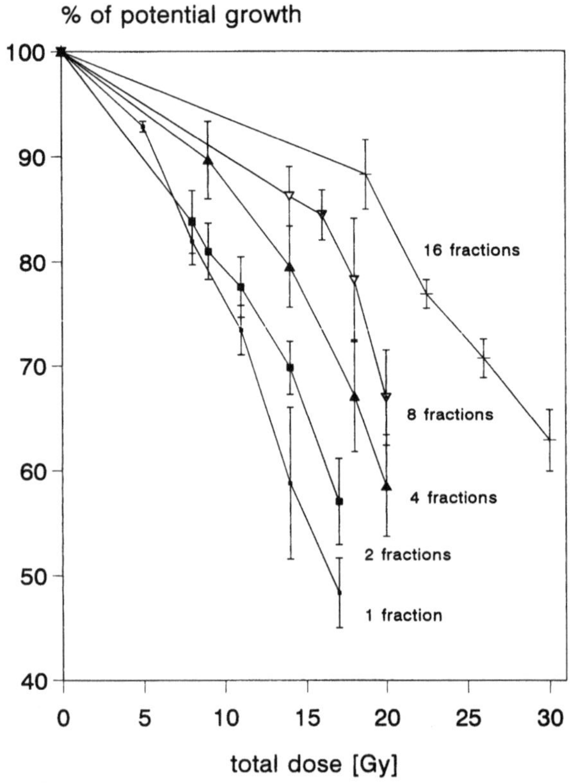

Fig. 1. Percentage of potential growth of irradiated rat tibia 14 weeks postirradiation dependent on total dose and number of fractions. Each data point represents the mean value for a group of 5–6 animals, *error bars* represent standard deviation

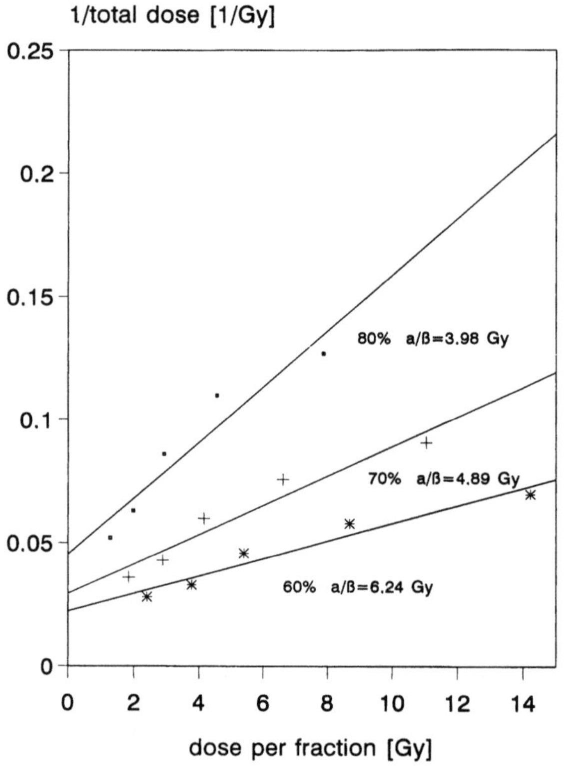

Fig. 2. Isoeffect curves (Fe plot) derived using a linear regression fit to the dose-response data shown in Fig. 1 (60%, 70%, or 80% of potential growth) and the graphically estimated α/β values

Table 1. Summary of α/β values estimated by several authors for various isoeffects of 80%–20% of potential growth

Isoeffect (% potential growth)	EIFFEL et al. 1990	MASUDA et al. 1990	ALHEIT[a] (rabbits 20 weeks postirradiation)	ALHEIT[a] (rats 14 weeks postirradiation)
80	4.51 Gy	4.6 Gy	4.0 Gy	3.98 Gy
70	4.92 Gy		5.2 Gy	4.89 Gy
60		4.4 Gy		6.24 Gy
40		6.1 Gy		
20		21.8 Gy		

[a] Unpublished data.

in each investigation, both in single dose irradiation and in the fractionation experiments. However, it can be recognized that by increasing the fractionation the curves are shifted to the right and become flatter. This means that in the higher fractionated irradiation schemes for the same effect on growing bones a higher dose is necessary. In a first approximation of these data we calculated isoeffective doses for 80%, 70% and 60% of potential growth by linear regression for each fractionation regimen.

These data are shown in Fig. 2 by using the Fe plot of DOUGLAS and FOWLER (1976). We estimated an α/β ratio of 3.98 Gy, 4.89 Gy and 6.24 Gy for a potential growth of 80%, 70% and 60%, respectively, by this graphical method. The α/β ratios for the radiation-induced delay of potential growth in the long extremities of laboratory animals, as reported by several authors, are shown in Table 1. For all authors we found the α/β ratio to be about 4–5 Gy, with an increase of the α/β ratio with a greater level of damage, i.e., a lower rate of potential growth. The last finding shows that by increasing the total dose and therefore the level of damage the repair potential decreases and the bone will be less sensitive to fractionation.

5 Summary and Therapeutic Recommendations

Since the earliest days of radiation therapy, radiotherapists have known the deleterious effects of ionizing radiation on growing bones. Irradiation in childhood must consider this effect. With the longer survival of children treated for tumors, radiation-induced damage of normal tissues such as growing bones has become of greater interest. Due to the fact that the radiation effect can clinically only be seen after a long interval between irradiation and manifestation of damage, knowledge of the relationships between dose, fractionation and time is very important. For clinical practice one must consider that there is a strong dependence of growth damage by irradiation upon the total dose and the dose per fraction. To minimize radiation-induced growth arrest, the radiotherapist should keep the dose administered to the epiphyseal plates to the absolute minimum by carefully planning the fields and shielding critical areas, if possible, and where not, to achieve a homogeneous dose distribution in the growth zone. Data from the more recent literature support the findings of a benefit of hyperfractionated radiation therapy for less damage to growing bones. This observation is supported by our own data, showing an intermediate α/β value for growth retardation in the long bones of rats. We agree with Eiffel (1988), Eiffel et al. (1990), Hartsell et al. (1989) and Masuda et al. (1990), that the growing cartilage is a late or intermediately responding tissue from the radiobiological point of view. Eiffel (1990) tried to explain this effect with a multicompartmental model made up of two or more cell lines of different radiation sensitivity. Such a simple model may consist of the following:

1. The fraction of chondrocytes in the proliferation zone of rapidly dividing cells with high sensitivity for irradiation and a low repair capacity (early reacting tissue) is damaged at first by low doses of about 5 Gy in a single fraction. This damage causes a temporary inhibition of growth if the chondrocytes are able to compensate the loss by further proliferation.
2. The fraction of chondroblasts in a narrow zone at the epiphyseal end of the growth plate with a lower mitotic rate is damaged later by higher doses, because they may have a higher radiation tolerance and a good capacity for repair of radiation injury. If the loss of proliferating chondrocytes cannot be compensated by proliferation, the chondroblasts will become a reserve pool for the proliferating chondrocytes and replace killed cells. If the dose per fraction is low enough to be repaired, this mechanism leads to a recovery of growth after some time. If repair is not possible because of high doses per fraction or such high total doses that the stem cell population is killed, an irreparable loss of growth potential occurs.
3. The metaphyseal vessels and the epiphyseal vasculature may play roles in modifying the radiation effect on the growth plate as a complex biological system. The observed effect of growth retardation is the summary of the response and the interrelationships of several tissue compartments.

In the range of tolerable damage, defined by radiooncologists as an α/β ratio of about 4–5 Gy, there is hope that hyperfractionated radiotherapy will have a protective effect on growing bones. If compared with a conventionally fractionated regimen of 20×2 Gy, for instance as usually administered for Wilms' tumor, the calculation of an isoeffective dose with doses per fraction of 1.2 Gy leads to 46 Gy by an α/β ratio of 4 Gy. For an α/β ratio of 10 Gy (early reacting tissues with side effects such as mucositis or skin erythema) we found an equivalent dose of 43 Gy and for an α/β ratio of 20 Gy (described in the literature for some tumors) of 41.5 Gy. That means for the same biological effect on the tumor one must give 1.5 Gy more with doses per fraction of 1.2 Gy and for the same effect in growth retardation one can deliver 6 Gy more. That means a 10% greater dose can be used for treating the tumor with the same risk of growth damage. Otherwise, with respect to growth damage, the equivalent of 10% of the dose can be spared with the same effect on tumor cure.

References

Barr JS, Lingley JR, Gail EA (1943) The effect of roentgen irradiation on epiphyseal growth. I. Experimental studies upon the albino rat. Am J Roentgenol 49: 104–115

Dahl B (1936) De l'effect des rayons X sur les os longs en dèveloppement et sur la fromation de cal. Étude radiobiologique et anatomique chez le rat. Skrifter der Norske Videnskaps-Akademi i Oslo 1936 I. Mathematisk-Naturvidenskapelig Klase 1. Bind Oslo, i Kommisjon Hos Jacob Byward 1937

Douglas BG, Fowler JF (1976) The effect of multiple small doses of X-rays on skin reactions in the mouse and a basic interpretation. Radiat Res 66: 401–426

Eiffel PJ (1988) Decreased bone growth arrest in weanling rats with multiple radiation fractions per day. Int J Radiat Oncol Biol Phys 15: 141–145

Eiffel PJ, Sampson Ch M, Tucker SL (1990) Radiation fractionation sensitivity of epiphyseal cartilage in a weanling rat model. Int J Radiat Oncol Biol Phys 19: 661–664

Gall EA, Lingley JR, Hilcken JA (1940) Comparative experimental studies of 200 and 1000 kV roentgen rays. I. The biological effects on the epiphysis of the albino rat. Am J Pathol 16: 605–618

Gauwerky F (1960) Über die Strahlenschädigung des wachsenden Knochens. I. Mitteilung. Strahlentherapie 113: 325–350

Gonzalez DG, van Dijk JDP (1983) Experimental studies on the response of growing bones to X-ray and neutron irradiation. Int J Radiat Oncol Biol Phys 9: 671–677

Hartsell WF, Hanson WR, Conterato DJ, Hendrickson FR(1989) Hyperfractionation decreases the deleterious effects of conventional radiation fractionation on vertebral growth in animals. Cancer 63: 2452–2455

Hinkel CL (1942) The effect of roentgen rays upon the growing bones of albino rats. I. Quantitative studies of the growth limitation following irradiation. Am J Roentgenol 47: 439–457

Hinkel CL (1943) The effect of irradiation upon the composition and vascularity of growing rat bones. Am J Roentgenol 50: 516–526

Kember NF (1967) Cell Survival and Radiation Damage in Growth Cartilage. Br J Radiol 40: 496–505

Kember NF, Sadek M (1970) Mitotic Suppression in Gut and Growth Cartilage by X-Irradiation in vivo Int J Radiat Biol 17: 19–23

Masuda K, Reid BO, Hunter N, Withers HR (1990) Bone growth retardation induced by single and multifractionated irradiation. Radiother Oncol 18: 137–145

Melanotte PL, Follis RH (1961) Early effects of X-irradiation on cartilage and bone. Amer J Pathol 39: 1–16

Neuhauser EBD, Wittenborg MH, Bermann CZ, Cohen J (1952) Irradiation effects of roentgen therapy on the growing spine. Radiology 59: 637–650

Perthes G (1903) Über den Einfluss der Röntgenstrahlen auf epitheliale Gewebe, insbesondere auf das Carcinom. Arch Klin Chir 79: 955–1000

Phillips RD, Kimeldorf DJ (1964) Acute and long-term effects of X-irradiation on skeletal growth in the rat. Am J Physiol 207: 1447–1451

Phillips RD, Kimeldorf DJ (1966) Age and dose dependence of bone growth retardation induced by X-irradiation. Radiat Res 27: 384–396

Probert JC, Parker BR (1975) The effects of radiation therapy on bone growth. Radiology 114: 155–162

Probert JC, Parker BR, Kaplan HS (1973) Growth retardation in children after megavoltage irradiation of the spine. Cancer 32: 634–639

Rausch L, Koch W, Hagemnn G (1964) Klinische und dosimetrische Untersuchungen zur Frage der kritischen Dosis und typischer Strahlenschäden am Skelett bestrahlter Angiom-Patienten. Strahlentherapie 55 (B): 198–214

Reidy JA, Lingley JR, Gail EA, Barr JS (1947) The effect of roentgen irradiation on Epiphyseal growth. II. Experimental Studies upon the dog. J Bone Joint Surg 29: 853–873

Riseborough EJ, Grabias St, Burton R, Jaffe N (1976) Skeletal alterations following irradiation for Wilms' tumor. J Bone Joint Surg 58A: 526–536

Rubin P, Casarett GW (1968) Growing cartilage and bone. In: Rubin P, Casarett GW (eds) Clinical radiation pathology, vol. 2 Saunders, Philadelphia, p 518 (Chap 14)

Schaefer P, Schumacher W, Krokowski E, Frost D (1965) Zeitabhängige Relation von Dosiseffekten. Strahlentherapie 128: 93–97

Shalet SM, Gibson B, Swindell R, Pearson D (1987) Effect of spinal irradiation on growth. Arch Dis Child 62: 461–464

Sissons HA (1955) Experimental study on the effect of local irradiation on bone growth. Progress in Radiobiology (ed. Mitchell, JS), p. 436, Edinburgh, Oliver and Boyd

Stasek V, Lokajicek M, Kolar J (1965) Zum Studium des Einflusses der ionisierenden Strahlen auf die wachsende Wirbelsäule. Strahlentherapie 126: 532–540

Vaeth JM, Levitt SH, Jones MD, Holtfreter Ch (1962) Effects of radiation therapy in survivors of Wilsms' Tumor. Radiology 79: 560–568

Wells AB (1969) The effect of acute and fractionated doses of X-rays on the growth of the mouse tibia. Brit J Radiol 42: 364–371

Whitehouse WM, Lampe I (1953) Osseous damage in irradiation of renal tumors in infancy and childhood. Am J Roentgenol 70: 721–729

8.2 Disturbances in Growth of Bone, Muscle, and Fat Tissue Following Irradiation in Childhood

Friedrich Kamprad

Combined therapy consisting of surgery, chemotherapy and irradiation has increased the number of children who survive their tumors. Therefore, the negative side effects of therapy have gained increasing significance. Apart from the problem of radiation-induced tumors, radiological damage of several juvenile tissues and organs must be considered. In order to prevent such injuries the tolerance of normal tissue in children to X-rays, alone or in combination with chemotherapy, needs to be investigated. For radiotherapy alone, the dose, volume dose and quality of radiation are important, but the degree of maturity and the particular irradiated organ also influence the extent of damage. In the case of combined radio- and chemotherapy the kind and dose of cytostatics and the timing of administration must be taken into consideration when investigating negative side effects. Furthermore, in many cases various organs are damaged, so that the negative effects are combined and the clinical symptoms are variable.

The biological mechanism of irradiation affecting the various organs differs. The decisive target cells in the juvenile skeleton are chondroblasts and osteoblasts. In a series of experiments, Cottier (1966) found signs of morphologic degeneration and distinct disturbance of the phosphatase activity in cartilage tissue in response to doses between 5.4 and 18.0 Gy. This results in a disturbed development in the region of the epiphysis. The destroyed cartilage is substituted by connective tissue.

Later, enhanced formation of bone material is visible at the margin of the connective tissue. In X-ray-images "lines of growth standstill" appear. In the human skeleton reactions in the region of the epiphysis begin after doses higher than 2–3 Gy. The simultaneous damage to osteoblastic cells is responsible for the disturbance of periostal bone growth. Regeneration after irradiation is normally incomplete.

Friedrich Kamprad, Prof. Dr., Universität Leipzig, Radiologische Klinik, Liebigstraße 20a, 0413 Leipzig, FRG

The result is a reduction of skeletal development during what should be the period of growth. Therefore, the extent of the damage is only visible after termination of growth in adolescence. The bones of the extremities show a decrease along their length growth and width. Also, in the skeleton of the trunk the cartilage regions of growth are endangered. Symmetrical irradiations, for example in the case of radiotherapy of the neuroaxis, produce symmetrical decreases in the growth of the vertebrae, which are responsible for the disproportion between the length of the extremities and the length of the trunk. Given equal doses of irradiation, the extent of growth reduction depends on the maturity of the skeleton during irradiation. For irradiation of the neuroaxis in children up to 1 year of age Shalet et al. (1987) calculated a reduction of 9 cm, in children 2–5 years of age 7 cm and in children 5–10 years of age 5.5 cm.

Special problems are connected with nonsymmetrical irradiations of the trunk because different doses produce various decreases in growth. Depending on the irradiated region asymmetries appear in the chest, pelvis or spinal column. Indirect radiation effects due to damage of the hormone-producing cells in the hypophysis act on the juvenile skeleton. Albertson-Wikland et al. (1987) showed this effect after radiation of the head with a dose of 40.0 Gy. An enhanced proportional reduction in case of simultaneous radiotherapy and chemotherapy was described by Leiper et al. (1987), Bushhouse et al. (1989) and Moell et al. (1988).

The simultaneous effects of irradiation on fat tissue and muscle are responsible for the magnitude of the clinical defects and symptoms. Based on animal experiments (Lewis 1954), a far-reaching resistance of muscle cells to clinical X-ray doses can be assumed. Alterations of muscle are likely to be due to lesions in the vessel endothelium. The combination of endothelial lesion and the development of hyaline material in vessel surroundings with local endothelial hypertrophy leads to the occlusion of the vessel lumen (Hopewell et al. 1986; Kwock et al. 1987; Rosen et al. 1989; Witte et al. 1989). This sequence of events is responsible for nutrient deficiency in the muscle leading to atrophy.

Experiments with juvenile animals (Smith and Loewenthal 1950) and clinical experiences, for example, with the central nervous system (Cantini et al. 1989), showed a distinctly enhanced radiosensitivity of the juvenile vessels. This may be the reason for more serious reactions of muscle in children. In computed tomography (CT) images, a decrease in muscle tissue and nonhomogeneous fibrosis and typical signs. In juvenile fat tissue the reactions of the endothelium to irradiation cause visible alterations. The direct radiation damage to juvenile fat cells influences the degree of disturbance. Experiments with animals (Cottier 1966) showed degeneration and atrophy of juvenile fat cells after irradiation with 6.0 Gy.

In the clinical use of X-rays, proper knowledge of the radiation tolerance of juvenile normal tissue is of great importance. All publications agree on the distinction of lesions depending on dose, volume dose, maturity of the irradiated organs and interval between irradiation and follow-up examination. The radiotherapist has to determine the best tumor therapy with respect to the possible occurrence of age-dependent lesions.

Our own results are based on a number of examinations, using clinical methods, X-ray images and CT images in children with malignant tumors treated with different therapies, i.e., surgery, radiotherapy and chemotherapy. Regarding the different quality of X-rays the actually absorbed dose in the investigated tissue was calculated. With the methods used the alterations in the irradiated region were compared with the normal status in the nonirradiated region of the opposite side of the body.

In our group 51 children were investigated at various intervals between irradiation and follow-up (Table 1). The evaluation of skeletal growth deficiency showed that the degree of damage was associated with the age at the time of irradiation.

Table 1. Patient characteristics

Age (years)	Number of patients	Absorbed average dose to soft tissue (Gy)	Follow-up (months) Minimum	Follow-up (months) Maximum
≤1	12	30.8	67	242
2–3	14	28.7	72	214
4–6	11	3.1	24	180
7–14	14	42.1	20	138

Table 2. Absorbed average dose (Gy) in soft tissue and degree of skeletal damage. Figures in parenthesis indicate absorbed doses in bone

Age (years)	Degree of skeletal damage 0	1	2	3
≤1	—	29 (38)	37 (48)	40 (51)
2–3	—	34 (43)	36 (50)	38 (52)
4–6	—	40 (40)	39 (59)	47 (57)
7–14	34 (34)	37 (47)	43 (50)	43 (54)

Degree of damage: 0, no visible alteration; 1, low disturbance without clinical significance; 2, clinical symptoms of damage; 3, interference with serious clinical significance.

Table 3. Frequency of skeletal damage

Age (years)	Degree of skeletal damage: *n* (%) 0	1	2	3
<1	—	4 (33)	6 (50)	2 (17)
2–3	—	4 (28)	6 (43)	4 (28)
4–6	—	1 (11)	6 (67)	2 (22)
7–14	6 (47)	2 (15)	3 (23)	2 (15)

Degree of damage: 0, no visible damage; 1, low disturbance without clinical significance; 2, clinical symptoms of damage; 3, interference with serious clinical significance.

Defects in growth which lead to clinical symptoms (stages 2 and 3) occur in approximately 65% of children younger than 7 years but in less than 40% of children between 7 and 14 years of age. With respect to lower doses near the margin of the irradiated region the first visible lesions were recognized in children up to 3 years of age at doses higher than 10.0 Gy, in children 4–6 years of age at doses higher than 20.0 Gy and in children older than 6 years of age, at doses higher than 35.0 Gy. When children between 1 and 3 years of age received 35.0 Gy or more, children up to 6 years of age received 40.0 Gy, and children older than 6 years received 48.0 Gy distinct effects appeared with high probability. The individual type of reaction differed, therefore, in spite of equal doses, and the extent of bone damage could vary (Tables 2, 3). The alterations of irradiated juvenile muscle were not uniform. In CT, some regions of muscle showed increased density, while others revealed a decreased density. Compared to the unirradiated region, the amount of muscle after irradiation was reduced, on an average by 35%; the individual variability was very high. The reduction of the amount of muscle also occur-

Table 4. Radiogenic alterations to fat tissue and striated muscle

Age (years)	Fat tissue						Striated muscle					
	Density[a]			Amount[b]			Density[a]			Amount[b]		
	Mean	Minimum	Maximum	Mean	Minimum	Maximum	Mean	Minimum	Maximum	Mean	Minimum	Maximum
<1	+23	+11	+40	−54	0	+40	−3	−33	+7	−33	0	−68
2–3	+12	−2	+40	−35	+5	−79	−1	−16	+8	−35	+5	−79
4–6	+13	−14	+36	−52	−20	−100	−2	−12	+4	−36	−2	−74
7–14	+18	−7	+33	−56	−7	−78	−4	−22	+20	−37	−4	−70

[a] Density alterations measured in change of Hounsfield units.
[b] Alterations in amount of tissue reported as percent in volume reduction.

red in babies who received only 65% of the average dose (Table 4). The same effects, with a dose dependence between age at time of radiation and extent of alteration, were also observed in fat tissue. In spite of the lower dose babies developed the most severe fibrosis. In all groups of irradiated children the amount of fat tissue was diminished by nearly 50% (Table 4). Based on the information in the literature and our own results some conclusions can be drawn. There is convincing evidence that therapeutic doses of X-rays produce lesions in the juvenile skeleton and muscle and fat tissue. The probability of such damage increases with the immaturity of the irradiated organ. Irradiation in childhood is tolerable only when compared to the great danger posed by the tumor and if the probability of cure with alternative therapeutic methods is distinctly lower. In these cases irradiation must be performed with CT planning using modern radiation equipment with protection of surrounding normal tissue. Radiation-induced damage is irreversible. Therefore, parents must be fully informed about the expected defects during the growth period. Radiation therapy in childhood contains a follow-up-program for diagnosis and therapy of radiogenic disturbances in the musculoskeletal system. Therapeutic possibilities in case of serious damage are limited.

Our current knowledge demonstrates the complexity of problems in radiation-induced growth disturbance. Further extensive investigations are required especially regarding lesions occurring during the period of childhood until adolescence.

References

Albertson-Wikland K, Lannering B, Marky I, Mellander L, Wannholt U (1987) A longitudinal study on growth and spontaneous hormone secretion in children with irradiated brain tumors. Acta Paediatr Scand 76(6): 966–973

Bushhouse S, Ramsay NK, Peskovitz OH, Kim T, Robinson LL (1989) Growth in children following irradiation for bone marrow transplantation. Am J Pediatr Hematol Oncol 11(2): 134–140

Cantini R, Giogetti W, Valleriani AM, Buchianti M, Amodeo C (1989) Radiation-induced cerebral lesions in childhood. Childs Nerv Syst 5: 135–139

Cottier B (1966) Histopathologie der Wirkung ionisierender Strahlen auf höhere Organismen. In: Diethelm L, Heuck F, Olsson O, Strnad F, Vieten H, Zuppinger A (eds) Handbuch der medizinischen Radiologie vol 2/2 Springer, Berlin, Heidelberg, New York

Hopewell JW, Campling D, Calvo W, Reinhold HS, Wilkinson JH, Yeung TK (1986) Vascular irradiation damage, its cellular basis and likely consequences. Br J Cancer 53 (suppl VII): 181–191

Kwock L, Davenport WC, Clark RL, Zarembra J, Lingle B, Chaney EL, Friedman M (1987) The effect of ionizing radiation on the pulmonary vasculature of intact rats and isolated pulmonary endothelium. Radiat Res 111: 276–291

Leiper AD, Stanhope R, Lau T, Grant DB, Blackloop H, Chessells JM, Plowman PN (1987) The effect of total body irradiation and bone marrow transplantation during childhood and adolescence on growth and endocrine function. Br J Hematol 67: 419–442

Lewis RB (1954) Changes in striated muscle following single intense doses of X-rays. Lab Invest 3: 48–55

Moell C, Garwicz S, Marky J, Mellander L, Karlberg J (1988) Growth in children treated for acute lymphoblastic leucemia with and without prophylactic cranial irradiation. Acta Paediatr Scand 77: 688–692

Rosen EM, Vinter DW, Goldberg JD (1989) Hypertrophy of cultured bovine aortic endothelium following irradiation. Radiat Res 117: 395–408

Shalet SM, Gibson B, Swindell R, Pearson D (1987) Effect of spinal irradiation on growth. Arch Dis Child 62: 461–464

Smith C, Loewenthal LA (1950) A study of elastic arteries in irradiated mice of different ages. Proc Soc Exp Biol (NY) 75: 854–861

Witte L, Fuks Z, Haimowitz-Friedman A, Vlodavsky I, De Witt S, Goodman B, Eldor A (1989) Effects of irradiation on the release of growth factors from cultured bovine, porcine and human endothelial cells. Cancer Res 49: 5066–5072

8.3 Growth Failure Secondary to Radiotherapy of Brain Tumors in Childhood

RICHARD H. GREINER, ERNST ARNOLD BLEHER, and PRIMUS E. MULLIS

CONTENTS

1 Introduction 255
2 Prospective Studies 255
2.1 Physiology of Growth Hormone 256
2.1.1 Physiology of the Hypothalamus and Pituitary Related to Growth Hormone 256
2.1.2 Physiology of Growth Hormone Related to Peripheral Organs 256
2.2 Altered Hypothalamo-pituitary Axis Secondary to Irradiation 256
2.3 Clinical Data 257
2.3.1 Follow-Up of Cranial Irradiation 257
2.3.2 Follow-Up of Craniospinal Irradiation 257
2.3.3 Follow-Up after Irradiation of Optic Glioma 258
2.4 Growth Hormone Replacement Therapy 258
2.4.1 Present Experience 258
2.4.2 Future Directions 258
3 Summary 259
References 259

1 Introduction

Intracranial tumors account for approximately 20% of all childhood malignancy, and therapy, given in about 50% of cases, consists of a combination of surgery and radiotherapy (HEIDEMANN et al. 1993). Improved techniques of radiotherapy coupled with the possibility of surgery have raised the 5 years disease-free survival figures in children with all types of brain tumors to nearly 50% (BIRCH et al. 1990). Therefore, an increasing number of children now survive malignant disease into adulthood, and it is important that children who have been cured of cancer are accepted as "normal" by their peers. Unfortunately, the intensive treatments necessary to achieve a potential cure have both neurodevelopmental and endocrine sequelae. Multiple pituitary deficiencies have been documented after surgery and/or radiotherapy directed to tumors lying within or close to the hypothalamo-pituitary axis. However, the occurrence of growth hormone (GH) deficiency/insufficiency as the earliest and often the only endocrine abnormality in children who have undergone cranial irradiation suggests that this axis is the most sensitive to the deleterious effects of irradiation. Furthermore, therapeutic irradiation in childhood may affect final height adversely for other reasons such as impaired spinal growth after spinal irradiation in childhood or early puberty.

2 Prospective Studies

It has been shown prospectively that hypothalamo-pituitary function is normal immediately after surgery and before radiotherapy (DACOU-VOUTETAKIS et al. 1975; DUFFNER et al. 1985); however a large proportion of patients cured of childhood brain tumors were short and GH deficient/ insufficient (ONOYAMA et al. 1975; BAMFORD et al. 1976; SHALET et al. 1976). As early as 3 months after radiotherapy, low serum GH levels and reduced GH stimulation tests have been reported (DACOU-VOUTETAKIS et al. 1975; DUFFNER et al. 1985). In order to define the GH deficiency/insufficiency we have to bear in mind that a search for a factor influencing the beginning and prevalence of radiation-induced GH deficiency/insufficiency will be the type of investigation used to assess GH secretion. GH responses to a pharmacological stimulus might be normal, although subnormal spontaneous GH secretion may exist. This phenomenon has been described as radiation-induced neurosecretory dysfunction. Endocrine test 2–10 years after irradiation showed consistently reduced serum GH levels (PERRY-KEENE et al. 1976; RICHARDS et al. 1976; SHALET et al. 1976), and the findings of reduced GH levels following stimulation tests (FRASIER 1974) support the concept of damaged hypothalamic centers causing the dysfunction (PERRY-KEENE et al. 1976).

RICHARD H. GREINER, Prof. Dr., ERNST ARNOLD BLEHER, Dr., Klinik für Radioonkologie der Universität Bern, Inselspital, 3010 Bern, Switzerland
PRIMUS E. MULLIS, Privatdozent, Dr., Pädiatrische Endokrinologie, Medizinische Kinderklinik der Universität Bern, Inselspital, 3010 Bern, Switzerland

2.1 Physiology of Growth Hormone

2.1.1 Physiology of the Hypothalamus and Pituitary Related to Growth Hormone

Growth hormone, the most abundant hormone produced in the somatotrope cells of the human pituitary gland, plays a major role in controlling postnatal growth. GH is secreted in a pulsatile fashion under coordinate regulation by hypothalamic somatostatin (SS) and GH releasing hormone and acts on multiple tissues to regulate metabolic functions and growth. Peripheral tissues produce insulin-like growth factor-1 (IGF-1) which is secreted into the circulation and acts as both an endocrine and a paracrine/autocrine factor. As a feedback mechanism, circulating IGF-1 inhibits GH secretion at the pituitary and/or hypothalamic level (SKLAR 1992). In addition, GH regulates its own secretion by a short-loop feedback. Estrogen stimulates GH secretion in humans; the mechanism is not clear, but the effect may be either to inhibit the action of GH peripherally or stimulate GH secretion at the hypothalamic level.

The pattern of GH secretion depends on a number of factors, including stage of development, nutritional state, sleep stage, stress and exercise (SKLAR 1992). The most consistent period of GH secretion, however, in both children and adults, is with the onset of the first slow wave of sleep (stages III and IV), which usually occurs within the first hour of sleep (TAKAAHASHI et al. 1968). During early childhood, in puberty and adulthood, GH is secreted in volleys of multiple secretory bursts. With increasing secretion of sexual hormones during puberty, the amplitude of GH secretion increases, resulting in overall increased GH production (ALBERTSSON-WIKLAND and ROSBERG 1988; MARTHA et al. 1989). The correlation between GH produced, height velocity and, therefore, stature and final height is obvious, whereas the secretion pattern and its effect on final height remains unclear (SKLAR 1992).

2.1.2 Physiology of Growth Hormone Related to Peripheral Organs

Based on studies on GH action in preadipocytes, a dual effector model of GH action has been proposed. GH first stimulates precursor cells to undergo differentiation, and somatomedins (IGF-I, etc.) then act as mitogens to stimulate clonal growth of the differentiated cells (ISAKSSON et al. 1987). Evidence supporting this hypothesis comes from experiments in which GH, injected into epiphyseal plates of hypophysectomized rats, yielded stimulated growth only in the injected limb. Furthermore, in growing tissues GH and IGF-I together influence protein synthesis and cell proliferation (GREEN et al. 1985).

2.2 Altered Hypothalamo-pituitary Axis Secondary to Irradiation

Impaired growth is evidenced by decreased height velocity, altered GH secretion and blunted GH responses to stimulation tests. As early as 3 months after completion of radiotherapy reduced serum GH levels can be measured (DUFFNER et al. 1985). Although there is a 100% incidence of GH insufficiency at 5 years (DUFFNER et al. 1985, LANNERING and ALBERTSSON-WIKLAND 1987; RAPPAPORT and BRAUNER 1989) the exact sequence of deficit is not predictable and varies widely in different patients (CHIN and MARUYAMA 1984; OBERFIELD et al. 1986). The 24 h serum GH profiles have shown that, though the diurnal rhythm is preserved, both the amplitude and frequency of secreted GH are reduced (BLATT et al. 1984; LANNERING and ALBERTSSON-WIKLAND 1987). Consequently, IGF-I levels are low (COSTIN 1988). All patients receiving ≥ 3000 cGy cranial irradiation presented a blunted peak GH response to insulin-induced hypoglycemia within 5 years of treatment for brain tumor, and in 65% of the children studied after a ≥ 3000 cGy irradiation dose similar stimulation patterns were found (CLAYTON and SHALET 1991a). Although the correlation between dose of irradiation received by the hypothalamo-pituitary axis and the degree of insufficient GH secretion is well established, a lowest acceptable dose has not yet been identified. Data from animal studies (CHROUSOS et al. 1982) support the idea that the increased irradiation sensitivity of the hypothalamic nuclei (PERRY-KEENE et al. 1976) causes the altered GH secretion pattern and that the amount of GH secreted following a simulation test might indicate the residual pituitary function. For example, GH releasing hormone (GHRH) yields excessive GH release which subsides parallelly to the time elapsed since irradiation (LUSTIG et al. 1985; LANNERING and ALBERTSSON-WIKLAND 1987). Interestingly before puberty, the altered GH secretion can be demonstrated using provocative tests even after a shorter period of time (ONOYAMA et al. 1975; DUFFNER et al. 1985; VOORHESS et al. 1986; ALBERTSSON-WIKLAND et al. 1987; BRAUNER et al. 1988) and/or after lower irradiation doses (SHALET et al. 1976; BRAUNER et al. 1986). Similarly, higher irradiation doses were reported to cause hormonal alteration earlier, whereas the opposite was found with lower doses (CLAYTON and SHALET 1991a). There have been reports of growth failure in as many as 70% of leukemic children treated with intensive chemotherapy and 2400 cGy cranial irradiation. Short-term data on 1800 cGy cranial irradiation, used since 1980, suggest that this dose causes no growth attenuation but long-term data are not available (POMAREDE et al. 1984; RAPPAPORT and BRAUNER 1989). In addition, DACOU-VOUTETAKIS et al. (1975) and OBERFIELD et al. (1986) reported that a "restitutio ad integrum" following low dose irradiation might be possible. Of clinical importance is that growth delay is usually documented only 2 years after radiotherapy, even if GH insufficiency was indicated much earlier (BRAUNER et al. 1986). The incidence of panhypopituitarism (additional lack of ACTH, TSH, FSH/LH) is irradiation dose-dependent and increases with time (DUFFNER et al. 1985; SHALET et al. 1988). The absence of these hormones has some impact on growth failure (TUNBRIDGE et al. 1973; CONSTINE et al. 1993).

2.3 Clinical Data

2.3.1 Follow-Up of Cranial Irradiation

Beginning at the time of diagnosis and thereafter on a regular basis (once a year) until the final height is reached, total body length, sitting height, leg length and bone age are to be followed carefully in order to control growth and height velocity (SHALET et al. 1987; DUFFNER et al. 1985). Already within the first year after radiotherapy of brain tumors there is a clear decrease in height velocity (DUFFNER et al. 1983; SULMONT et al. 1990), especially if irradiation started before the onset of puberty (DUFFNER et al. 1985; VOORHESS et al. 1986; ALBERTSSON-WIKLAND et al. 1987). In addition, 2 and 5 years after radiotherapy height differs one and three standard deviations, respectively, from normals (VOORHESS et al. 1986), bone maturation is retarded (DUFFNER et al. 1985; SHALET et al. 1988) and body weight reduced (ONOYAMA et al. 1975). A complicating issue in the follow-up of growth, however, is the tendency of early puberty, particularly in females. To the inexperienced eye, it may appear that children may grow at a normal velocity and do not require investigation. But one has to bear in mind that an early pubertal spurt due to sex steroids may mask GH insufficiently, resulting in a blunted growth spurt, accelerated skeletal maturation and, therefore a, compromised final height. As a rule of thumb, the younger the child is at the beginning of treatment, the greater the divergence from normal development appears; the span, however, cannot be fully judged until the end of growth period after puberty (SHALET et al. 1988).

2.3.2 Follow-Up of Craniospinal Irradiation

The analysis of growth following craniospinal irradiation of tumors metastasizing in the meninges, e.g., medulloblastomas, revealed that short stature is further aggravated if spinal irradiation is given. Spinal irradiation damages both vertebral epiphyseal growth plates and the bony matrix (SHALET et al. 1987), thus limiting the potential for spinal growth, a component particularly important to height achieved during the pubertal growth spurt. It is during puberty when most of the impairment in spinal growth occurs, irrespective of the age at irradiation. Consequently, the prognosis for spinal growth in an irradiated child who is still prepubertal should not be too optimistic. Whereas a growth deficit after exclusive brain irradiation can be determined conclusively only after 2 years, a definite reduction in height can already be found 1 year after irradiation of the entire CNS (BROWN et al. 1983; OBERFIELD et al. 1986; ALBERTSSON-WIKLAND et al. 1987; DARENDELILER et al. 1990). Furthermore, skeletal disproportion (CHIN and MARUYAMA 1984; SULMONT et al. 1990) due to the impaired spinal growth, resulting in a deficit in sitting height (BROWN et al. 1983), becomes obvious. The younger the child is at treatment, the more severe is the restriction on spinal growth and the shorter and more disproportionate the child becomes as he/she approaches adulthood (SHALET et al. 1987). After a dose of spinal irradiation of 3000 cGy and more (as usually given in medulloblastomas) the estimated height loss is 9 cm, 7 cm and 5.5 cm if irradiation is given at the ages of 1, 5 and 10 years, respectively (SHALET et al. 1987). The growth deficit at the end of the first year of treatment can already reach as much as 3 cm (BROWN et al. 1983).

As mentioned earlier, growth loss is less definitely more influenced by age at the beginning of cranial radiotherapy than is the case in spinal irradiation. In either case, the gradual loss in sitting height, independent of age at the time of radiotherapy, is less in the prepubertal than in the pubertal and/or postpubertal growth period (SHALET et al. 1988). After exclusive spinal irradiation the impairment in spinal growth, and therefore loss in sitting height, is even more significant during puberty (PROBERT and PARKER 1975; DONALDSON et al. 1988; CLAYTON and SHALET 1991b). Growth failure after craniospinal irradiation may be aggravated by thyroid dysfunction which, unexpectedly, is significantly more prevalent in children after treatment with a combination of chemotherapy and spinal irradiation than after spinal irradiation alone (OLSHAN et al. 1992). The prevalence of primary thyroid dysfunction is about 30% compared with 3% for secondary dysfunction. The mechanism of thyroid disturbance requires further studies. It has been suggested that postirradiation thyroid damage might be an autoimmune phenomenon. Nevertheless, it reinforces the need for lifelong surveillance of thyroid function in children who have received chemotherapy and craniospinal irradiation (BROWN et al. 1983; OBERFIELD et al. 1986; PASQUALINI et al. 1987). In addition, early or precocious puberty has been reported in some children who have received cranial irradiation, with an impact on growth and development as already mentioned earlier (WINTER and GREEN 1985; PASQUALINI et al. 1987; DARENDELILER et al. 1990; SULMONT et al. 1990).

2.3.3 Follow-Up after Irradiation of Optic Glioma

Optic glioma are often associated with precocious puberty. The onset of puberty in children with radiation-induced GH insufficiently occurs at a significantly earlier chronological age and bone age than in children with isolated idiopathic GH deficiency and may affect both sexes (SHALET et al. 1988). It are, therefore, the youngests at irradiation who are likely to have the most profound disturbances in timing of puberty. Clinically, children with precocious puberty might retain a sufficient height velocity due to the increased levels of sexual hormones which mask the GH insufficiency.

2.4 Growth Hormone Replacement Therapy

2.4.1 Present Experience

To determine if GH had a significant impact on growth in children with radiation-induced GH insufficiency the height velocity during the first year of GH therapy was compared with the pretreatment height velocity. Daily subcutaneous injections of human GH over at least 1 year definitely increased the rate of growth (RICHARDS et al. 1976). During the first year of treatment a well defined increase in height velocity occurred which again slowed down in the second year (WINTER and GREEN 1985; SHALET et al. 1992). To achieve a maximal response, GH should be substituted early so that children might catch up on the loss (LIVSEY et al. 1990; KANEV et al. 1991). Development stimulated before puberty, however, favors leg length (LIVSEY et al. 1990) and, thus, after craniospinal irradiation the difference between the upper and lower segment of the lower extremities (OBERFIELD et al. 1986; CLAYTON et al. 1988; SULMONT et al. 1990). Final heights studies (CLAYTON et al. 1988) indicated that GH substitution was of significant benefit in children with radiation-induced GH insufficiency. But the height gained, or rather the height loss which had been prevented, was disappointingly small and much less than that seen in GH-treated children with idiopathic GH deficiency and in short normals (SULMONT et al. 1990; LANNERING and ALBERTSSON-WIKLAND 1989; SHALET et al. 1992). Most interestingly, the benefit of GH therapy correlates negatively with the spontaneous secretion of GH (LANNERING and ALBERTSSON-WIKLAND 1989). After craniospinal irradiation, GH replacement therapy may not alter the growth of an irradiated spine when compared with the spinal growth of GH deficient children without radiotherapy (CLAYTON et al. 1988; SULMONT et al. 1990). Rather it might exaggerate body disproportion which already exists (SHALET et al. 1988; DARENDELILER et al. 1990; LIVSEY et al. 1990). Studies are currently underway analyzing height prognosis for this form of radiation-induced skeletal dysplasia increasing the dose of GH from 0.5 up to 1 U/kg per day (CLAYTON et al. 1988a, b; LANNERING and ALBERTSSON-WIKLAND 1989; SHALET et al. 1992). Thus, an 8.2 cm increase in height was reported during the first year of treatment with a scarcely smaller gain in the second year (LANNERING and ALBERTSSON-WIKLAND 1989). The theoretical risk that GH may predispose to recurrence of malignancy remains unproven (OGILVY-STUART et al. 1992).

2.4.2 Future Directions

The impact of early puberty in a child with radiation-induced growth failure is to reduce the time available for GH treatment. Consequently, pubertal development may be stopped using a gonadotrophin releasing hormone (GnRH) analogue and additional GH treatment. It is relatively straightforward to halt the progression of puberty, but it is too early to judge the effect on final height (SHALET et al. 1992).

3 Summary

Irradiation to the hypothalamo-pituitary axis may lead to pituitary hormone deficits. The greater the radiation dose the earlier GH insufficiency will occur after therapy. Furthermore, 100% of children receving ≥ 3000 cGy presented with subnormal GH secretion and, therefore, a decrease in height velocity. Simultaneous spinal irradiaton increases the growth failure by local suppression of the chondrocytic stem cells and a reduction of the number of chondrocytes in the epiphysis itself. Thus, a very important clinical message would be to treat all children with brain tumors treated by standard radiation programs with GH 2 years after their primary treatment. It is an established fact that after 2 years of primary radiotherapy, either cranial or craniospinal, the majority of children will be GH insufficient. Thus, the policy should be to treat the children with GH without any preceding testing procedures. In order to follow the function of the hypothalamo-pituitary growth axis, height, sitting height, leg length, weight, bone age and IFG binding protein-3 should be assessed regularly (KANEV et al. 1991; SHALET et al. 1992). Puberty might mask a GH insufficiency and present an early pubertal spurt due to sexual hormones resulting in a blunted growth spurt, accelerated skeletal maturation and, therefore, compromised final height (CLAYTON et al. 1991b). In children who have had spinal irradiation, GH therapy results in disproportionate growth and an apparently less favorable response to treatment. However, with adequate dosage, sitting height can improve by treatment implying that some spinal growth does occur. The growth response in the leg is similar to that of children treated for idiopathic GH deficiency. In some cases, optimal treatment might make children achieve the predicted midpercentile height. Early treatment is particularly suitable for the craniospinally treated child of short parents.

References

Albertsson-Wikland K, Rosberg S (1988) Analyses of 24-hour growth hormone profiles in children: relation to growth. J Clin Endocrinol Metab 67: 493–500

Albertsson-Wikland K, Lannering B, Màrky I, Mellander L, Wannholt U (1987) A longitudinal study on growth and spontaneous growth hormone (GH) secretion in children with irradiated brain tumors. Acta Paediatr Scand 76: 966–973

Bamford FM, Morris-Jones P, Pearson D, Ribeiro GG, Shalet SM, Beardwell CG (1976) Residual disabilities in children treated for intracranial space-occupying lesions. Cancer 37: 1149–1151

Birch JM, Hartley AL, Teare MD, Blair V, McKinney PA, Mann JR, Stiller CA, Draper GZ, Jonston HE, Cartwright RA (1990) The inter-regional epidermiological study of childhood cancer (IRESCC): Case-control study of children with central nervous system tumors. Br J Neurosurg 4: 17–25

Blatt J, Bercu BB, Gillin JC, Mendelson WB, Poplak DG (1984) Reduced pulsatile growth hormone secretion in children after therapy for acute lymphoblastic leukemia. J Pediatr 104: 182–186

Brauner R, Czernichow P, Rappaport R (1986) Greater susceptibility to hypothalamo pituitary irradiation in younger children with acute lymphoblastic leukemia. J Pediatr 108: 332

Brauner R, Malandry F, Rappaport R, Zucker JM, Kalifa C, Pierre-Kahn A, Bataini P, Dufier JL, Tar A (1988) Sequential occurrence of endocrine disturbances in children treated for optic gliomas. Pediatr Res 23: 111

Brown IH, Lee TJ, Eden OB, Bullimore JA, Savage DCL (1983) Growth and endocrine function after treatment for medulloblastoma. Arch Dis Child 58: 723–727

Chin HW, Maruyama Y (1984) Age at treatment and long-term performance. Results in medulloblastoma. Cancer 53: 1952–1958

Chrousos GP, Poplak D, Brown T, O'Neill D, Schwade J, Bercu BB (1982) Effects of cranial radiation on hypothalamic-adenohypophyseal function: abnormal growth hormone secretory dynamics. J Clin Endocrinol Metabol 54: 1135–1139

Clayton PE, Shalet SM (1991a) Dose dependency of time of onset of irradiation-induced growth hormone deficiency. J Ped 118: 226–228

Clayton PE, Shalet SM (1991b) The evolution of spinal growth after irradiation. Clin Oncol 3: 220–222

Clayton PE, Shalet SM, Price DA (1988a) Growth response to growth hormone therapy following craniospinal irradiation. Eur J Pediatr 147: 593–596

Clayton PE, Shalet SM, Price DA (1988b) Growth response to growth hormone therapy following craniospinal irradiation. Eur J Pediatr 147: 597–601

Constine LS, Woolf PD, Cann D, Mick G, McCormick K, Raubertas RF, Rubin P (1993) Hypothalamic-pituitary dysfunction after radiation for brain tumors. N Engl J Med 328: 87–94

Costin G (1988) Effects of low-dose cranial radiation on growth hormone secretory dynamics and hypothalamic pituitary functions. Am J Dis Child 142: 847–852

Dacou-Voutetakis C, Haidas ST, Zannos-Mariolea L (1975) Radiation and pituitary function in children. Lancet 2: 1206–1207

Darendeliler F, Livsey EA, Hindmarsh PC, Brook CGD (1990) Growth and growth hormone secretion in children following treatment of brain tumors with radiotherapy. Acta Paediatr Scand 79: 950–956

Donaldson S, Kleeberg P, Cox R (1988) Growth abnormalities associated with radiation in children with Hodgkin's disease. Proc Am Soc Clin Oncol 7: 224

Duffner PK, Cohen ME, Anderson SW, Voorhess ML, MacGillivray MH, Panahon A, Brecher ML (1983) Long-term effects of treatment on endocrine function in children with brain tumors. Ann Neurol 14: 528–532

Duffner PK, Cohen ME, Voorhess ML, MacGillivray MH, Brecher ML, Panahon A, Gilani BB (1985) Long-term effects of cranial irradiation on endocrine function in children with brain tumors. A prospective study. Cancer 56: 2186–2193

Frasier SD (1974) A review of growth hormone stimulation tests in children. Pediatrics 53: 929–937

Green H, Marikawa M, Nixon T (1985) A dual effector theory of growth-hormone action. Differentiaion 29: 195–198

Heideman RL, Freeman RC, Packer RJ, Rorke LB, Albright LA (1993) Tumors of the nervous system. In: Pizzo PA, Poplak DG (ed) Principles and practice of pediatric oncology. 2nd edn. Lippincott, Philadelphia, pp 633–681

Isaksson OGP, Lindhahl A, Nilsson A, Isgaard J (1987) Mechanism of stimulatory effect of growth hormone on longitudinal bone growth. Endocrinol Rev 8: 426–438

Kanev PM, Lefebvre JF, Mauseth RS, Berger MS (1991) Growth hormone deficiency following radiation therapy of primary brain tumors in children. J Neurosurg 74: 743–748

Lannering B, Albertsson-Wikland K (1987) Growth hormone release in children after cranial irradiation. Horm Res 27: 13–22

Lannering B, Albertsson-Wikland K (1989) Im-proved growth response to growth hormone treatment in irradiated children. Acta Paediatr Scand 78: 562–567

Livsey EA, Hindmarsh PC, Brook CGD, Whitton AC, Bloom HJG, Tobias JS, Godlee JN, Britton J (1990) Endocrine disorders following treatment of childhood brain tumors. Br J Cancer 61: 622–625

Lustig RH, Schriock EA, Kaplan SL, Grumbach MM (1985) Effect of growth hormone-releasing factor on growth hormone release in children with radiation-induced growth hormone deficiency. Pediatrics 76: 274–279

Martha RM, Rogol AD, Veldhuis JD (1989) Alterations in the pulsatile properties of circulating growth hormone concentrations during puberty in boys. J Clin Endocrinol Metab 69: 563–570

Oberfield SE, Allen JC, Pollack J, New MI, Levine LS (1986) Long-term endocrine sequelae after treatment of medulloblastoma: prospective study of growth and thyroid function. J Pediatr 108: 219–223

Ogilvy-Stuart AL, Ryder WDJ, Gattamaneni HR, Clayton PE, Shalet SM (1992) Growth hormone and tumor recurrence. Br Med J 304: 1601–1605

Olshan JS, Gubernik J, packer RJ, D'Angio GJ, Goldwein JW, Willi SM, Moshang GT (1992) The effect of adjuvant chemotherapy on growth in children with medulloblastoma. Cancer 70: 2013–2017

Onoyama Y, Abe M, Takahashi M, Yabumoto E, Sakamoto T (1975) Radiation therapy of brain tumors in children. Radiology 115: 687–693

Pasqualini T, Diez B, Domene H, Escobar ME, Gruneiro L, Heinrich JJ, Martinez A, Iorcansky S, Sackmann-Muriel F, Rivarola M (1987) Long-term endocrine sequelae after surgery, radiotherapy and chemotherapy in children with medulloblastoma. Cancer 59: 801–806

Perry-Keene DA, Connelly JF, Young RA, Wettenhall HNB, Martin FIR (1976) Hypothalamic hypopituitarism following external radiotherapy for tumors distant from the adenohypophysis. Clin Endocrinol 5: 373–380

Pomarede R, Czernichow P, Zucker JM, Schlienger P, Haye C, Rosenwald JC, Lab BA, Rappaport R (1984) Incidence of anterior pituitary deficiency after radiotherapy at an early age: study in ratinoblastoma. Acta Paediatr Scand 73: 115–119

Probert JC, Parker BR (1975) The effects of radiation therapy on bone growth. Radiology 114: 155–162

Rappaport R, Brauner R (1989) Growth and endocrine disorders secondary to cranial irradiation. Pediatr Res 25: 561–567

Richards GE, Wara WW, Grumbach MM, Kaplan SL, Sheline GE, Conte FA (1976) Delayed onset of hypopituitarism: sequelae of therapeutic irradiation of central nervous system, eye, and middle ear tumors. J Pediatr 89: 553–559

Shalet SM, Beardwell CG, Morris-Jones P, Bamford GN, Ribeiro GG, Pearson D (1976) Growth hormone deficiency in children with brain tumors. Cancer 37: 1144–1148

Shalet SM, Gibson B, Swindell R, Pearson D (1987) Effect of spinal irradiation on growth. Arch Dis Child 62: 461–464

Shalet SM, Clayton PE, Price DA (1988) Growth and pituitary function in children treated for brain tumors or acute lymphoblastic leukemia. Horm Res 30: 53–61

Shalet SM, Ogilvy-Stuart AL, Crowne EC, Clayton PE (1992) Indications for human growth hormone treatment of radiation-induced growth hormone deficiency. In: Green DM, D'Angio GJ (ed) Late effects of treatment for childhood cancer. Wiley-Lyss, New York, pp 71–79

Sklar CA (1992) Physiology of growth hormone production and release. In: Green DM, D'Angio GJ (eds) Late effects of treatment for childhood cancer. Wiley-Lyss, New York, pp 49–54

Sulmont V, Brauner R, Fontoura M, Rappaport R (1990) Response to growth hormone treatment and final height after cranial or craniospinal irradiation. Acta Paediatr Scand 79: 542–549

Takaahashi Y, Kipnis DM, Daughaday WH (1968) Growth hormone secretion during sleep. J Clin Invest 47: 2079–2090

Tunbridge WMG, Marshall JC, Burke CW (1973) Primary hypothyroidism presenting as pituitary failure. Br Med J 1: 153–154

Voorhess ML, Brecher ML, Glicksman AS, Jones B, Harris PM, Krischer J, Boyett J, Forman E, Freeman A (1986) Hypothalamic-pituitary function of children with acute lymphocytic leukemia after three forms of central nervous system prophylaxis. A retrospective study. Cancer 57: 1287–1291

Winter RJ, Green OC (1985) Irradiation-induced growth hormone deficiency: blunted growth response and accelerated skeletal maturation to growth hormone therapy. J Pediatr 106: 609–612

9 Cancerogenesis

9.1 Experiments on the Carcinogenic Potential of Antineoplastic Agents

MARTIN R. BERGER

CONTENTS

1 Long-Term Toxic Risk of Antineoplastic Agents 263
2 Strategies to Reduce the Carcinogenic Risk of Cytostatic Agents Based on Bioassay Evaluation 264
2.1 Detoxification of Noxious Metabolites 264
2.2 Chemical Modification of Carcinogenic Cytotoxic Drugs 264
2.2.1 2-Chloroethyl-*N*-nitrosoureas 264
2.2.2 Mustard Derivatives 265
2.2.3 Triazene Derivatives 267
2.3 Modulation of Carcinogenic Expression 267
2.3.1 Ilmofosine 267
2.3.2 Dinaline 269
3 Are These Strategies Applicable to the Human Situation? 269
References 270

1 Long-Term Toxic Risk of Antineoplastic Agents

The carcinogenic potential of antineoplastic agents can be viewed as a long-term toxic risk, first identified in animal experiments 25 years ago. In 1967, SCHMÄHL was reported on the carcinogenic activity of cyclophosphamide and triazichone in rats. His group, as well as others, extended this field of research during the following years (SCHMÄHL 1986). The findings were later paralleled by the clinical experience that antineoplastic treatment induced second tumors in patients who had been treated for cancer or for other diseases such as autoaggressive diseases, benign hyperproliferations, contracture of Dupuytren, or multiple sclerosis (KORNHUBER et al. 1987). Thus, the predictive value of earlier animal experiments was corroborated. Today, as a result of large epidemiologic studies, the carcinogenic risk to humans of antineoplastic agents has been ranked into different categories of carcinogenicity, as shown in Table 1

Table 1. Anticancer drugs classified according to the International Agency for Research on Cancer (IARC): carcinogenicity categories (FRASER and TUCKER 1989)

Generic name	Class
Carcinogenic to humans	
Busulfan	Alkylating agent
Chlornaphazine[a]	Alkylating agent
Chlorambucil	Alkylating agent
Cyclophosphamide	Alkylating agent
Phenylalanine mustard	Alkylating agent
MOPP[b]	
Treosulphan	Alkylating agent
Semustine/methyl CCNU	Alkylating agent
Probably carcinogenic to humans	
Higher degree of certainty	
Carmustine/BCNU	Alkylating agent
Cisplatin	Alkylating agent
Doxorubicin	Antitumor antibiotic
Lomustine/CCNU	Alkylating agent
Nitrogen mustard	Alkylating agent
Pipobroman	Alkylating agent
Procarbazine	Alkylating agent
Triethylene thiophosphoramide	Alkylating agent
Lower degree of certainty	
Dacarbazine	Alkylating agent
Uracil mustard	Alkylating agent
Cannot be classified as to carcinogenicity to humans	
Dactinomycin	Antitumor antibiotic
Methotrexate[c]	Antimetabolite
5-Fluorouracil[d]	Antimetabolite

[a] No longer in clinical setting.
[b] MOPP, nitrogen mustard (alkylating agent) vincristine, procarbazine (alkylating agent), prednisone.
[c] Not currently on IARC list, but should be added.
[d] Data currently available suggest compound is not carcinogenic.

(KALDOR et al. 1988, 1990a, b; FRASER et al. 1989; SCHMÄHL 1987). Interestingly, these categories very closely reflect the risk classification of anticancer agents obtained from animal studies, which can be summarized as follows: A high risk of inducing second cancer is associated with the use of alkylating agents or cisplatin, the continuous administra-

MARTIN R. BERGER, Privatdozent, Dr., Deutsches Krebsforschungszentrum, Institut für Toxikologie und Chemotherapie, Im Neuenheimer Feld 280, 69120 Heidelberg, FRG

tion of relatively low dosages of antineoplastic agents and regimens inducing high immunosuppression. A low second cancer risk is given with the use of antimetabolites, vinca alkaloids, the intermittent administration of relatively high ("pulse") doses and regimens inducing low immunosuppression. Having identified the hazard of second cancer induction and largely estimated the current risk to humans, toxicologic research currently mainly concentrate on strategies in limiting this risk. This chapter will focus on some strategies to reduce this risk, as conducted at the Institute of Toxicology and Chemotherapy of the German Cancer Research Center during the last 15 years (Berger 1991).

2 Strategies to Reduce the Carcinogenic Risk of Cytostatic Agents Based on Bioassay Evaluation

The strategies that have been identified can be grouped as follows:

1. Detoxification of noxious metabolites
2. Chemical modifications of carcinogenic cytotoxic drugs resulting in less hazardous analogues
3. Modulation of carcinogenic expression by new agents

Each of these aspects is addressed separately below.

2.1 Detoxification of Noxious Metabolites

Coadministration of cyclophosphamide and mesna (sodium 2-mercaptoethane sulfonate, Fig. 1) is the only example of cancer prevention by successful detoxification of noxious metabolites. Administration of the alkylating agent cyclophosphamide constitutes a well-known risk of inducing second tumors such as leukemias and urinary bladder carcinomas. The latter neoplasms probably result from the generation of urotoxic metabolites of cyclophosphamide such as acrolein. Urotoxic side effects, particularly hemorrhagic cystitis, have therefore been a limiting factor in the use of cytostatic oxazaphosphorines and the protracted local irritation probably is the basis of urinary bladder cancer development.

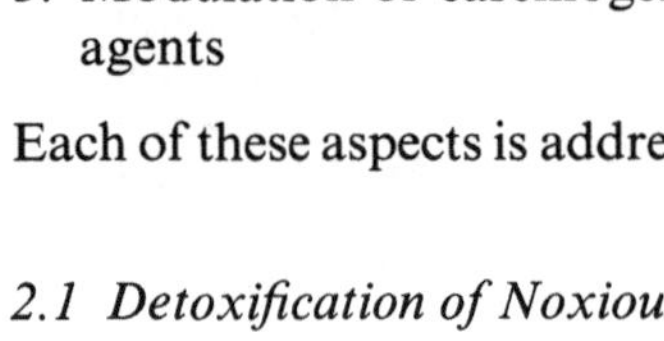

Fig. 1. Chemical structure of sodium 2-mercaptoethane sulfonate (mesna)

By using mesna it has become possible to regionally detoxify urotoxic metabolites in the kidneys and the urinary tract and to prevent urotoxic side effects. In the body, mesna is rapidly converted to the biologically inactive disulfide (dimesna). After glomerular filtration, dimesna is reduced by the glutathione system of renal tubular cells and is excreted in the urine as mesna, the free thiol compound, which then detoxifies oxazaphosphorine metabolites (Brock and Pohl 1986). When the uroprotector was administered concomitantly with cyclophosphamide to rats over 20 months (Table 2), a dose-related reduction of cyclophosphamide-induced urinary bladder carcinomas and papillomas was achieved (Habs and Schmähl 1983; Schmähl et al. 1984). Other cyclophosphamide-induced neoplasms such as those of the nervous system or the hematopoietic and lymphatic tissue remained uninfluenced. Thus, an organ-specific risk of cyclophosphamide was reduced by giving a specific antidote which does not interfere with its therapeutic potency in other organs. It is noteworthy that the protective ability of mesna against urinary tract cancers is not restricted to toxic effects of cyclophosphamide but also applies to the urinary tract toxicity of certain *N*-nitrosamines (Tacchi et al. 1984) and cisplatin (Kempf and Ivankovic 1987).

2.2 Chemical Modification of Carcinogenic Cytotoxic Drugs

2.2.1 2-Chloroethyl-*N*-nitrosoureas

2-Chloroethylnitrosoureas are highly active anticancer agents in experimental systems (Eisenbrand et al. 1989). They decompose to yield two electrophilic reactants: a bifunctional alkylating 2-chloroethyldiazonium intermediate and a carbamoylating isocyanate. Representatives of the first generation of this class such as *N*,*N'*-bis(2-chloroethyl)-*N*-nitrosourea (BCNU) were introduced into the clinic in the early 1960s; their use, however, was limited because of delayed and cumulative side effects resulting in part from their carbamoylating activity which does not significantly contribute to their anticancer activity (Stahl and Eisenbrand 1991).

Subsequent analogue development was aimed at good solubility in water and at equivalent thera-

Table 2. The influence of mesna (sodium 2-mercaptoethane sulfonate) on cyclophosphamide-induced urinary bladder tumors

Treatment	Tumor incidence (%)			
	Urinary bladder	Nervous tissue	Hematopoietic and lymphatic tissue	Other organs
Control	0	5	1	3
Mesna	0	4	0	6
Cyclophosphamide[a]	32	20	5	16
Cyclophosphamide + mesna (low dose)[b]	24	20	10	28
Cyclophosphamide + mesna (high dose)[c]	2	20	8	22

[a] 2.5 mg/kg × 5/week for 20 months.
[b] 5 mg/kg × 5/week for 20 months.
[c] 15 mg/kg × 5/week for 20 months.

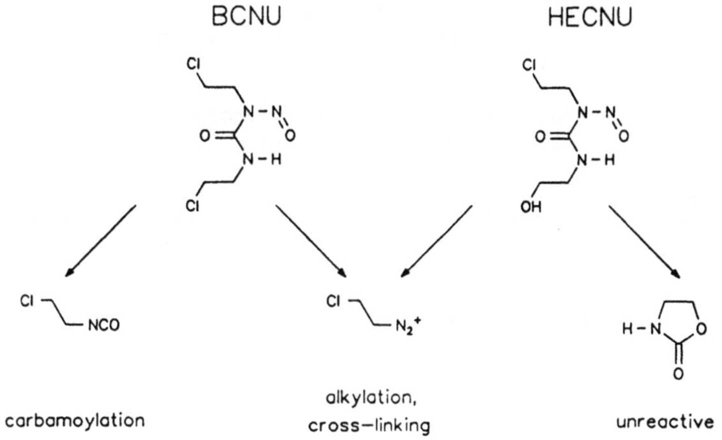

Fig. 2. Decomposition of *N,N'*-bis(2-chloroethyl)-*N*-nitrosourea (*BCNU*) and *N*-(2-chloroethyl)-*N'*-(2-hydroxyethyl)-*N*- nitrosourea (*HECNU*)

peutic activity but reduced rates of side effects. One of these second generation analogues resulted from exchanging a chlorine atom in the chloroethyl group at *N'*-position of BCNU for a hydroxyl group. This compound-*N*-(2-chloroethyl)-*N'*-(2-hydroxyethyl)-*N*-nitrosourea (HECNU), which has no carbamoylating activity, was evaluated for its carcinogenic potential in comparison with BCNU (see Fig. 2). In an additional experiment the long-term efficacy of *N*-(2-chloroethyl)-*N'*-(4-amino-2-methyl-5-pyrimidinyl)methylnitrosourea hydrochloride (ACNU) which is a further, water soluble, second generation compound was assessed (Schmähl and Habs 1982; Berger et al. 1988).

The administration schedules were based on i.v. injections of doses of 150–9.5 mg/m^2 and repeated every 6 weeks for up to ten cycles, thus mimicking clinical regimens. As summarized in Table 3, BCNU had a considerable carcinogenic potential whereas its close congener HECNU was less carcinogenic in rats. This can partly be explained by the carbamoylating activity of BCNU effecting, e.g., glutathione reductase in lung tissue (Stahl and Eisenbrand 1991). HECNU, which has no influence on this defense system against oxidative stress, does not induce either pulmonary fibrosis in patients or lung cancer in rats, as was observed for BCNU (Weiss et al. 1981; Fiebig et al. 1984). Since ACNU induced neoplasms comparable to BCNU, it has to be assumed that this water soluble analogue is less advantageous than HECNU with respect to its long-term toxicologic potential. The results observed favor the use of HECNU in those chemotherapeutic studies in which 2-chloroethyl-*N*-nitrosoureas are to be included, as, e.g., for the treatment of brain tumors.

2.2.2 Mustard Derivatives

Carcinogenicity reduction was also observed in an investigation on prednimustine (the prednisolone

Table 3. Overview on organ-specific tumor incidences following regular i.v. administration of three 2-chloroethyl-*N*-nitrosoureas in male Wistar rats

Tissue of tumor incidence	BCNU[a]	HECNU[b]	ACNU[c]
Neurogenic tissue	+	+	(+)
Lung	+	0	+
Hematopoietic and lymphatic tissue	0	0	0
Mammary gland	0	0	(+)
Forestomach	0	(+)	0
Adrenal gland	0	0	(+)
Dosage[d,e]	9.5–75	9.5–75	9.5–150

+, proven evidence of carcinogenicity; (+), clear indication of carcinogenicity; 0, no evidence of carcinogenicity.
[a]BCNU: *N,N'*-bis(2-chloroethyl)-*N*-nitrosourea.
[b]HECNU: *N*-(2-chloroethyl)-*N'*-)(2-hydroxyethyl)-*N*-nitrosourea.
[c]ACNU: *N*-(2-chloroethyl)-*N'*-(4-amino-2-methyl-5-pyrimidinyl)methyl-nitrosourea hydrochloride.
[d]Dose escalation: 9.5, 19, 39, 75, 150 mg/m^2.
[e]Schedule: i.v. injection every 6 weeks for up to ten cycles.

Table 4. Summary of organ-specific tumor incidences following regular p.o. administration of prednimustine, chlorambucil, prednisolone and chlorambucil plus prednisolone to female Sprague-Dawley rats

Tissue of tumor incidence	Prednimustine	Chlorambucil	Prednisolone	Chlorambucil + prednisolone
Mammary gland	0	+	0	+
Nervous tissue	0	+	0	+
Hematopoietic and lymphatic tissue	0	+	0	0
External auditory canal	(+)	+	0	+
Dosage[a]	12	3	3	3+3
Molecular weight	647	304	361	301 + 361
Gastrointestinal absorption	40%–60%	70%	80%	70%–80%

+, proven evidence of carcinogenicity; (+), clear indication of carcinogenicity; 0, no evidence of carcinogenicity.
[a]Schedule: 9, 4.5, 2, or 1 po administration/month for 18 months.

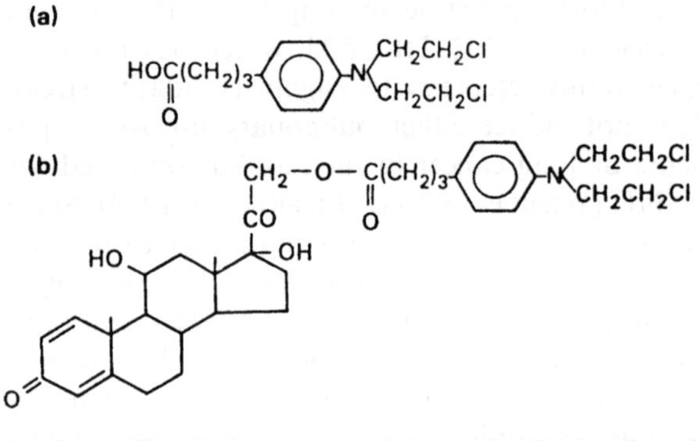

Fig. 3a,b. Chemical structures of chorambucil (**a**) and prednimustine (**b**)

ester of chlorambucil) compared to chlorambucil, prednisolone, and chlorambucil plus prednisolone in female Sprague-Dawley rats (see Fig. 3). The oral doses were selected according to molecular weight and specific gastrointestinal absorption. Thus prednimustine was given at a dose four times higher than that of chlorambucil on a milligram per kilogram basis (Table 3) to balance therapeutic and toxic activities. Body weight development during treatment indicated at least equal toxicity of the respective agents. As shown in Table 4, no carcinogenic activity was found following administration of prednisolone. Chlorambucil was highly carcinogenic in four target organs, and the simultaneous administration *mixture* of chlorambucil plus prednisolone was nearly as carcinogenic as chlorambucil alone. Prednimustine, however, was distinctly less toxic over the long-term at equivalent dosages. Assuming a therapeutic efficacy of prednimustine which is at least comparable or even superior to that of the physical mixture, the data suggest that prednimustine is to be preferred over the combination of chlorambucil plus prednisolone or chlorambucil alone (Berger 1985b).

Table 5. Summary of carcinogenicity testing with selected triazenes at equimolar doses administered i.v. to male Sprague-Dawley rats

Compound[a]	Tumor-bearing animals (%) Total	Malignant	Carcinogenicity
3,3-Dimethyl-1-phenyltriazene	27	20	+
1-(4-Chlorophenyl)-3,3-dimethyltriazene	17	10	(+)
1-(4-Bromophenyl)-3,3-dimethyltriazene	10	3	(+)
1-(2,4,6-Trichlorophenyl)-3,3-dimethyltriazene	10	10	(+)
1-(2,4,6-Tribromophenyl)-3.3-dimethyltriazene	10	10	(+)
3-Methyl-1-phenyltriazene	48	38	+
1-(4-Chlorophenyl)-3-methyltriazene	10	8	(+)
1-(4-Bromophenyl)-3-methyltriazene	13	8	(+)
1-(2,4,6-Trichlorophenyl)-3-methyltriazene	8	3	0
1-(2,4,6-Tribromophenyl)-3-methyltriazene	8	3	0

+, proven evidence of carcinogenicity; (+), clear indication of carcinogenicity; 0, no evidence of carcinogenicity.
[a] Intravenous administration of 0.1 mmol/kg every 2 weeks (maximum 20 injections).

2.2.3 Triazene Derivatives

The carcinogenicity of triazene compounds is well documented (Kolar 1986; Berger 1986). Selected agents, e.g., dacarbazine, have been introduced into clinical trials because of their cytostatic activity (Kolar 1986). In an approach to separate carcinogenic and cytostatic properties, 3,3-dimethyl-1-phenyltriazene and its corresponding *N*-monomethyltriazene congener were progressively ring-halogenated to yield the respective 4-chloro, 4-bromo, 2,4,6-trichloro and 2,4,6-tribromo derivatives. Three of the ten structures are depicted in Fig. 4. These compounds were investigated for their carcinogenic properties in a comparative study. The results are detailed in Table 5. They show that the nonhalogenated reference compounds exhibited distinct carcinogenic effects and that the long-term toxic potential of the ring-halogenated congeners was distinctly reduced with increasing ring halogenation. Thus, the cytostatic effects of triazenes are not rigidly correlated with their carcinogenic properties (Kolar and Habs 1984; Berger and Kolar 1986).

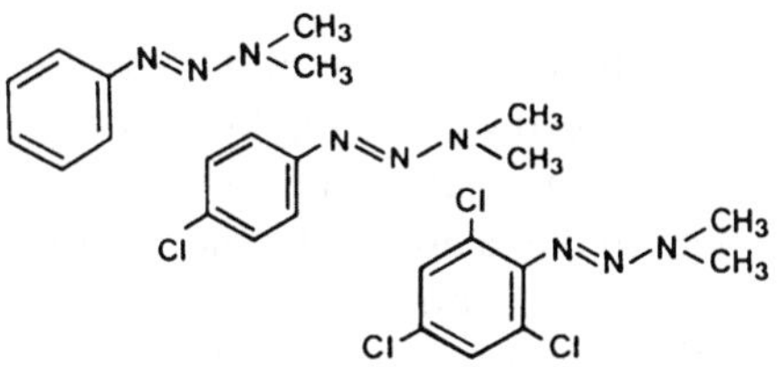

Fig. 4. Chemical structures of three representative triazene derivatives

2.3 Modulation of Carcinogenic Expression

2.3.1 Ilmofosine

The alkyllysophospholipid 1-hexadecylmercapto-2-methoxymethyl-rac-propyl-3-phosphocholine (TLP, ilmofosine; Fig. 5) was used to modulate the carcinogenic expression of the chemical carcinogen methylnitrosourea (MNU). MNU was injected i.v. to female Sprague-Dawley rats at doses of 50 or 25 mg/kg on day 50 of life. Thereafter TLP was administered p.o. for 12 weeks to groups of rats starting either 1 day, 21 days, or 42 days after carcinogen injection (Fig. 6). Two doses of TLP were given in order to administer both a low immunomodulatory and a high cytocidal dose of the alkyllysophospholipid.

The tumor occurrence at week 40 following MNU alone was 98% after 50 mg/kg and 85% after 25 mg/kg. The low dose of TLP had no influence on manifestation of mammary lesions and did not suppress tumor growth during the 12 week administration period. In contrast, the higher dose of TLP suppressed tumor occurrence and tumor growth

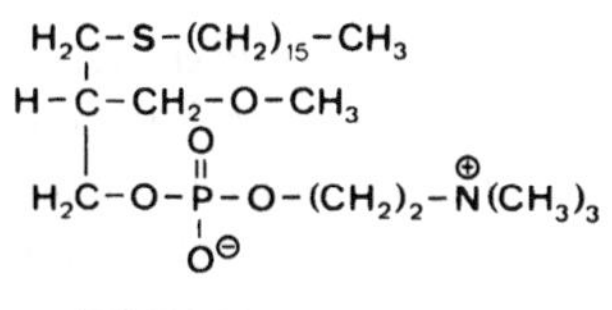

Fig. 5. Chemical structure of ilmofosine (TLP, BM 41.440)

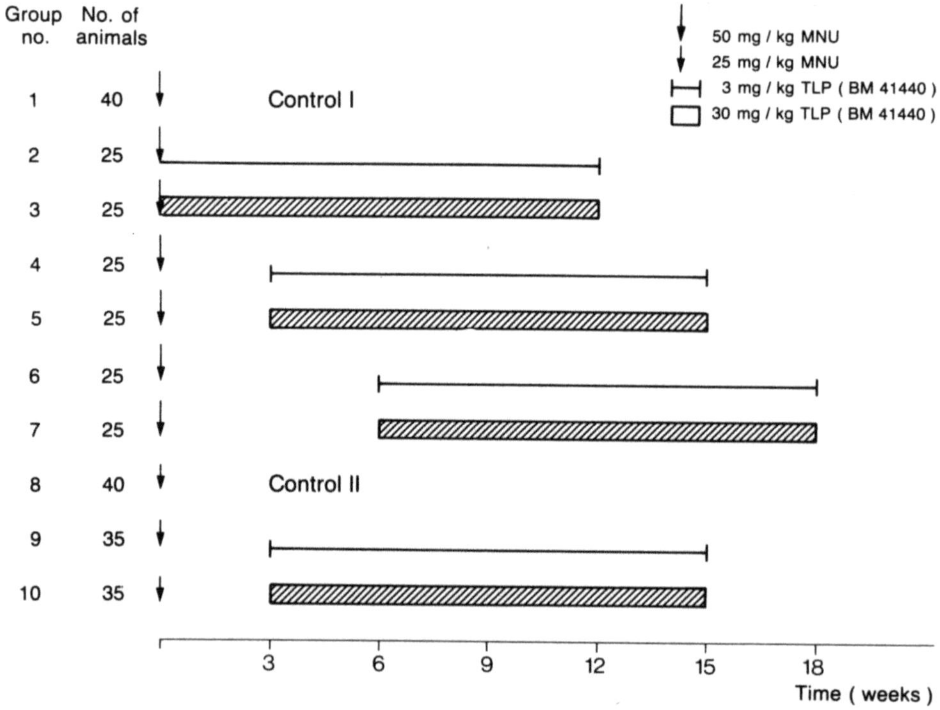

Fig. 6. Experimental design of administering TLP to groups of female Sprague-Dawley rats induced with methylnitrosourea (*MNU*)

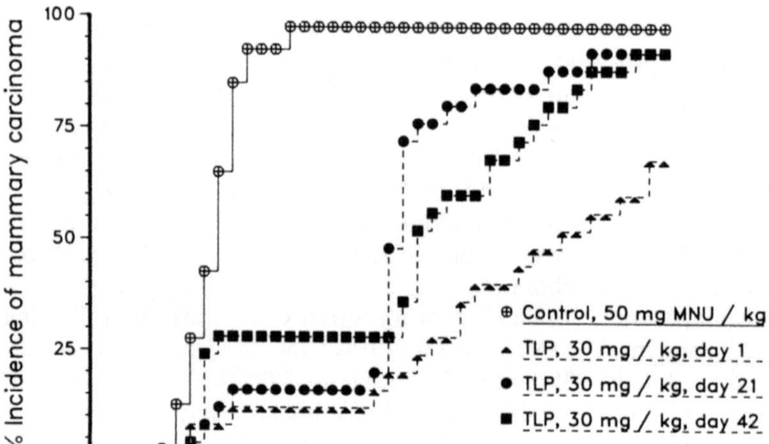

Fig. 7. Influence of TLP (30 mg/kg) on the increase in mammary carcinoma incidence of Sprague-Dawley rats induced with 50 mg/kg methylnitrosourea (*MNU*)

following 50 mg/kg MNU for a considerable time (Fig. 7). This inhibition was dependent on the start of TLP administration since the lowest tumor incidence was seen following the earliest start of TLP administration and vice versa. Moreover, the growth inhibition was maintained for 3–7 weeks after the end of the respective treatment period. An even longer delay in tumor manifestation was seen when the higher dose of TLP was administered to rats induced with 25 mg/kg MNU (Fig. 8). At week 40, a 68% reduction in tumor incidence was seen as compared to a 30% difference following the optimal treatment of animals induced with the high dose of MNU. The low dose of TLP, however, did not effect any tumor growth suppression (Berger and Schmähl 1987). These data clearly show that the

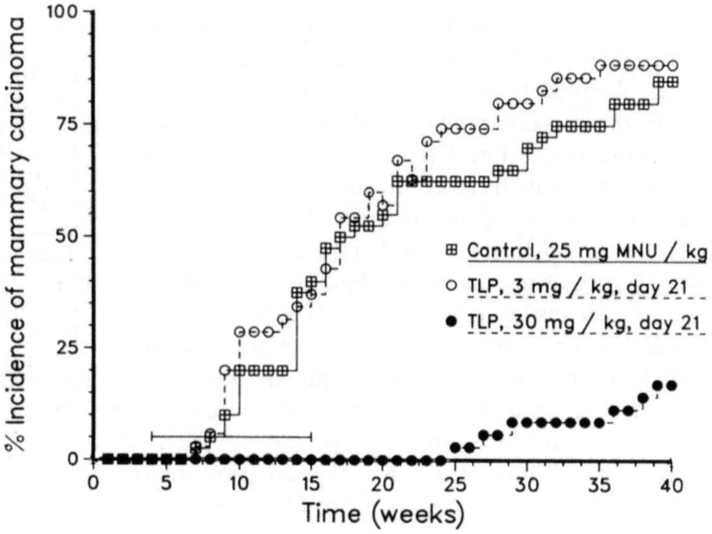

Fig. 8. Influence of TLP (3 or 30 mg/kg) on the increase in mammary carcinoma incidence of Sprague-Dawley rats induced with 25 mg/kg methylnitrosourea (*MNU*)

expression of malignancies can be suppressed by certain compounds to a considerable extent, although the genetic basis of tumor development already exists and probably remains unaffected by the treatment used (PAHLKE 1987).

2.3.2 Dinaline

Dinaline (Fig. 9) is a recently developed compound which has not yet been used clinically but is gaining interest because of its high antineoplastic activity in preclinical systems (BERGER et al. 1985). It belongs to a new class of cytostatic agents with a hitherto unknown mechanism of action. Dinaline was evaluated for possible carcinogenic potential in a rat bioassay. Surprisingly, the spontaneous cancer incidence was reduced regarding neoplasms of the hematopoietic and lymphatic tissue, the mammary gland, the pituitary gland, and the liver. Reduction of tumor occurrence allowed female animals to live significantly longer than untreated controls of the same sex (BERGER and SCHMÄHL 1991). However,

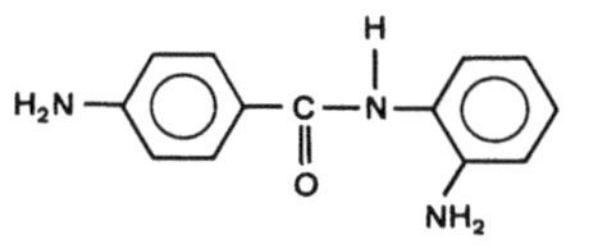

Fig. 9. Chemical structure of dinaline

Table 6. Summary of carcinogenic response to dinaline in Sprague-Dawley rats

Tissue of tumor incidence	Males	Females
Hematopoietic and lymphatic tissue	(−)	−
Mammary gland	0	−
Pituitary gland	(−)	−
Liver	(−)	0
Adrenal gland	(+)	0
Gonads	+	+
Vagina		+
All malignant tumors	−	−
All benign tumors	+	0

+, proven evidence of carcinogenicity; (+), clear indication of carcinogenicity; 0, no evidence of carcinogenicity; (−), clear indication of reduced cancer incidence; −, proven evidence of reduced cancer incidence.

slightly increased tumor rates were assessed in the adrenal gland, the male and female gonads, and the vagina. It has to be noted that the overall incidence of malignant tumors was considerably decreased as a net effect in both sexes, whereas the overall incidence of benign tumors was increased in males only (Table 6). Thus, the compound is the first cytostatic agent which effectively reduced the spontaneous tumor incidence and prolonged the life expectancy of animals used in a bioassay.

3 Are These Strategies Applicable to the Human Situation?

The results presented demonstrate that three strategies can be followed experimentally to successfully reduce the carcinogenic risk of cytostatic chemotherapy. They include the use of specific antidotes, chemical modifications of cytostatics to yield less hazardous compounds, and modulation of carcinogenic expression. Certainly, the first two strategies will be much easier to transfer into the clinic, since they can be subsumed under "primary prevention" of a given hazard. It is therefore not surprising that the use of mesna as a protecting agent against urotoxic effects has entered clinical routine relatively quickly. Similarly, exchanging more carcinogenic with less carcinogenic drugs will quickly be acceptable, if the anticancer efficacies are comparably high. Such considerations also pertain to the exchange of carcinogenic drugs in combination treatment as, for instance, replacement of carcinogenic cyclophosphamide in the CMF regimen by the noncarcinogenic agent vincristine (HABS et al. 1981; BERGER et al. 1983).

Modulation of carcinogenic expression, however, will be more difficult to translate to the clinical situation, since an active measure with an as yet unknown mechanism of action is to be taken. Certainly, some reserve is advisable, in particular since side effects have to be expected and drug metabolism might differ between the different species in addition to host factors. More research will be necessary to elucidate these problems and the principal mechanisms of the modulation of tumor expression. If such strategies could be followed in patients, some day the therapeutic gain would be important since successful modulation of tumor expression would help to limit the risk of anticancer treatment also in those patients who cannot profit from primary prevention approaches.

References

Berger MR (1986) Carcinogenicity of alkylating cytostatic drugs in animals. In: Schmähl D, Kaldor JM (eds) Carcinogenicity of alkylating cytostatic drugs. IARC, Lyon, pp 161–176 (IARC scientific publications, vol 78)

Berger MR (1991) Strategies of reducing the carcinogenic risk of cytostatic agents on the basis of bioassay evaluation. Neoplasma 38: 369–378

Berger MR, Kolar GF (1986) Comparative carcinogenicity of ring-halogenated 3-methyl-1-phenyltriazenes and their 3,3-dimethyl analogs at equimolar dose levels in male Sprague-Dawley rats. J Cancer Res Clin Oncol 111: 129–132

Berger MR, Schmähl D (1987) Modulation of chemical carcinogenesis in rats by alkyllysophospholipids. Lipids 22: 935–942

Berger MR, Schmähl D (1991) On the long-term toxic risk of dinaline. Cancer Lett 60: 237–243

Berger MR, Habs M, Schmähl D (1983) Noncarcinogenic chemotherapy with a combination of vincristine, methotrexate and 5-fluorouracil (VMF) in rats. Int J Cancer 32: 231–236

Berger MR, Bischoff H, Fritschi E, Henne T, Hermann M, Pool BL, Satzinger G, Schmähl D, Weiershausen U (1985a) Synthesis, toxicity and therapeutic efficacy of 4-amino-N-(2′-aminophenyl)benzamide: a new compound preferentially active in slowly growing tumors. Cancer Treat Rep 69: 1415–1424

Berger MR, Habs M, Schmähl D (1985b) Comparative carcinogenic activity of prednimustine, chlorambucil, prednisolone and chlorambucil plus prednisolone in Sprague-Dawley rats. Arch Geschwulstforsch. 55: 429–442

Berger MR, Petru E, Schmmähl D (1988) Carcinogenicity of ACNU and three related N-nitroso derivatives following repeated intervenous administration to male Wistar rats. Oncology 45: 127–133

Brock N, Pohl J (1986) Prevention of urotoxic side effects by regional detoxification with increased selectivity of oxazaphosphorine cytostatics. In: Schmähl D, Kaldor JM (eds) Carcinogenicity of alkylating cytostatic drugs. IARC, Lyon, pp 269–279 (IARC scientific publications, vol 78)

Eisenbrand G, Berger MR, Brix HP, Fischer JE, Mühlbauer K, Nowrousian MR, Przybilski M, Schneider MR, Stahl W, Tang W, Zelezny O, Zeller WJ (1989) Nitrosoureas: modes of action and perspectives in the use of hormone receptor affine carrier molecules. Acta Oncol, 28: 203–211

Fiebig HH, Henss H, Schuckardt C, Arnold H, Löhr GW, Eisenbrand G (1984) Phase I and II study of the new water soluble nitrosourea HECNU. J Cancer Res Clin Oncol 107 [Suppl]: 47

Fraser MC, Tucker MA (1989) Second malignancies following cancer therapy. Semin Oncol Nurs 5: 43–55

Habs M, Schmähl D (1983) Prevention of urinary bladder tumors in cyclophosphamide-treated rats by additional medication with the uroprotectors sodium 2-mercaptoethane sulfonate (mesna) and disodium 2,2′-dithio-bisethane sulfonate (dimesna). Cancer 51: 606–609

Habs M, Schmähl D, Lin PZ (1981) Carcinogenic activity in rats of combined treatment with cyclophosphamide, methotrexate and 5-fluorouracil. Int J Cancer 28: 91–96

Kaldor JM, Day NE, Hemminki K (1988) Quantifying the carcinogenicity of antineoplastic drugs. Eur J Cancer Clin Oncol 24: 703–711

Kaldor JM, Day NE, Pettersson F, Clarke EA et al (1990a) Leukemia following chemotherapy for ovarian cancer. N Engl J Med 322: 1–6

Kaldor JM, Day NE, Clarke EA, van Leuwen FE et al (1990b) Leukemia following Hodgkin's disease. N Engl J Med 322: 7–13

Kempf SR, Ivankovic S (1987) Nephrotoxicity and carcinogenic risk of cis-platin (CDDP) prevented by sodium 2-mercaptoethane sulfonate (mesna): experimental results. Cancer Treat Rev 14: 365–372

Kolar GF (1986) Carcinogenicity of cytostatic triazenes. In: Schmähl D, Kaldor JM (eds) Carcinogenicity of alkylating cytostatic drugs. IARC, Lyon, pp 111–126 (IARC scientific publications, vol 78)

Kolar GF, Habs M (1984) Comparative metabolism and carcinogenicity of ring-halogenated 3,3-dimethyl-1-phenyltriazenes. J Cancer Res Clin Oncol 108: 71–75

Kornhuber H, Mauch E, Petru E, Schmähl D (1987) Zum Malignitätsrisiko bei Cyclophosphamid-Therapie der multiplen Sklerose. Dtsch Med Wochenschr 112: 530

Pahlke W (1987) Präklinische Untersuchungen des neuen Thioätherphospholipids BM 41.440. In: Unger C, Eibl H, Nagel GA (eds) Die Zellmembran als Angriffspunkt der Tumortherapie. Zuckschwerdt, Munich, pp 65–76 (Aktuelle Onkologie, vol 34)

Schmähl D (1967) Karzinogene Wirkung von Cyclophosphamid und Triazichon bei Ratten. Dtsch Med Wochenschr 92: 1150–1152

Schmähl D (1986) Carcinogenicity of anticancer drugs and especially alkylating agents. In: Schmähl D, Kaldor JM (eds) Carcinogenicity of alkylating cytostatic drugs. IARC, Lyon, pp 29–36 (IARC scientific publications, vol 78)

Schmähl D (1987) Zweittumoren nach Chemotherapie maligner Tumoren. Arzneimittelforschung/Drug Res 37: 288–290

Schmähl D, Habs M (1982) Cancer after the use of alkylating and non-alkylating cytotoxic agents in animals. Cancer Surv 1: 585–597

Schmähl D, Habs M, Tacchi AM (1984) Prophylaxe der Tumorentstehung in der Harnblase durch Natrium-2-mercaptoethansulfonat (Mesna). Urologe 23: 291–296

Stahl W, Eisenbrand G (1991) Comparative study on the influence of two 2-chloroethylnitrosoureas with different carbamoylating potential towards glutathione and glutathione-related enzymes in different organs of the rat. Free Radic Res Commun 14: 271–278

Tacchi AM, Schmähl D, Habs M (1984) Delay of bladder cancer induction in rats treated with N-nitroso-N-butyl-N-(4-hydroxybutyl)amine by administration of sodium 2-mercaptoethane sulfonate (mesna). Cancer Lett 22: 89–94

Weiss RB, Poster DS, Penta JS (1981) The nitrosoureas and pulmonary toxicity. Cancer Treat Rev 8: 111–124

9.2 Secondary Malignancies Following Cytotoxic Chemotherapy

HANS JOSEF WEH

CONTENTS

1 Introduction 273
2 Hodgkin's Disease 273
3 Non-Hodgkin's Lymphomas 275
4 Multiple Myeloma 275
5 Breast Cancer 275
6 Ovarian Cancer 276
7 Germ Cell Tumors in Men 276
Conclusions 276
References 276

1 Introduction

As more and more patients with malignant diseases are either cured by chemotherapy or surviving longer, long-term complications of cytotoxic treatment have become increasingly evident. Among them, the occurrence of secondary malignancies is the most feared. Malignancies following successful chemotherapy of various malignant diseases, such as Hodgkin's and Non-Hodgkin's lymphomas, multiple myeloma, breast cancer, ovarian cancer and germ cell tumors are well-known and documented. However, there are also patients with nonneoplastic diseases in whom secondary malignancies develop after chemotherapy (KYLE 1982), for example, rheumatoid arthritis, nephropathy and multiple sclerosis. In this chapter an overview of the incidence of these secondary malignancies and their association with clinical parameters with respect to the above mentioned primary neoplastic diseases is given.

2 Hodgkin's Disease

Secondary malignancies following chemotherapy have been studied most extensively in Hodgkin's disease, since most patients can be cured or are at least long-term survivors. In Hodgkin's disease the high incidence of so-called secondary (therapy-induced) myelodysplastic syndromes (MDSs) and acute leukemias (ALs) was noted first. During the last 10 years there have been many reports on this late complication (Table 1). Several risk factors for the development of secondary MDS and AL are known: Preceding radiotherapy almost never leads to this complication (GLICKSMAN et al. 1982; COLTMAN and DIXON 1982; ZARRABI and ROSNER 1989). PEDERSEN-BJERGAARD et al. (1987) have reported on an increased incidence of MDS and AL in patients older than 40 years, and others (VAN DER VELDEN et al. 1988; VAN LEEUWEN et al. 1987) in patients after splenectomy. The most important risk factor, however, is undoubtedly prior chemotherapy (GLICKSMAN et al. 1982; VALAGUSSA et al. 1982; COLTMAN and DIXON 1982; BLAYNEY et al. 1987; PEDERSEN-BJERGAARD et al. 1987; TUCKER et al. 1988; VAN LEEUWEN et al. 1989; AMAR et al. 1990; ANDRIEU et al. 1990; CIMINO et al. 1991; ZARRABI and ROSNER 1989), particularly:

1. Type of chemotherapy: the regimens most frequently used are the ABVD scheme (adriamycin, bleomycin, vinblastine and DTIC) and the MOPP (nitrogen mustard, oncovin = vincristin, procarbazine, prednisone) or MOPP-like schemes. In patients treated with ABVD chemotherapy, MDS or AL are extremely rare (VALAGUSSA et al. 1982; ZARRABI and ROSNER 1989). MOPP chemotherapy is associated with an AL risk ranging from 1.8% to 13% (Table 2). The substances responsible for this high leukemic risk are procarbazine, cyclophosphamide and nitrogen mustard.
2. Dose of chemotherapy: generally, leukemia risk increases with increasing doses of the above mentioned chemotherapeutic agents. In PEDERSEN-BJERGAARD et al.'s study (1987), for example, the risk of leukemia after 9 years was 6.4% in patients who had received up to six courses of

HANS JOSEF WEH, Prof. Dr., Universitätskrankenhaus Eppendorf, Abteilung Onkologie/Hämatologie, Martinistraße 52, 20251 Hamburg, FRG

Table 1. Reported cases of secondary MDS/AML following Hodgkin's Disease

References	Study group	Number of patients with Hodgkin's disease ($n = 7681$)	Number of patients with MDS/AML ($n = 168$)
GLICKSMANN et al. (1982)	Cancer Leukemia Group B	798	10
VALAGUSSA et al. (1982)	Milan	1032	10
COLTMAN et al. (1982)	SWOG	659	21
BLAYNEY et al. (1987)	NCI	192	12
PEDERSEN-BJERGAARD et al. (1987)	Finsen Institute	391	20
TUCKER et al. (1988)	Stanford	1507	28
VAN LEEUWEN et al. (1989)	Amsterdam	774	22
HENRY-AMAR et al. (1990)	EORTC	1449	12
ANDRIEU et al. (1990)	Paris	462	10
CIMINO et al. (1991)	Rome/Bologna/Florence	947	23

MDS, myelodysplastic syndromes; AML, acute myeloid leukemias.

Table 2. Cumulative risk of AML/MDS after MOPP or MOPP-like chemotherapy for Hodgkin's disease

Reference	Cumulative risk (%)
CIMINO et al. (1991)	1.8 after 10–19 years
VALAGUSSA et al. (1982)	2.3 after 10 years
COLTMAN et al. (1982)	6.2 after 5–7 years
TUCKER et al. (1988)	3 after 5 years
PEDERSEN-BJERGAARD et al. (1987)	11.5 after 15 years
	13 after 10 years

MOPP, but it was increased to a 10 year risk of 24.6% in those who had received more courses.

3. Combination with radiotherapy: in Hodgkin's disease – in contrast to other malignancies – MDS/AL is increased in patients after combined chemoradiotherapy compared to chemotherapy alone. In the study of CIMINO et al. (1991), AL risk was 1.8% 10–19 years after chemotherapy alone. After combined chemoradiotherapy it increased from 3.1% after 10 years to 8.1% after 19 years. VALAGUSSA et al. (1982) reported a leukemic risk after 10 years of 2.3% in patients treated with MOPP only and 6.5% in those treated with MOPP and radiotherapy.

The risk of developing AL increases shortly after the end of treatment (BLAYNEY et al. 1987; PEDERSEN-BJERGAARD et al. 1987) and reaches a maximum after about 6 years. PEDERSEN-BJERGAARD et al. (1987) and BLAYNEY et al. (1987) did not find any more leukemias after 10 and 11 years, respectively.

Clinically these leukemias show some peculiarities compared to primary (de novo) leukemias:

1. They are almost exclusively acute myeloid leukemias (AML), acute lymphocytic leukemias or chronic leukemias are the exception.
2. These AMLs are frequently preceded by MDS and many patients die due to MDS-specific complications without developing overt AML.
3. AML often is characterized morphologically by trilineage anomalies, i.e., morhpological anomalies of erythrocytes, neutrophils and megakaryocytes.
4. Anomalies of chromosomes 5 and 7 (-5, $5q-$, -7, $7q-$) (PEDERSEN-BJERGAARD et al. 1990) are typical (Fig. 1).
5. Prognosis is extremely poor.

Non-Hodgkin's lymphomas are another malignancy occurring after treatment of Hodgkin's disease. Their incidence is lower than that of MDS/AML and ranges between <1% and 5.9% after 15 years (TUCKER et al. 1988; VAN LEEUWEN et al. 1989; CIMINO et al. 1991). Some of the clinical characteristics are given in Table 3. In many respects these

Table 3. Clinical characteristics of 114 patients with non-Hodgkin's lymphomas following treatment for Hodgkin's disease (From ZARRABI and ROSNER 1989)

Preceding treatment (*n*)
Radiotherapy (51)
Chemotherapy (21)
Combined chemoradiotherapy (30)
High-grade non-Hodgkin's lymphomas ($n = 75$)
Frequent extranodal involvement (gastrointestinal tract, CNS)
Poor prognosis
Occurrence later than MDS/AML

MDS, myelodysplastic syndromes; AML, acute myeloid leukemias.

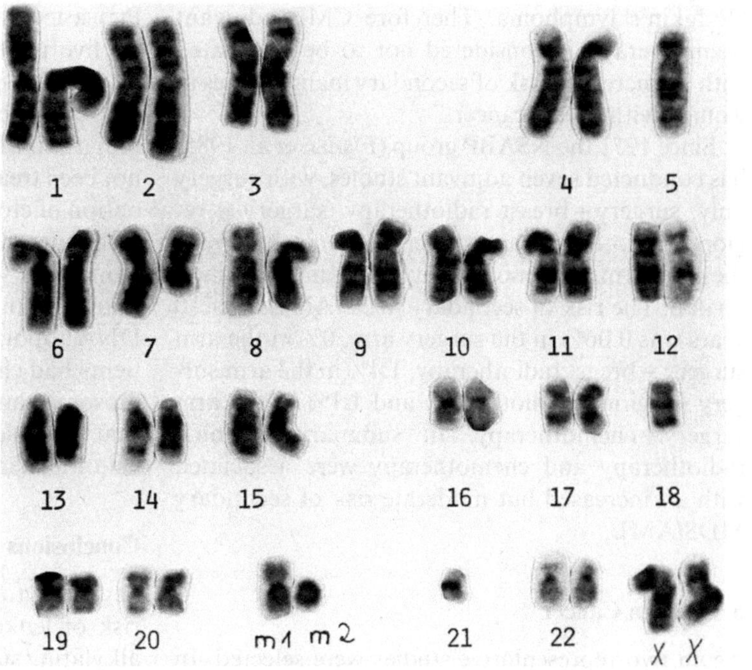

Fig. 1. Representative G-banded karyotype of a patient with secondary acute myeloid leukemia showing 45, XX, −5, −18, −21, del (7) (*q*2), +*m*1, +*m*2

lymphomas resemble those found in patients with AIDS.

The most frequent malignancies after treatment of Hodgkin's disease are solid tumors. In these cases, radiotherapy rather than chemotherapy is considered to be the causative treatment modality and therefore is not the subject of this review.

3 Non-Hodgkin's Lymphomas

Secondary malignancies are reported in large series from the Finsen Institute (602 patients) (PEDERSEN-BJERGAARD et al. 1985), the NCI (517 patients) GREEN et al. (1983) and the NCI Surveillance, Epidemiology, and End Results Program (29,153 patients) (TRAVIS et al. 1991). The risk of developing AML was 6.3% after 7 years (PETERSEN-BJERGAARD et al. 1985) and 7.9% after 10 years (GREEN et al. 1983). The influence of treatment was not as clear as in Hodgkin's disease. It correlated with alkylating agents, notably cyclophosphamide, but radiotherapy alone was also followed by leukemia.

4 Multiple Myeloma

The incidence of secondary MDS/AML has been studied in depth by the Medical Research Councils Working Party on Leukaemia in Adults (CUZICK et al. 1987). Between 1964 and 1975, 648 patients were randomized into various treatment arms, such as melphalan, cyclophosphamide and melphalan/prednisone. Twelve patients developed MDS/AML. The risk of developing MDS/AML was 3% after 5 years, 10% after 8 years and 20% after 10 years. In this study it was shown that the risk of developing MDS/AML was significantly correlated with the length of melphalan treatment. The 12 patients with subsequent MDS/AML received melphalan for an average of 25.9 months, whereas controls received the drug for an average of only 18.4 months ($p = 0.05$). Duration of cyclophosphamide administration however did not influence the risk of secondary malignancy.

5 Breast Cancer

Two representative studies on adjuvant treatment in breast cancer were selected for this review. In the Milano study (VALAGUSSA et al. 1987), conducted between 1973 and 1978, 845 patients were randomized to either follow-up (179 patients), 12 courses of CMF (cyclophosphamide, methotrexate, 5-fluorouracil) chemotherapy (451 patients) or six courses of CMF chemotherapy (216 patients). The risk of developing a second malignancy was 4.0% in the control group and 4.2% in the CMF group. No patient developed MDS/AML or non-Hodgkin's lymphoma. Therefore CMF adjuvant chemotherapy is considered not to be associated with an increased risk of secondary malignancies in women with breast cancer.

Since 1971 the NSABP group (FISHER et al. 1985) has conducted seven adjuvant studies, with surgery only, surgery + breast radiotherapy, surgery + regional radiotherapy and surgery + chemotherapy as the main arms. Chemotherapy always included melphalan. The risk of secondary MDS/AML after 10 years was 0.06% in the surgery arm, 0% in the arm surgery + breast radiotherapy, 1.4% in the arm surgery + regional radiotherapy and 1.1% in the arm surgery + chemotherapy. In summary, regional radiotherapy and chemotherapy were associated with an increased but moderate risk of secondary MDS/AML.

6 Ovarian Cancer

Again two representative studies were selected. In the study of GREENE et al. (1986) 3,363 patients were postoperatively treated with (a) no radiation or chemotherapy, (b) radiation only, (c) chemotherapy only and (d) radiation + chemotherapy. Some 35 patients developed MDS/AML. The cumulative risk at 10 years of developing MDS/AML was 0%, 0.1%, 8.6% and 8.3%, respectively. The risk was therefore significantly increased in the chemotherapy group. The main chemotherapy agents were melphalan and cyclophosphamide. The leukemic risk was significantly higher in the melphalan treated patients (11.2%) than in the cyclophosphamide group (5.4%). In both groups the risk increased with increasing doses of the drugs. Nearly identical findings were reported by KALDOR et al. (1990). Reviewing population-based cancer registries in Europe and Canada he identified 99,113 patients of whom 114 developed MDS or AML. Again the relative risk was significantly elevated in patients treated postoperatively with chemotherapy only (12.0) or combined chemoradiotherapy (9.8) compared to the groups with only surgery (1.0) or radiotherapy (1.6). Within the chemotherapy group the highest risks were found for chlorambucil, melphalan and treosulfan and for all three drugs the risk was dose-dependent.

7 Germ Cell Tumors in Men

Whereas only occasional cases of secondary leukemia following germ cell tumor have been reported so far (overview in REDMAN et al. 1984) PEDERSEN-BJERGAARD et al. (1991) recently reported on five patients with secondary MDS/AML in a total of 212 patients. The cumulative risk of leukemic complication was 4.7% after 5.7 years. The remarkable fact of this report was that patients had not been treated with alkylating agents but a combination of etoposide, cisplatin and bleomycin, drugs so far not considered to be leukemogenic. All patients with secondary leukemia had received more than 2000 mg/m^2 etoposide, an inhibiting agent of DNA topoisomerase II, and three of the five patients had chromosomal anomalies involving chromosome bands 11*q*23 and 21*q*22. It therefore seems that etoposide in high doses has to be added to the list of leukemogenic drugs.

Conclusions

Several cytostatic agents undoubtedly increase the risk of leukemic complications. Among these the alkylating substances melphalan, procarbazine and cyclophosphamide, and etoposide in high doses are most leukemogenic. The leukemogenic potential is closely dose-dependent. However, so far, there is no explanation, why these drugs are leukemogenic and why others, e.g., the anthracyclines, are not.

Secondary MDS and AML differ from primary MDS and AML with respect to morphological, cytogenetic and prognostic features. The maximal incidence of secondary MDS/AML is about 5 years after the primary malignancy. Additional radiotherapy increases the leukemic risk only in Hodgkin's disease, but not in other malignancies.

In secondary non-Hodgkin's lymphomas, the exact etiological role of chemotherapy is unknown. Chemotherapy does not increase the risk of secondary solid tumors.

The reason why chemotherapy causes secondary MDS and AML but not solid tumors is probably due to the rapid proliferation of bone marrow cells and hence their increased vulnerability compared to cells of other organs.

References

Andrieu JM, Ifrah N, Payen C, Fermanian J, Coscas Y, Flandrin G (1990) Increased risk of secondary acute nonlymphocytic leukemia after extended-field radiation therapy combined with MOPP chemotherapy for Hodgkin's disease. J Clin Oncol 8: 1148–1154

Blayney DW, Longo DL, Young RC et al (1987) Decreasing risk of leukemia with prolonged follow-up after chemotherapy and radiotherapy for Hodgkin's disease. N Engl J Med 316: 710–714

Cimino G, Papa G, Tura S et al (1991) Second primary cancer following Hodgkin's disease: updated results of an Italian multicentric study. J Clin Oncol 9: 432–437
Coltman CA Jr, Dixon DO (1982) Second malignancies complicating Hodgkin's disease: a southwest oncology group 10-year follow-up. Cancer Treat Rep 66: 1023–1033
Cuzick J, Erskine S, Edelman D, Galton DAG (1987) A comparison of the incidence of the myelodysplastic syndrome and acute myeloid leukaemia following melphalan and cyclophosphamide treatment for myelomatosis. Br J Cancer 55: 523–529
Fisher B, Rockette H, Fisher ER et al (1985) Leukemia in breast cancer patients following adjuvant chemotherapy or postoperative radiation: the NSABP experience. J Clin Oncol 1985, 3, 1640–1658
Glicksman AS, Pajak TF, Gottlieb A, Nissen N, Stutzman L, Cooper MR (1982) Second malignant neoplasms in patients successfully treated for Hodgkin's disease: a cancer and leukemia group B study. Cancer Treatm Rep 66: 1035–1044
Greene MH, Young RC, Merrill JM, De Vita VT (1983) Evidence of a treatment dose response in acute nonlymphocytic leukemias which occur after therapy of non-Hodgkin's lymphoma. Cancer Res 43: 1891–1898
Greene MH, Harris EL, Gershenson DM et al (1986) Melphalan may be a more potent leukemogen than cyclophosphamide. Ann Intern Med 105: 360–367
Henry-Amar M, Hayat M, Meerwaldt JH et al (1990) Causes of death after therapy for early stage Hodgkin's disease entered on EORTC protocols. Int J Radiation Oncology Biol Phys 19: 1155–1157
Kaldor JM, Day NE, Pettersson F et al (1990) Leukemia following chemotherapy for ovarian cancer. N Engl J Med 322: 1–6
Kyle RA (1982) Second malignancies associated with chemotherapeutic agents. Semin Oncol 9: 131–142
Pedersen-Bjergaard J, Ersböll J, Sörensen HM et al (1985) Risk of acute nonlymphocytic leukemia and preleukemia in patients treated with cyclophosphamide for non-Hodgkin's lymphomas. Ann Intern Med 103: 195–200
Pedersen-Bjergaard J, Specht L, Larsen SO et al (1987) Risk of therapy-related leukaemia and preleukaemia after Hodgkin's disease. Relation to age, cumulative dose of alkylating agents, and time from chemotherapy. Lancer II: 83–88
Pedersen-Bjergaard J, Philip P, Larsen SO, Jensen G, Byrsting K (1990) Chromosome aberrations and prognostic factors in therapy-related myelodysplasia and acute nonlymphocytic leukemia. Blood 76: 1083–1091
Pedersen-Bjergaard J, Daugaard G, Hansen SW, Philip P, Larsen SO, Rörth M (1991) Increased risk of myelodysplasia and leukaemia after etoposide, cisplatin, and bleomycin for germ cell tumors. Lancet II: 359–363
Redman JR, Vugrin D, Arlin ZA et al (1984) Leukemia following treatment of germ cell tumors in men. J Clin Oncol 2: 1080–1087
Travis LB, Curtis RE, Boice JD Jr, Hankey BF Fraumeni JF Jr (1991) Second cancers following non-Hodgkin's lymphoma. Cancer 67: 2002–2009
Tucker MA, Coleman CN, Cox RS, Varghese A, Rosenberg SA (1988) Risk of second cancers after treatment for Hodgkin's disease. N Engl J Med 318: 76–81
Valagussa P, Santoro A, Fossati Bellani F, Franchl F, Banfi A, Bonadonna G (1982) Absence of treatment-induced second neoplasms after ABVD in Hodgkin's disease. Blood 59: 488–494
Valagussa P, Tancini G, Bonadonna G (1987) Second malignancies after CMF for resectable breast cancer. J Clin Oncol 5: 1138–1142
Van der Velden JW, van Putten WLJ, Guinee VF et al (1988) Subsequent development of acute non-lymphocytic leukemia in patients treated for Hodgkin's disease. Int J Cancer 42: 252–255
Van Leeuwen FE, Somers R, Hart AAM (1987) Splenectomy in Hodgkin's disease and second leukemias. Lancet II: 210–211
Van Leeuwen FE, Somers R, Taal BG et al (1989) Increased risk of lung cancer, non-Hodgkin's lymphoma, and leukemia following Hodgkin's disease. J Clin Oncol 7: 1046–1058
Zarrabi MH, Rosner F (1989) Second neoplasms in Hodgkin's disease: current controversies. Hematol Oncol Clin North 3: 303–318

9.3 Secondary Malignancies After Radiotherapy

SEYMOUR H. LEVITT

CONTENTS

1 Introduction 279
2 Radiation Exposure and the Mechanism of Carcinogenesis 279
3 Incidence of Radiation-Induced Secondary Malignancies 281
3.1 Radiation-Induced Breast Carcinogenesis 282
3.2 Secondary Cancers Following Radiation for Cervical Cancer 283
3.3 Secondary Cancers Following Hodgkin's Disease 284
3.4 Pediatric Second Primary Tumors 285
4 Discussion 285
References 287

1 Introduction

Since Roentgen's discovery of X-ray in 1895 and its early use in medicine, there have been numerous reports of the harmful effects of radiation. As early as 1896, dermatitis of the hands was reported by Grubbe. The first cancer in an X-ray ulcer was reported in 1902 by Frieben. Blood changes were noted by Milchner and Mosse in 1904, bone marrow changes by Warthin in 1906, and leukemia in five radiation workers by Jagic in 1911 (UPTON 1986). Numerous similar reports have appeared in the literature since those early years confirming that radiation does have a carcinogenic effect and is, indeed, a carcinogen. The development of secondary malignancies following the use of radiation to treat either benign or malignant disease therefore raises important questions and concerns over the use of radiotherapy. This chapter will address these concerns by assessing the actual dangers and risks of radiation.

SEYMOUR H. LEVITT, Prof. Dr., Department of Therapeutic Radiology – Radiation Oncology, Box 494, UMHC, University of Minnesota, Minneapolis, MN 55455-0110, USA

2 Radiation Exposure and the Mechanism of Carcinogenesis

Exposure to radiation comes from many sources, including natural background, cosmic rays, and radionuclides. Natural background is the most frequent cause of radiation carcinogenesis. Less than half of the exposure comes from the healing arts, the primary role of which is played by diagnostic radiology (JABLON 1984). Fewer than 3% of the total cancer mortalities are estimated to be due to all forms of radiation, and less than 1.5% of total cancer is due to the healing arts.

Factors that influence the risk of carcinogenesis include age at time of exposure, length of observation of the population, characteristics of the radiation (electromagnetic or particulate), source and type of exposure (external vs internal, single dose vs fractionated vs continuous), rate of exposure, total dose, and characteristics of the population (e.g., racial and environmental risk of nonradiogenic neoplasia) (FAJARDO 1986).

The mechanism of carcinogenesis is complex. Current theories break this development into three phases of transformation: initiation, promotion, and progression. In the first phase, initiation, a factor, such as radiation or a chemical, usually causes an irreversible genetic mutation of the normal cell that then primes the cell for uncontrolled growth. Some initiators are radiations, urethane, and nitrosamines. In the second phase, promotion, a substance encourages the initiated cells to reproduce faster than normal cells whereby the probability of malignant transformation increases. The effects of promotion may be reversible. Some promoters are DDT, saccharin, phenobarbitol, many chemicals in cigarette smoke, an irradiation. The third and final phase is progression, in which some of the altered cells undergo a second genetic mutation, which allows them to grow uncontrollably, without the stimulus of promoters, and progress to full malignancy. In the mechanism of radiation oncogenesis, irradiation can act as an initiator, a promoter, or both so that ionizing radiation is classified as a complete carcinogen. Experimental data indicate that it may play each of these roles depending on the neoplasm (FARBER 1984).

UPTON (1987) has stated that it is possible that only one change induced by radiation in an appropriate cell may increase the probability of neoplasia, even though the process of carcinogenesis appears to require a multiplicity of changes in the affected cancer-forming cell (such as may be associated with successive stages of tumor initiation, promotion, and progression). Consequently, carcinogenic effects of radiation, like mutagenic effects of radiation, are considered for purposes of protection to have no threshold and to behave as a stochastic phenomenon. Upton also noted that certain other effects of radiation, such as cataracts of the lens, decreased fertility and depression of the bone marrow, require the killing of many cells in the affected organs, indicating that the effects of radiation vary with the severity of cell loss. Detecting the threshold of radiation effects therefore requires sensitive measuring of the consequences of cell loss. The nonthreshold, or stochastic, effects are viewed as probabilistic phenomenon varying in frequency but not in severity with dose, while the nonstochastic effects are viewed as determinate phenomenon with thresholds varying both in frequency and severity according to dose.

Based on the available information on the mechanism of carcinogenesis, Upton states that it can be assumed that the frequency of initiation increases as a linear nonthreshold function of low linear energy transfer (LET) irradiation dose. This is considerably higher per unit dose than the frequency of mutations at any one genetic locus implicating multiple oncogenic sites, damage of the genome at sites unlikely to be repaired, or genetic damage other than point mutations (CLIFTON et al. 1985; KENNEDY and LITTLE 1984). The specific genes involved have not yet been identified, but conceivably may include anti-oncogenes and oncogenes (GARTE et al. 1985; GUERRERO et al. 1984; KNUDSON 1985). Although it appears that more than one oncogene must be activated to induce neoplastic transformation, data imply that the initiation may require only one hit.

Additional studies cited by UPTON (1987) report various theories on the phases of promotion and progression of carcinogenesis. WEINSTEIN et al. (1984) stated that the molecular mechanism of promotion remains to be determined, but traditionally it has been thought that tumor promoting chemicals act predominantly through epigenetic mechanisms. Numerous authors, including CERUITTI et al. (1983), UPTON et al. (1984) and LIEHR et al. (1985), have noted that recently many chemicals have been found to be capable of inducing damage to chromosomes and DNA via free radicals or other indirect mechanisms. It has been postulated that the cells killed by radiation promote regenerative hyperplasia. MARSHALL and GROER (1977) implicate such a mechanism in the induction of osteosarcomas by bone-seeking α emitters, while KAPLAN (1967) implicates this mechanism in the induction of thymic lymphomas, ovarian tumors, and thyrotropic pituitary tumors through abscopal effects. Tumor promotion may involve more than one step and typically requires repeated and prolonged exposure to promoting stimuli. Tumor progression remains to be explained in molecular terms. However, studies by NOWELL (1976) and FARBER (1984) indicate that mutations in chromosome aberrations implicate that the process may be accelerated by repeated exposure to radiation or other carcinogens, or by selection pressures that favor the outgrowth of increasingly autonomous clonal derivatives.

In his book on radiobiology, HALL (1988) also looks at the mechanism of carcinogenesis induced by radiation. He points out that radiation is highly efficient at breaking chromosomes and that broken chromosomes can rejoin to produce either a dicentric and acentric fragment or a translocation. The dicentric fragments, likely to be lethal translocations, can result in an oncogene being expressed if, after the rejoining, it is close to an active regional piece of another chromosome. Burkitt's lymphoma is a human tumor associated with the activation of a *myc* oncogene by a specific translocation.

Another study, by WEICHSELBAUM et al. (1989) noted that the loss of genetic material may result in predisposition to malignant disease and noted that deletion or tanscriptional inactivation of a specific gene is associated with tumor development in retinoblastoma. They hypothesized that when hereditary retinoblastoma patients are treated with radiation, the incidence of osteosarcoma within the treatment field is extremely high compared to other cancer patients treated with radiotherapy. This suggested that radiation-induced deletions of critical DNA sequences may be an important event in radiation carcinogenesis. It was proposed that radiation-induced tumors may result from deletion of tissue-specific regulatory genes and that base alterations caused by radiation and dominantly transforming oncogenes may also contribute to radiation carcinogenesis.

Looking at oncogenic mechanisms in 1991 data of radiation-induced cancer, a National Cancer Institute workshop followed up on some of Weichselbaum's claims, that the suppression of tumor genes through activation or loss are due to the effect of ionizing radiation on the suppressor genes. The participants of the workshop further noted that people who have a family history of cancer or have more than one type of cancer should be considered at high risk for radiation-induced cancer (ELKIND et al. 1991).

3 Incidence of Radiation-Induced Secondary Malignancies

Reports of the incidence of neoplasms secondary to radiation are relatively low. However, they do occur and it is important to attempt to evaluate their actual risk. FAJARDO (1986) defined factors that must be present in order to determine whether irradiation has induced a human neoplasm. These include tumors that occur in tissues exposed to ionizing radiation, that are different from any local neoplasm present, and that appear after a period of latency (probably more than 2 years for leukemias and 6 years for solid tumors). A sufficient number of cases must be available to suggest a possible causal relationship. Human tumors that are possibly radiation-induced include lymphomas, leukemias (usually granulocytic), bone sarcomas, osteochondromas, and second neoplasm in childhood bone and soft tissue sarcoma.

Tumors that provide satisfactory evidence of radiation-induction are those that show statistically significant differences in incidence between the irradiated and a comparable control population. Human tumors satisfactorily proved to be radiation-induced include bone sarcomas, soft tissue sarcomas, cavitary mesotheliomas, paranasal sinus tumors, skin cancers (basal and squamous), pulmonary carcinoma, esophagial carcinoma, gastric carcinoma, colonic carcinoma, thyroid, cancer, leukemia, breast carcinoma, liver tumors, and multiple myeloma. The majority of these are tumors reported as secondary to radiation of atomic bomb exposure.

BOICE (1988) recently published a paper showing that recent studies of populations irradiated for diagnositc reasons had increased excess cancers; prenatal irradiation, irradiation for tuberculosis, and excessive dental or diagnostic X-rays were all implicated (Tables 1, 2). Recent studies of populations irradiated for benign disease showed excess cancers for ankylosing spondylitis, tinea capitis, thymus enlargement, benign head and neck disease, benign breast conditions, and benign gynecologic disease. Populations irradiated for malignant disease showed excess secondary cancers for cervical cancer, childhood cancer, Hodgkin's disease, non-Hodgkin's lymphoma, and uterine corpus, ovary, and breast cancers.

It is important to note that most of these studies reporting radiation carcinogenesis are epidemiologic studies and are problematic primarily because the populations studied were exposed for a particular reason and therefore may not be representative of the population at large. The reasons why those exposed to radiation are not typical of the general population may not affect radiation sensitivity, but, nevertheless, an appropriate comparison group is required. A secondary problem arises because most of the studies are retrospective, that is, exposure to radiation occurred in the distant past so that the

Table 1. Recent studies of populations irradiated for benign disease (BOICE 1988)

Population	Excess cancers
Spondylitis (SMITH and DOLL 1982; DARBY et al. 1985, 1987)	Leukemia, lymphomas, lung, esophagus, stomach, central nervous system
Tinea capitis (RON and MODAN 1980, 1984; RON et al. 1988; SHORE et al. 1984)	Thyroid, brain, skin
Thymus enlargement (HILDRETH et al. 1985; SHORE et al. 1985)	Thyroid, breast, skin
Benign head and neck disease (MAXON et al. 1980; SANDLER et al. 1982: SCHNEIDER et al. 1985)	Thyroid, salivary gland, neural tumors
Benign breast conditions (BARAL et al. 1977; SHORE et al. 1986)	Breast
Benign gynecological disease (SMITH and DOLL 1976; WAGONER 1984)	Leukemia, intestine, rectum, uterus, urinary organs

Table 2. Recent studies of populations irradiated for malignant disease (BOICE 1988)

Population	Excess cancers
Cervical cancer (KLEINERMAN et al. 1982; BOICE et al. 1985, 1987; CURTIS et al. 1985b; STORM and BOICE 1985)	Leukemia, bladder, rectum, uterus, ovary, stomach, bone, connective tissue, thyroid, kidney
Childhood cancer (LI 1977; MIKE et al. 1982; KAPLAN et al. 1983; DRAPER et al. 1986; TUCKER et al. 1984, 1986, 1987a, 1987b)	Bone, thyroid, connective tissue, breast, possibly brain; no leukemia
Hodgkin's disease (BOIVIN et al. 1984; CURTIS et al. 1985b; BOLVIN and HUTCHISON 1984; TUCKER et al. 1988)	Possibly breast, stomach, thyroid, oral cavity, lung; no leukemia
Non-Hodgkin's lymphoma (GREENE et al. 1983)	Leukemia
Uterine corpus cancer (CURTIS et al. 1985b; BOIVIN et al. 1986)	Rectum, leukemia
Ovarian cancer (CURTIS et al. 1985b)	Colon, rectum, bladder
Breast cancer (CURTIS et al. 1985a; HANKY et al; FISHER et al. 1985; EWERTZ et al. 1984, BOIVIN et al. 1986)	Uterus; possibly leukemia, lung, second breast

exact dose of radiation delivered to individuals or to a group is not known (National Academy of Sciences 1980).

Finally, to interpret the percentage increase and cancer risk above the naturally occurring rate, the following example may be helpful: If the natural lifetime risk is 160000 cases per 1 million persons, the rate if 16%. An increase due to radiation equal to 0.5% of the natural rate would result in an increase of 160000 × 0.005 or 800 cases. This means that 160800 total cases will occur at the natural lifetime risk rate of 16.08% after radiation, thus pointing out the difficulties involved in the data analysis and risk assessment (JABLON 1984).

3.1 Radiation-Induced Breast Carcinogenesis

One area of great interest is radiation-induced breast carcinogenesis. The evidence for this is based on atomic bomb data, fluoroscopy data, patients treated for postpartum mastitis with orthovoltage irradiation, patients treated with radiation for cystic disease, and patients treated for cancer of the contralateral breast (LEVITT 1989). BOICE et al. (1979) noted that radiation-induced breast cancer does not appear in any of these groups until the age of breast cancer risk, i.e., the development of cancer is influenced by hormonal or other age-related factors occurring later in life. This latency, however, appears unrelated to dose. For example, radiogenetic breast cancers induced by large doses do not appear to occur earlier than those induced by lower doses.

In previously published evaluations of the trials related to radiation breast carcinogenesis, we have concluded that there are a number of problems with each of these studies (LEVITT and MANDEL 1983, 1985). We noted that major studies implicating a significant risk to breast cancer secondary to radiation suffer from one or more methodologic flaws: the absence of appropriate comparison groups, greater diagnostic surveillance in irradiated groups, the overinterpretation of relative risk, and the inability to separate the risk of breast cancer associated with the original disease from the additional risk of radiation. We also noted that in none of the studies has it been possible to accurately evaluate the effect of other known risk factors in breast cancer, including geographic area of residence, social class, age at first birth, history of benign disease, family history of cancer, and menstrual history. We concluded that breast cancer in women is a complex disease involving predisposing and epidemiologic factors.

There is no doubt that radiation is a carcinogenic agent and no question that the incidence of breast cancer increases in individuals who are treated with radiation during the perimenarchial ages of 10–19. A recent study found that women younger than 30 years of age treated with radiation for Hodgkin's disease were at an increased risk of developing breast cancer, with a dramatic increase in risk more than 15 years after radiotherapy (HANCOCK et al. 1993). Other reports have evaluated the potential biases on the risk of breast cancer among women who received radiotherapy for acute postpartum mastitis (PRINCE and HILDRETH 1986; SHORE et al. 1986). These reports did not assess all potential biases but did find that patients who had mastitis and who did not receive radiation developed a similar incidence of nonneoplastic breast tumors as did patients who received radiation. The studies also noted that the relative risk for neoplastic breast tumors secondary to radiation declined to 2.6 (95% confidence level of 1.1–4.5) from higher previous estimates of the same patient material.

For women treated with radiation for breast cancer, the risk of developing secondary primary contralateral breast cancer does not appear to increase. A study that looked at 14 000 breast cancer patients treated between 1946 and 1982 found that 194 of these women developed secondary primary tumor in the contralateral breast more than 1 year after diagnosis of first primary. No evidence of radiation-induced carcinogenesis to the contralateral breast was indicated when comparing groups treated with radiation with those not treated with radiation (BASCO et al. 1985). Similarly, a recent report of the Stockholm trial of a 13–19 year follow-up of patients treated with adjuvant radiotherapy for breast cancer found no increase in secondary primary cancer, particularly contralateral breast cancer, associated with the use of radiation (RUTQVIST 1993). Although forthcoming data from studies that have just been completed will help confirm these reports, it appears that secondary contralateral breast cancer is not significantly increased following radiation for primary breast disease.

Recently, the increased risk of carcinogenesis has been one of the arguments generated to refute the use of conservation surgery and radiation therapy to treat breast cancer. We evaluated this risk and noted that if we assume the highest risk, an approximate sixfold increase from 1 to 300 rads to the opposite breast, 36 cases of breast cancer per 1 million women would result from exposure to radiation following a 10 year latent period (LEVITT and MANDEL 1985). Therefore, among the 20 000 patients per year usually undergoing radiation therapy in our country following lumpectomy, fewer than one additional case of breast cancer would occur after 10 years. The risk is probably overestimated since exposure to radiation at an older age is associated with a lower risk of exposure than at an early age.

One study, reported by HANKY et al. (1983), showed an increased incidence of second breast cancer following mastectomy and radiation therapy. We evaluated this study and noted that when the data were stratified by age, stage, and length of follow-up there was no consistent pattern of elevated relative risk. In fact, for the majority of the risk estimates the 90% confidence interval includes 1.0, thus indicating a nonsignificant result. Furthermore, selection of the therapeutic regiment for patients with breast cancer was not random. Radiation therapy was used in conjunction with surgery more frequently when nodes were involved suggesting more frequently advanced stage of tumor and perhaps a greater likelihood of developing a second cancer. We also noted that the 90% confidence interval was used rather than the usual 95% confidence interval, which significantly increases the risk of a false-positive conclusion (LEVITT and MANDEL 1984).

A very recent study by BOICE and colleagues (1992) analyzed 41 109 women with breast cancer treated between 1935 and 1982 in Connecticut to evaluate the effect of irradiation on the development of second breast cancer in the contralateral breast. They found that "radiotherapy for breast cancer contributes little to the already high risk of a second cancer in the opposite breast. Fewer than 3% of all second breast cancers in this study could be attributed to previous radiation treatments" (BOICE et al. 1992). They did note, however, that the risk of developing second breast cancer following irradiation significantly increased in women less than 45 years of age (95% confidence level of 1.07–2.36). The significance of this statistic is questionable, however, because the data show that for women less than 35 years of age there was no significance risk (95% confidence interval of 0.89–5.74), nor was there significant risk for women between the ages of 35 and 44 years of age (95% confidence interval of 0.94–2.26). Only by combining these two intervals did the authors arrive at a statistically significant increase for women less than 45 years of age (BOICE et al. 1992). This study confirms the conclusions we made in our earlier reports.

3.2 Secondary Cancers Following Radiation for Cervical Cancer

In a recently reported study by BOICE et al. (1988) of radiotherapy for cervical cancer, 4188 women with multiple cancers and 6880 controls out of 150 000 patients irradiated had individual dose determinations of 20 irradiated organs. Several cancers were noted to be related to high doses of radiation on the order of several hundred gray, including cancers of the rectum, bladder, vagina, and all female genital organs taken together. This linkage was suggestive, but not conclusive, for cancers of the ovary, rectum, bone, connective tissue, uterine corpus, and non-Hodgkin's lymphoma. Conversely, high doses of radiation did not appear to increase the risk of cancer of the small intestine, colon, vulva, Hodgkin's disease, multiple myeloma, and chronic lymphocytic leukemia. The authors noted surprise at the lack of radiation effect for colon cancer because the number of cases was large and the doses were high. They hypothesized that the high doses perhaps experienced by the colon were sufficient to cause cell killing rather than transformation. The authors further noted that excess tumors occurred only after doses of greater than 10 Gy and that no study, including those on the Japanese atomic bomb survivors, has reported increased risk at levels below several gray.

It was also found that there was a suggested radiation association for non-Hodgkin's lymphoma, but not for Hodgkin's disease, multiple myeloma, or chronic lymphocytic leukemia. The authors hypothesized that if non-Hodgkin's lymphoma is radiation-induced, it appears to occur only after very high doses. No suggestion of an increased risk of multiple myeloma following irradiation was found. Cancer of the bladder was increased following an average dose of several hundred gray. Cancer of the pancreas, however, was not convincingly linked to radiotherapy, whereas renal cancer was significantly elevated among 15 year survivors. A twofold risk of stomach cancer was associated with average organ dose of 2 Gy.

Direct information on low dose risk was obtained from the large number of breast cancers associated with radiation doses from 0.01 to 0.98 Gy (0.31 Gy average) scattered from the radiation delivered to the cervix. Overall no radiation risk was found and there was no evidence of dose response. The authors felt that perhaps irradiating the ovaries may have lowered the risk. They noted that scatter from the patients's body introduced a low dose of radiation to the thyroid, and leakage through the collimator was associated with a twofold risk; however, statistical significance was not found.

The authors conclude that for most cancers linked to radiation of the cervix, risk appeared to be highest 20 or more years after exposure. For leukemia, however, the risk was highest 1–4 years after treatment, especially for women under 55 years when irradiated. The authors noted that radiation is a known carcinogen and that it is not surprising that elevated risks are seen following radiotherapy. However, they further stated that, despite the large number of women studied, only a few second cancers were convincingly linked to radiation. Clearly the large radiation doses experienced by the patients with cervical cancer did not dramatically alter the risk of developing a second cancer. It was estimated in a former cohort series that, at most, only about 5% of all second cancers are attributed to radiation (Boice et al. 1985).

3.3 Secondary Cancers Following Hodgkin's Disease

Recent reports in the literature have noted an increased number of secondary cancers following Hodgkin's disease, including lung cancer, melanomas, non-Hodgkin's lymphoma, thyroid cancer, and acute nonlymphocytic leukemia. The recent review of 18 major clinical series reported 662 secondary cancers rising in more than 14000 patients (Kaldor and Lasset 1990). Relative risk was most elevated for acute leukemia and its association with chemotherapy was noted to be stronger than its association with radiotherapy. Hodgkin's disease itself carries with it a substantially increased risk of lung cancer, non-Hodgkin's lymphoma, and other cancers, but, apart from leukemia, none of these cancers appear to be clearly associated with therapy. In the reported study of 662 second cancers, 249 were leukemias and 44 were non-Hodgkin's lymphomas. The authors noted that no study reported a sufficient number of cases of any particular type of solid tumor to permit a clear evaluation of differences and risks among treatment categories.

List et al., quoted in an article authored by Kaldor and Lasset (1990), noted a high frequency of supradiaphragmatic radiation and in-field tumors among the reported lung cancer cases, but were unable to conclusively implicate radiotherapy as a causative factor in an increased incidence of lung cancer among Hodgkin's disease survivors. The authors further looked at incidence studies in cancer registries and noted an increased incidence of acute leukemia, lung cancer, and non-Hodgkin's lymphoma compared to the normal population. There were also significantly elevated risks for breast, cervix, and skin cancers. There seemed to be an increase of cancer of the salivary glands, nasopharynx, pharnyx, and bone in women with moderate increase in risk of thyroid cancer and melanoma. These increases cannot be attributed with any degree of certainty to Hodgkin's disease or to its therapy. However, they are unlikely to be artifactual consequences of increased medical surveillance following Hodgkin's disease.

An international workshop in 1989 developed a detailed analysis of risk for all tumor types combined, leukemia, non-Hodgkin's lymphoma, and all solid tumors combined (KALDOR and LASSET 1990). The risk of leukemia was greatly increased when MOPP-type chemotherapy (mechlorethamine, vincristine, procarbazine, pednisone) was given alone or with radiation. There was also an increased risk associated with splenectomy. Chemotherapy had no effect on the risk of solid tumors, whereas total nodal irradiation increased risk by 80%. For non-Hodgkin's lymphoma, no association with any treatment category was evident. It was concluded that the risk for leukemia is clearly related to chemotherapy. Different combinations of chemotherapy may be more leukemogenic than others – the MOPP-like combinations, such as COPP, in which cyclophosphamide replaces the nitrogen mustard of MOPP, appear to be more leukemogenic than the new type of combination chemotherapy known as ABVD. There is no evidence that radiotherapy enhances the leukemogenic effect of chemotherapy. The risk of leukemia appears to be maximal 4–8 years after the diagnosis of Hodgkin's disease. The risk of solid tumors appears to be related to radiotherapy rather than chemotherapy, although studies of individual sites have not yet confirmed the role played by radiotherapy in inducing solid tumors after Hodgkin's disease. The risk of solid tumors increases steadily both in absolute and relative terms for over 15 years, particularly among patients who are treated with total nodal irradiation. An important question yet to be measured is whether Hodgkin's disease itself (or in addition to its therapy) increases the risk of second cancer in surviving patients (Table 3).

3.4 Pediatric Second Primary Tumors

A recent paper by HAWKINS (1990) evaluated 9279 survivors of childhood neoplasms other than retinoblastoma treated in Britain before 1980. The cumulative risk of second primary tumors by 25 years from 3 years survival was 3.7%. This corresponded to about five times the number expected from radiocancer occurring in the general population. In the absence of both radiotherapy and chemotherapy there was four times the expected number of subsequent risk. The risk of second primary tumor associated with radiotherapy was six times as expected and the risk for both radiotherapy and chemotherapy was nine times as expected. There was evidence that radiotherapy was involved in the development of many of the second primary tumors observed. However, case control investigations were required to examine the relationship between the relative risk of second primary tumors and therapy in detail. Secondary leukemia appeared to occur more frequently among more recently diagnosed children with cancer. The authors noted it was important to continue to monitor the occurrence of second primary tumors with a view to identify the least carcinogenic therapy consistent without compromising survival prospects (Table 4).

A recent study by CUMBERLIN et al. (1989) presents a model for evaluating isolated contributions of scattered ionizing radiation in inducing second malignancies in the cancer patients. The authors presented estimates of the expected number of second malignancies induced in selective sensitive sites by scatter radiation during radiotherapy for cancer. They estimated that in the year 1987, 192 761 new cancer patients received radiotherapy as part of their initial plan. Their models predicted that radiation may induce 63–84 secondary breast cancers, 64–72 secondary thyroid cancers, 94–157 secondary lung cancers, and 489–707 secondary leukemias over the remaining lifetime of this patient population. It was noted that this represented a lifetime incidence of 0.7% for leukemia and 0.3% for solid tumors. Thus, the incidence should be placed in perspective with the current concept of cancer management, such as combined modality therapy, which carries a risk of carcinogenesis greater than either modality alone, and when the alternatives to radiotherapy are nonexistent or may be cosmetically or functionally undesirable.

4 Discussion

In the Helen Woodward symposium, JOHN BOICE (1988) noted that recent studies on medically irradiated populations have increased our understanding of radiation carcinogenesis. These studies have shown that: (1) low doses of radiation may increase the risk of cancer (investigations of prenatal X-ray exposures, especially in twins, show that very low doses of ionizing radiation may cause cancer in humans; and low-dose exposures of about 10 cGy may increase the risk of thyroid cancer); (2) fractionated doses and single exposures of the same total dose appear to be as effective in causing breast cancer, but less effective for lung cancer; (3) radiation to young patients can produce later cancers

Table 3. Proportional hazards model on second cancer risk[a] for 12411 patients who survived at least 1 year after Hodgkin's disease diagnosis: results for a model allowing all the variables simultaneously (SOMERS et al. 1990)

Variables	Regression coefficient	Standard error	RR[b]
Sex			
Males	0		1.0[c]
Females	−0.23	0.09	0.79**
Age (years)			
15–19	0		1.0
20–29	0.06	0.19	1.06
30–39	0.49	0.19	1.64**
40–49	1.19	0.19	3.28***
50–59	1.98	0.19	7.24***
60+	2.32	0.20	10.18***
Histology			
Lymphocytic predominance	0		1.0
Nodular sclerosing	−0.17	0.14	0.85
Mixed cellularity	−0.26	0.15	0.77+
Lymphocytic depleted	−0.39	0.32	0.68
Unclassified	0.30	0.30	1.35
Bone marrow involvement			
No	0.30		1.0
Yes	−0.12	0.30	0.88
Response to initial treatment			
Complete remission	0		1.0
No complete remission	0.20	0.21	1.22
Initial treatment type			
Splenectomy			
No	0		1.0
Yes	0.19	0.09	1.20*
If irradiation alone	0		1.0
Mantle or inverted Y radiotherapy alone	0.08	0.18	1.08
Subtotal nodal irradiation or total nodal irradiation alone	0.37	0.18	1.44*
MOPP-like chemotherapy	0.51	0.19	1.67**
Other chemotherapy	0.56	0.37	1.75
Irradiation (any type)			
+MOPP-like	0.68	0.17	1.97***
+other chemotherapy	0.53	0.37	1.70
Clinical outcome[d]			
No relapse	0		1.0
First relapse treated with:			
Radiotherapy	0.47	0.28	1.60+
Chemotherapy	0.78	0.14	2.18***
Both	0.59	0.12	1.81***
Global χ-square	572.58		
p value (df)	<0.0001	22	

p value: + <0.10, * <0.05, ** <0.01; *** <0.001; two-sided test; MOPP, mechlorethamine, vincristine, procarbarine, prednisone.
[a]ICDO-9 173, 180, and 195–199 excluded.
[b]Relative risk: RR = exp(regression coefficient).
[c]Reference category.
[d]Time-dependent covariates.

(excess breast cancers can occur among women exposed under age 10 indicating that immature breast is susceptible to carcinogenic effect of radiation; moderate doses on the order of 1 Gy to the brains of children can cause tumors later in life; moderately high doses to the skin can cause cancer when followed by frequent exposure to ultraviolet light; and bone cancer occurs after high-dose radiotherapy for childhood cancer, but children with retinoblastoma are not more susceptible to

Table 4. Risk of second primary tumors after all first primary tumors except retinoblastoma: association with treatment (adapted from HAWKINS 1990)

Treatment group	Number	Mean follow-up period (years)	Observed	Expected	Observed/ expected	Confidence interval (95%)
Neither radiotherapy nor chemotherapy	1495	9.5	10	2.6	3.9	1.9, 7.1
Radiotherapy but no chemotherapy	2668	9.8	29	5.1	5.6	3.8, 8.1
Both radiotherapy and chemotherapy	2699	3.8	10	1.1	9.3	4.5, 17.0

radiation-induced cancers than are children with other malignancies; (4) radiotherapy may not significantly increase the risk of leukemia following childhood cancer, whereas chemotherapy with alkylating agents is a major risk factor; (5) radiotherapy for cervical cancer can increase the rate of subsequent leukemia and the risk of radiation-induced second malignancies for cervical cancer patients follows a time-response model consistent with a constant multiplication of the underlying background incidence, i.e., the relative risk model seems to hold for adjusting risk forward in time; (6) second cancers following radiotherapy for a variety of cancers occur primarily among long-term survivors; and (7) high-dose external beam therapy can cause thyroid cancer, whereas high-dose radioactive^{131}I probably does not.

From this increased knowledge of radiation carcinogenesis, we have attempted to place in perspective the actual risk of developing second malignant neoplasms following radiation therapy. Analysis of the literature and of the assumptions and statistical methods used to evaluate carcinogenesis reveals that, although there is indeed a risk of second malignant neoplasms following radiation, the risk is not significant enough to avoid the use of radiation in situations in which radiation is curative or organ preserving. Also, the incidence of second malignant neoplasms following radiation alone is substantially less than that following a combination of radiation and chemotherapy. This must be kept in mind in situations in which radiation is effective without the addition of chemotherapy.

Consider of the risk of second malignant neoplasms must be part of every treatment choice. Determining the degree of risk must be intelligently weighed with the benefits of treatment. Radiation is a proven effective treatment carrying a reasonably small risk of second malignant neoplasms. While there is substantial evidence of this, radiation-induced carcinogenesis remains somewhat misunderstood. Jablon states well this confusion: "It is perhaps ironic that, despite this knowledge, and in the face of widespread public concern and apprehension about radiation-induced cancer, only a very small part of the cancer burden which afflicts humanity – less than 3% – may actually be attributable to radiation. Moreover, more than half of this hypothetical burden is caused by radiation that we cannot do anything about – that resulting from natural background. It is, of course, necessary to reduce radiation exposures where this can be done without paying an exorbitant price. Nevertheless, if our object is to lessen appreciably the impact of environmentally induced cancer, ionizing radiation is not a promising target" (JABLON and BAILOR 1980). In placing the actual risk of radiation carcinogenesis in this proper perspective, it is similarly important to acknowledge that, since there is a small but present risk of radiation carcinogenesis, it is important that the radiation oncologist be diligent in appropriately using radiation. This requires careful attention to and precision of detail in administering radiation appropriately to the appropriate sites, while avoiding unnecessary irradiation to areas not requiring treatment. Radiation is an effective treatment when used properly; increasing our understanding of the minimal risk of secondary malignant neoplasms, while remaining attentive to reducing the risk, is important in improving the effective use of radiotherapy.

References

Baral E, Larrsson LE, Mattsson B (1977) Breast cancer following irradiation of the breast. Cancer 40: 2905–2910

Basco V, Coldman A, Elwood J, Young M (1985) Radiation dose and second breast cancer. Br J Cancer 52: 319–325

Boice JD Jr (1988) Carcinogenesis: a symposis of human experience with external exposure in medicine. Health Physics 55(4): 621–630

Boice JD Jr, Land CE, Shore RE et al (1979) Risk of breast cancer following low-dose radiation exposure. Radiology 131: 589–597

Boice JD Jr, Day NE, Andersen A et al (1985) Second cancers following radiation treatment for cervical cancer: an international collaboration among cancer registries. J Natl Cancer Inst 74: 955–975

Boice JD Jr, Blettner M, Kleinerman RA et al (1987) Radiation dose and leukemia risk in patients treated for cancer of the cervix. J Natl Cancer Inst 79: 1295–1311

Boice JD Jr, Engholm, G, Kleinerman RA et al (1988) Radiation dose and second cancer risk in patients treated for cancer of the cervix. Radiat Res 116: 3–55

Boice JD Jr, Harvey EB, Blettner M et al (1992) Cancer in the contralateral breast after radiotherapy for breast cancer. N Engl J Med 326(12): 781–784

Boivin JF, Hutchison GB (1984) Second cancers after treatment for Hodgkin's disease: a review. In: Boice JD Jr, Fraumeni JF Jr (eds) Radiation carcinogenesis: epidemiology and biological significance. Raven, New York, pp 181–189

Boivin JF, Hutchison GB, Lyden M et al (1984) Secondary primary cancers following treatment of Hodgkin's disease. J Natl Cancer Inst 72: 233–241

Boivin JF, Hutchison GB, Evans FB et al (1986) Leukemia after radiotherapy for first primary cancers of various anatomic sites. Am J Epidemiol 123: 993–1003

Cerutti PA, Amstad P, Emerit I (1983) Tumor promoter phorbol-myristate-acetate induced membrane-mediated chromosomal damage. In: Nygaard OF, Simic MG (eds) Radioprotectors and anticarcinogens. Academic, New York

Clifton KA, Kamiya K, Mulcahy RT, Gould MN (1985) Radiogenic neoplasia in the thyroid and mammary clonogens: progress, problems, and possibilities. In: Woodhead AD, Shellabarger CJ, Bond V, Hollaender (eds) Assessment of risk from low-level exposure to radiation and chemicals. A critical review. Plenum, New York, pp 329–342 (Basic life science series, vol 33)

Cumberlin RL, Dritschilo A, Mossman KL (1989) Carcinogenic effects of scattered dose associated with radiation therapy. Int J Radiat Oncol Biol Phys 17: 623–629

Curtis RE, Boice JD, Jr, Kleinerman RA et al (1985a) Summary: multiple primary cancers in Connecticut, 1935–82. Natl Cancer Inst Monogr 68: 219–242

Curtis RE, Boice JD Jr, Kleinerman RA et al (1985b) Summary: multiple primary cancers in Connecticut, 1935–82. Natl Cancer Inst Monogr 68: 113–137

Darby SC, Nakashima E, Kato H (1985) A parallel analyses of cancer mortality among atomic bomb survivors and patients with ankylosing spondylities given X-ray therapy. J Natl Cancer Inst 75: 1–21

Darby SC, Doll R, Gill SK, Smith PG (1987) Long-term mortality after a single treatment course with X-rays in patients treated for ankylosing spondylitis. Br J Cancer 55: 179–190

Draper GJ, Sanders BM, Kingston JE (1986) Second primary neoplasms in patients with retinoblastoma. Br J Cancer 53: 661–671

Elkind MM, Benjamin SA, Sinclair SW et al (1991) Oncogenic mechanisms in radiation-induced. Cancer Res 51: 2740–2747

Ewertz M, Machado SG, Boice JD Jr, Jensen OM (1984) Endometrial cancer following treatment for breast cancer: a case-control study in Denmark. Br J Cancer 50: 687–692

Fajardo LF (1986) Ionizing radiation and neoplasia. In: Fenoglio-Preiser (M, Weinstein A, Kaufman B (eds) New concepts in neoplasis as applied to diagnostic pathology. Williams and Wilkins, Baltimore

Farber E (1984) Cellular biochemistry of the stepwise development of cancer with chemicals: G.H.A. Clowes memorial lecture. Cancer Res 44: 5463–5474

Fisher B, Rockette H, Fisher ER et al (1985) Leukemia in breast cancer patients following adjuvant chemotherapy or postoperative radiotherapy: the NSABP experience. J Clin Oncol 3: 1640–1658

Garte SJ, Hood AT, Hochwalt AE et al (1985) Carcinogen specificity in the activation of transforming genes by direct-acting alkylating agent. Carcinogenesis 6: 1709– 1712

Greene MH, Young RC, Merrill JM, DeVita VT (1983) Evidence of a treatment dose response in acute non-lymphocytic leukemias which occur after therapy of non-Hodgkin's lymphoma. Cancer Res 43: 1891–1898

Guerrero I, Calzada P, Mayer A, Pellicer A (1984) A molecular approach to leukemogenesis: mouse lymphomas contain an activated c-ras oncogene. Proc Natl Acad Sci USA 81: 202–205

Hall EJ (1988) Radiobiology for the radiologist, 3d edn. Lippincott, Philadelphia

Hancock SL, Tucker MA, Hoppe RT (1993) Breast cancer after treatment of Hodgkin's disease. J Natl Cancer Inst 85: 25–31

Hanky BF, Curtis RE, Naughton MD et al (1983) A retrospective cohort analysis of second breast cancer risk for primary breast cancer patients with an assessment of the effect of radiation therapy. J Natl Cancer Inst 70: 197–204

Hawkins MM (1990) Second primary tumors following radiotherapy for childhood cancer. Int J Radiat Oncol Biol Phys 19: 1297–1301

Hildreth NG, Shore RE, Hempelmann LH, Rosenstein M (1985) Risk of extrathyroid tumors following radiation treatment in infancy for thymic enlargement. Radiat Res 102: 378–391

Jablon S (1984) Epidemiologic perspectives in radiation carcinogenesis. In: Boice JD Jr, Fraumeni JF Jr (eds) Radiation carcinogenesis: epidemiology and biological significance, vol 26. Raven, New York, pp 1–8

Jablon S, Bailar JC III (1980) The contribution of ionizing radiation to cancer mortality in the United States. Prev Med 9: 219–226

Kaldor JM, Lasset C (1990) Second malignancies following Hodgkin's disease. In: Somers R, Henry-Amar M, Meerwaldt JK, Carde P (eds) Treatment strategy in Hodgkin's disease. Libbey, London

Kaplan HS (1967) On the natural history of the murine leukemias: Presidential address. Cancer Res 27: 1327–1340

Kaplan MM, Garnick MB, Gelber R et al (1983) Risk factors for thyroid abnormalities after neck irradiation for childhood cancer. Am J Med 74: 272–280

Kennedy AR, Little JB (1984) Evidence that a second event in X-ray-induced oncogenic transformation in vitro occurs during cellular proliferation. Radiation Res 99: 228–248

Kleinerman RA, Curtis RE, Boice JD Jr, Flannery JT, Fraumeni JF Jr (1982) Second cancers following radiotherapy for cervical cancer. J Natl Cancer Inst 69: 1027–1033

Knudson AG (1985) Hereditary cancer, oncogenes, and antioncogenes. Cancer Res 45: 1437–1443

Levitt SH (1989) Radiation carcinogenesis. In: Vaeth JM, Meyer JL (eds) Radiation tolerance of normal tissues. Karger, Basel, pp 408–416 (Frontiers of radiation therapy and oncology, vol 23)

Levitt SH, Mandel JS (1983) Breast irradiation and future risk of carcinogenesis. In: Vaeth JM (ed) Conservation surgery and radiation therapy in the treatment of operable breast cancer. Karger, Basel, pp 131–142 (Frontiers of radiation therapy and oncology, vol 17)

Levitt SH, Mandel JS (1984) Benefits versus risks in conservation surgery with irradiation for breast cancer. Am J Med 77: 93–100

Levitt SH, Mandel JS (1985) Breast carcinogenesis: risk of radiation. Int J Radiat Oncol Biol Phys 11: 1421–1423

Li FP (1977) Second malignant tumors after cancer in childhood. Cancer 40; 1899–1902

Liehr JG, Randerath K, Randerath E (1985) Target organ-specific covalent DNA damage preceding diethylstilbestrol-induced carcinogenesis. Carcinogenesis 6: 1067–1069

Marshall JM, Groer PG (1977) A theory of the induction of bone cancer by alpha radiation. Radiat Res 71: 149–192

Maxon HR, Saenger EL, Thomas SR et al. (1980) Clinically important radiation-associated thyroid disease. A controlled study. JAMA 244: 1802–1805

Mike V, Meadows AT, D'Angio GJ (1982) Incidence of second malignant neoplasms in children. Results of an international study. Lancet 2: 1326–1331

National Academy of Sciences (1980) The effects of populations of exposure to low levels of ionizing radiation. National Academy, Washington DC

Nowell PC (1976) The clonal evolution of tumor cell populations. Science 194: 23–28

Prince MM, Hildreth NG (1986) The influence of potential biases on the risk of breast tumors among women who received radiotherapy for acute postpartum mastitis. J Chron Dis 39(7): 553–560

Ron E, Modan B (1980) Benign and malignant thyroid neoplasms after childhood irradiation from tinea capitis. JNCI 66: 7–11

Ron E, Modan B (1984) Thyroid and other neoplasms following childhood scalp irradiation. In: Boice JD Jr, Faumen JF Jr (eds) Radiation carcinogenesis: epidemiology and biological significance. Raven, New York, pp 139–151

Ron E, Modan B, Boice JD Jr (1988) Mortality from cancer and other causes following radiotherapy for ringworm of the scalp. Am J Epidemiol 127: 713–725

Rutqvist LE (1993) Radiation therapies for breast cancer: current knowledge on advantages and disadvantages In: Höffken K (ed) Peptides in oncology II. Somatostatin analogues and bombesin antagomists. Springer, Berlin Heidelberg New York, pp 119–127 (Recent results in cancer research, vol 127)

Sandler DP, Comstock GW, Matanoski GM (1982) Neoplasm following childhood radium irradiation of the nasopharynx. JNCI 68: 3–8

Schneider AB, Shore-Freedman E, Ryo UY et al (1985) Radiation-induced tumors of the head and neck following childhood irradiation. Prospective studies. Medicine 64: 1–15

Shore RE, Albert R, Reed M et al (1984) Skin cancer incidence among children irradiated for ringworm of the scalp. Radiat Res 100: 192–204

Shore RE, Woodard E, Hildreth N et al (1985) Thyroid tumors following thymus irradiation. JNCI 74: 1177–1184

Shore RE, Hildreth N, Woodard W et al (1986) Breast cancer among women given X-ray therapy for acute postpartum mastitis. J Natl Cancer Inst 77: 689–696

Smith PG, Doll R (1976) Late effects of X-irradiation in patients treated for metropathia haemorrhagica. Br J Radiol 224–232

Smith PG, Doll R (1982) Mortality among patients with ankylosing spondylitis after a single treatment course with X-rays. Med J 284: 449–460

Somers R, Henry-Amar M, Meerwaldt JK, Carde P (1990) Treatment strategy in Hodgkin's disease. Libbe London, p 367

Storm HH, Boice JD Jr (1985) Leukemia after cervical cancer irradiation in Denmark. Int J Epidemiol 14: 363–368

Tucker MA, Meadows AT, Boice JD et al (1984) Cancer risk following treatment of childhood cancer. In: Boice JD Jr, Fraumeni JF Jr (eds) Radiation carcinogenesis: epidemiology and biological significance. Raven, New York, pp 211–224

Tucker MA, Meadolos AT, Boice JD Jr et al (1986) Therapeutic radiation at young age linked to secondary thyroid cancer. Proc Am Soc Clin Oncol 5: 827 (Abstract)

Tucker MA, D'Angio GJ Jr et al (1987a) Bone sarcomas linked to radiotherapy and chemotherapy in children. N Engl J Med 317: 588–593

Tucker MA, Meadows AT, Boice JD Jr et al (1987b) Leukemia after therapy with alkylating agents for childhood cancer. JNCI 78: 459–464

Tucker MA, Coleman CN, Cox RS, Varghese A et al (1988) Risk of second malignancies treatment for Hodgkin's disease. N Engl J Med 318: 76–81

Upton AC (1986) Historical perspectives on radiation carcinogenesis. In: Upton AC, Albert RE, Burns FJ, Shore RE (eds) Radiation carcinogenesis. Elsevier, New York

Upton AC (1987) Cancer induction and non-stochastic effects. B J Radiol 60: 1–16

Upton AC, Clayson DG, Jansen JD et al (1984) Report of ICPEMC task group 5 on the differentiation between genotoxic and nongenotoxic carcinogens. Mutat Res 133: 1–49 (ICPEMC publ 9)

Wagoner JK (1984) Leukemia and other malignancies following radiation therapy for gynecological disorders. In: Boice JD Jr, Fraumeni JF Jr (eds) Radiation carcinogenesis: epidemiology and biological significance. Raven, New York, pp 153–159

Weichselbaum RR, Becket MA, Diamond AA (1989) An important step in radiation carcinogenesis may be inactivation of cellular genes. Int J Radiat Oncol Biol Phys 16: 277–282

Weinstein IB, Gatto-Celli S, Kirschmeier P et al (1984) Cellular targets and host genes in multistage carcinogenesis. Fed Proc 43: 2287–2294

Subject Index

abscess 124
ABVD 51, 164–165, 171, 192, 227, 273, 285
α-β-value
see linear-quadratic model
acetylcyteine 146–148
ACNU 265
acral crythema 128
acrolein 207, 211, 264
ACTH 59, 62, 65, 67
actinomycin D 8, 127, 128
acyclovir 210
adrenoceptor up-regulation 183
adriamycin 112, 127–129, 153, 156, 176, 273
age
and radiosensitivity of tissues 8
AIDS 7, 275
-related Kaposi's sarcoma 128
alcohol
and mucositis 5, 115
alkylating agents 263
allopurinol 13, 115
alopecia 127
alveolar edema 153
amenorrhea 236
α-1-microglobulin 209
aminoglycoside therapy and ototoxicity 84
amphoterecin B 210
analgetica abuse 222
anaphylactic shock 129
anastomotic leak 122–125
angioedema 129
angiotensin-converting enzyme inhibitors 178
anthracyclines 13, 175
antibiotics 210, 222
antimetabolites 264
Ara C
see cytarabin
asparaginase 13, 29, 129
ataxia telangiectasia, AT 5, 17
avalanche-effect 216
axonal neuropathy 54
azoospermia 229, 236

BCNU 144, 148, 152, 219, 264
biorhythm 17
bleeding 122–125
bleomycin 16, 53, 54, 273, 276
-induced lung fibrosis 8, 96, 141, 146, 152, 153, 157
skin reactions 128
bolus injections versus continuous infusions
of adriamycin, and cardiotoxicity 177
of cisplatin, and ototoxicity 84
of ifosfamide, and nephrotoxicity 211
bone density 227
bone marrow transplant
and pneumonitis 136
TBI and gonadal toxicity 236
TBI and renal toxicity 219, 222
bone necrosis 107
breast cancer
and lymphedema 99–103
after radiotherapy 282, 283
bronchiolitis 153
bronchoalveolar lavage 145–146
Brown-Sequard-syndrom 37
busulfan 128, 152

calcitonin 230, 232
carbacholine 116
carboplatin 56
mucositis 113
ototoxicity 81
nephrotoxicity 210
carboxylators 15
cardiomyopathy 8, 168, 171, 193, 199
CCNU 152
chlorambucil 266, 276
chlorhexidine 116
CHOP 51
chromosomal aberrations 15
cisplatin 8, 14, 30, 153, 209–211, 219, 263, 264, 276
mucositis 112
ototoxicity 74, 75, 81–84
peripheral neurotoxicity 51, 53–56
CMF 275, 276
Cockayne's syndrome 5
cognitive dysfunctions 25
collagen 95
combined modality therapy
and mucositis 111–116
conduction defects 199
congestive heart failure 176
continuous infusion
versus bolus injections, see bolus injections
COPP 51, 164–165, 227, 228, 232, 285
coronary artery disease 168, 170, 192
corticosteroids 24
corticotropins 55
craniospinal irradiation 257, 258
creatinine clearance 218
cryoconservation of sperm 238
cryotherapy 116
cyclophosphamide 30, 127, 141, 152, 153, 238, 263, 273, 275, 276
cyclosporin 219, 222
cystinosis 207
cytarabine 13, 30–32, 127, 128, 152, 238
cytokines
and mucositis 90
and fibrosis 93

dactinomycin
see actinomycin D
daunorubicin 127–129, 153, 176, 177
dental care 115
dental prophylaxis 109
dermatitis 106–109
diabetes 8, 39, 62, 221
-insipidus 70
diarrhea 112–114
diet 9
diffusion capacity 144
dinaline 269
diuretics
and ototoxicity 84
Down's syndrome 15
doxorubicin
see adriamycin
DTIC 273

ECG-abnormalities 167
echocardiography 178, 199
EEG 29
electronystagmography, ENG 76
EMG 44, 45, 48, 52
emphysema 8
encephalopathies 29
enzyme defects 16
epiphyseal plate 245
erythema multiforme 129
erythropoetin deficiency 218
estrogen
deficiency 227
replacement, substitution therapy 229, 230
ethacrynic acid
see diuretics
etoposide 53, 54, 276
evoked otoacoustic potentials 84

Fanconi's syndrome 5, 207–209
fat tissue reduction after radiotherapy 253
fertility 237
fibroblasts
differentiation 94–95
postmitotic fibrocytes 93–96
progenitor fibroblast cells 93–96
radiosensitivity 5
fibrosis 90, 106–109, 253
lung fibrosis 138, 141
fistula 114, 124
fludarabine 13
folinic acid 14, 113–115
fractional shortening 167, 168, 176, 183
fragile X-syndrome 15
FSH 59, 62, 67, 228, 229, 232
5-FU, 5-Fluorouracil 8, 16, 17, 31, 275
mucositis 112–114
skin reactions 128
stomatitis 127
functional subunits 216
furosemide
see diuretics

galactosemia 207
Gardner's syndrome 5
gastric outlet obstruction 124
germ cell aplasia 230
gluthathione system 141, 265
gout nephritis 221
growth hormone
deficiency 59, 255
secretion 67, 256
therapy 60, 61, 258, 259

head and neck cancer 105–109, 113–115
hearing loss
after radiotherapy 73–76
heavy particle therapy 68
HECNU 265
hemoglobin level 8
hidradenitis 129
high resolution computed tomography 153
hydroxyurea 13, 129
hyperaminoaciduria 208
hyperfractionation 105, 113, 247, 249
hyperpigmentation 127
hyperprolactinemia 68
hypersensitivity reaction 152
hypertension 8, 39, 167, 215, 218–221
hyperthyroidism 8
hypogonadism 236
hypophosphatemia 208
hypothyroidism 236

ICRF-187
and anthracycline cardiotoxicity 178–179
idiosynchratic X-ray reaction 5
ifosfamide 30, 128, 148
ilmofosine 267
immunoglobulin G excretion 209
immunosuppression 152
infusion therapy 153
insulin tolerance test 60
interferon 113
interleukin 152
interstitial edema 153
interstitial nephritis 215
interstitial pneumonia 138
intraoperative radiotherapy, IORT 44–48, 121–125
ischemic heart disease 198–201
see also myocardial infarction
isotope techniques
for detecting radiation nephritis 218, 220

left ventricular ejection fraction 183, 198, 199
LET 280
leukemias 273–276
Leydig cell function 230, 237
LH 59, 62, 67, 228, 229, 232
Lhermitte's sign 37
linear-quadratic model
cardiotoxicity 182, 198
growth disturbances 248, 249
mucositis 109
nephrotoxicity 218
neurotoxicity 45
radiation myelitis 39
loperamide 116
LQ-model
see linear-quadratic model

mantle irradiation, mediastinal irradiation 170–171, 176, 193, 194
mastitis 282
melphalan 275, 276
membrane enzymes
and ototoxicity 83
6-mercaptopurine 13, 16
Mesna 30, 207, 211, 264
metabolic polymorphism 15
methotrexate 8, 13, 14, 30–32, 127, 144, 152, 153, 211, 275, 276
methylnitrosourea 267
microalbuminuria 218
miliary tuberculosis 157
mitochondria 83
mitomycin C
mucositis 114–115
and lung toxicity 141–148, 152
mixed functional oxidative enzyme system, MFOS 15
MOPP 51, 171, 192, 227, 285
mucositis 89, 106–109
multiple drug resistence 14
multiple myeloma 275
mycotic lung infections 157
myelodysplastic syndromes 273, 274, 276
myocardial infarction 170–171, 192, 199–201
myocardial scintigraphy 199

N-acetyl-βD-glucosaminidase 209
N-acetylcyteine 146–148, 178
naevi, melanocytic 129
nail disorders 128
nephrectomy 209, 211, 219
nephritis 8
neuropathy 43–48
neuropsychological changes 32
nitrogen mustard 273
nitrosoureas 141
nitrous oxide 16
nominal standard dose 25
normal tissue complication probability 217

obstruction
see gastric outlet obstruction 124
octreotide 116
oligospermia 236
opportunistic lung infections 153–157
Org 2766 55
oropharyngeal cancer
mucositis 105–109
osteocalcin 230, 232
osteomalacia 209
osteosarcoma 176, 280
otitis media 74
ovarian failure 229
ovaropexy 240
5-oxoprolinuria 5

palmar-plantar erythro-dysesthesia 128
pancreatic complications 125
panhypopituitarism 257
parathormone 230
pentoxifylline 116
perforation
of small bowel 112
pericardectomy 170
pericardial thickening 167–168, 170
pericarditis 169, 181, 198–199
photosensitivity reactions 128
pilocarpine 116
platinum compounds
see cisplatin, carboplatin
plethysmometry
in lymphedema 99
pleural pain 144
plexopathy 43
pneumocytes 138, 143
pneumonitis 6, 136–138, 152
positron emission tomography, PET 25
prednimustine 265, 266
pregnancy 238, 241
procarbazine 153, 191, 273, 276
prostaglandin E 115
proteinuria 208–209, 215
pseudoallergies 129

puberty
  precocious puberty 61, 258
pulmonary hemorrhage 157
pyridinemia 16

radiation-induced brain neoplasms 26
radionecrosis of brain tissue 24, 25
radionuclide ventriculography 178
recall-phenomenon 114, 128, 157
releasing hormones 65
renal failure 39
respiratory distress syndrome, RDS 152
retinoblastoma 280
retinol-binding protein 218
rickets 208, 211

salivary gland hypofunction 116
saturation effect 246
scoliosis 246, 247
semen analysis 229
semicastration 237
silver nitrate solution 115
smoking
  mucositis 5, 115
  pneumonitis 139
  radiation myelitis 39
sodium thiosulfate 14
somnolence syndrome 24
splenectomy 273, 285
spermatogenesis 236, 237
steroids
  and lung toxicity 145, 148
  see also corticosteroids
stomatitis 112–113, 127
stunting dose 246
sucralfate 115
surfactant 143

tannin 115
telangiectasia 4–6
TGF-β
  see transforming growth factor β
thio-tepa 129
thyroid dysfunction 258
TNF
  see tumor necrosis factor
transferrin 209
transforming growth factor β
  and fibrosis 93, 96
  and mucositis 90
treosulfan 276
triazene derivate 267
triazinate 129
TSH 59, 65, 67
tumor necrosis factor 116

ulcers, ulceration 107, 127

valvular thickening 167–168
verapamil 14
vinblastine 53, 128, 146, 273
vinca alkaloids 51, 53, 54, 264
vincristine 51
vitamin D 230
vitamin E 178

Whipple's operation 124
white matter changes 24, 36
Wilm's tumor 219
WR 2721 56

xerostomia 116

List of Contributors

Dr. HORST ALHEIT
Universitätsklinikum Carl Gustav Carus
Klinik und Poliklinik für Strahlentherapie
Fetscherstraße 74
01307 Dresden
FRG

Prof. Dr. MICHAEL BAMBERG
Radiologische Universitätsklinik
Abteilung für Strahlentherapie
Hoppe-Seyler-Straße 3
72076 Tübingen
FRG

Dr. MICHAEL BAUMANN
Radiologische Klinik, Abteilung für
Strahlentherapie
Universitätsklinikums Eppendorf
Martinistraße 52
20251 Hamburg
FRG

Prof. Dr. JÖRN D. BECK
Klinik für Kinder und Jugendliche
Pädiatrische Hämatologie und Onkologie
Loschgestraße 15
91054 Erlangen
FRG

Dr. CHRISTIAN BEHLES
Klinik für Innere Medizin
des Universitätsklinikums Steglitz
Abteilung Hämatologie/Onkologie
Hindenburgdamm 30
12203 Berlin
FRG

PD Dr. WERNER BERBERICH
Institut für Strahlentherapie
Städtisches Klinikum St. Marien
92224 Amberg
FRG

PD Dr. MARTIN R. BERGER
Deutsches Krebsforschungszentrum
Institut für Toxikologie und Chemotherapie
Im Neuenheimer Feld 280
69120 Heidelberg
FRG

Dr. ANGELA BESSERER
Universitätsklinikum Steglitz
Abteilung Radiologie
Hindenburgdamm 30
12203 Berlin
FRG

Dr. STEFAN BIELACK
Abteilung für pädiatrische
Hämatologie und Onkologie
Universitätskinderklinik
Martinistraße 52
20251 Hamburg
FRG

Dr. ANKE BINDER
Universität Tübingen
Abteilung Strahlenbiologie
Röntgenstraße 11
72076 Tübingen
FRG

Dr. STEFAN BIRKENHAKE
Klinik und Poliklinik für
Strahlentherapie der Universität
Universitätsstraße 27
91054 Erlangen
FRG

Prof. Dr. ERNST ARNOLD BLEHER
Klinik für Radioonkologie
der Universität Bern
Inselspital
3010 Bern
Switzerland

Dr. Carsten Bokemeyer
Zentrum für Innere Medizin und Dermatologie
Abteilung Hämatologie/Onkologie
Konstanty-Gutschow-Straße 8
30623 Hannover
FRG

Dr. Joachim Boos
Universitätskinderklinik Münster
Pädiatrische Hämatologie/Onkologie
Albert-Schweitzer-Straße 33
48129 Münster
FRG

PD Dr. Michael Buchfelder
Neurochirurgische Klinik der Universität
Schwabachanlage 6
91054 Erlangen
FRG

PD Dr. Helmuth G. Dörr
Klinik für Kinder und Jugendliche
Loschgestraße 15
91054 Erlangen
FRG

Prof. Dr. Jürgen Dunst
Strahlentherapeutische Klinik
Martin-Luther-Universität Halle-Wittenberg
Dryanderstr. 4–7
06097 Halle/Saale
FRG

Dr. Dr. Michael Engel
Abteilung für Mund-, Kiefer- und Gesichtschirurgie
der Universitäts-Zahn-, Mund- und Kieferklinik
66421 Homburg/Saar
FRG

Prof. Dr. Rudolf Erttmann
Abteilung für pädiatrische
Hämotologie und Onkologie
Universitätskinderklinik
Martinistraße 52
20251 Hamburg
FRG

Dr. Dieter Felsenberg
Klinik für Innere Medizin
des Universitätsklinikum Steglitz
Abteilung Radiologie
Hindenburgdamm 30
12203 Berlin
FRG

Prof. Dr. Michael Flentje
Klinik und Poliklinik für Strahlentherapie
Josef-Schneider-Straße 11
97080 Würzburg
FRG

Dr. Bernd Frank
Universitätsklinikum Magdeburg
Abteilung Neurologie
Leipziger Straße 44
39120 Magdeburg
FRG

Prof. Dr. Hermann Frommhold
Radiologische Universitätsklinik
Abteilung Strahlentherapie
Hugstetter Straße 55
79106 Freiburg
FRG

Prof. Dr. Michael Galanskti
Zentrum Radiologie der Medizinischen Hochschule
Abteilung für Diagnostische Radiologie I
Konstanty-Gutschow-Straße 8
30625 Hannover
FRG

Dr. Ulrich Gatzemeier
Lungenfachklinik
Onkologische Abteilung
Wöhrendamm 80
22927 Großhansdorf
FRG

Dr. Joachim Grab
Chirurgische Klinik
Klinikum Großhadern
Marchioninistraße 15
81377 München
FRG

Dr. Gerhard Grabenbauer
Klinik und Poliklinik für Strahlen-
therapie der Universität
Universitätsstraße 27
91054 Erlangen
FRG

Prof. Dr. Richard H. Greiner
Direktor
Klinik für Radioonkologie
der Universität Bern
Inselspital
3010 Bern
Switzerland

Dr. Sabine Hartmann
Klinik für Phoniatrie und
Pädiatrische Audiologie
Universität Münster
Kardinal-von-Galen-Ring 10
48129 Münster
FRG

Dr. Karl Henne
Radiologische Universitätsklinik
Abteilung Strahlentherapie
Hugstetter Straße 55
79106 Freiburg
FRG

Prof. Dr. Thomas Herrmann
Medizinische Akademie Carl Gustav Carus
Abteilung Strahlentherapie
Fetscherstraße 74
01307 Dresden
FRG

Prof. Dr. Clemens F. Hess
Radiologische Universitätsklinik
Abteilung für Strahlentherapie
Hoppe-Seyler-Straße 3
72076 Tübingen
FRG

Dr. rer. nat. Norbert Hodapp
Klinik für Strahlentherapie
Robert-Koch-Straße 40
37075 Göttingen
FRG

Prof. Dr. Friedrich Kamprad
Universität Leipzig
Radiologische Klinik
Liebigstraße 20a
04103 Leipzig
FRG

Dr. Ludwig Keilholz
Klinik und Poliklinik für Strahlentherapie
der Universität
Universitätsstraße 27
91054 Erlangen
FRG

Dr. Andreas Koch
Klinik für Kinder und Jugendliche
Loschgestraße 15
91054 Erlangen
FRG

PD Dr. Armand Koch
Universitäts-HNO-Klinik
und Poliklinik
66421 Homburg/Saar
FRG

Prof. Dr. Rudolf Korinthenberg
Universitätskinderklinik
Abteilung Neuropädiatrie
und Muskelerkrankungen
Mathildenstraße 1
79106 Freiburg
FRG

Dr. Rolf D. Kortmann
Radiologische Universitätsklinik
Abteilung für Strahlentherapie
Hoppe-Seyler-Straße 3
72076 Tübingen
FRG

PD Dr. Hans-Jörg Krämling
Chirurgische Klinik
Klinikum Großhadern
Marchioninistraße 15
81377 München
FRG

Prof. Dr. Ernst-D. Kreuser
Abteilung Innere Medizin
mit Schwerpunkt Hämatologie und Onkologie
Universitätsklinikum Steglitz
Hindenburgdamm 30
12203 Berlin
FRG

Prof. Dr. Michael Landthaler
Dermatologische Klinik und Poliklinik
der Universität
Franz-Josef-Strauß-Allee 11
93053 Regensburg
FRG

Seymour H. Levitt, MD
Professor, Department of Therapeutic Radiology
University of Minnesota Medical School
Box 494, UMHC
Harvard St. at East River Parkway
Minneapolis, MN 55455-0110
USA

Prof. Dr. Michael Molls
Institut und Polliklinik für
Strahlentherapie und Radiologische
Onkologie der TU München
Ismaninger Straße 15
81675 München
FRG

Gisela Moog
Radiologische Universitätsklinik
Abteilung Strahlentherapie
Hugstetter Straße 55
79106 Freiburg
FRG

Prof. Dr. R.-P. Müller
Medizinische Einrichtungen der Universität Köln
Klinik und Poliklinik für Strahlentherapie
Joseph-Stelzmann-Straße 9
50924 Köln
FRG

PD Dr. Primus E. Mullis
Pädiatrische Endokrinologie
Medizinische Kinderklinik
der Universität Bern
Inselspital
3010 Bern
Switzerland

Dr. Marcus Niewald
Abteilung für Strahlentherapie
Radiologische Universitätsklinik
66421 Homburg/Saar
FRG

Dr. med. Ludwig Plasswilm
Klinik und Poliklinik für Strahlentherapie
der Universität
Universitätsstraße 27
91054 Erlangen
FRG

Dr. Regine Rathmann
Zentrum Radiologie der Medizinischen Hochschule
Abteilung für Diagnostische Radiologie I
Konstanty-Gutschow-Straße 8
30625 Hannover
FRG

Dr. Silvia Reitz
Institut und Poliklinik für
Strahlentherapie und Radiologische
Onkologie der TU München
Ismaninger Straße 15
81675 München
FRG

Dr. Michaela Riepl
Kilinik und Poliklinik für Strahlentherapie
der Universität Erlangen-Nürnberg
Universitätsstraße 27
91054 Erlangen
FRG

Prof. Dr. H. Peter Rodemann
Universität Tübingen
Abteilung Strahlenbiologie
Röntgenweg 11
72076 Tübingen
FRG

Dr. Rainer Rossi
Universitätskinderklinik
Pädiatrische Hämatologie/Onkologie
Albert-Schweitzer-Straße 33
48129 Münster
FRG

Dr. Christian Rübe
Radiologische Klinik Großhadern
Abteilung Strahlentherapie
Marchioninistraße 15
81377 München
FRG

Prof. Dr. Hansjörg Sauer
Ludwig-Maximilians-Universität München
Medizinische Klinik III des
Universitätsklinkum Großhadern
Marchioninistraße 15
81377 München
FRG

Dr. Thorsten Sauerwald
Klinik für Kinder und Jugendliche
Loschestraße 15
91054 Erlangen
FRG

Dr. MARTIN SCHABET
Radiologische Universitätsklinik
Abteilung für Neurologie
Hoppe-Seyler-Straße 3
72076 Tübingen
FRG

Dr. CORNELIA SCHAEFER-PROKOP
Zentrum Radiologie der Medizinischen Hochschule
Abteilung für Diagnostische Radiologie I
Konstanty-Gutschow-Straße 8
30625 Hannover
FRG

Dr. CHRISTOPH SCHLICHTING
Marienkrankenhaus
54293 Trier-Ehrang
FRG

Prof. Dr. HANS-JOACHIM SCHMOLL
Zentrum für Innere Medizin und Dermatologie
Abteilung Hämatologie/Onkologie
Konstanty-Gutschow-Straße 8
30623 Hannover
FRG

Prof. Dr. KLAUS SCHNABEL
Abteilung für Strahlentherapie
Radiologische Universitätsklinik
66421 Homburg/Saar
FRG

PD Dr. JOHANNES SCHORCHT
Medizinische Akademie Carl Gustav Carus
Abteilung Strahlentherapie
Fetscherstraße 74
01307 Dresden
FRG

Dr. HEINRICH SCHÜNEMANN
Klinik Bad Trissl
Abteilung für Gynäkologie I und Lymphtherapie
83080 Oberaudorf
FRG

PD Dr. SUSANNE SCHULTZ-HECTOR
GSF-Forschungszenrun für
Umwelt und Gesundheit GmbH
Institut für Strahlenbiologie Neuherberg
85764 Oberschleißheim
FRG

Prof. Dr. JOACHIM SLANINA
Radiologische Universitätsklinik
Abteilung Strahlentherapie
Hugstetter Straße 55
79106 Freiburg
FRG

Dr. VRATISLAV STRNAD
Klinik und Poliklinik für
Strahlentherapie der Universität
Universitätsstraße 27
91054 Erlangen
FRG

Prof. Dr. ECKHARD THIEL
Abteilung für Innere Medizin
mit Schwerpunkt Hämatologie und Onkologie
Universitätsklinikum Steglitz
Hindenburgdamm 30
12203 Berlin
FRG

Prof. Dr. KLAUS-RÜDIGER TROTT
Professor Department of Radiation Biology
St. Bartholomew's Medical College
Charterhouse Square
London EC1M 6BQ
England

Dr. ALEXANDER UHRIG
Klinik für Innere Medizin
mit Schwerpunkt Kardiologie
Universitätsklinikum Steglitz
Abteilung Kardiologie
Hindenburgdam 30
12203 Berlin
FRG

Dr. HEINZ VÖLLER
Klinik für Innere Medizin
mit Schwerpunkt Kardiologie
Universitätsklinikum Steglitz
Hindenburgdamm 30
12203 Berlin
FRG

Prof. Dr. HANS JOSEF WEH
Universitätskrankenhaus Eppendorf
Abteilung Onkologie/Hämatologie
Martinistraße 52
20251 Hamburg
FRG

Dr. Ralf Wilkowski
Klinik für Strahlentherapie der
Ludwig-Maximilians-Universität
Marchioninistraße 15
81377 München
FRG

Prof. Dr. Norman Willich
Klinik und Poliklinik
für Strahlentherapie/Radioonkologie
Westfälische-Wilhelms-Universität Münster
Albert-Schweitzer-Straße 33
48129 Münster
FRG

MIX
Papier aus verantwortungsvollen Quellen
Paper from responsible sources
FSC® C105338

If you have any concerns about our products,
you can contact us on
ProductSafety@springernature.com

In case Publisher is established outside the EU,
the EU authorized representative is:
Springer Nature Customer Service Center GmbH
Europaplatz 3, 69115 Heidelberg, Germany

Printed by Libri Plureos GmbH
in Hamburg, Germany